Cued Speech and Cued Language for Deaf and Hard of Hearing Children

EDITED BY

Carol J. LaSasso
Kelly Lamar Crain
Jacqueline Leybaert

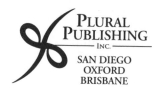
PLURAL
PUBLISHING
INC.

SAN DIEGO
OXFORD
BRISBANE

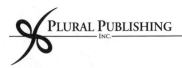

5521 Ruffin Road
San Diego, CA 92123

e-mail: info@pluralpublishing.com
Web site: http://www.pluralpublishing.com

49 Bath Street
Abingdon, Oxfordshire OX14 1EA
United Kingdom

FSC
Mixed Sources
Product group from well-managed
forests and other controlled sources

Cert no. SW-COC-002283
www.fsc.org
© 1996 Forest Stewardship Council

Copyright © by Plural Publishing, Inc. 2010

Typeset in 10½/13 Palatino book by Flanagan's Publishing Services, Inc.
Printed in the United States of America by Bang Printing
Second printing, August 2010 by McNaughton and Gunn

Library of Congress Cataloging-in-Publication Data

Cued speech and cued language for deaf and hard of hearing children / [edited by] Carol J.
LaSasso, Kelly Lamar Crain, and Jacqueline Leybaert.
        p. ; cm.
    Includes bibliographical references and index.
    ISBN-13: 978-1-59756-334-5 (alk. paper)
    ISBN-10: 1-59756-334-X (alk. paper)
    1. Deafness—Treatment. 2. Deaf children—Rehabilitation. 3. Hearing impaired children
—Rehabilitation. 4. Speech therapy. I. Leybaert, Jacqueline. II. LaSasso, Carol J. III. Crain,
Kelly Lamar.
    [DNLM: 1. Deafness—therapy. 2. Child. 3. Hearing Impaired Persons—education.
4. Hearing Impaired Persons—rehabilitation. 5. Language Therapy. 6. Manual Communication. 7. Speech Therapy. WV 271 C965 2010]
    RF290.C78 2010
    617.80083—dc22
                                                                                2009044429

Cued Speech and Cued Language for Deaf and Hard of Hearing Children

Cover image of Nefitiri Fellows and Lawrence LaSasso.

CONTENTS

FOREWORD

Why is this book about Cued Speech needed now, more than 40 years after R. Orin Cornett invented it and first suggested its use in educating deaf children? The incidence of children born with hearing impairment is still relatively high, representing between one and six in 1,000 live births, of whom about 10% have a profound hearing loss. The large majority of these children are born to hearing parents whose own language and communication skills are based on their previous and current experience with heard speech. We now know that early experiences of children with their caregivers are vital to the development of language and communication, and that if this is not optimal, children will not be able to make effective use of their skills, and risk isolation. Hearing parents of a deaf child are unlikely to share an effective environment for developing these skills. This is the challenge faced by the parents and support community of a deaf child. How can the deaf child, born into a home that uses spoken language, develop so that she or he reaches their full potential in a world that depends more and more on communicating effectively through language—whether speaking, signing, reading, or writing? Some believe that the advances in cochlear implant technology have solved, or "cured," deafness, or are on the verge of doing so. Indeed, these technologies continue to improve, and cochlear implantation is now occurring as early as during the first

year of life—but this would be to overestimate the "cure." Cochlear implants are devices that enhance the perception of sound: they suit many, but not all patients; they do not yet mirror the perceptual experience of hearing individuals. Further, implants can fail, and years of intensive aural habilitation therapy are necessary to maximize the benefit of the device. Cochlear implants promise to be an ever improving part of a solution, but may never constitute the (or a) solution, in and of themselves.

In most developed countries, the parents of a child born deaf today face a bewildering array of choices and strategies in relation to communication and language access. Should they try amplification devices and teach the child to listen and speak? Should they opt for a cochlear implant and "make do" with gestural communication and speechreading until the surgery (or surgeries) can be performed and appropriate interventions can be initiated? Should they: take a crash course in a signed language, such as American Sign Language (ASL); learn signs borrowed from signed languages and apply those signs to their own spoken language; or call on the services of a skilled signer to help develop early communication with their child—and support the child's own developing communication skills? Should parents attempt some combination of these options? Which should they try first, and when should they "give up and move on" to another? As the reader will learn from this volume, Cued Speech offers a further possibility: show the child the traditional spoken language of the home in its entirety, and allow the child to integrate whatever hearing (augmented or not) is available. Unlike speechreading, which cannot offer the full range of spoken language contrasts available by ear (for example, "ma," "pa," and "ba" all look the same on the lips of the speaker), Cornett's system allows the speaker to make absolutely clear *which* utterance was meant by including a disambiguating hand gesture synchronized with the mouth patterns to indicate the speech segment intended. That is, using the two visible articulating systems of mouth and hand together, a clear, complete, "purely visual" version of the spoken language can be delivered in the absence of either speech or hearing. This is very different from a signed language, where although mouth movements often accompany manual gestures, the relative roles of mouth and hand do not perform this function.

Although Cornett's attempts persuaded some parents, educators, and administrators, the use of Cued Speech has been sporadic in deaf education, and it is only within the last twenty or so years that research has been conducted in Europe and the United States on its efficacy and utility in relation to the child's developing cognitive skills. In this edited volume, the reader will discover from multiple perspectives (linguistics, cognition, neuropsychology, speech science, hearing science, transliteration, computer science, education) how effective Cued Speech can be in developing traditionally spoken language skills and in making speech and spoken language available to the deaf child.

Because Cued Speech makes speech segments (phonemes) visible and dis-crete, it can be of special use in the earliest stages of reading (e.g., decoding) which require the child to develop automated abilities in isolating and identifying speech segments and mapping them to letter forms. This is where the deaf child who does not have access to the full phonological structure of the spoken language faces a significant and fundamental hurdle. Does the privileged access to the segmental structure of speech afforded by Cued Speech help the deaf child to clear this obstacle to fluent reading and spelling? This was Cornett's goal, and that goal has been supported empirically by the work that Alegria and Leybaert, with colleagues led by Périer, started in Belgium 20 years ago. That body of work, with French speakers, has shown conclusively that children exposed consistently to Cued Speech gained and maintained a headstart over deaf children of similar intelligence and skill who did not have Cued Speech. Those who started using Cued Speech before school were even more likely to forge ahead, often with literacy levels and styles indistinguishable from hearing children. In this volume, this original research project is discussed and findings are brought up to date, in addition to recent findings related to the early language and literacy development of deaf children in English- and Spanish-language environments.

It is becoming increasingly clear that all children (not just those with hearing loss) are sensitive to the sight as well as the sound of speech in the first year of life, and that these experiences lay the foundation for developing native language skills. It is in these early months that the deaf child is likely to tune in to each and every available means of communicating and tracking the intentions of his or her caregivers, including the structure of the child's speech and the spoken language it represents. Cueing is a skill that parents can learn quickly and can use with relative ease as they speak. Perhaps when they do so with their very young deaf child, we should consider cueing to be a special kind of infant-directed speech? The importance of Cued Speech is that it opens up the world of spoken language to the deaf child in a clear and simple way, from the outset. This has, as Cornett envisioned, the potential to allow a form of the traditionally spoken language to develop naturally in a deaf child, via a communication modality that the child and the child's caregiver can use easily, fluently, and collaboratively. This edited volume, with its 24 chapters written by 42 scholars in the United States and Europe, is a fitting memorial to Cornett's vision, in showing just how effective Cued Speech can be in making spoken languages visible and fully accessible for a deaf child in preparation for formal reading instruction and academic achievement.

Ruth Campbell, Ph.D.
Professor Emeritus, Department of Cognitive, Perceptual and Brain Sciences
Division of Psychology and Language Sciences,
University College London
October 30, 2009

Dr. Campbell is an experimental psychologist and neuropsychologist with interests in deafness and cognition, and the neural bases of cognitive processes in relation to developmental plasticity. One of her long-time research interests relates to how speechreading (lipreading) works in hearing and deaf people. She has held faculty posts at the University of Oxford and the University of London, and cofounded the Deafness, Cognition, and Language Centre at University College London in 2005.

CONTRIBUTORS

Jesus Alegria, Ph.D.
Honorary Professor, Laboratoire
  Cognition, Langage et
  Développement (LCLD)
Université Libre de Bruxelles (U.L.B.),
  Belgium

Dr. Alegria has made a career as an academic in the Université Libre de Bruxelles (Belgium) as a member of the Laboratory of Experimental Psychology (now Laboiratoire Cognition, Langage & Développement), where he has taught courses on cognitive and linguistic development. At the age of 70, Dr. Alegria became involved in psycholinguistic research related to spoken and written language acquisition. He became fascinated with deaf children's linguistic development and the potential of Cued Speech as a tool to provide them a complete model of their surrounding language(s). A research program was then established with his colleagues of the Laboratory, Brigitte Charlier, Catherine Hage, Josiane Lechat and Jacqueline Leybaert, and a collaboration was formed with the Ecole Integrée, a school in Brussels, which had adopted Cued Speech in the early 1980s.

Chapter 5

Mario Aparicio, Ph.D.
Postdoctoral Research Fellow,
  Laboratoire Cognition, Langage et
  Développement (LCLD)
Université Libre de Bruxelles (U.L.B.),
  Belgium

Dr. Aparicio received his Ph.D. in Neuropsychology from University Louis Pasteur in Strasbourg, France. His doctoral research focused on brain activity during phonological processing in oral deaf readers. He is currently a postdoctoral research fellow at the Laboiratoire Cognition, Language & Development in the Université Libre de Bruxelles (Belgium). His current interests focus on the patterns of neuronal activation during speech perception in deaf users of Cued Speech and sign language.

Chapter 24

Michelle L. Arnold, Au.D. Candidate
Clinical Doctoral Student in
  Audiology
University of South Florida, Tampa

Ms. Arnold is currently completing requirements for a Doctorate of Audiology (Au.D.) in the Department of Communication Sciences and Disorders at the University of South Florida in Tampa. She is working under the tutelage of Dr. Charles I. Berlin, a key figure in the discovery and understanding of Auditory Neuropathy/Auditory Dys-synchrony (AN/AD), and has worked closely with Dr. Kelly Lamar Crain on research related to Cued Speech usage among deaf adults.

Chapter 15

Virginie Attina, Ph.D.
Postdoc Research Fellow, Brain
   Dynamics and Cognition Unit (U821)
National Institute of Health and
   Medical Research, Lyon, France

Dr. Attina received her Ph.D. in Cognitive Sciences from Grenoble Institute of Technology, France, in 2005. Her doctoral research focused on the temporal organization of French Cued Speech, where she investigated the relationship between production and perception in the processing of Cued Speech. In 2006, she became a postdoctoral research fellow with the University of La Laguna, Tenerife, Spain, where she is focusing on psycholinguistics and word recognition in deaf people. She is currently a postdoctoral research fellow at the Brain Dynamics and Cognition unit (U821) (National Institute of Health and Medical Research), Lyon, France. Her current interests include neurological temporal processing of information and brain-computer interfaces.

Chapter 19

Edward T. Auer, Jr., Ph.D.
Assistant Professor, Department of
   Speech-Language-Hearing
University of Kansas, Lawrence

Dr. Auer's interest in Cued Speech stems from his investigations into how signals (artificial and biological) combine with visual speech to result in accurate speech perception. His current research projects relate to perception of signals associated with communication in adults with normal hearing, profound hearing loss, auditory neuropathy, and cochlear implants. His projects focus on the interface between the phonetic information and lexical processing, as well as individual differences in perceptual ability. He investigates both spoken and manual communication using a wide range of methods, including functional magnetic resonance imaging, electrophysiology, computational modeling, and behavioral testing.

Chapter 18

Gerard Bailly, Ph.D.
Director of Research, ICP Talking
   Machines Team, GIPSA Lab and
Director of the Research Federation
   PEGASUS
Grenoble, France

Dr. Bailly joined the Institut de la Communication Parlée (ICP) Grenoble, France in 1986 as Chargé de Recherche with the French National Center for Scientific Research, after two years as postdoctoral fellow with INRS Telecommunications in Montréal. Director of Research since 2002, he is now the head of the ICP Talking Machines team at GIPSA-Lab and director of the research federation PEGASUS. He co-organized the first speech synthesis conference in 1991 and co-chaired the first international conferences on smart objects and ambient intelligence in 2003 and 2005. Editor of three books and author of 25 international journal articles, 15 book chapters, and more than 150 international conference papers, his current interest is audiovisual synthesis and multimodal interaction with conversational agents in situated face-to-face communication.

Chapter 19

Denis Beautemps, Ph.D.
Researcher, French National Center on
   Research
Grenoble, France

Dr. Beautemps received his Ph.D. in Signal, Image, and Speech Processing from the Grenoble Institute of Technology, France in 1993. He has been a Permanent Researcher of the Center National of Research (the French

CNRS) since 1998 at the ICP, "Département Parole et Cognition de GIPSA-lab (Grenoble Image Parole Signal Automatique laboratory)," Dr. Beautemps specializes in the modeling of the adaptability in speech, from perception to speech production. Since 2000, he has focused on Cued Speech. He is currently involved in several projects that address fundamental questions related to Cued Speech, particularly related to control, hand-lip co-articulation, and integration.

Chapter 19

Charles I. Berlin, Ph.D.
Professor, Louisiana State University
(Ret.) Research Professor, University
of South Florida, Tampa

Dr. Berlin retired in 2002 as Professor of Otorhinolaryngology, Head and Neck Surgery, and Physiology, and Director of the world-renowned Kresge Hearing Research Laboratory at LSU Medical School in New Orleans. He is the first audiologist and hearing scientist to have an Academic Chair named after him (the $1 Million Charles I. Berlin, Ph.D. Chair in Molecular and Genetic Hearing Science, created by the Louisiana Board of Regents). In 2005, Dr. Berlin was invited to be a Research Professor at the University of South Florida's Department of Otolaryngology Head and Neck Surgery and the Department of Communication Sciences and Disorders, where he coordinates one of its Pediatric Research Units.

Chapter 15

Lynne E. Bernstein, Ph.D.
Senior Scientist, House Ear Institute,
Los Angeles CA
Adjunct Professor, University of
Southern California, Los Angeles

Dr. Bernstein's interest in Cued Speech began during her research years at Gal-

laudet University where she carried out studies of visual speech perception in deaf students. She currently has research projects on speech perception in adults with normal hearing, profound hearing loss, auditory neuropathy, and cochlear implants. An ongoing focus on visual speech perception includes developing a synthetic talking face. Multisensory speech perception experiments include visual, auditory, and vibrotactile stimuli. Dr. Bernstein's projects use a wide range of methods, including functional magnetic resonance imaging, electrophysiology, computational modeling, and psychophysics.

Chapter 18

Louis D. Braida, Ph.D.
Professor of Electrical Engineering and
Health Science and Technology
Massachusetts Institute of Technology,
Cambridge, MA

Dr. Braida received B.E.E. degree in Electrical Engineering from the Cooper Union, New York, NY and M.S. and Ph.D. degrees in Electrical Engineering from the Massachusetts Institute of Technology. He is currently Henry Ellis Warren Professor of Electrical Engineering and Health Science and Technology at the Massachusetts Institute of Technology, Cambridge. His research focuses on auditory perception and the development of improved hearing aids and other aids for deaf individuals.

Chapters 20 and 21

Maroula S. Bratakos, B.S., M.Eng.
Systems Engineer, NextWave
Broadband Inc.
San Diego, California

Ms. Bratakos received the B.S. and M.Eng. degrees in Electrical Engineering from the Massachusetts Institute of Technology, Cambridge, in 1993 and 1995, respectively. She is currently a systems engineer focused on the fields of wireless and VoIP. She previously worked at Nuera Communications leading their VoIP gateway product. She currently works on WiMAX base station development at NextWave Wireless.

Chapter 20

Miguel A. Carreira-Perpiñán, Ph.D.
Assistant Professor, Electrical
  Engineering and Computer Science
University of California, Merced

Dr. Carreira-Perpiñán is an assistant professor in Electrical Engineering and Computer Science at the University of California, Merced. He received a Ph.D. in Computer Science from the University of Sheffield, UK, and did postdoctoral work at Georgetown University and the University of Toronto. He is the recipient of an NSF CAREER award for machine learning approaches to articulatory inversion. His research interests lie in machine learning, with applications to speech processing, computer vision and computational neuroscience.

Chapter 22

Marie-Agnès Cathiard, Ph.D.
Maître de Conférences' in Phonetics
  and Cognition
Stendhal University, Grenoble, France

Dr. Cathiard received her Ph.D. in Cognitive Psychology in 1994. She is currently Maître de Conférences' in Phonetics and Cognition, at Stendhal University (Grenoble, France). Her research interests are currently focused on the multimodal integration of speech, with a special focus on perceptuomotor interactions, and more recently speech working memory. Since 2001, she has been working on the production and perception of le Langage Parlé Complété (LPC).

Chapter 19

Brigitte L. Charlier, Ph.D.
Headmaster, Centre Comprendre et
  Parler de Bruxelles
Professor, Université Libre de
  Bruxelles, Belgium, Laboratoire
  Cognition, Langage et
  Développement (LCLD)

Dr. Charlier is Headmaster of the Centre Comprendre et Parler de Bruxelles, which serves 300 deaf and hearing impaired children, and is a Professor at the Université Libre de Bruxelles. She holds a master's degree in Speech Therapy and a doctoral degree in Psychology. Dr. Charlier has been a Cued Speech user for more than 27 years. She conducts research on Cued Speech, particularly concerning the development in deaf children of cognitive abilities related to linguistic acquisition and phonological development, such as working memory, short-term memory, acquisition of phonological features, normative evaluations, and neurologic development. She also is interested in the same topics related to sign language acquisition and in sign writing systems.

Chapter 24

Cécile Colin, Ph.D.
Assistant Professor
Université Libre de Bruxelles (U.L.B.),
  Brussels, Belgium

Dr. Colin's research interests focus on speech perception in adults and children, with a particular focus on the integration between auditory and visual inputs, which she investigates with behavioral and electrophysiologic techniques. She is particularly familiar with the recording of the Mismatch Negativity (MMN), an event-related potential indexing the automatic detection of a deviant auditory stimulus occurring in a sequence of standard stimulations. Part of her time is devoted to the study of the best acquisition and computation parameters of the MMN, in order to improve its intrinsically low signal-to-noise ratio, with the final objective to use it as a clinical tool aimed at objectively assessing speech discrimination abilities in children. She currently is involved in a research program examining audiovisual speech perception in children fitted with a cochlear implant, as a function of the implantation moment and of the use of Cued Speech.

Chapter 6

Stéphanie Colin, Ph.D.
Assistant Professor
Institute of Science and Practice of Education and Training, University of Lyon, France

Dr. Colin received her Ph.D. in Psychology from the Free University of Brussels (Belgium, Laboratory of Experimental Psychology) and the University of Lyon 2 (France, EMC/DDL Laboratory). Her Ph.D. thesis was a longitudinal study of the relationships between early phonological abilities in kindergarteners and acquisition of written language in the first and second grades in deaf children. She is interested in Cued Speech as a predictor of reading acquisition. Current research focuses on the combined effect of cochlear implants and Cued Speech on literacy development in deaf children and youth and the various factors that could promote reading acquisition in deaf pre-readers and beginning readers: phonological training and effect of early print exposure.

Chapter 11

Kelly Lamar Crain, Ph.D.
Assistant Professor, Aural Habilitation/Deaf Education
University of South Florida, Tampa

Dr. Crain holds a bachelor's degree in Speech-Language Pathology and Audiology from the University of Southern Mississippi, and master's and doctoral degrees in Deaf Education from Gallaudet University. His interest in Cued Speech began during his graduate education at Gallaudet. While working as a research associate at Gallaudet, Dr. Crain collaborated with the Center for the Study of Learning at Georgetown University, where he contributed to neuroimaging studies of language and cognition with hearing and deaf individuals from oral, signing, and cueing backgrounds. Dr. Crain's current research interests include the development of cued language by deaf infants, the role of visually acquired phonology in the decoding and reading comprehension abilities of deaf children, and the evolving role of Cued Speech and cued language in the lives of deaf adults.

Chapters 2, 8, 9, 12–14, and 17

Paul Duchnowski, Ph.D.
Core Software Technology Developer
Nuance Communications, Inc., Burlington, MA

Dr. Duchnowski received S.B., S.M, and Sc.D. degrees in Electrical Engineering from the Massachusetts Institute of Technology where his research concentrated on human audition, automatic speech recognition, and communication aids for deaf individuals. He currently develops core software technology for the automatic dictation products of Nuance Communications, Inc. in Burlington, MA.

Chapters 20 and 21

Guinevere F. Eden, D. Phil.
Associate Professor, Department of Pediatrics
Director, The Center for the Study of Learning
Georgetown University, Washington D.C.

Dr. Eden received her D.Phil. in Physiology from Oxford University and has since focused on the application of functional neuroimaging techniques to study the neural basis of developmental dyslexia. As Director of the Center for the Study of Learning, at Georgetown University, Dr. Eden oversees federally supported research related to the neural representation of reading and how it may be altered in individuals with developmental disorders or altered early sensory experience. She and her colleagues are researching how reading is impacted by instructions or mode of communication and are utilizing functional MRI to study the neurobiological correlates of reading remediation. Dr. Eden also serves as a scientific co-director for the Science of Learning Center on Visual Language and Visual learning (VL2) at Gallaudet University. She currently is president of the International Dyslexia Association and serves on the editorial boards of the Annals of Dyslexia, Dyslexia, and Human Brain Mapping.

Chapter 13

Earl Fleetwood, M.A., CI, CT, TSC
Staff Interpreter, Sign Language Associates, Inc.
Instructor and Consultant, Language Matters, Inc.

Mr. Fleetwood holds a master's degree in ASL-English Interpretation from Gallaudet University. He co-authored curriculum for the original cued language transliterator training programs at Gallaudet. He is a cofounder of the TECUnit, the national certifying body in the United States for practitioners who transliterate between cued English and spoken English. Mr. Fleetwood is dually certified, holding national certifications as both a cued language transliterator and signed language interpreter. He is co-author of the TECUnit's cued language transliterator (CLT) Code of Conduct, CLT National Certification Examination, and CLT State Level Assessment as well as of Language Matters Inc.'s (LMI) graduate and undergraduate coursework comprising the Cued Language Transliterator Professional Education Series. He has written or co-authored a variety of instructional audio and video materials related to cueing, and numerous books and articles related to cued language linguistics, cued language transliteration, signed language linguistics, and ASL-English interpretation.

Chapter 3

Guillaume Gibert, Ph.D.
Postdoctoral Research Associate, Brain Dynamics and Cognition Unit
National Institute of Health and Medical Research

Dr. Gibert received his Ph.D. in Signal, Image and Speech processing from the Grenoble Institute of Technology, France, in 2006. Through his doctoral research, he implemented and evaluated the first complete 3D Text-to-(French) Cued Speech synthesizer. This system was used to watermark hand and face gestures of a virtual animated agent in a broadcasted audiovisual sequence. He is currently a postdoctoral research associate in the Brain Dynamics and Cognition Unit (U821) of National Institute of Health and Medical Research (INSERM). His present work focuses on the development of novel and efficient signal processing techniques for brain-computer interfaces and neurofeedback.

Chapter 19

Catherine Hage, Ph.D.
Speech Therapist, Centre Comprendre et Parler
Associate Professor, Université Libre de Bruxelles, Laboratoire Cognition,

Langage et Développement (LCLD), Belgium

Dr. Hage teaches university students about the acquisition of language by deaf children. She has a master's degree in Speech Therapy and a Ph.D. in Psychology. Her research interests focus on the effect of Cued Speech on the acquisition of some morphophonological aspects of French oral language, such as grammatical gender and prepositions. She introduced Cued Speech into Belgium, where she was the first speech therapist to use it. Currently, she works with both very young deaf children with cochlear implants, and hard of hearing children. She is interested in the development of oral language by children with cochlear implants and in oral bilingualism in very young deaf children.

Chapter 6

Jintao Jiang, Ph.D.
Senior Research Engineer
Division of Communication and
 Auditory Neuroscience, House Ear
 Institute,
Los Angeles, California

Dr. Jiang received his Ph.D. degree in Electrical Engineering from the University of California at Los Angeles, California, in 2003. His doctoral research focused on audiovisual speech processing, perception, and recognition. Since 2003, he has been a senior research engineer at the House Ear Institute, where his research interest is in the areas of audiovisual processing, perception, synthesis, and recognition and developing and evaluating a concatenative Cued Speech synthesis system. Dr. Jiang's interest in Cued Speech originated from his research in audiovisual speech perception and research in visual speech synthesis.

Chapter 18

Judy Kegl, Ph.D.
Professor, Director of the Signed
 Language Research Laboratory
University of Southern Maine,
 Portland, Maine

Dr. Kegl oversees several research projects on the cross-linguistic comparison of signed languages and the emergence of a new signed language in Nicaragua. She coordinates the training of ASL/English interpreters under a grant to the University from the Maine Department of Education. She received her Ph.D. in linguistics from the Massachusetts Institute of Technology in 1985 and has completed extensive postdoctoral studies in neuroscience at Rutgers, the State University of New Jersey. She has published extensively on the linguistics of signed languages as well as spoken and signed language aphasia.

Chapter 23

Claire Klossner, TSC
ASL Interpreter and Cued Language
 Transliterator, Sign Language
 Associates
Adjunct Instructor, Gallaudet
 University, Washington, D.C.

Ms. Klossner learned how to cue at a young age as a member of a cueing family. She is a nationally certified Cued Language Transliterator and works as both a Cued Language Transliterator and Signed Language Interpreter in the Washington, DC area. She is an instructor for the Cued Language Transliterator Professional Education Series for Language Matters, Inc., and has taught Cued Speech classes and transliterator training classes to groups across the United States. She also teaches Cued Speech at the graduate level for the Department of Hearing, Speech and Language Sciences at Gallaudet University.

Chapter 17

Daniel S. Koo, Ph.D.
Assistant Professor, Department of
  Psychology
Gallaudet University, Washington, D.C.

Dr. Koo holds a master's degree in Linguistics from Gallaudet University and a Ph.D. in Brain and Cognitive Sciences from the University of Rochester. He completed a postdoctoral fellowship in the Center for the Study of Learning, Georgetown University Medical Center. Born deaf to hearing parents, Dr. Koo's interest in Cued Speech stems from his own personal experience growing up with the system. He is interested in how the visual language-learning experience of deaf individuals shapes their linguistic representations and processes, particularly those who use Cued Speech. Currently, he is using functional MRI technology to explore the neural bases of reading and phonological processes in deaf individuals of different communication backgrounds to better understand the relationship between phonology, linguistic modality, and the neural substrates underlying language processes in the brain.

Chapters 4 and 13

Jean C. Krause, Ph.D.
Assistant Professor, Communication
  Sciences and Disorders
University of South Florida, Tampa

Dr. Krause holds a B.S.E.E. degree in Electrical Engineering from Georgia Institute of Technology (1993) and an SM degree (1995) and Ph.D. degree (2001) in Electrical Engineering from Massachusetts Institute of Technology (MIT). She is co-inventor of an "automatic cueing of speech" system and has extensive expertise in Cued Speech transliteration and the evaluation of Cued Speech transliterators. She is certified as an Instructor of Cued Speech by the National Cued Speech Association (NCSA) and also is chair of the NCSA's Instructor Certification Committee and Testing Committee. In addition, she is certified (OTC) in oral transliteration by the Registry of Interpreters for the Deaf. Her research is concerned with the perception of languages and visual communication systems used in the education of deaf children (i.e., American Sign Language, sign systems, and Cued Speech), as well as the perception of speech by normal hearing listeners and listeners with hearing loss.

Chapter 20, 21, and 23

Kitri Larson Kyllo, M.Ed., Ed.S.
Assistant Director, Intermediate
  District 917
Program for Learners Who Are Deaf
  and Hard of Hearing
Rosemount, Minnesota

Ms. Kyllo holds a masters degree in Special Education: Deaf/Hard of Hearing (D/HH) and Education Specialist degree in Educational Administration. She has worked in the field of Deaf Education for over 30 years as a special education administrator, a teacher of learners who are D/HH, and a nationally certified sign language interpreter. Ms. Kyllo has served in her current position since 1991 supervising programming for learners who are D/HH, visually impaired, and physically and health disabled. Ms. Kyllo continues language and literacy data-collection efforts supporting the benefits of immersion in cued languages for the development of skills in language, literacy, spoken language, and auditory development for learners who are D/HH.

Chapter 10

Carol J. LaSasso, Ph.D.
Professor, Department of Hearing,
  Speech and Language Sciences
Gallaudet University, Washington D.C.

Dr. LaSasso is a Professor of Hearing, Speech, and Language Sciences at Gallaudet University. She is an affiliated researcher with the Center for the Study of Learning at Georgetown University, which is conducting neuroimaging studies of language and cognition with hearing and deaf individuals from oral, signing, and cueing backgrounds. In addition, Dr. LaSasso is affiliated with the Science of Learning Center on Visual Language and Visual Literacy (VL2) at Gallaudet University. She has served as President of the Special Interest Group in Reading and Deafness for the International Reading Association and has published extensively in the areas of phonological abilities, vocabulary, reading comprehension, and test-taking abilities of deaf childen and youth. For 10 years, Dr. LaSasso directed diagnostic reading clinics for more than 400 deaf and hard of hearing children and their parents from ASL, manually coded English, oral-aural, and Cued Speech backgrounds in Washington D.C., W. Hartford, CT, and Wilson NC. Dr. LaSasso currently teaches Ph.D. seminars and directs federal personnel preparation grants from the U.S. Department of Education.

Chapters 1, 9, and 11–14

Jacqueline Leybaert, Ph.D.
Professor of Psychology
Laboratoire Cognition, Langage, et Développement (LCLD), Université Libre de Bruxelles (U.L.B.), Belgium

Dr. Leybaert teaches courses on language acquisition, cognitive development, sensory deficits and neural plasticity, and dyscalculia. Her doctoral dissertation related to the use of phonological codes by deaf children in reading, spelling and short-term serial memory. Since then, her research interests have focused on the effect of Cued Speech on "the three Rs."

More recently, she directed research about audiovisual integration and speech perception in noise in children with a cochlear implant and children with specific language impairment. She also is interested in numerical cognition in children with deafness and children with specific language impairment (SLI). She has co-edited two books in French about linguistic and cognitive development in deaf children and has written numerous articles and book chapters about these topics.

Chapters 6, 11, and 24

David S. Lum, S.B., M.Eng.
Software Developer and Designer, Amdocs, Inc.
Dulles, Virginia

Mr. Lum received the S.B. and M.Eng. degrees from the Massachusetts Institute of Technology, Cambridge, in 1994 and 1995, respectively. He currently works as a software developer and designer for Amdocs, Inc. He contributes to open source software projects as often as he can.

Chapter 20

Dominic W. Massaro, Ph.D.
Professor of Psychology and Computer Engineering
University of California, Santa Cruz

Dr. Massaro is a Professor of Psychology and Computer Engineering, director of the Perceptual Science Laboratory, and Chair of Digital Arts and New Media M.F.A. program at the University of California, Santa Cruz. He received a B.A. in Psychology (1965) from UCLA and an M.A. (1966) and a Ph.D. (1968) in Psychology from the University of Massachusetts-Amherst. He has been a Guggenheim Fellow, a University of Wisconsin Romnes Fellow, a James McKeen Cattell Fellow, and an NIMH Fellow. He is past president of the Society for Computers in Psychology, and is currently the book review editor of the *American Journal of Psychology* and founding co-editor of the journal *Interpreting*. He has published numerous academic journal articles, written and edited several books. His research uses a formal experimental and theoretical approach to the study of speech perception, reading, psycholinguistics, memory, cognition, learning, and decision-making.

Chapter 22

David J. Merrill, Ph.D.
Postdoctoral Fellow
MIT Media Laboratory, Cambridge, Massachussetts

Dr. Merrill is a graduate of the Fluid Interfaces Group at the MIT Media Lab, where he worked with professor Pattie Maes. He received a B.S. in Symbolic Systems (2000) and an M.S. in Computer Science (2002) from Stanford University. Dr. Merrill's research is focused on physical interfaces and ubiquitous computing. His work has produced novel interaction techniques for music and digital sound that leverage people's existing knowledge and expressive gestures, systems for mobile, attention-sensitive browsing of information in the physical world, and the first general purpose, distributed, inch-scale tangible user interface platform.

Chapter 22

Melanie Metzger, Ph.D.
Professor, Department of Interpretation
Gallaudet University, Washington D.C.

Dr. Metzger holds a master's degree in ASL Linguistics from Gallaudet University and a doctoral degree in Sociolinguistics from Georgetown University. She co-authored the curriculum for the original cued language transliterator training programs at Gallaudet. She also is a cofounder of Language Matters, Inc. (LMI) and TECUnit and co-author of the TECUnit's cued language transliterator (CLT) Code of Conduct and the CLT national and state level examinations. Dr. Metzger is nationally certified as both a CLT and signed language interpreter. Dr. Metzger has written or co-authored a variety of instructional audio and video materials related to cueing, as well as numerous books and articles reflecting her interest in researching cued language discourse, cued language transliteration, signed language discourse and ASL-English interpretation.

Chapter 3

Ignacio Moreno-Torres, Ph.D.
Professor, Departamento de Filología Española (Spanish Language Department)
Universidad de Málaga, Spain

Dr. Moreno-Torres received a Ph.D. in Spanish Language from the Autonomous University of Barcelona (Spain) in 1994. He now teaches and conducts research in language acquisition at the Universidad de Málaga, Spain, where he collaborates with Dr. Santiago Torres-Monreal in the Método Oral Complementado (MOC) lab, a research center dedicated to investigations of Cued Speech. Dr. Moreno-Torres' current research interests include phonological, lexical, and grammatical acquisition in prelingually deafened children fitted with cochlear implants.

Chapter 7

Donna A. Morere, Ph.D.
Associate Professor, Clinical Psychology Program
Department of Psychology, Gallaudet University, Washington D.C.

Dr. Morere has been on the faculty of the doctoral program in Clinical Psychology at Gallaudet University since 1990. She became interested in Cued Speech when her son was born deaf in 1992. Being aware of the literacy challenges of deaf children, she investigated options and discovered Cued Speech. In addition to her faculty position, Dr. Morere has a private practice in Clinical Neuropsychology in which she evaluates deaf children with special needs using signs, Cued Speech, and oral communication and consults with schools and parents on services to deaf children with additional challenges. Her research interests include language and literacy in deaf children and language development of deaf children with special needs.

Chapter 16

Philippe Peigneux, Ph.D.
Professor of Psychology
Université Libre de Bruxelles (U.L.B.),
   Belgium

Dr. Peigneux was trained in Psychological Sciences (M.Sc., Ph.D.) at the University of Liège in Belgium. His research interests focus on the dynamic cognitive and neural processes that subtend the creation and consolidation of novel memories in the human brain. During his research career at the Cyclotron Research Centre of the ULg, he conducted pioneering functional neuroanatomical studies showing relationships between sleep, circadian rhythms, cognition and memory consolidation processes. Since 2006, he has been a Professor of Clinical Neuropsychology at the Faculty of Psychological Sciences, and Director of the Neuropsychology and Functional Neuroimaging Research Unit at the Université Libre de Bruxelles.

Chapter 24

Brenda Schick, Ph.D.
Associate Professor, Department of
   Hearing Speech and Language Sciences
University of Colorado, Boulder

Dr. Schick studies the development of signed and spoken languages as well as its relationship to cognition in deaf children. Her recent work has focused on the development of a Theory of Mind in deaf children and how it relates to language skills. Dr. Schick is the co-developer of the Educational Interpreter Performance Assessment (EIPA), a tool designed to evaluate the skills of K to 12 interpreters. With colleagues, she has published data on the performance skills of interpreters who work in the K to 12 setting. Dr. Schick has served as the school board president for Rocky Mountain Deaf School, a bilingual charter school for deaf children in metro Denver. In addition, she is a CODA (child of a deaf adult), having grown up in a deaf family.

Chapter 23

Matthew G. Sexton, S.B., M.Eng.
Technical Director, Mercury Computer
   Systems
Chelmsford, Massachusetts

Mr. Sexton received the S.B. and M.Eng. degrees from the Massachusetts Insitute of Technology, Cambridge, in 1994 and 1995, respectively. He is currently a technical director at Mercury Computer Systems, Inc., accelerating real-time applications through parallel processing and algorithm optimization.

Chapter 20

Thomas F. Shull, TSC
Cued Language Transliterator, Cued
   Speech Instructor, Transliterator
   Trainer
Language Matters, Inc.

Mr. Shull learned to cue in 1989 and was immediately interested in the potential of Cued Speech for natural language development and visual communication. He began facilitating communication between deaf and hearing consumers as a cued language transliterator and is nationally certified by the TECUnit. Since 1990, he has worked in a variety of educational settings from preschool through doctoral programs. Additionally, he works for Language Matters, Inc. as a transliterator instructor. He presents nationally and internationally on issues pertaining to transliteration, expressive and receptive cueing technique, and instructional practices. He has devised numerous curricula for Cued Speech instruction to a variety of populations. He is particularly interested in issues of equal access in education and the instruction of foreign languages via the modality of cueing.

Chapter 2

Ted Supalla, Ph.D.
Associate Professor, Brain and
   Cognitive Sciences and Linguistics
University of Rochester, New York

Dr. Supalla was born Deaf to Deaf parents and learned ASL at home. He received his Ph.D. in Psychology at the University of California, San Diego. Dr. Supalla's research involves the study of signed languages of the world, particularly those which have emerged naturally within communities of deaf people. He is also interested in online psycholinguistic and neurolinguistic processing research, including studies of sentence comprehension and memory as well as fMRI studies on visual-gestural language processing. To determine whether such overarching linguistic properties are optimized for use in visual-manual code systems, Dr. Supalla is interested in learning about how Cued Speech in particular operates in terms of bimodal structure and processing by groups of users.

Chapter 4

Santiago Torres-Monreal, Ph.D.
Professor, Departamento de Psicología
   Básica (Dept. of Basic Psychology)
Universidad de Málaga, Spain

Dr. Torres-Monreal received a Ph.D. degree in Psychology from the University of Murcia (Spain) in 1987. As part of his doctoral dissertation, he adapted Cued Speech for Spanish (La Palabra Complementada, LPC). He now teaches and carries out research in experimental psychology at the University of Málaga (Spain), where he founded the Método Oral Complementado (MOC) lab, a research center dedicated to investigations of Cued Speech and its effect in several areas. Dr. Torres-Monreal's research interests include language acquisition in deaf children, reading and writing skills of deaf children, and the role of Cued Speech in relation to oral language and literacy.

Chapter 7

This book is dedicated to:

Dr. R. Orin Cornett, (1913–2002)
Vice President, Gallaudet University
Whose invention of Cued Speech has far surpassed even what
Dr. Cornett could have envisioned;

The first generation of adult cuers of American English,
and their pioneering parents, siblings, and teachers;

Our Families
Especially Jim, Gina, Tony, and Lauren
Without whose love, support, and encouragement, this book
would not have been possible;

Dr. Sadanand Singh (1934–2010), who understood and appreciated the
value of Cued Speech for children who are deaf or hard of hearing and
encouraged us throughout our journey to complete this book;

and

Dr. Virginia A. Heidinger (1920–2006)
Professor Emerita, Gallaudet University.

Section I

CUED SPEECH AND CUED LANGUAGE

Chapter 1

WHY A BOOK ABOUT CUED SPEECH AND CUED LANGUAGE AND WHY NOW?

Carol J. LaSasso

Viewing Deaf Children as Capable Instead of Disabled

Currently, children who are deaf or hard of hearing in the United States are viewed as *disabled* and in need of costly government-supported special education services. These services include: individual education plans (IEPs), segregated classes, special teachers, special reading programs, adapted curricula, sign-supported speech communication methods, standardized test accommodations, and in some programs, American Sign Language (ASL) instead of English as the instructional language. Unfortunately, despite all of these services, the average reading comprehension level of deaf[1] stu-dents exiting the educational system today is comparable to that of 9-year-old hearing students (Karchmer & Mitchell, 2003). This statistic, virtually unchanged for the past 50 years, has led some to conclude that English is neither a *visual language* nor a *natural language* for deaf children and that only signed, or sign, languages are natural languages for deaf children (Johnson, Liddell, & Erting, 1989).

Contributors to this volume view deaf children differently. Deaf children are viewed as capable of learning English naturally in the same ways and at the same rates as hearing peers. English and other traditionally spoken languages[2] are viewed as being both *visual* and *natural* languages for deaf children when children are provided

---

[1]The term "deaf" is used in this chapter to refer to individuals who are deaf or hard of hearing.
[2]The existence of cued languages provides evidence that consonant-vowel and tonal languages can be used interactively, in real time, without employing speech or sound, and completely in the visual mode. In light of this evidence, use of the term "traditionally spoken language" within this book underscores the reality that "spoken" is a conventional mode rather than a required one. See Chapter 3.

clear, complete, visual access to the language of the home. Deaf children who come to school with cued English skills comparable to the spoken English skills of hearing peers are viewed as being capable of progressing through the *same* reading and content area curricula with unmodified instructional materials, instructional procedures, and achievement tests when they are provided *functionally equivalent visual access* to the language of instruction. Deaf children who come to school with another cued language (e.g., cued Spanish) are viewed capable of learning to read and progress through the English as a Second Language (ESL) curriculum with hearing peers when they have functionally equivalent, clear, complete, visual access to the ESL curriculum via cued English.

What is proposed in this book is a paradigm shift[3] in Deaf Education—away from viewing deaf children in terms of a traditional *deficiency model*, in which deaf children are automatically considered to be *disabled* or *communication disordered* in terms of acquiring English naturally, learning to read with the same materials and procedures as hearing peers, and progressing through academic curricula with far fewer accommodations, including modified tests.[4] The shift in perspective proposed here is for deaf children to be viewed as: (1) *capable* visual learners, (2) *capable* of acquiring English (and other traditionally spoken languages) in the same ways and at the same rates as hearing peers,

and (3) *capable* of learning to read and progress through the curriculum in the same ways and at the same rates as hearing peers. As will be demonstrated in the various chapters of this book, the shift in perspective proposed here not only is a feasible, cost-effective alternative for educating deaf children, but it also is practical, as well as theoretically and empirically supportable.

Language and Communication Options in the United States for Deaf Children

Readers of this book are expected to vary in terms of their familiarity with deafness, Deaf Education in the United States, ASL, manually coded English (MCE) sign systems, Cued Speech, and cued language; thus, this chapter begins with a discussion of key terminology that will appear in the various chapters of this book. It is important for readers to keep the distinction between *communication* and *language* clear: *communication* includes any means of conveying information, including traffic lights, noises, and nonlinguistic getures; a *language* is a socially constructed system of arbitrary symbols and rules that evolves within a community over time for the purpose of communicating. Cued Speech

---

[3]"Paradigm shift" is an oft-used phrase in academic literature, but the comprehensive and holistic change in perspective and thinking proposed in this volume can only truly be defined as a paradigm shift. In order for the reader to fully appreciate the arguments herein, virtually all commonly held and preconceived notions of many about deafness, communication, language, and the education of deaf individuals must be reexamined.

[4]See Cawthon (2008) for a summary of test accommodations used with deaf students in the United States.

is a system of *communication* that includes a set of visible symbols. The use of those symbols to visually convey the phonology, morphology, syntax, and prosodic features of English or other traditionally spoken languages in natural interaction, results in the emergence of a cued language. Cued languages employ certain visual features found in signed languages, structural features of spoken languages, and articulatory features unique to the cued mode (see Chapters 2 through 4).

Language Options for Parents of Deaf Children

Given the fact that sign-supported speech, or MCE sign systems, do not constitute language, traditional language options for parents of deaf children in the United States have been a spoken language (i.e., English) or a signed language (i.e., ASL). In this book, cued language, including *cued English* (see Chapter 10) and *cued Spanish* (see Chapter 17), is proposed as a third option. Some of the advantages and limitations of each option are discussed below.

Spoken Language Option

Spoken language options, variously referred to as oral-aural methods, typically are composed of speech, speechreading, and use of hearing enhancement devices (see Beattie, 2006 for an overview of the range of oral-aural options). The major advantage of a spoken language option, compared to signed or cued language options, is that typically it requires the least adaptation and effort for hearing parents. Parents focus on speaking clearly

and making sure that the child is looking at them in order to lipread, or speechread, what is being said (Charlier, Hage, Alegria, & Perier, 1990; Nicholls & Ling, 1982). Use of residual hearing and reliance on amplification are key features of spoken language/oral-aural methods.

The major limitation of oral-aural methods is that only about 30% of syllables or words can be visually distinguished via lipreading (Nicholls & Ling, 1982). For example, the phonemes /p/, /b/, and /m/ look identical on the lips and cannot be distinguished solely by vision. Language acquisition is challenging, at the very least, where the input is only 30% accessible. Children who tend to benefit most from a spoken language option are those who either have a cochlear implant or have a lesser degree of hearing loss (Blamey et al., 2001; Geers, 2006).

Signed Language Option

Prior to the work of Stokoe (1960), signed languages were not considered to be languages in their own right. Stokoe, however, demonstrated that ASL is a complete visual language, structurally independent from spoken English, with which it coexists. The syntax and grammar of ASL are independent from English. Regardless, ASL is as functional as English or any other traditionally spoken language (Stokoe, 1960). More than 120 signed languages have been identified (Gordon, 2005; retrieved February 9, 2009 from http://www.ethnologue.com). Signed languages currently being studied for their structure and use by sign language researchers around the world include: Mexican Sign Language, Italian Sign Language, French Sign Language, Swedish Sign Language, Norwegian Sign Language, British Sign Language,

Australian Sign Language (Auslan), New Zealand Sign Language, German Sign Language, Dutch Sign Language, Indo-Pakistan Sign Language, Japanese Sign Language, Vietnamese Sign Language, Irish Sign Language, Flemish Sign Language, and Argentine Sign Language (personal communication, Ceil Lucas, Linguistics Department, Gallaudet University, February, 2009).

The major advantage of signed languages for children who are deaf is that they are visual and exist and function fully in the absence of either speech or hearing. The major disadvantages for nonsigning hearing parents relate to the availability of language models and the difficulties inherent in learning a new language in a timely manner to be effective language models for children. More than 95% of children who are deaf or are born to nonsigning hearing parents (Mitchell & Karchmer, 2004). The difficulty that hearing parents have in learning ASL vocabulary and syntactic rules in a timely manner to be effective language models for their child during the critical language learning years is well known (Kemp, 1998).

Cued Language Option

Cued languages, including cued French (Langage Parlé Complété), cued Spanish (La Palabra Complementada), cued American English, cued Thai, and the other 59 cued languages and dialects to date, are visual forms of traditionally spoken languages that exist and function fully in the absence of speech or hearing.

Cued languages consist of elements of both signed and spoken languages, but have features that are unique to cued languages (see Chapters 2 through 4).[5] In this book, unless otherwise noted, cued language is discussed in the context of English.

There are two primary advantages of cued language over signed language for the 95% of parents of deaf children who are themselves hearing (Mitchell & Karchmer, 2004). First, learning to cue a language that one already knows can be accomplished in a weekend. Parents who do so can be fluent visual language models of English and other traditionally spoken languages for their deaf child in a very short period of time. Torres, Moreno-Torres, and Santana (2006) found that the mother in their study became a fluent cuer of Spanish in less than 3 months. The author of this chapter has supervised numerous graduate students who had completed a basic cueing class and were assigned to do their 6 weeks' student teaching in a cued English class with deaf children.[6] In each situation, at the beginning of the student teaching practicum, the student teacher was judged by the cooperating teacher as not yet a fluent cuer (i.e., able to cue at the same rate as or slightly slower than speech would normally occur); however, by the end of 6 weeks, each of the graduate students was judged by their cooperating teacher as being fluent.

A second advantage of cued English over ASL is that it offers the same advantage in learning to read that English-speaking children have, compared to chil-

---

[5]Although a cued language and a traditionally spoken language can co-occur, neither speech nor hearing is required for the reception or expression of cued language.
[6]Deaf students in these classes ranged in age from 8 to 14 years.

dren who are learning English as a Second Language. That is, learning to read a language is much simpler for children who are familiar with the conversational form of that language *before* formal reading instruction than it is for children who are learning to read while *simultaneously* learning the language.

Visual Communication Systems Used with Deaf Students in the United States

In an attempt to convey English to, from, and among deaf students, at least three approaches employ the visual mode. These include: fingerspelling, signing MCE sign systems, and cueing English.

Fingerspelling

Fingerspelling systems vary from country to country; however, in all forms, fingerspellers convey the letters of the alphabet (i.e., graphemes) used to spell words in that language. Fingerspelling in many countries, including the United States, uses 26 discrete handshapes on a single hand to represent the 26 letters of the alphabet. Fingerspelling in other countries, including England, is a two-handed system. Fingerspellers can spell out each word, sentence, paragraph, or longer unit of discourse being conveyed. The information conveyed by fingerspelling about English is neither phonemic nor morphemic, but rather is *graphemic*.

As a code for spelling the words of a language that one already knows, one advantage of fingerspelling is that the

handshapes can be learned quickly; many of the handshapes are iconic so they are easy to remember; and once learned, English or any other alphabetic language can be conveyed to and among users fluent in that language. Disadvantages of fingerspelling include that it can be slower for face-to-face interaction. Fingerspelling has remained a component of both MCE sign systems and ASL, but it is not considered an independent means of language acquisition and is not currently used as a communication system unto itself by any language group.

Manually Coded English (MCE) Sign Systems

MCE sign systems, such as Seeing Essential English, or SEE I (Anthony, 1971); Signing Exact English or SEE II (Gustason, Pfetzing, & Zawolkow, 1972); Linguistics of Visual English (Wampler, 1971); and Signed English (Bornstein, Saulnier, & Hamilton, 1973–1984), are *hybrids*, meaning that they are motivated by elements of both ASL and English. MCE sign systems combine visually accessible, manual, and nonmanual signs from ASL with English syntax,[7] and use invented manual signs in an attempt to visually convey subword, morphological elements such as English prefixes and suffixes. The major difference between a cued language and an MCE sign system is that cueing conveys English and other cued languages beginning at the *phoneme* level, whereas the most fundamental unit of English that MCE sign systems even attempt to convey is *morphemic*. Compared to fingerspelling or cueing, MCE sign systems require the

---

[7]English syntax differs from ASL syntax.

most memory on the part of the expressive communicator who needs to learn an extensive sign vocabulary[8] and make translation decisions regarding which ASL (or invented) sign to pair with which English word. MCE sign systems have been in widespread use by parents and schools in the United States since the early 1970s. Despite their widespread usage, reading levels of deaf students today are the same as they were before the MCE sign systems were created.

Cued Speech

Cued Speech, developed in 1967, is a manual communication system designed to convey English visually at its most fundamental (phoneme) level. Cued Speech has been adapted to 63 languages and dialects (see Figure 1–1).

Cued American English, the first cued language, includes eight handshapes and four placements combined with nonmanual information on the mouth[9] to convey English beginning at the *phoneme* level, the same fundamental level that traditionally spoken languages convey via speech. Figure 1–2 illustrates the handshapes and placements for cued American English. Phonemes, the most fundamental component of a language, combine to form syllables and morphemes, which can either be bound (e.g., prefixes) or free (e.g., words). Morphemes, the smallest *meaningful* unit of language, combine syntactically in a rule-driven system for word order to form phrases and sentences and longer units of discourse.

Cued symbols vary slightly from country to country; however, in all forms, cuers convey languages, alphabetic or tonal, at their most fundamental (i.e., phoneme) level. Cuers present each phoneme of each cued word with the same specificity and distinction that speakers present each phoneme of each spoken word. In this way, it is possible for hearing and deaf cuers to convey any dialect of English (e.g., *pahk the cah* for *park the car*, with a Boston accent) or other traditionally spoken languages. Cued language transliterators (CLTs) can, to a certain degree, convey languages they do not understand. By listening to and visually recoding the phonemes of each spoken syllable, the transliterator leaves it to the deaf individual to group the phonemes (into words) and comprehend the text, a task that must also be undertaken by their hearing classmates (see Chapter 17 for a description of this process as it is used in foreign language instruction). Cuers of English and other traditionally spoken languages also can convey *prosody* to reflect rhythm, intonation, stress, and related attributes of the given language.

The Timeliness of a Book About Cued Speech and Cued Language

A number of factors are converging at this time to support the timeliness of a book about Cued Speech and cued language. These include: (1) the continued

---

[8]Compared to ASL, some might consider MCE sign systems easier to learn because the signer does not need to learn syntactic rules of ASL. Instead, ASL words are signed in the same word order as English.

[9]Additional manual and nonmanual features carry prosodic information.

Afrikaans	Hausa	Polish
Alu	Hawai'ian	Portuguese (Brazilian)
American English	Hebrew	Portuguese (European)
Arabic	Hindi	Punjabi (Lahore Region)
Australian English	Hungarian	Russian
Bengali	Idoma Nigerian	Scottish English
British English	Igbo	Setswana
Byelorussian	Indonesian	Shona
Cantonese	Italian	Somali
Catalan	Japanese	South African English
Croatian-Serbian	Kiluba-Kituba	Spanish
Czech	Korean	Swahili
Danish	Lingala	Swedish
Dutch	Malagasy	Swiss-German
Filipino/Tagalog	Malay	Telegu
Finnish	Malayalam	Thai
French	Maltese	Trinidad-Tobago (English)
French-Canadian	Mandarin	Tshiluba
German	Marathi	Turkish
Greek	Navajo	Urdu
Gujarati	Oriya	Yoroba Nigerian

Figure 1–1. The 63 languages and dialects to which Cued Speech has been adapted to date. Adapted with permission from a chart available on the National Cued Speech Association's Web site (http://www.cuedspeech.org).

CUED SPEECH FOR AMERICAN ENGLISH

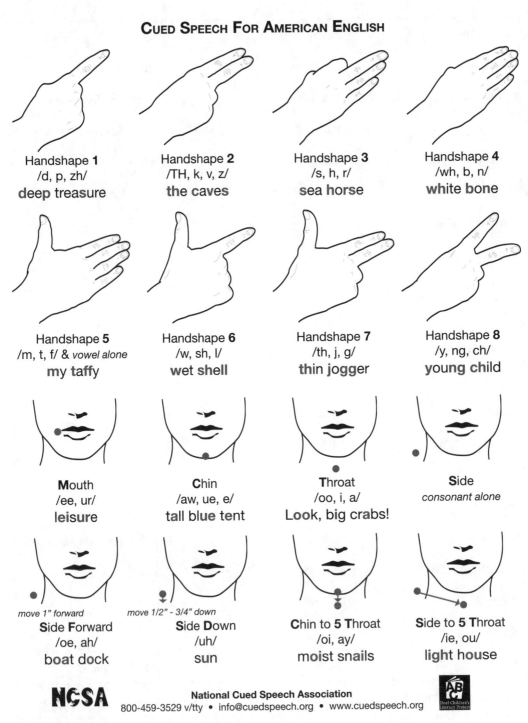

Handshape **1**
/d, p, zh/
deep trea**s**ure

Handshape **2**
/TH, k, v, z/
the caves

Handshape **3**
/s, h, r/
sea horse

Handshape **4**
/wh, b, n/
white bone

Handshape **5**
/m, t, f/ & *vowel alone*
my taffy

Handshape **6**
/w, sh, l/
wet shell

Handshape **7**
/th, j, g/
thin jogger

Handshape **8**
/y, ng, ch/
young child

Mouth
/ee, ur/
leisure

Chin
/aw, ue, e/
tall blue tent

Throat
/oo, i, a/
Look, big crabs!

Side
consonant alone

move 1" forward
Side **F**orward
/oe, ah/
boat dock

move 1/2" - 3/4" down
Side **D**own
/uh/
sun

Chin to **5 T**hroat
/oi, ay/
moist snails

Side to **5 T**hroat
/ie, ou/
light house

NCSA

National Cued Speech Association
800-459-3529 v/tty • info@cuedspeech.org • www.cuedspeech.org

Figure 1–2. American English cue chart with IPA symbols.

low reading achievement levels of deaf students; (2) recent advances in our knowledge of factors impacting the development of reading; (3) increased accountability of schools to develop students' phonological and reading abilities; (4) evidence that English and other traditionally spoken languages are *visual languages* when cued; (5) economic factors as an impetus for examining current instructional practices; and (6) advances in technology related to early identification and hearing enhancement, including cochlear implants.

Continued Low Reading Levels

The major factor promoting the timeliness of a book about Cued Speech and cued language at this time relates to the continued low reading achievement levels of deaf students despite more than 35 years of widespread use of MCE sign systems by parents and teachers of deaf students. The average reading level of deaf high school seniors is third to fourth grade, comparable to that of 9-year-old hearing children (Mitchell & Karchmer, 2004). This remains virtually unchanged since before the MCE sign systems were created to address the low reading achievement levels in the early 1970s. Drasgow and Paul (1995) discuss two hypotheses for the limited effectiveness of MCE sign systems for conveying English: the structural limitation hypothesis and the degraded input hypotheses (see Chapter 12). In the view of the editors of this book, the major limitation of MCE sign systems is that they do not convey any information about the phonology of English; therefore, deaf children are not afforded clear and complete access to the "continuous phoneme stream" of English which is considered essential for natural language acquisition (see Chapter 12).

Recent Advances in our Knowledge of Factors Impacting the Development of Reading

The timeliness of a book about Cued Speech and cued language is also supported by recent advances in our knowledge about factors that impact the development of reading. The federally appointed National Reading Panel (National Reading Panel [NRP], 2000) conducted a met-analysis of the research literature related to reading comprehension. The NRP (2000) identified five variables that are critical to the development of reading, including: phonemic awareness, vocabulary, phonics, fluency, and comprehension strategies. Readers of this book will learn that linguistic access via Cued Speech, compared to communication access via oral-aural methods or MCE sign systems, is the most theoretically and empirically supportable mode for developing *each* of these abilities in deaf students. Refer to Chapter 12 for a description of how Cued Speech addresses each of these areas needed for literacy development of deaf students.

Increased Accountability of Schools to Develop Students' Phonological and Reading Abilities

The timeliness of a book about Cued Speech and cued language is also supported by the ever increasing accountability of schools for improving reading achievement of all students in the United States, including deaf students (see Cawthon & Wurtz, 2008, 2009 for a discussion of increased accountability in schools). The No Child Left Behind (NCLB) legislation (2001) restricts federal funds to schools that fail to meet student accountability measures, including reading achievement measures. Less punitive federal measures designed to improve reading achievement have included the lucrative NCLB Reading First and Early Reading First grants to states for educational programs to address, among other things, phonological abilities of students. Increasingly, educational programs serving deaf students are seeking ways to develop students' phonological needs. Visual-kinesthetic sensory approaches to phonics instruction for deaf students, such as Visual Phonics (Trezak, Wang, Wood, Gampp, & Paul, 2007), are gaining in popularity. The advantage of Cued Speech over Visual Phonics is that Cued Speech not only addresses the same phonics needs of deaf students, but it also serves the broader purpose of providing a visually complete mode for conveying and receiving English unambiguously, in the absence of speech or hearing. Furthermore, because cued English produced by deaf students does not depend on speech intelligibility, their cueing teachers can be more accurate in their educational diagnoses, and provide more appropriate instruction (see Chapter 12).

Economic Factors as Impetus for Examining Current Instructional Practices

Historically, special education in the United States has placed an enormous financial burden on shrinking state and federal budgets. The use of Cued Speech has the potential for greatly reducing the financial burden of educating deaf students. Specifically, when deaf children from English-speaking homes come to school with cued English abilities comparable to English abilities of hearing peers, they can be fully mainstreamed with hearing peers as long as they have clear, complete visual access to cued English. Furthermore, deaf children from homes where a cued language other than cued English is used (e.g., cued Spanish), can be mainstreamed with other ESL learners and can be expected to function as well as hearing peers when they have clear, complete visual access to the language(s) of instruction, including cued English and cued Spanish (see Chapter 17 for a description of a public school program in the United States that offers cued Spanish to parents of deaf children).

Deaf children who are afforded clear complete visual access to the curriculum via a cued language can be expected to learn to read with the same reading materials and procedures as used with hearing peers; thereby eliminating the need for special reading materials. Furthermore, deaf cuers who come to school with cued English language abilities comparable to the spoken English abilities of hearing peers and who have teachers who are fluent cued English users can be expected to progress as effectively and at the same rate as hearing peers through the normal curriculum and perform comparably on standardized tests normed on hearing students. This reality has been shown to eliminate the need to provide the deaf student with: (1) segregated special classes, (2) adapted curricula, and (3) modified standardized tests. Because consistent use of cued language allows deaf students to be educated in the same places with the same instructional materials, procedures, and tests, and on the same timeline as their hearing peers, it greatly reduces the cost of special education services. Given increasing demands that special education resources be used judiciously, the time is right for a close examination of Cued Speech and cued language.

Increasing Evidence That Signed Languages Are Not the Only Complete Visual Languages for Deaf People

Another factor promoting the timeliness of a book about Cued Speech and cued language is increasing evidence from deaf cuers of English, French, Spanish, and other traditionally spoken languages that natural signed languages are not the only complete visual languages for deaf people (Johnson et al., 1989). The belief that signed languages are the only natural languages for deaf people was the impetus for a paradigm shift in Deaf Education that began in the 1990s in many of the day and residential schools away from English and toward ASL as the instructional language. By 1999, between 36 to 40% of deaf children in day and residential schools were in programs that described themselves as ASL-written English bilingual (formerly referred to as bilingual-bicultural, or BiBi programs) (LaSasso & Lollis, 2003). In these programs, ASL is typically reported to be the instructional language, both spoken English and signed English are typically discouraged, and English is developed via fingerspelling and print. LaSasso and Lollis found that the reported impetus for these programs was: (1) dissatisfaction with continued low reading levels of deaf students; and (2) belief in the views expressed by Johnson et al. (1989) that English *cannot* be acquired naturally by

deaf children, that English-based signing (i.e., MCE sign systems) is ineffective, and that the only alternative is a separate instructional language, one that is a complete visual language (i.e., ASL). In a more recent reflection of many of those same views, Gallaudet University, the world's only liberal arts university for deaf people, also has recently declared itself to be an ASL-English bilingual university. At Gallaudet, spoken or signed-based English is discouraged by many in favor of ASL.

Evidence from the first generation of adult native cuers of English (see Chapter 9) and the first deaf children of native cuers of English (see Chapter 8), coupled with more than 25 years of research related to the impact of Cued Speech on natural language acquisition and the development of reading (see Chapters 11 and 12), support the positions that: (1) cueing is an effective communication mode for conveying English and other traditionally spoken languages clearly and completely in the absence of either speech or hearing, and (2) the natural acquisition of English and other traditionally spoken languages is within the realm of possibilities, and even likely, for deaf children consistently exposed to a cued language during the critical language learning years.

Advances in Technology Related to Early Identification and Hearing Enhancement

Recent advances in technology for early identification of hearing loss, coupled with hearing enhancement technology, including cochlear implants and digital hearing aids, are another factor, converging with others, to promote the timeliness of a book about Cued Speech and cued language. Although technological advances have dramatically enhanced the potential of spoken language options for deaf children (Ackley & Decker, 2006; Harkins & Bakke, 2003; Watson, Hardie, Archbold, & Wheeler, 2008), none of these devices is yet capable of providing clear, complete access to English and other traditionally spoken languages (Bradham & Jones, 2008), and none is projected to do so in the foreseeable future (personal communication, Robert Ackley, Chair, Hearing Speech and Language Sciences Department, Gallaudet University, February, 2009). Specifically, as discussed in Chapter 6, available hearing enhancement devices do not yet provide sufficient acoustic information about the fine-grained phonology of English and other traditionally spoken languages; because they do not provide sufficient acoustic phonological contrasts provided by spoken language, these devices cannot supplant the visual phonological contrasts provided via cued language. Leybaert, Colin, and Hage (Chapter 6) describe findings from a recent study showing that Cued Speech enhances phonological perception of children with cochlear implants.

What Readers Will Learn from This Book

Readers will learn that Cued Speech has made contributions to numerous other fields of study, particularly in terms of cross-disciplinary research. Our understanding of visual language and communication has been enhanced by the inclusion of Cued Speech in academic dialogues by highlighting the similarities and differences among spoken, signed, and cued language. Readers will learn of the latest computer-generated aids to communication, which are either being developed for use with Cued Speech or were conceived because of Cued Speech. Readers also will learn of the expanding role of Cued Speech in the lives of hearing and deaf individuals (e.g., developmental, social, academic). Finally, readers of this book will understand how the case of Cued Speech lends further support to the notion that children, regardless of hearing status, have an irrepressible predisposition to acquire language, whether signed, spoken, *or cued*, whether alphabetic or tonal.

Contributions to Other Fields

Readers of this book will learn that cueing has moved far beyond Orin Cornett's 1966 invention of Cued Speech. This is true in terms of its use (by whom, how, and for what purposes); its status as a means of first-order language transmission; and contributions to the fields of speech science, hearing science, cognition, linguistics, reading, and deaf education.

Speech Science

Cueing has influenced the field of speech science by demonstrating that phonological perception by those who have access to the visual and acoustic modes is not uniquely an *auditory* perceptual process, but rather, it is a *bi-* or *multimodal* process, heavily influenced by visual information.

Hearing Science

Despite the tremendous advances in hearing enhancement technology, most notably in cochlear implants, none is yet capable of providing full auditory access to spoken language. In Chapter 6, results of recent research illustrating how Cued Speech enhances speech perception of children with cochlear implants are described.

Cognition

Our understanding of sensory perception via exposure to co-occurring cued and spoken information has informed studies of perception, memory, and cognition. Several contributors to this volume report novel research related to phonetic and phonological perception (see Chapter 3 by Metzger & Fleetwood, Chapter 5 by Alégria, and Chapter 18 by Bernstein, Auer, & Jiang). For a discussion of how phonological information is processed in memory by deaf individuals perceiving Cued Speech, see Chapter 24.

Linguistics

The existence of cued language has influenced the fields of linguistics and psycholingustics by demonstrating that well-established notions such as minimal pairs, allophones, phonemes, stress, and prosody can exist independently of acoustic information. Linguistic terms (e.g., phonemes, phonology, phonological recoding, phonics, rhyming, and phonemic awareness), that are traditionally defined in terms of "speech sounds," need to be redefined to account for the fact that in cued languages, these constructs exist in the absence of either speech or hearing (see Chapters 2 through 4).

Reading

Readers of this book will learn that phonics, which has traditionally been considered to require "auditory feedback" to "sound out" novel print words that are in readers' conversational vocabulary, can

be used by deaf children who cue. Prelingually, profoundly deaf children from cued language backgrounds illustrate that one does not need to be able to hear or speak to be able to phonically attack novel print words. Deaf cuers can be observed to "cue out" novel print words in ways similar to hearing people sounding out novel words. It is well established that children who come to the task of learning to decode print with a fully formed language base and age-appropriate phonological awareness skills are better equipped to apply that foundation to the phonics decoding process by the first grade and reading comprehension by the fourth grade (Juel, 1988). Research related to the natural acquisition of cued language by deaf children indicates that this phenomenon can apply to deaf as well as hearing children.

Deaf Education

Cued Speech has expanded our concept of where deaf students go to school and how they are educated. For example, whereas "bilingual deaf education" once only meant an ASL-written English model in which ASL is promoted as the instructional language and spoken or signed English is discouraged (LaSasso & Lollis, 2003), an alternative model now exists (described in Chapter 10) in which both ASL and English are conveyed conversationally and visually, and deaf students are exposed to English *prior* to reading instruction. Another application of Cued Speech to foreign language instruction for deaf students is described by Klossner and Crain in Chapter 17, where they also describe an effective Spanish-language parent education program for Spanish speaking parents of deaf children in a large public school program in the United States.

Interdisciplinary Nature of Cued Speech and Cued Language Research

Readers may be surprised to find that so many authors contributing chapters to a book about Cued Speech and cued language are not researchers in deaf education and/or reading, but rather are scientists from the fields of linguistics, psycholinguistics, neurolinguistics, cognition, speech science, hearing science, and computer science as well as service providers for deaf children and youth, including audiologists, cued language transliterators, teachers of deaf students, and teacher educators. The chapters in this book reflect *recent advances* in our understanding and application of Cued Speech and cued language as well as how they will be useful in the *near future*. What the contributing authors and editors of this volume have in common is a shared admiration and respect for cued language, beginning with the development of Cued Speech, for not only addressing the need of deaf children to naturally acquire English or other traditionally spoken languages in preparation for reading, but also for providing insights into the nature of language, be it in signed or traditionally spoken modalities. The invention of Cued Speech and the subsequent emergence of cued language has provoked more research in more academic disciplines than Cornett (or anybody else) could have envisioned.

Cornett understood that exposure to spoken language and/or invented sign systems does not provide deaf children sufficient input for learning to use or read any language. Cornett's original invention of a *visual* communication system, first characterized as an aid to speechreading, has evolved into cued language counterparts for 63 of the world's spoken languages and dialects. Cornett could not have envisioned that one day other scholars of cueing, including those who are themselves deaf, would reciprocate and inform further study of both *spoken* and *signed* language. For example, in Chapter 4 of this volume, psycholinguists Koo and Supalla, each of whom is deaf (one a native signer of ASL; the other a native cuer of American English), describe and discuss their research findings related to the structure of cued language, which provide insights into the nature of both signed language and spoken language.

Synergistic Relationships Between and Among Spoken, Signed, and Cued Language

Advances in the knowledge of signed languages in the 1960s greatly influenced Cornett's creation of Cued Speech. Cornett was particularly influenced by Stokoe's (1960) seminal work that established ASL as a fully developed language with phonological, morphological, semantic, syntactic, and pragmatic elements that exist in the absence of speech and hearing. Stokoe's findings challenged the thinking of the time, including Cornett's, that human languages are inextricably linked to speech. If Stokoe were correct, Cornett reasoned, and languages could be conveyed entirely in the visual mode without speech or hearing, perhaps there were manual alternatives for conveying *English* clearly and completely beginning at its most basic (i.e., phonemic) level to deaf people. As a result, cued English shares characteristics with both signed ASL and spoken English; it is a visual gestural language, and it transmits information about the phonology, morphology, syntax, and prosody of English.

Alignment of Cueing with Computer Technology

Readers of this book will learn that technological advances related to cueing also have moved far beyond Cornett's original Autocuer, which consists of eyeglasses and a wearable computer that is capable of analyzing incoming speech and translating that acoustic input into visual cues that were superimposed on the face of the speaker. Today, there are at least four teams of researchers on both sides of the Atlantic, which are employing computer technology to address phonologic access and perceptual needs of deaf individuals, including (1) a computer-based spoken-to-cued synthesis system integrated with a lexical analysis tool, (2) a complete 3-dimensional text-to-cued French synthesizer for television access for individuals who are deaf or hard of hearing, and (3) computer-based language supplement devices which have the potential to address visual access needs of deaf individuals in face-to-face conversations with hearing individuals. The technological devices related to cueing described in this volume demonstrate how great the possibilities are for technology to overcome communication barriers related to sensory differences, as well as opportunities for private industries that are interested in automatic cued language translation.

Expanding Applications of Cueing

Cornett initially envisioned Cued Speech as a bimodal tool for developing English language abilities in children who are deaf rather than as a self-contained and wholly visible phenomenon. This initial conceptualization was one of hearing parents simultaneously cueing and speaking with deaf children receiving the cues (and perhaps, some of the auditory message), but likely only speaking in response. Today, this can and does happen; but also common are deaf children who cue expressively to their parents and peers; some choose to simultaneously speak, others do not. As the reader will see in Chapter 9, the first deaf children growing up with cued English have now grown into deaf adults who continue to cue expressively for a variety of personal, academic, and professional reasons. Readers will learn about the views of these deaf adults, related to communication, language, literacy, academic, social, and professional attainments. Their views illustrate the direct and indirect positive effects that exposure to cued language can have on individuals who are deaf and can help counter claims of some that deaf children growing up with cued language suffer from social isolation, a lack of deaf identity, or inability to communicate with hearing or deaf individuals from varied communication backgrounds.

Quite recently, the first generation of deaf native cuers of English have married, begun families of their own, and for the first time, have become cued language models for their own children, whether deaf or hearing. In Chapter 8, readers will learn about the language development and pre-literacy development of deaf twin daughters of two deaf native cuers of English who use cued English with their daughters.

The Irrepressible Predisposition for Language

Finally, readers of this book will learn that the example of deaf children from cued language backgrounds supports the prevalent view that children are biologically predisposed to acquire the language of their home as their first language (L1) *naturally*. Previous support for this view has been limited to the observations that children in all parts of the world tend to acquire their home language in similar ways and rates, regardless of the complexity or nature (alphabetic or tonal) of the language. Prior to the emergence of cued language, the one group of children for whom this theory did not seem to apply were deaf children of nonsigning hearing parents. It is demonstrated in this volume that it is not *deafness*, per se, that prevents deaf children from naturally acquiring traditionally spoken home languages; rather, it is the *communication method* selected by adult language models that promotes or precludes the natural acquisition of the English and other traditionally spoken languages by deaf children. In this book, we provide evidence from research conducted in Europe and North America that cueing provides clear, complete, *visual* access to the continuous phoneme stream of alphabetic and tonal languages such that deaf children can acquire English and other traditionally spoken languages *naturally* in preparation for formal reading instruction and academic achievement, in much the same ways and rates as hearing peers.

Historically, the debate in the United States about the optimum L1 for a deaf child, in preparation for formal reading instruction, has been limited to the perspectives of those who support either *English* or *ASL*. The perspective of Cornett and this volume's editors is that given the important role of parents during the critical language learning years, the *home language* is the optimum L1 for a deaf child. Where the home language is a natural signed language, that language should be the child's L1. Where the home language is a traditionally spoken language, the viability of that language as L1 and cueing as a mode for conveying that language (e.g., English, Spanish, and other traditionally spoken languages) is a theme that figures prominently in this volume.

Organization of the Book

The 24 chapters in this book are organized into six sections: Section I: Cued Speech and Cued Language; Section II: Cued Speech for Phonological Perception; Section III: Cueing for Natural Language Acquisition; Section IV: Cued Language for the Development of Reading; Section V: Cued Speech for Atypical Populations; and Section VI: Cued Speech/Cued Language on the Horizon.

Section I: Cued Speech and Cued Language

This introductory chapter is followed by three chapters that address cueing from a linguistic point of view. In Chapter 2, Shull and Crain describe the history of Cued Speech and the scientific challenges Cornett faced in designing a system to fully represent phonology visually for American English and 62 other languages and dialects, demonstrating that cueing is appropriate for more than only English or French. They describe eight common features, or universals, in the various cueing systems. They explain how discrete phonemes are formed into meaningful units of language, including syllables, words, and longer units of literal and nonliteral discourse without speech. They distinguish

Cued Speech and cued language, including their inextricable, but separate, features and internal linguistic variation. Finally, they discuss different categories of cuers and distinguish between cued language transliterators and sign language interpreters.

In Chapter 3, Metzger and Fleetwood frame the discussion of the relationship between Cued Speech and cued language. The authors make the case that, because the linguistic decisions of deaf native cuers in their study seemed unaffected by linguistically dissociated spoken messages that co-occurred with cued messages, cued languages are truly unimodal despite their roots in Cued Speech, a bimodal system. The authors discuss how the emergence of cued languages has contributed to linguists' knowledge about the nature of traditionally spoken languages and language in general; specifically that the most basic unit of language (i.e., phonemes) can be fully specified, or distinguished, visually without speech or hearing. The authors' findings provide further evidence that the ability of cued language to provide this visual specificity makes it a viable visible option for deaf children.

Chapter 4, by Koo and Supalla, describes results of two experimental studies that were designed to examine the linguistic outcome of lifelong experience with Cued English in terms of a theoretical nativization model. The nativation model proposes that language learners go through an internal structuring process in which they initially construct a unique linguistic system (nativization) using presumed innate linguistic abilities and gradually re-adapt their system (denativization) to match the target environment language. As deaf native cuers of English presumably have unambiguous visual access to their language environment, the question investigated by Koo and Supalla is whether

deaf native cuers depend more on their own internal mechanism or undergo a denativization process toward a complete phonological representation of the target language. The first study is a linguistic analysis of cued sentence production by adult native cuers of English. The second examines the internalization of English allomorphs in adult native cuers of English.

Section II: Cued Speech for Phonological Perception

Section II has two chapters. In Chapter 5, by Alégria, the reader will learn about the audiovisual, or multimodal, nature of phonological perception and the role cueing has played in understanding this nature. Alégria focuses on how cueing is processed, specifically how lipreading and hand cues articulate with one another to produce visual phonetic information. He discusses pioneering research which provides evidence that cueing improves lipreading, thereby permitting elaborate linguistic representations to be conveyed, which are equivalent to those elaborated via spoken language. Finally, Alégria discusses the effects of early (versus later) exposure to cued language in the context of native cuers, citing the first generation of deaf children who have developed linguistic competence sharing the phonemic structure of spoken language, on the basis of a purely visual input.

In Chapter 6, Leybaert, Colin, and Hage discuss findings from recent studies, which show that children fitted with a cochlear implant rely much more on speechreading and are better at audiovisual integration than children with normal hearing. The authors then describe their recent research with the McGurk paradigm, which demonstrates that children with a cochlear implant are influenced more by the visual information read on the lips than auditory information in the case of incongruent stimuli. They reason that it seems probable that children who first develop a phonological system through exposure to a cued language will benefit more from the auditory information delivered by the cochlear implant than those without exposure to a cued language. They further reason that consistent exposure to a cued language will facilitate the development of morphosyntax, which could be at risk for children who rely only on auditory information delivered by the implant.

Section III: Cueing for Natural Language Acquisition

This section has four chapters. In Chapter 7, Moreno-Torres and Torres summarize findings from their research related to the nature and quality of linguistic input provided by cueing. Findings suggest that mothers are able to learn to cue their home language and provide a rich linguistic input to their deaf child in a very short period of time without a negative impact on the amount of language conveyed by mothers, nor on the use of natural gestures.

In Chapter 8, Crain reports findings from the first study of the expressive and receptive language development of deaf children born to deaf native cuers of English. The longitudinal study tracked prereading language development milestones of twin girls from 10 to 36 months, finding phonological, morphological, lexical, and syntactic developmental trajectories within the ranges expected of hearing children born to hearing parents. Preliteracy behaviors such as nursery rhymes, letter naming, and print letter recognition were observed

by the age of 3 years, suggesting normal preliteracy development.

In Chapter 9, Crain and LaSasso report findings from a national survey of deaf adults who self-identify as cuers. Questions in this study explore the effects of being raised with cued language in terms of deaf cuers' self-identity and perceptions of hearing and deaf communities, as well as the current respective roles of cued and signed communication in their lives. Findings from this study reflect that these deaf adults perceive themselves as confident, academically successful, and highly literate and suggest that individuals raised with cued language do not appear to suffer from isolation at home, school, or with peers, and that these deaf adults generally consider themselves highly capable of moving between and among various hearing and deaf groups and subgroups, adapting communication modality and language usage to match their environments.

In Chapter 10, Kyllo describes a prototype Cued English and ASL bilingual program in the United States, which reports reading achievement scores of deaf students immersed in cued American English to be comparable to hearing peers. This chapter should be particularly interesting to parents and educators of deaf children.

Section IV: Cued Language for the Development of Reading

Section IV has four chapters. The first two chapters of this section are the result of a lengthy "dialogue" among the three editors of this book regarding the nature of reading and, consequently, the role of Cued Speech in its development, instruction, and assessment. Ultimately, it was decided to discuss separately: (1) the role of Cued Speech in reading defined narrowly as mastery of the alphabetic principle and (2) the role of Cued Speech in reading more broadly as: comprehension or measured comprehension (i.e., performance on reading comprehension tests). Leybaert and Colin, with strong backgrounds in experimental psychology, have focused much of their research on a more narrow view of reading—decoding. LaSasso and Crain, with backgrounds in Speech and Hearing Sciences and Deaf Education, tend to view reading more broadly as comprehension or measured comprehension (test performance).

In Chapter 11, Leybaert, Colin, and LaSasso focus on reading in a narrow sense (i.e., decoding). Most of the cueing research related to reading of deaf students has focused on phonological factors impacting reading, including: phonemic awareness, phonological recoding, and phonics. While acknowledging that the ultimate goal of reading instruction is comprehension and demonstrating comprehension on tests, the authors of this chapter guide the reader through the research related to deaf students' phonological awareness, decoding and recoding, and spelling abilities.

In Chapter 12, LaSasso and Crain discuss reading in a broader context: reading comprehension and measured reading comprehension (i.e., performance on reading comprehension tests). Comprehension is conceptualized as a process that either moves forward or is impeded based on the reader's own questions regarding code, language, content, and the nature of the reading task. In this view, knowledge of the language used in print material read by readers is viewed as important, if not more important than phonological knowledge related to phonemic awareness, phonological recoding, and phonics (i.e., the alphabetic principle). In this chapter, the theoretical supportability of Cued Speech compared to MCE sign systems for the natural acquisition of English is emphasized and the relative advantages of Cued Speech over Visual Phonics for the development of reading abilities are described.

In Chapter 13, Koo, Crain, LaSasso, and Eden report findings from a first of its kind study that compares groups representing combinations of *hearing status* (i.e., deaf and hearing), *language* (i.e., ASL and English), and *communication modality* (i.e., oral, signing, cueing). The study is also the first of its kind to employ a new test of phoneme detection, a computer-based phoneme recognition test for use with all hearing and communication backgrounds. One of the most important findings from this study relates to measured word fluency of deaf (including cueing) readers. This is of particular interest, considering that measures of written English fluency reliable for use with deaf readers are not commercially available (see Chapter 12). Furthermore, fluency is one of the five areas identified impacting reading in the 2000 NRP report. The finding that deaf cuers' word fluency was superior to that of oral or signing deaf participants and comparable to that of hearing peers is intriguing.

In Chapter 14, Crain and LaSasso report results of a study of the phonological awareness and reading comprehension of 10- to 14-year-old deaf developing readers from oral and cueing backgrounds, utilizing a generative rhyming task and a standard silent reading measure. Despite a more severe degree of deafness and lower rated speech intelligibility, deaf participants from the cueing group demonstrated a higher degree of phonological awareness than did deaf participants from the oral group, generating more correct rhyming responses, and more importantly, more correct responses which bear no orthographic similarity to test stimuli, therefore requiring an internalized phonological representation.

Section V: Cued Speech for Atypical Populations

This section contains three chapters. In Chapter 15, audiologists Arnold and Berlin present a discussion of the differential diagnosis of auditory neuropathy/auditory dys-synchrony (AN/AD) as a temporal disorder of hearing distinct from the traditional view of deafness. The authors overview the common approaches to visual supports for spoken language development for children with AN/AD and argue for the application of Cued Speech for this underestimated and largely misdiagnosed population.

In Chapter 16, psychologist Morere discusses the diagnosis of secondary disabilities in deaf children, including: primary language disorder, nonverbal language disorder, attention deficit hyperactivity disorder, autism, and the benefits of cueing for language development and teaching with these special populations. Morere describes practical strategies for using cueing in therapies and interventions with these populations.

In Chapter 17, Klossner and Crain discuss how the home language can be L1 for deaf children of parents who do not speak the dominant spoken language of a community, such as Spanish-speaking parents in the United States The chapter provides a detailed description of one school program's development of a Spanish-language version of parent cueing instruction, as well as the theoretical basis for the use of cued symbols specific to the target languages.

Section VI: Cued Speech/Cued Language on the Horizon

The final section of this volume contains four chapters discussing exciting technological initiatives designed to enhance phonological perception and literacy of deaf individuals. In Chapter 18, Bernstein, Auer, and Jiang, at the Neuroscience Department at the House Ear Institute, describe an innovative training system comprised of a computer-based cued symbol synthesis system integrated with a lexical analysis tool. This system is being designed to effectively provide early and extensive exposure to cueing, assist children with profound hearing losses to achieve phonological representations of traditionally spoken words, provide cochlear implant recipients with visible and augmented inputs in the format of visible language to facilitate their auditory habilitation, and adequately and efficiently train teachers and parents to cue. The use of this technical system has potential for contributing to the development of children's reading proficiency, and parents could have an effective, efficient, and affordable method to assist their deaf child in acquiring traditionally spoken home languages during the critical period of language development.

In Chapter 19, Attina, Beautemps, Gibert, Cathiard, and Bailly, at the Institut de la Communication Parlée (ICP, Institute of Speech Communication) in Grenoble, France, describe the results of their analysis of the temporal features of Cued Speech needed for their design of their complete three-dimensional text-to-(French) cueing synthesizer for television access for individuals who are deaf or hard of hearing. This system watermarks hand and face gestures of a virtual animated cueing agent (ARTUS) in a broadcast audiovisual sequence and shows great promise for tel-evised spoken language access for deaf and hard of hearing individuals in France as well as in other countries, including the United States.

In Chapters 20 and 21, Duchnowski, Krause, and colleagues discuss recent advances at the Massachussetts Institute of Technology (MIT) in the Autocuer that was originally developed by Cornett. The current version of the Autocuer employs two computers: one computer prepro-cesses the acoustic waveform and handles the capture of images of the talker and a second computer performs phonetic recognition and produces best-matched cue sequences. The images are stored in the computer's memory for 2 seconds prior to superposition of a hand image correspon-ding to the cue indicated by the second computer and playback for the cue receiver, which allows enough time for the cue to be identified by the recognizer. During the past decade, there have been signifi-cant advances in the development of the Autocuer, which enhance its potential for addressing auditory access needs of deaf individuals in face-to-face conversations.

In Chapter 22, Massaro and colleagues describe an innovative language supple-ment device that is currently being devel-oped in the Perceptual Science Laboratory at the University of California in Santa Cruz. Influenced by Cued Speech, Mas-saro's device combines speech information available via audition and speechreading with other *visual* cues. In Massaro's device, three bars, or rectangles, on in the viewer's eyeglasses indicate how much of the sound coming in is voiced, nasalized, or fricative by lighting up one or more of the bars. Massaro's device, coupled with the other technological devices related to cueing described in this volume, demonstrate how great the possibilities are for technology

to overcome limitations associated with sensory deficits, including deafness.

In Chapter 23, Krause, Schick, and Kegl detail the recent adaptation of the Educa-tional Interpreter Performance Assessment (EIPA) to assess the abilities of cued lan-guage transliterators in educational settings. Incorporation of cueing into the EIPA rep-resents a significant advancement for the field of cued language transliteration and illustrates the growing visibility and recog-nition of cueing in the mainstream educa-tion of deaf students.

In the concluding chapter, Leybaert, Charlier, and colleagues address whether and how the brain processes nonmanual lip movements; manual cues also are dis-cussed in the framework of neural plastic-ity. Recent neuroimaging studies show that the auditory cortices can be rewired to process visual information, including lipread or signed information in the case of deafness. Behavioral studies have shown that information from the nonmanual and manual symbols that comprise cueing is processed as linguistic information by those deaf individuals who are early cued language users. Early cuers also show a left hemispheric specialization for the processing of cued dynamic stimuli, while late cuers show an atypical hemispheric dominance. Leybaert and Charlier currently are engaged in a funded research program involving neuroimaging studies of indi-viduals from cued language backgrounds.

Rationale for an Edited Versus an Authored Book About Cued Speech and Cued Language

The editors of this book originally were contacted by another publishing company to "author" a book about advances in cueing. Our 80 years' combined experience researching language and reading of deaf students certainly prepared us for that task; however, we believed that the story we could and *should* tell about Cued Speech and cued language would be best told by those who have researched cueing, used it in educational programs, and/or have begun developing computer technological applications for fully accessible face-to-face or televised phonological perception. Accordingly, we proposed to Plural Publishing, Inc. to tell our story in this edited format. We are grateful to Dr. Sadanand Singh and his team for their enthusiastic support of this volume as well as the 42 authors from the United States and Europe who accepted our invitation to contribute to the 24 chapters of our book and help us counter the claim that cueing is merely a research interest of a handful of specialists. Through the various chapters in this book, readers will learn that Cued Speech and cued language are lively subjects of research in numerous academic fields; are being applied in educational settings from early intervention (0 to 3) through postgraduate and doctoral study; and that Cued Speech continues to serve a role in the natural acquisition of language and daily communication needs of many deaf individuals in both the United States and Europe.

References

Ackley, R., & Decker, T. (2006). Audiological advancement and the acquisition of spoken language in deaf children. In P. Spencer & M. Marschark (Eds.), *Advances in the spoken language development of deaf and hard of hearing children* (pp. 64–84). New York, NY: Oxford University Press.

Anthony, D. (1971). *SEE I (Vols. 1–2)*. Anaheim, CA: Educational Services Division, Anaheim Union School District.

Beattie, R. (2006). The oral methods and spoken language acquisition. In P. Spencer & M. Marschark (Eds), *Advances in spoken language development of deaf and hard of hearing children* (pp. 103–135). New York, NY: Oxford University Press.

Blamey, P., Sarant, J., Paatsch, L., Barry, J., Bow, C., Wales, R., . . . Tooher, R. (2001). Relationships among speech perception, production, language, hearing loss, and age in children with impaired hearing. *Journal of Speech, Language, and Hearing Research, 44*, 264–285.

Bornstein, H., Saulnier, K., & Hamilton, L. (1973–1984). *The Signed English series*. Washington, DC: Gallaudet College Press.

Bradham T., & Jones, J. (2008). Cochlear implant candidacy in the United States: Prevalence in children 12 months to 6 years of age. *International Journal of Pediatric Otorhinolaryngology, 72*, 1023–1028.

Cawthon, S. (2008). Accommodations use for statewide standardized assessments: Prevalence and recommendations for students who are deaf or hard of hearing. *Journal of Deaf Studies and Deaf Education, 13*, 55–76.

Cawthon, S., & Wurtz, K. (2009). Alternate assessment use with students who are deaf or hard of hearing. *Journal of Deaf Studies and Deaf Education, 14*(2), 155–177.

Charlier, B., Hage, C., Alegría, J., & Périer, O. (1990). Evaluation d'une pratique prolongé du LPC sur la compréhension de la parole par l'enfant atteint de déficience auditive [Evaluation of the effects of prolonged Cued Speech practice upon the reception of oral language in deaf children]. *Glossa, 22*, 28–39.

Cornett, R. O. (1967). Cued Speech. *American Annals of the Deaf, 112*, 3–13.

Drasgow, E., & Paul, P. (1995). A critical analysis of the use of MCE systems with deaf students: A review of the literature. *Association of Canadian Educators of the Hearing Impaired, 21*, 80–93.

Geers, A. (2006). Spoken language in children with cochlear implants. In P. Spencer & M. Marschark (Eds.), *Advances in spoken language development of deaf and hard of hearing children* (pp. 244–270). New York, NY: Oxford University Press.

Gordon, R. (Ed.). (2005). *Ethnologue: Languages of the world* (15th ed.). Dallas, TX: SIL International. Retrieved February 9, 2009, from http://www.ethnologue.com/

Gustason, G., Pfetzing, D., & Zawolkow, E. (1972). *Signing exact English.* Rossmore, CA: Modern Signs Press.

Harkins, J., & Bakke, M. (2003). Technologies for communication: Status and trends. In P. Spencer & M. Marschark (Eds.), *Advances in spoken language development* (pp. 406–419). New York, NY: Oxford University Press.

Johnson, R., Liddell, S., & Erting, C. (1989). *Unlocking the curriculum: Principles for achieving access in deaf education (Working Paper #89-3).* Washington DC: Gallaudet University.

Juel, C. (1988). Learning to read and write: A longitudinal study of fifty-four children from first through fourth grade. *Journal of Educational Psychology, 80,* 437–447.

Karchmer, M., & Mitchell, R. (2003). Demographic and achievement characteristics of deaf and hard-of-hearing students. In M. Marschark & P. Spencer (Eds.), *Handbook of deaf studies, language, and education* (pp. 21–37). New York, NY: Oxford University Press.

Kemp, M. (1998). Why is learning American Sign Language a challenge? *American Annals of the Deaf, 143,* 255–259.

LaSasso, C., & Lollis, J. (2003). Survey of residential and day schools for deaf students in the United States that identify themselves as bilingual-bicultural programs. *Journal of Deaf Studies and Deaf Education, 8,* 79–91.

Mitchell, R., & Karchmer, M. (2004). Chasing the mythical ten percent: Parental hearing status of deaf and hard of hearing students in the United States. *Sign Language Studies, 4,* 138–163.

National Reading Panel. (2000). *Teaching children to read.* United States Department of Health and Human Services, Public Health Service, National Institutes of Health, National Institute of Child Health and Human Development, NIH Pub. No. 00-4769.

Nicholls, G., & Ling, D. (1982). Cued speech and the reception of spoken language. *Journal of Speech and Hearing Research, 25,* 262–269.

No Child Left Behind Act of 2001. 20 U.S.C. 6301 et seq (2002).

Rasinski, T. (2004). *Assessing reading fluency.* Honolulu, HI: Pacific Resources for Education and Learning.

Stokoe, W. (1960). *Sign language structure.* Silver Spring, MD: Linstok Press.

Torres, S., Moreno-Torres, I., & Santana, R. (2006). Quantitative and qualitative evaluation of linguistic input support to a prelingually deaf child with Cued Speech: A case study. *Journal of Deaf Studies and Deaf Education, 11,* 438–448.

Trezak, B., Wang, Y., Woods, D., Gampp, T., & Paul, P. (2007). Using visual phonics to supplement beginning reading instruction for students who are deaf or hard of hearing. *Journal of Deaf Studies and Deaf Education, 12,* 373–384.

Wampler, D. (1971). *Linguistics of Visual English: An introduction.* Santa Rosa, CA: Early Childhood Education Department, Aurally Handicapped Program, Santa Rosa City Schools.

Watson, L., Hardie, T., Archbold, S., & Wheeler, A. (2008). Parents' views on changing communication after cochlear implantation. *Journal of Deaf Studies and Deaf Education, 13,* 104–116.

Chapter 2

FUNDAMENTAL PRINCIPLES OF CUED SPEECH AND CUED LANGUAGE

Thomas F. Shull and Kelly Lamar Crain

In this chapter we describe the history of Cued Speech and the scientific challenges involved in designing a system to represent phonology visually for American English and 62 other languages and dialects (http://www.cuedspeech.org/sub/cued/language.asp#dialects) (see Figure 1–1). We describe eight common features, or universals, of the various Cued Speech systems. We explain how discrete phonemes combine into meaningful units of language, including syllables, words, and longer units of literal and nonliteral discourse. We distinguish Cued Speech and cued language, including their interdependent but separate features and internal linguistic variation. Finally, we discuss different categories of cuers and distinguish between Cued Speech transliterators and sign language interpreters.

Gallaudet University) in Washington, DC. Cornett learned that deaf students at Gallaudet struggled with the written form of English and sought to develop a solution to this problem (Cornett, 1967). Through his investigation, Cornett concluded that insufficient access to the phonology of a spoken language prevented development of literacy within that language. He believed that clear, complete access to phonology is a prerequisite to develop proficiency with the written form. Cornett, a physicist by training, set out to develop a system whereby the phonology of English and other traditionally spoken languages would be wholly visible, the information on the mouth would play a role in accurately sending (and receiving) the message being conveyed, and the users could communicate directly in real time (Cornett, 1985).

Historical Context

Cornett invented Cued Speech in 1966 while serving as Vice President for Long-Range Planning at Gallaudet College (now

Phonology

Phonology is the study of a language's smallest distinctive units and the rules that govern their assembly. Once considered solely in the domain of spoken languages, linguists and other scholars now also consider and study the phonologies of signed languages, such as American Sign Language (Brentari, 1998).

Phonemes function as the building blocks of human languages. Although individual phonemes do not inherently convey meaning, they can be combined to form meaningful units (morphemes). In order for a language to make use of phonemes, these functional units must be rendered distinctly and recognized by receivers. When speaking a language, the distinctiveness of a phoneme is represented by a unique composition of acoustic features. For example, the spoken representations of /p/ and /b/ are nearly identical in their production except for vibration of vocal folds. This feature, called voicing, uniquely identifies /b/ from its voiceless cognate /p/. The presence or absence of vocal fold vibration is one distinctive feature that makes it possible to render and perceive different phonemes distinctly and thus to build a variety of English words: *pin* and *bin* or, as in French, *peau* (skin) and *beau* (handsome).

Cornett recognized that the contrast between English phonemes relies on the acoustic properties found in their spoken representations. However, certain essential contrastive features, such as voicing, are lost to the deaf receiver. The visual information seen on the face that occurs as an artifact of spoken English (speechreading) is insufficient for rendering the language reliably. Phonemes become indistinguishable when their uniquely identifying features are reduced solely to the visual by-products of their articulation through speech. Words such as *tin*, *din*, *dill*, *lid*, *lint*, *dent*, *dull*, *lull*, and *ton* become

difficult (if not impossible) to distinguish through speechreading alone. Context assists to narrow the guesswork necessary when speechreading. However, it is important to remember that deaf children who are learning a language may be attempting to recognize words they already know. They also will encounter words for the first time through an ambiguous visual channel and sometimes without the essential and varied world experiences necessary to supply context. The degree of ambiguity that is deemed acceptable within a language-learning context can be argued. However, Cornett decided that access to phonology through a visual channel must be reliable and generally unambiguous if deaf and hard-of-hearing people are to acquire native competence in a consonant-vowel language and if they are to become literate its written form. Cornett concluded that in order to represent English phonology visually, he would need to invent manual features to replace the distinctive acoustic features that might be imperceptible to or insufficient for the deaf receiver.

Designing a System to Represent Phonology Visually

The Cued Speech system consists of three components: the mouth movements typically associated with the speaking of a given language, the shape of the hand, and the placement or movement of the hand about the face. When cueing, the individual synchronizes mouth movements with the manual cues from a single hand. Each manual cue consists of two parameters: the handshape and the hand placement or movement.

Cues for American English

Cornett invented Cued Speech for use with American English, and described the system as having exactly eight handshapes (numbered 1–8 for ease of reference) and four placements (referred to as side, mouth, chin, and throat) (Cornett, 1985). He later added two movements to his system to clarify the vowel system further. The current "Cued Speech Chart," as disseminated by the National Cued Speech Association, is displayed in Chapter 1, Figure 1–2.

It may be worth noting that Cornett was a physicist by training, as he relied heavily on his mathematics and science background to calculate algorithms and matrices in his attempt to make the Cued Speech system as economical as possible. This is how he was able to arrive at the original eight handshapes and four placements, using no more elaborate, time-consuming, or mentally taxing a system than was necessary. From basic physics, Cornett decided that the hand is too large an articulator to make movements small enough or quickly enough to mirror those of the speech mechanism. Therefore, the system would rely as much as possible on that information on the mouth that is visibly accessible, reducing the requirement placed on the hand.

He decided that the information conveyed by the hand must co-occur in a systematic way with the information conveyed by the mouth, resulting in a double, two-dimensional matrix (one matrix for consonant phonemes and one for vowel phonemes, with the two dimensions for each being mouth and hand). In other words, the identification of a group of lookalike consonants on the mouth (e.g., /m/, /b/, /p/) with the simultaneous identification of a group of consonants by handshape (e.g., handshape 5, representing /m/, /f/, /t/) provides only one point of intersection. In this example, bilabial compression produced simultaneously with handshape 5 (all five fingers extended) results in a single point of overlap—the consonant phoneme, /m/, uniquely and unambiguously identified from all others. Similarly, the identification of a group of look-alike vowels on the mouth (e.g., /ʌ/, /i/, /ɛ/, /ɪ/) with the simultaneous identification of a group of vowel phonemes by hand placement (e.g., the throat placement, representing /ɪ/, /æ/, /ʊ/) provides only one point of intersection (in this case, /ɪ/), resulting in the identification of a single vowel phoneme (Cornett, 1994).

It is extremely important to note that Cued Speech does not attempt to encode specific, distinctive features of speech (e.g., voice, manner, placement); there is no cue for "voice" and no cue for "voiceless." Instead, contrast is supplied by the combination of information on the hand with information of the mouth so that each and every phoneme of the target language is uniquely identified. In his earliest attempts at designing the system, Cornett grouped consonants by acoustic properties (e.g., voiced/voiceless, stops/plosives) to illustrate certain phonetic properties of speech, but such iterations failed to achieve more than 70% accuracy of discrimination in his early tests. He therefore abandoned this approach in favor of the present phonemic system (Cornett, 1994).

Cornett classified consonant phonemes into eight groups based on the highest average visual contrast. So for instance, consider the following groups of consonants that look similar on the mouth when they are lipread: /m b p/, /f v/, and /t d n l/. Cornett redistributed these consonants (as well as the other consonants of

American English) into new groups, which are distinguishable on the lips. The consonants /m/, /f/, and /t/ were deemed sufficiently contrastive on the mouth so they were grouped together. He then assigned each new group of consonants to a handshape. When cued, phonemes that look alike on the mouth would look different on the hand, and conversely, phonemes that look alike on the hand would look different on the mouth. So, the phoneme /f/ is contrasted from /v/ by their different handshapes. Conversely, /f/ and /m/ are represented by the same manual cue, but are readily differentiated by information on the mouth. The receiver must then attend to both the hand and the mouth.

Cornett took other considerations into account when assigning phonemes to manual cues. Consonant phonemes that occur relatively more frequently in English were assigned handshapes that required less energy to form and execute. Adjustments to these initial groupings were made to account for the most frequently occurring consonant clusters. In this way, common consonant clusters in English (e.g., /st/, /ts/, /rt/, /tr/) would be cued via handshape transitions that could be executed relatively quickly.

Cornett followed the same principles of frequency and visual contrast to group the vowel phonemes, resulting in four placements (i.e., mouth, chin, throat, and side) with one placement having two movements (i.e., side-down and side-forward). One challenge regarding vowels in English emerged in determining how to represent diphthongs. A diphthong is a single vowel phoneme that starts at or near the articulatory position for one vowel and moves to or toward the position of another (Loos et al., 2004). Cornett accommodated four English diphthongs

(i.e., /ɔɪ/ as in *boy*, /aɪ/ as in *buy*, /au/ as in *bough*, and /eɪ/ as in *bay*) and his system mirrors this definition. That is, a cued diphthong is a single cued vowel phoneme that starts at the articulatory position for one vowel placement and moves to the position of another. One example of this, as illustrated in Figure 2–1, is the cued diphthong /eɪ/, which starts at the /e/ position (the chin) and moves to the /ɪ/ position (the throat) in one fluid gesture. When viewing the figures in this chapter (or any static representation of cueing) it is important to note that the appropriate articulatory gestures on the mouth must be produced and synchronized with the manual cues.

Incorporating information found on the mouth is integral to the Cued Speech system. In Cornett's design, the phonemes of English are distributed among groups of manual cues whereby the information on the mouth combined with the information on the hand constitutes a unique feature-bundle to signify a specific pho-

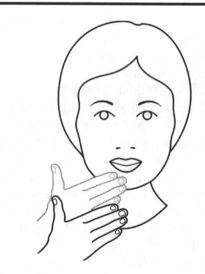

Figure 2–1. Cues for the diphthong /eɪ/.

neme. This stipulation simplifies learning to cue since there are fewer symbols to learn and contributes to efficiency in production (i.e., there is not a unique cue for every phoneme of a language, and as we discuss, some cues can be rendered simultaneously). Further benefits from this aspect of the design of Cued Speech are discussed in later chapters in terms of its impact on lipreading/speechreading abilities among deaf and hard-of-hearing cuers.

It is worth noting that while the information found on the mouth is the same among cuers despite their hearing status, the associations with this information may not be. That is, information seen on the mouth is often described by cueing advocates as "the natural mouth movements that accompany speech" (NCSA, 2006). At the time Cued Speech was created, the first individuals to cue expressively were hearing, native speakers of English. For these individuals, the process of learning to cue involved learning particular hand movements to coincide with the natural mouth movements they made while speaking English (i.e., the visual information available on their mouths was a byproduct of the act of speaking). However, Fleetwood and Metzger (1998) point out that although the visual information on the mouth occurred as a function of speech, this is a historical reality, but not a prerequisite to using Cued Speech. Proponents of Cued Speech continue to describe the system in terms of its serving as a supplement to speechreading or in conjunction with the natural mouth movements produced while speaking a language. However, although we refer to the information visible on the mouth as that which is generally associated with speaking a language, our operational definition is not meant to

suggest that all Cued Speech users must vocalize in order to cue, nor that any audition is required to receive cueing.

Adaptations to Other Languages

Subsequent adaptations for the cueing of English in England and Australia draw from the same manual signals, but differ from the American system in that they include phonemes specific to those dialects and distribute those phonemes differently to ensure sufficient contrast within those phonological systems. Initially, Cornett attempted to group the phonemes of any given language to the same eight handshapes (for consonants) and four placements (for vowels) used in his original system; however, he occasionally found it necessary to introduce novel handshapes or placements to accommodate a greater number of phonemes than are found in English, or a particular set of phonemes that could not otherwise be fully distinguished (Cornett, 1994). An early example of this is the addition of a vowel placement on the cheekbone ("pommette"), which is used in the cueing of French. French has a number of nasalized vowels that closely resemble their nonnasalized counterparts when speechread; therefore, an additional placement was necessary for the French adaptation of Cued Speech— le Langage Parlé Complété (or LPC).

At the time of this publication, Cued Speech, in all of its adaptations, draws from an inventory of 17 handshapes, five hand placements about the face, and at least five movements (e.g., rising, falling, rotating) to identify each phoneme of more than 63 languages and dialects uniquely (http://www.cuedspeech.org/sub/cued/

language.asp#dialects). To our knowledge, the greatest number of handshapes is required for the cueing of Polish, and the greatest number of placements (5) is shared by a number of languages.

Similarities Across Languages

Adaptations to subsequent languages have necessitated variations in handshape placement, and/or movement assignments. Additionally, cultural implications have played a role in divergent views of the role of Cued Speech and its applications for individuals who are deaf or hard of hearing. For example, Cued Speech in Spain is viewed largely as a clinical application (as opposed to a communication modality for educational purposes), and as an augment to oral communication (as opposed to a distinct communication modality). However, a number of statements can be made about Cued Speech, irrespective of the language for which it is used or the ways in which it can be implemented. Cued Speech is always composed of handshapes, placements, and synchronized mouthshapes, with the manual portion requiring the use of a single hand. The adaptations of Cued Speech can be acquired, taught, and learned by similar learners in remarkably similar ways and time frames, regardless of the complexity or nature of the language. Once fluency is achieved, cueing can be produced in real time. Cued Speech is a phonemic, not phonetic system, and bears no more or less direct relationship to orthography (the writing system of a language) than does speech. Cued Speech can be expressed and received with or without audition or the use of vocal speech.

Cued Speech Consists of Mouth Movements, Handshapes, and Placements

In all Cued Speech systems to date, the consonants of a spoken language are grouped so that consonants that are easily distinguishable from one another on the mouth are assigned to a common handshape, consonants that are visually similar on the mouth are assigned to different handshapes, and the minimal number of handshapes is used. Similarly, in all Cued Speech systems to date, the vowels of a spoken language are grouped so that vowels that are easily distinguishable from one another on the mouth can be assigned to a common placement (location); vowels that are visually similar on the mouth are assigned to different placements; and the minimal number of placements is used. Although not an exception to the rule, one qualification related to this discussion concerns the cueing of tonal languages such as Chinese and Thai. Tammasaeng (1985) documented the successful application of Cued Speech to the Thai language in which the inclination and movement of the hand is used to indicate tone (simultaneous to the hand's shape and placement). Also noteworthy is the Cued Speech adaptation to Malagasy. The vowels spoken in Malagasy were deemed sufficiently distinguishable on the mouth alone and therefore all handshapes are produced at a single placement (the side).

Cued Speech Requires the Use of a Single Hand

Even to the inexperienced observer, this characteristic readily distinguishes Cued Speech from signed languages and manually coded English (MCE) systems, which make use of both hands. The cuer is free to use the other hand simultaneously to perform other tasks, such as using natural gestures commonly used by speakers of languages (e.g., pointing). Although the cueing of any given utterance is achieved by use of a single hand, cuers (especially cued language transliterators who cue expressively for long periods of time) may utilize both hands, alternating from one hand to the other to avoid fatigue (Fleetwood & Metzger, 1990). Alternating hands can also be used while transliterating to distinguish between two speakers or to differentiate the linguistic message of a speaker from environmental sounds (such as the whir of an air conditioner, or the closing of a door). The use of two hands simultaneously producing the same manual cues while accompanying a single mouth movement has been documented as a natural prosodic feature of native deaf cuers, typically for emphasis (Fleetwood & Metzger, 1998).

Cued Speech Can Be Learned in a Relatively Short Period of Time

The cues of Cued Speech and the rules governing their production (often likened to learning the placement of the keys on the keyboard for typing) can be learned in a relatively short period of time, typically less than a week (Cornett & Daisey, 2001). Some individuals learn Cued Speech in weekend workshops or "Cue Camps." Other individuals acquire Cued Speech via self-instruction that may take several weeks. Still others learn Cued Speech at a college or university, with instruction spanning the length of a school semester. The goal of each of these types of instruction is for the cuer, with the aid of a chart,

to be able to cue anything in the target language (Henegar & Cornett, 1971). It should be noted that the range of time cited here for learning Cued Speech presupposes that students already know the language and are not learning both the mode (Cued Speech) and the language (English) simultaneously. Deaf children who acquire English through Cued Speech are not taught the system of cues, per se. Rather, they acquire the language through the cues in a similar manner as children who learn English through speech or ASL through signing (see Crain, this volume). For these children the language and modality are acquired simultaneously over the course of years. For adolescents and adults who already speak English, learning to cue simply requires learning the associations between the cues and the target phonemes they represent. In this case, adults with linguistic competence do not acquire the language and mode simultaneously; rather, they learn a finite set of cues that are applied to the language they already know. For this reason, it is relatively simple and, for adults who know a language, to learn Cued Speech only requires only a short amount of time. Learning Arabic Cued Speech, a system of nine handshapes and four placements, is not the same as learning cued Arabic (the entire language expressed through Cued Speech). Individuals can learn a foreign adaptation of Cued Speech by learning its inventory of phonemes and the associated cues that represent them without knowing how to arrange the cues in meaningful ways (phonology, morphology, syntax, semantics, pragmatics). Furthermore, learning Cued Speech does not imply fluency (i.e., cueing at or near the normal conversational rate). The time needed to become fluent varies between individuals. Observation and documentation of graduate students completing a student teaching experience with deaf children in cueing environments were judged (by themselves and the cueing cooperating teacher) to be less than fluent at the beginning of a 6-week student teaching experience and to be fluent at the end of the 6 weeks (see Chapter 12). Henegar and Cornett (1971) noted that the development of skill in expressive cueing sufficient for easy, natural communication takes months of actual use.

Signing deaf adults who are motivated to learn Cued Speech can do so; however, the time required and the level of success depends greatly on a number of factors, including language background (e.g., English, ASL), communication background (e.g., experience with spoken language, ASL, MCE systems), and auditory history (degree of hearing loss, onset of deafness, benefit of amplification) (C. Klossner, personal communication, January 2009). Deaf adults with an already complete or fairly complete phonological inventory of the target language (the language to be cued) can be taught in a manner and time frame similar to that of hearing learners. Conversely, deaf adults with relatively little previous access to the phonological structure of the target language need to learn to cue, but must also learn the phonology, lexicon, and/or grammar of English. This process would more closely resemble the teaching of English as a Second Language (ESL), and would therefore take considerably longer (Mitchell & Myles, 2004). Cued Speech can benefit adult learners by serving as an unambiguous language model for those seeking English proficiency. The processes of learning to cue and building fluency can differ for hearing adults, deaf adults, and deaf children, and are highly influenced by linguistic history, quality and

quantity of interactions and use, and so forth. It is important to remember that this process is different for deaf children who naturally and passively acquire English through Cued Speech for whom no previous linguistic exposure is required or expected. Obviously, the greatest benefit of exposure to Cued Speech is found when it is applied to a complete language for natural communication with infants (see Chapter 8 for a discussion of the natural acquisition of cueing and the English language by deaf children). Currently, there is no evidence to support that intelligence is a salient factor in learning to cue anymore than it is in learning other linguistic modalities like speaking or signing.

Cued Speech Can Be Produced in Real Time

The rate at which cues can be produced is made possible by two important features of Cornett's design. The first was the decision to encode the vowels by hand locations and the consonants by hand placements. Vowels average longer duration times acoustically than consonants (Blamey, et al., 2001), which corresponds to the relatively longer time it takes the cuer to move from one location to another. Inversely, consonants represent shorter acoustic events, and it is also possible for cuers to transition rapidly from one handshape to another. The second feature of Cornett's design was for Cued Speech to allow the possibility of transmitting a consonant and a vowel in a single gesture of combined manual cues. This contributes to the ease and conversation rate of delivery associated with fluent cueing. The production of cues seems to slow the speech rate by about 30%, that is, from six syllables per second to four syllables per second (Duchnowski et al., 2000). See Chapter 20 for an in-depth discussion of timing effects in expressive cueing.

Cued Speech is a Phonemic System

As has been stated, Cued Speech was designed to render the phonology of traditionally spoken languages through visual, rather than acoustic means. Although the reasoning for conveying a language, like English, in a visual channel may be evident, the significance of doing so at the phonological level may not be as obvious. Other attempts to convey spoken languages visually have relied on the use of signs borrowed from signed languages or invented signs that are arranged to represent English grammar at the morphological level.

Cueing, on the other hand, conveys English at a phonological level, which enables it to convey features of English that cannot be conveyed via MCE systems. Different manually coded English (MCE) sign systems vary in the ways that they attempt to show English. For example, some adopt an invented sign to represent the past tense. In English, one such past tense marker is the suffix "-ed." This meaningful segment, or morpheme, is added to a number of English verbs to convey that the action occurred in the past (e.g., *called, walked, wanted*). At a morphological level, an invented sign could be added to operate in place of the morpheme "-ed." However, the realization of the "-ed" morpheme in these previous examples is not phonemically identical. If the same examples are considered at a phonological level, one finds that there are variations in the English pronunciation of the morpheme: called /d/, walked /t/, and wanted /ɪd/. Although MCE systems might represent these morphemes identically, Cued Speech does not. When cueing each of these words, each segment is represented. Therefore, their pronunciations are also conveyed: /kald/, /wɔkt/, and /wantɪd/. Aspects of English words such as the rhyme that occurs between *played/maid* and *raft/laughed* remain intact when they are cued. Furthermore, internal morphemic changes are revealed through cueing. Verbs that have irregular past tense forms such as *dig/dug*, *freeze/froze/frozen*, and *leave/left* rely on changes to the consonant and vowel phonemes in altering the root form. Although these same internal changes can be cued (by changing the appropriate hand placement and final handshapes), no such comparable internal changes can be made to a sign to reflect changes to the English phonological form. Attempts to represent English reliably at a morphological level ignore the reality that English grammar, its associations between words like rhyme, and its written form all rely on knowledge of its phonology.

Cued Speech Is Not Phonetically Based

Cued Speech visually conveys English and other traditionally spoken languages by fully specifying *phonemic* contrasts (which simultaneously have *phonetic* features). The terms phonemic and phonetic are often used interchangeably, when in fact there are important differences between them. Take, for instance, the phoneme /t/. This segment is contrastive from other segments that, in spite of being acoustically similar when spoken, can be used to make different words. For example, the words *ten* and *den* are perceived as different words despite the similarity of the underlying /t/ and /d/. The distinguishing features in their spoken forms contribute to the perception of contrastive segments. Spoken output of the phoneme /t/ can vary depending on its phonetic environment, or the surrounding sounds. All of the possible spoken forms of a phoneme are referred to as allophones. While discussing phonemes and allophones in writing, we adopt the convention to place phonemes in slashes (e.g., /t/) and allophones in brackets (e.g., [t]). The [t] in *top*, the [t] in *star*, and the [t] in *hot* do not sound the same when spoken.

The design of Cued Speech, however, was not intended to represent the phonetic properties of speech; it conveys the broader phonemic category of /t/. All the various spoken instances of /t/ are cued the same. In only a few cases are allophonic variation discriminated by Cued Speech. One example is the schwa (/ə/) in English which is an unstressed vowel occurring in many English words, such as in the first syllable of *above*, the second syllable of *independent*, and the third syllable of *unnecessary*. The schwa is a predictable variation of several English vowels. It is generally represented in adaptations of Cued Speech as a short, quick downward movement from the side placement.

The distinction between phonetics and phonemics becomes important to our discussion in light of the differences in how hearing cuers and deaf cuers likely process visual linguistic information. It is true that Cued Speech is phonemically based, in that the cues disambiguate or fully specify each of the phonemes of a language. In the actual practice of cueing, Cued Speech *can* be influenced by an individual's knowledge of or access to certain phonetic properties of speech, however, that knowledge or access is not necessary to cue a linguistic message accurately.

Although Cued Speech was not designed to do so, attempts to represent phonetic properties of speech are some-times made. Speech-language pathologists sometimes use cues in novel ways to evoke target speech sounds from deaf clients. For example, if a child is able to produce the target sounds [t] and [ʃ] through speech, the clinician could cue a word like *much* as /mʌtʃ/ in order to prompt the student to correctly produce [tʃ]. The sound [tʃ] in its spoken form is categorized as an affricate. That is, a sound that is made is a composite of two sounds: a stop and a fricative; in this case /t/ and /ʃ/. So in a clinical setting, one might make use of the cues for /t/ and /ʃ/ as prompts to assist the child who can produce these sounds in isolation to produce them as part of the sounds [tʃ]. It is important to remember, however, that productive qualities like voicing are not encoded in cues. Also, although some of the articulatory gestures within the oral tract are visible to the deaf receiver (e.g., bilabial compression for /m/, /b/, and /p/) some are not available through vision (/k/, /g/, and /ŋ/). Concepts of placement (i.e., front or back sounds) are not encoded in the manual information of the cues.

Cueing Does Not Directly Correlate to Orthography

When applied to a language, Cued Speech serves to represent the phonology of a language. In other words, the cues serve to represent the pronunciation of an utterance in its primary form, rather than to reflect its spelling in its written form. In English, the words *hair* and *hare* are likely to be pronounced identically despite their different spelling. Because these words share a common pronunciation, they are cued identically. On the other hand, the words *dove* (the past tense of dive) and *dove* (a white bird) are pronounced differently despite their spelling and accordingly are cued differently. Cued Speech, therefore, has no more or less a connection to spelling than does speech. The degree to which the cueing of a word reflects its spelling is a function of the phonological transparency of the traditionally spoken language for which Cued Speech has been adapted. Therefore, the cueing of words such as *hit*, *dug*, and *lad* closely resemble the way in which they are spelled. However, the words *sugar*, *tomb*, and *knight* are cued as they are pronounced regardless of their phonically irregular spelling. Refer to Chapters 11 and 12 for a discussion of the impact of Cued Speech on the acquisition and development of reading abilities.

Cued Speech Exists With or Without Audition or Vocal Speech

Cued Speech is a visual communication system mapped onto a phonology that may or may not interface with speech or sound. For hearing individuals, the phonology of a language is so closely related to the sounds of that language, they are nearly inextricable. In fact, however, the phonemes of a language can be considered independently of speech sounds. That is, phonemes are not the sounds themselves. Rather, they are the underlying mental representations or categories of contrastive units activated by the sounds (Liberman & Mattingly, 1985). These contrastive units are very commonly related to speech sounds, but are not synonymous with them.

For individuals who can hear and learn to cue, the existing sound-to-phoneme associations are available and convenient for assigning handshapes and placements to the "sounds" of speech. For these individuals, Cued Speech may indeed be a sound-based system. In fact, this paradigm has been long held, at least in part, because

the first expressive cuers were hearing adults. For cuers who are deaf, however, depending on degree of deafness and previous auditory linguistic experience, the entire internal phonological system can be established solely through the relationships among contrastive features of mouthshape, handshape, and placement. Depending on an individual's access to audition, the sounds of speech could be a factor in these associations, but not necessarily so.

The term *sound-based*, although not necessarily accurate, is also often used to emphasize the fact that cueing has no direct relationship with the spelling of words, as well as to emphasize Cued Speech's relationship to phonology (rather than to actual sound). Understanding and appreciating the role of Cued Speech in making phonology visible is essential in understanding the capacity of Cued Speech to convey traditionally spoken languages visually at every level.

From Discrete Phonemes to Meaningful Units of Language

Cued Speech is often described in terms of isolated phonemic values or as a means of disambiguating a small set of phonemes whose spoken representations look similar on the mouth (e.g., /m/, /b/, and /p/). However, descriptions limited to isolated phonemes fall short in their ability to illustrate the breadth of linguistic information that can be conveyed via cueing. Readers of such descriptions might incorrectly conclude that Cued Speech use is limited to disambiguation of lone phonemes for speechreading. However, cues can be arranged in an infinite number of meaningful ways.

English, like many spoken languages, is a consonant-vowel language. This means that syllables contain as their nucleus a vowel (V) with a place on either end for a consonant (C). The acronym CVC, then, refers to a syllable with a consonant, followed by a vowel, followed by a consonant (as in the English words *cat* /kæt/ and *wish* /wɪʃ/). Many variations of the CVC structure are possible, including consonant clusters appearing before or after the vowel (e.g., the CCCVCCC monosyllabic English word *strengths* /strɛŋθs/), and instances where consonants are absent on either side of the nucleus (e.g., the VCC monosyllabic English word *ant*), and cases in which the vowel constitutes the entire syllable, without consonants before or after (e.g., the V monosyllabic English word *a*.)

The Cued CV Syllable

First, we examine the basic cued syllable, a consonant-vowel syllable (CV). The handshape (that represents a particular consonant phoneme) contacts a hand placement (that represents the following vowel phoneme). These manual cues are rendered simultaneously with the appropriate articulatory gestures on the mouth to signal the production of the syllable. For every cued dyad (a handshape and hand placement pair), any phonemic value represented by the handshape always precedes any phonemic value represented by the hand placement. So, for example, the syllable /rɪ/, as illustrated in Figure 2–2, is cued with the handshape representing /r/ (handshape 3) contacting the placement for /ɪ/ (which is represented by contacting a location on the throat) while simultaneously rendering the appropriate articulatory gestures on the mouth.

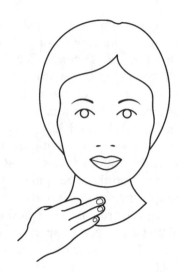

Figure 2–2. Cues for the CV syllable /rɪ/.

As discussed, not every handshape and hand placement combination yields a syllable. This distinction is language dependent. The cueing of English requires the ability to deliver consonant clusters or blends, while the cueing of Japanese does not.

Variations of the CV syllable

In the absence of a preceding consonant phoneme, a null handshape is used to signal that no preceding consonant is present (e.g., the English letter name for "E"). In such cases, handshape 5 is used to contact the appropriate vowel placement. This assignment of the null consonant to handshape 5 occurs in most of the current adaptations of Cued Speech. An exception to this rule is found in cued Polish, which employs a handshape that resembles a loosely formed fist to signify the lack of a preceding consonant.

Within other syllables, a consonant phoneme may not be immediately followed by a vowel phoneme. When this occurs, the handshape for that consonant is placed at the null placement (near the side of the face). To illustrate these two phenomena, let us examine a VC syllable that exhibits both: the word *ease* (/iz/). The first segment is the vowel /i/ which is represented near the corner of the mouth (mouth placement) but in order to contact it, one must use the null handshape, handshape 5, to indicate that no consonant precedes the vowel. Despite the spelling, the next phoneme is the consonant /z/, which is represented by handshape 2. This handshape is not immediately followed by another vowel phoneme (again, in spite of spelling) so the hand is placed at the null placement for vowels, which is near the side of the face (the side placement), as illustrated in Figure 2–3. These manual gestures must also be synchronized with articulatory gestures for each segment on the mouth.

In addition to hand placements to represent vowel phonemes, hand movements also exist in several adaptations of Cued Speech. In American English, move-

ments from the side placement proceed forward for the vowels /o/ and /a/ or down for the vowels /ə/ and /ʌ/. In cued Portuguese the word "sim" /sĩ/ (yes) is represented with handshape 3 (for /s/) rendered at the cheekbone placement (for /ĩ/) with a slight rotation of the hand to further distinguish the vowel phoneme from others that reside at that placement.

Consonant Clusters and the CV Syllable

The preceding basic rules serve as the foundation that governs how handshapes and placements are combined. For the sake of thoroughness, let us continue to examine how phonemes build into various types of syllables and how Cued Speech handshapes and placements build in an analogous manner. Using the previous CV example of /rɪ/ (see Figure 2–2) we can construct a variety of words around it. By adding a consonant to the end of our syllable /rɪ/, we create the CVC word "rip" (/rɪp/), illustrated in Figure 2–4. This is cued with handshape 3 at the throat

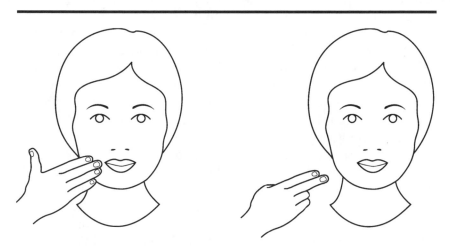

Figure 2–3. Cues for the English word *ease*.

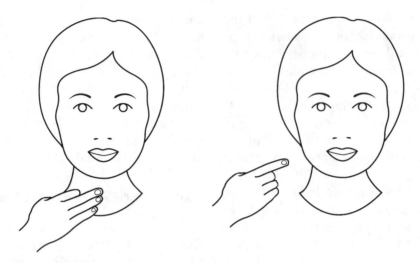

Figure 2–4. Cues for the English word *rip*.

placement, followed by handshape 1 at the neutral/null, side placement because no vowel follows it (with the assumption that the accompanying articulatory gestures are available on the mouth and are rendered synchronously with the appropriate accompanying gesture on the hand.)

Here we have now moved from the realm of nonsense syllable to morpheme, the English word *rip* (which could refer either to a verb which means "to tear," a noun which refers to "the tear" itself, or a number of figurative meanings).

The CVCC word *rips* (/rɪps/), as illustrated in Figure 2–5, is cued with the 3 handshape at the throat placement, followed by the 1 handshape at the neutral (side) placement, but then is followed by the 3 handshape at that same placement to represent the addition of the phoneme /s/.

By adding another morphological unit (the suffix –s), we provide additional information—denoting pluralization of the noun or, perhaps, placing a verb in the present tense, while also supplying some grammatical information about person and number. The CCVCC word *trips* /trɪps/, as illustrated in Figure 2–6, is cued by simply adding handshape 5 at the neutral (side) position to the production used above.

The addition of the initial consonant /t/ changes the semantic association of the morpheme entirely. Interestingly, there are several possible associations for the word *trips* in English. This word refers to the plural form of the English noun synonymous with the English word *journeys*. It also serves as the third person singular form of the present tense verb similar to *stumbles*. The same form indicts both meanings. Without sufficient context, the receiver cannot be sure which is being referenced. This ambiguity in meaning is found in the spoken, cued, and written forms of the word in isolation. It is advantageous that the rendering of the cued word *trips* is equally unclear in both the cued and spoken form. The same strategies used to provide clarification in spoken English can be used in cued English.

Following the same logic in patterning, the CCCVCC word *strips* /strɪps/,

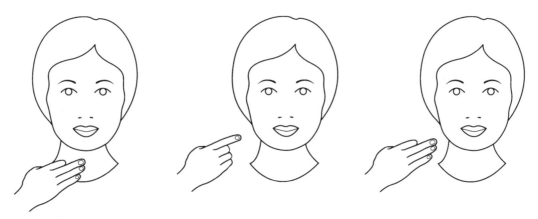

Figure 2–5. Cues for the English word *rips*.

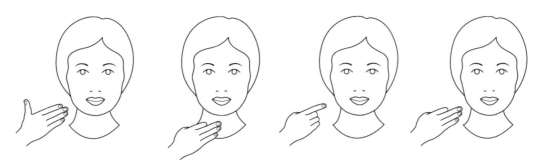

Figure 2–6. Cues for the English word *trips*.

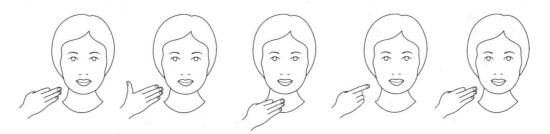

Figure 2–7. Cues for the English word *strips*.

as illustrated in Figure 2–7, is cued be beginning with handshape 3 for /s/ at the neutral (side) position, followed by handshape 5 in the same position for /t/, followed by the 3 handshape at the throat placement for /rɪ/, followed by the 1 handshape at the neutral (side) placement for /p/, followed by the 3 handshape at that same placement for /s/. These gestures and their transitions can be made quickly because of the relatively small articulatory space of cueing and can be produced within complete utterances and at a rate allowing for conversational discourse.

Note that there are an equal number of phonemic representations in the cued form as in the spoken, with the handshape for /r/ occurring at the hand placement for /ɪ/ allowing for economy of motion. Also, for each consonant in a blend or cluster, there will be a separate handshape. This ensures that the deaf receiver is provided with access to each phoneme sequentially presented. For each syllable in a word, there either will be a hand movement or contact made to a placement on the face.

From Phonemes to Morphemes and Words

Cued Speech renders visible the patterning rules of syllables and, ultimately, allows for the internalization of the morphological structure and associations of language in the minds of its users. Every human language relies on morphemes (meaningful units). Morphemes may be free (standing independently as words) or bound (which must be joined with another morpheme and cannot stand alone). In the case of free morphemes, an example is the Spanish word, *perro* (dog), which is both a word and a single meaningful unit, or morpheme. However, if we add the letter –*s*, the single Spanish word *perros* now comprises two morphemes: the free morpheme *perro* (dog) and the bound morpheme –*s* (more than one). This morphological structure is intact in the cued form of the Spanish word. Additional variations in the morphological affixes can also be conveyed. For example, in English, a common way to pluralized nouns involves

the addition of the suffix "–s." The words *lips*, *eyes*, and *noses* demonstrate this phenomenon. However, despite the uniform addition of the letter "s" in their written forms, the suffix is not pronounced the same when added to these different root words: *lips* ends with the consonant phoneme /s/, *eyes* ends with the consonant phoneme /z/, and *noses* ends with the added VC syllable /ɪz/, to be pronounced /nozɪz/. The variations among morphemes (allomorphy) like those previously discussed in the example of the suffix "-ed" can be cued accurately and acquired naturally by deaf children. This holds true for cases of plural forms and those in which the base root word changes in the plural form, such as in the English examples of *ox/oxen*, *man/men*, *mouse/mice*, and *woman/women*.

Words and word parts (i.e., affixes and inflections) are represented fully in both their cued forms. As we have seen, the morphology of spoken languages (in its various inflected forms) relies on changes at a phonological level. With this ability of Cued Speech to preserve both meaning and form faithfully, the associations between morphemes are available to the language user. In other words, the association between the cued word *cat* and its semantic meaning (to a classification of animals) is available to the receiver. Furthermore, the structure of the morpheme *cat* is also available—as a one syllable word comprising three English phonemes /k æ t/. Other associations between words (and parts of words), such as homophones, heteronyms, word roots, and affixes are also readily available to cued language users. *Site* and *sight* are homophones. *Polish* (from Poland) and *polish* (to buff to a shine) are heteronyms. *Impede* and *pedestal* derive from the same root word. The word *trunk* may have semantic associations to an elephant's nose, a case used for traveling, the back storage compartment of a car, as well as the base of a tree. Rules that govern the joining of morphemes are also available to the cuer. The morpheme "un-" must be attached to another morpheme and cannot occur alone (e.g., *unmarried*)

The words language-users employ not only serve to convey a particular meaning; words have many other semantic associations. As we have discussed, one form may have multiple meanings, and words which differ in meaning may be associated due to their similarities in form. Cued Speech is unique in that these semantic associations of both form and meaning are preserved. When cued, the words *bell* and *bowl* use the same initial and final handshapes, but the hand placement for the vowel differs. When cueing the words *bat* and *pat*, the initial handshapes indicating the initial consonant differ between these words, but the hand placement indicating the vowel and the final handshape indicating the final consonants do not. Thus, the words *pat* and *bat* not only rhyme in the spoken form, they also rhyme visually. This ability on the part of Cued Speech to convey onsets, rimes, and syllables accurately makes it ideal for the development of phonological awareness for deaf and hard of hearing children (see Chapter 14 for a discussion of the relationship between phonological awareness and reading comprehension).

This is a marked difference between Cued Speech and systems that attempt to encode spoken languages at a morphologic level using invented and borrowed signs. Manually Coded English systems such as Signing Exact English attempt to represent English at a morphologic level, and are vulnerable to the limitations inherent

in such an approach (see Chapter 12 for a comparison of communication modalities typically used in attempts to convey English visually).

Joining Syllables

The process of joining syllables to convey words, phrases, and sentences is similar to the process by which phonemes are sequenced and produced via Cued Speech. Regardless of whether syllables are entire monosyllabic words or are segments of multisyllabic words, syllables are assembled according to the language of the cuer.

Connected discourse, in which syllable boundaries often occur across word boundaries, is common in traditionally spoken languages and in the cueing of languages as well. This generally occurs in order to save time and energy, and to reduce the range of motion required of the articulators. An example of this phenomenon in spoken English is the phrase *jump across*. Parsed at the word boundary, the phrase is obviously jump/across. Parsed at the syllable boundary (more common in connected speech), the phrase might be uttered as jum/pa/cross. The parsing of the words, in spite of their production, is possible by the experienced language user. The design of Cued Speech readily lends itself to connected discourse, which may yield benefits to deaf cuers in producing English in a natural manner with typical rhythm and cadence.

In rare occurrences, connected discourse can lead to some confusion. Take for example, the unlikely but illustrative examples of the sentences *He's a nice man* and *He's an ice man*. In spoken English, these sentences might be said identically. Likewise, these sentences might be cued identically. The determination of semantic meaning is left to the interpretation of the receiver in both the spoken and cued versions based on context and probability. On the other hand, for an interpreter or transliterator to convey these sentences via a signed language or MCE system, the intended meaning must be known *before* it can be conveyed. This does not illustrate any weakness on the part of signed languages. The same problem in interpretation would occur between any two languages.

Joining Words

As discussed, the cueing of a language allows the contrastive building blocks (phonemes) to be combined into meaningful words and parts of words (morphemes). These units can be further combined so that all levels of the linguistic hierarchy can be conveyed clearly. As discussed in Chapter 12, modern attempts to explicitly teach these skills deaf child during the school age years have proven ineffective. It is through the consistent exposure to the phoneme stream of a language that the deaf child is afforded the opportunity to acquire the many subtle rules, generalizations, and exceptions that govern language use. This becomes especially important when we consider how word order affects the meaning. The following English sentences have very different meanings, despite comprising the same three words: Claire sees Lauren. Lauren sees Claire. The following French sentence would seem odd to an English speaker if translated literally: *Jean m'a vu dans la voiture rouge* (*Jean me saw in the car red*), but to an individual who has acquired the rules of French syntax, the sentence is grammatically acceptable (*Jean saw me in the red car*).

The rules that govern the joining of words (syntax) are not taught explicitly;

they develop naturally with repeated exposure to the common and acceptable forms used in a given language, as well as to the occasional (and often jarring) violations of those rules one encounters while communicating with others. Although users of a language do not have difficulty discriminating allowable from unacceptable forms, they may not be consciously aware of the underlying grammatical rules that determine acceptability within their own language. Take, for example, the following pairs of sentences:

The cold soup is on the table.

The soup that is cold is on the table.

In the previous two sentences, the adjective *cold* can be placed before the subject or it can be placed after the verb as part of the predicate. Both forms are acceptable in English. However, now consider the following:

My former husband is unreasonable.

My husband who is former is unreasonable.

In these sentences, we find that the adjective *former* can occur before the noun it modifies but not in the predicate. The second sentence is considered linguistically unacceptable. Conversely, some adjectives operate differently.

My alone children need supervision.

My children who are alone need supervision.

Here, we see that the adjective *alone* may not occur immediately preceding the noun it modifies (as in the first sentence) and must occur in the predicate to be deemed acceptable in English. Most native English users would not have difficulty identifying the inappropriate syntactic versions of the above examples. They might be hard pressed, however, to state a rule for these adjectives or to provide other adjectives that follow the same pattern. These examples are intended to illustrate just a narrow sliver of the subconscious, internal grammar afforded to competent users of a language, including deaf native cuers of that language. It also serves to illustrate the extreme, often painstaking, difficulty of teaching English to nonnative users. The necessity of explaining these rules rather than providing opportunities for natural interaction within the language can make the process laborious, inefficient, and often ineffective.

Making Literal and Nonliteral Meaning

Similar to the effect of language exposure and experience on syntactic competence is the effect of language exposure and experience on an individual's ability to comprehend and appreciate the difference between literal meaning and nonliteral (i.e., figurative) meaning. To appreciate how someone can be *tickled pink* (in American English) without being touched and without physically changing color, one needs to have experienced the phrase a number of times and within contexts of someone being quite pleased. Similarly, in order to appreciate that someone can *jeter l'éponge* (in French, literally *to throw the sponge*) without actually manipulating a sponge, an individual needs to have experienced that specific phrase, in the context of someone quitting or conceding. It has been estimated that as much as 23% of spoken English is figurative (Conley, 1976).

Again, the process of explicitly teaching figurative language (e.g., idioms, metaphors, hyperbole) to nonnative language learners consumes an inordinate amount of time and energy that individuals with sufficient exposure to the target language and all its complexity do not require, and therefore, can to devote to other cognitive tasks.

Cued Speech and Cued Language

Previously, we have focused on the rules of Cued Speech, which govern how handshapes and hand placements or movements are articulated to convey language. We have also discussed rules that determine verb inflection and pluralization. These rules also define how we cue, but are based on different parameters—the rules that govern language use. In *Cued Language Structure: An Analysis of Cued American English Based on Linguistic Principles* (1998), Fleetwood and Metzger were the first to write extensively about Cued Speech and cued language as separate phenomena. Fleetwood and Metzger point out that, prior to the work of William Stokoe in the early 1960s, which asserted that the signing of Deaf communities in the United States was neither a visually represented variant of English nor a pidgin, *language* had long been accepted as a sound-based/spoken phenomenon. The study of signed languages in the 1970s raised this issue among linguists, leading Noam Chomsky to revise his discussions of the *sound-meaning correspondence* to that of a *signal-meaning correspondence*. This distinction recognizes that language resides in the mind while the signal (which can be spoken, signed, cued, written, etc.) is the physical actualization of the language.

Communication and Language: Inextricable But Separate

Fleetwood and Metzger argue that if neither language and speaking nor language and signing are one and the same, then by extension, language and cueing (i.e., cued language and Cued Speech) are not the same. The logic is simple, yet fundamental. The structure of a language (e.g., its phonology, morphology, syntax) must not be confused with the modalities for conveying language (e.g., cueing, signing, speaking). Signed languages, spoken languages, and cued languages can be quite similar in terms of their structure, in that they all consist of basic units that can be parsed or combined, and are ordered in various ways to create words and sentences to express a seemingly limitless number of ideas. These three classes of languages (i.e., signed, spoken, cued) differ a great deal, however, in terms of form. Signed languages rely on manual signs, facial expression, and mouth movements specific to signed languages, which may or may not resemble the mouth movements associated with spoken languages. Spoken languages rely on speech (including vocal inflection), facial expression, and natural gestures. Cued languages rely on manual cues, the mouth movements typically associated with speech, facial expression, and natural gestures. Fleetwood and Metzger (1998) coined the term *cuem* (pronounced /kyoom/) to refer to the composite of manual cues and the artifacts of articulatory gestures seen on the mouth independent from vocalization and any requisite audition. Cued Speech handshapes and placements, however, even when coupled with the requisite information on the mouth, do not necessarily constitute language. This is clear in contexts where cues from the Cued Speech system are used in therapeutic settings to provide visual referents for single speech sounds or to provide visual feedback to deaf children attempting to produce speech. Although this approach may be effective for its purpose, a deaf child with this limited exposure would not be expected to acquire or develop language unless those discrete segments were arranged into more complex and complete utterances and the child has sufficient opportunities to interact using the language. It is for this reason that a distinction should be made between Cued Speech (the finite system of cues) and cued language (which denotes whole, natural language conveyed via Cued Speech).

The distinction between cueing and language is made clear when comparing the cases of cueing, speaking, and signing. Cueing, signing, and speaking are all modalities for conveying language, but none are languages themselves. Cued English is a language; Cued Speech is the communication modality. Spoken English is a language, whereas speech is the communication modality. American Sign Language is a language, signing is the communication modality. Opponents of Cued Speech sometimes point at the fact that Cued Speech is not a language as a reason for its being inappropriate for use with deaf children. However, although Cued Speech is not a language, it can serve as a modality for language. The quality of language exposure provided to a deaf child is neither determined nor limited by Cued Speech. Cued Speech is neither a methodology nor a set, prescriptive educational approach. However, claims that Cued Speech is unsound because it is not a language fail to take into account that Cued Speech operates independently of the language being cued. Signing and speaking are not languages; however, their viability for conveying language is not questioned. Within some educational systems, signing is used in ways that do not adequately support language acquisition; this is not an inherent fault of the modality of signing, but a flaw in its application. Similarly, in cases where Cued Speech is used inappropriately for adequate language acquisition and academic instruction, the flaw is in its application, not inherent to the system itself.

Fleetwood and Metzger (1997) note that languages are not always bound to a single communication modality. In the case of deafblind users of American Sign Language, the visual channel is supplanted by a tactual one. Although ASL is a traditionally signed language, it is not limited to one channel provided that it may be rendered unambiguously in another. This is indeed the case, for deafblind users who rely on American Sign Language, but access it through touch rather than vision. Likewise, traditionally spoken languages, like Japanese or English, are not limited to an acoustic channel provided that they may be rendered unambiguously in another. This is the case for deaf cuers who access these languages not through audition, but through vision via Cued Speech.

This relatively new case of cued languages has necessitated a paradigm shift from referring to *spoken languages* to referring to *traditionally spoken languages*. The term *cued language*, as first described by Fleetwood and Metzger (1998), also refers to a class of languages (similar to the term *spoken language*) and referring to a subset of languages for which an adaptation of Cued Speech has been devised. The need to distinguish between cued and spoken languages emerged not when Cornett invented his system, but when hearing and deaf individuals began using that system as a way to communicate linguistic infor-

mation (i.e., began to share language via cueing). Fleetwood and Metzger define a cued language, then, as any traditionally spoken consonant-vowel language in which the visual symbols of Cued Speech (e.g., mouth movements, manual cues, facial expression) serve as the foundation for conveying independently of audition all of the features constituting a language. Therefore, the terms *Cued Speech* and *cued language* are not synonymous or interchangeable; Cued Speech is the communication modality through which cued languages are expressed.

Internal Linguistic Variation

Languages exhibit internal variation in the form of dialects (Parker & Riley, 2005). All human languages exhibit dialectal variation, both signed and spoken. The phonological nature of Cued Speech makes it nearly impossible for the cuers to avoid reflecting their own accents in their cueing. As has already been mentioned, some dialects have their own adaptation of Cued Speech. For example, distinct Cued Speech systems exist for English in England, Australia, and the United States. Differences exist among the Cued Speech adaptations for these English language dialects; however, there is considerable overlap, as well. Some additions have been made. For example, English in England contains vowels that American English does not have. Although adjustments must be made when cuers of one dialect encounter cuers from another, it is unlikely that they would be mutually unintelligible. Speakers of American English, however, realize that there is a great deal of variation within the boundaries of their own country. Speakers from Maine do not sound like speakers from New York, Virginia, Georgia, Texas, or

Chicago. Dialectal variation can be exhibited in numerous ways, including: pronunciation, as in, *Let's walk down by the* /krɪk/ versus /krik/ (creek); vocabulary, as in, *I've shlepped this all over town*; and syntax, as in, *Can I come with?* Language variation exhibited at the level of phonemes and beyond can be readily cued through Cued Speech. Although one might suppose that this would be confusing to the deaf receiver, it is likely to be as confusing as it is for hearing people. Some confusion may occur that requires clarification. However, unambiguous exposure to a variety of pronunciations through Cued Speech could prove advantageous to those deaf individuals who may encounter similar pronunciations when speechreading.

Suprasegmentals in Cued Language

So far, we have discussed the C-V combinations that serve to create meaning in spoken and cued languages (i.e., segments). Other elements above the level of the segment, known as suprasegmentals, can color an utterance and shade its meaning. The retort, "It's not *what* you said, but *how* you said it" might be apt in describing the nature and importance of suprasegmentals in language. We look at such features as rhythm, intensity, inflection, prominence, and mood and how each is actualized in the spoken form of a language and the cued form.

Rhythm

Rhythm involves the alterations in speed —the speeding up, slowing down, holding, or pausing to affect meaning. This can occur to group elements as in the following:

You can have strawberry, banana, or chocolate.

You can have strawberry-banana or chocolate.

In these examples, the use of rhythm distinguishes the first sentence in which three flavors are available and the second sentence where only two choices are available, one being a blend of both strawberries and bananas. Experienced cuers can also alter the speed at which they deliver cues in order convey an intended meaning. Duration of consonants and vowels can show emphasis:

No, I don't want to go.

Nooooooooooo, I don't want to go.

In this example, note that although we might commonly say that the word *no* was held for emphasis, in actuality only part of the word is held. The duration (and possibly exaggeration) of the vowel is the salient feature in this example. The increased duration (and possible exaggeration) of the side-forward movement in cueing can be used to signify the extended vowel segment. This technique can also be used to highlight segments. In clinical settings, speech-language pathologists lengthen and exaggerate segments to call a particular segment to the attention of their clients.

Intensity

The term *intensity* refers to the amount of energy, which in speech translates to the perception of volume. In cueing, however, manual cues have no acoustic volume, but they can vary in intensity. Cueing parents are keenly aware of intensity in cueing. The visual equivalent of yelling involves more forcefully delivered handshapes against placements, sharper transitions between cues, and an increase in the spatial area in which the cues occur. Additionally, the eyes may be widened and accompanying facial expression may evoke a sense of anger. In contrast, what might be deemed a cued form of whispering involves a decrease in the area of the cueing space, positioning of the body to reduce visibility to others, lowering or shielding of the manual cues from those not participating in the conversation. Interestingly, the act of whispering in speech generally involves a reduction in intensity but also an omission or reduction in vocal fold vibration. As there is no single correlate for voicing in cueing comparable visual strategies are used to reduce the transmission area of the cued message. One would be unlikely, however, to find cuers replacing voiceless for voiced phonemes, although it is possible to do so.

Inflection

Changes in pitch have already been discussed in reference to tone languages. Inflectional differences can distinguish statements from questions even in cases where the words in each sentence are identical. In languages like French and English, inflection can be used in this way:

Il veut que je l'aide à porter les valises.

Il veut que je l'aide à porter les valises?

He wants me to help him carry the suitcases.

He wants me to help him carry the suitcases?

In these examples, the indication of a declarative sentence is made by the relative steady (but not flat) rise and fall in pitch. In the second sentence of each pair, however, we find that a rise in pitch signals an interrogative form. The interrogative form when cued involves the raising or furrowing of the eyebrows and may involve other visual cues such a slightly thrusting the head forward depending on the question type and context.

Prominence

Changes in rhythm and duration, intensity, and inflection contribute to making some words and parts of words more prominent than others. Take for example the statement, "No, she was wearing a green skirt." By varying the question that prompts this response, we are able to see the changes in prominence likely to result:

Was he wearing a green skirt?
No, SHE was wearing a green skirt.

She is wearing a green skirt?
No, she WAS wearing a green skirt.

Was she buying a green skirt?
No, she was WEARING a green skirt.

Was she wearing two green skirts?
No, she was wearing A green skirt.

Was she wearing a blue skirt?
No, she was wearing a GREEN skirt.

Was she wearing a green shirt?
No, she was wearing a green SKIRT.

In the above examples, one word is highlighted by an increase in intensity, duration, and possibly inflection. In the example of the question "Was she wearing two green skirts?" one might find that the pronunciation of the word *a* differs between this response and the others. In previous examples, the word *a* is likely to have been pronounced simply as the unstressed schwa as in the first vowel in the word *above*. However, when that word became stressed it is likely to be pronounced as /eɪ/ as in the first vowel in the word *acorn*. These distinctions in prominence and pronunciation are produced via Cued Speech. Perhaps, more significantly, Cued Speech conveys prominence not only at the word level, but at the syllable level as well. This distinction means that the stress of a word can also be conveyed via cueing. By changing the speed, duration, and intensity of the cues and by incorporating a slight head-thrust, differences in stress can be cued. These elements might be combined with changes in the quality of the vowels. Consider the following words in terms of changes in stress and vowel production.

Bio	/**baɪ** oʊ/
Biology	/baɪ **a** lə dʒi/
Biological	/baɪ ə **la** dʒə kəl/

The tendency of certain multisyllabic English words to make use of schwas in unstressed syllables is available to the deaf cued English user. Additionally, there are cases in English where syllabic stress differentiates parts of speech in spite of the fact that the segments within each of the words are identical:

Noun	Verb
PERmit	perMIT
INsult	inSULT
IMport	imPORT

In each of these cases, the cued versions for each pair are readily distinguishable through stress as they are in their spoken forms in spite of the fact that the handshapes and placements for each pair are identical.

Mood

Many of the prosodic elements found in spoken English have analogous visual correlates. However, how would one cue sarcasm, anger, glee, disapproval, or disgust? Again, many of the tones speakers of a language take with one another have observable, reproducible visual qualities: duration, intensity, inflection, and so forth. In addition, facial expression must be used when cueing to supply mood. Furrowed eyebrows, frowning, smiling, rolling eyes, engaged or disengaged eye gaze, and other similar behaviors can be used to convey mood. Facial expression plays a significant role in both signed and spoken languages. Likewise, facial expression is an essential component of cued English as well.

The prosodic features we have discussed are rarely seen in typical descriptions of Cued Speech, despite the fact that analogous visual prosodic information is necessary for the English meaning to be cued faithfully. Again, for this reason and others, specification between references to the invented articulatory system (Cued Speech) and the union of Cued Speech and a consonant-vowel language (cued language) may be necessary in some cases.

Conclusion

We have described the history of Cued Speech and its use among deaf and hearing populations in countries around the world. We have provided a means of discussing separately three inextricably linked yet discrete phenomena: (1) the invented communication system Cued Speech; (2) the expressive and receptive communication modality known as cueing; and (3) the natural language form known as cued language. We have explained how, via cueing, discrete visible phonemes combine into meaningful units of language, including syllables, words, and longer units of literal and nonliteral language usage. Finally, we have discussed different applications of Cued Speech and cueing, as well as general categories of cuers, including deaf native cuers, hearing cuers, and Cued Speech/ cued language transliterators. Cued Speech and cued language are truly complex phenomena which are only beginning to be fully understood. We hope that the information and ideas presented in this chapter will provide a lens through which the reader can better understand and appreciate the chapters that follow.

References

Blamey, P., Barry, J., Bow, C., Sarant, J., Paatsch, L., & Wales, R. (2001). The development of speech production following cochlear implantation. *Clinical Linguistics and Phonetics, 15,* 363–382.

Brentari, D. (1998). *A prosodic model of sign language phonology.* Cambridge, MA: MIT Press.

Conley, J. (1976). The role of idiomatic expressions in the reading of deaf children. *American Annals of the Deaf, 12,* 381–385.

Cornett, R. O. (1967). Cued Speech. *American Annals of the Deaf, 112,* 3–13.

Cornett, R. O. (1985). Update on Cued Speech. *Cued Speech Annual, 1,* 3–8.

Cornett, R. O. (1994). Adapting Cued Speech to additional languages. *Cued Speech Journal, 5,* 19–29.

Cornett, R. O., & Daisey, M. (2001). *The Cued Speech resource book for parents of deaf children.* Cleveland, OH: National Cued Speech Association.

Duchnowski, P., Lum, D., Krause, J., Sexton, M., Bratakos, M., & Braida, L. (2000). Development of speechreading supplements based on automatic speech recognition. *IEEE Transactions on Biomedical Engineering, 47,* 487–496.

Fleetwood, E., & Metzger, M. (1990). *Cued Speech transliteration: Theory and application.* Silver Spring, MD: Calliope Press.

Fleetwood, E., & Metzger, M. (1997). *Does Cued Speech entail speech: A comparison of cued and spoken information in terms of distinctive features.* Unpublished manuscript. Gallaudet University, Washington, DC.

Fleetwood, E., & Metzger, M. (1998). *Cued language structure: An analysis of cued American English based on linguistic principles.* Silver Spring, MD: Calliope Press.

Henegar, M., & Cornett, R. (1971). *Cued Speech handbook for parents. Cued Speech program.* Washington DC: Gallaudet College.

Liberman, A., & Mattingly, I. (1985). The motor theory of speech perception revised. *Cognition, 21,* 1–36.

Loos, E., Day, D., Jordan, P., & Wingate, J. (2004). *Glossary of linguistic terms.* Retrieved January 20, 2006, from http://www.sil.org/linguistics/GlossaryOfLinguisticTerms/WhatIsADiphthong.htm

Mitchell, R., & Myles, F. (2004). *Second language learning theories.* New York, NY: Oxford University Press.

National Cued Speech Association. (2006). *Cued Speech for American English.* Downloaded January 20, 2006, from http://www.cuedspeech.org/PDF/NewChart8.5X11.pdf

Parker, F., & Riley, K. (2005). *Linguistics for non-linguists* (4th ed.). New York, NY: Allyn & Bacon.

Tammasaeng, M. (1985). *The effects of Cued Speech upon tonal reception of the Thai language by hearing-impaired children.* Unpublished doctoral dissertation. Gallaudet University, Washington, DC.

Chapter 3

CUED LANGUAGE: WHAT DEAF NATIVE CUERS PERCEIVE OF CUED SPEECH

Melanie Metzger and Earl Fleetwood

Background

Cued Speech or Cued Language

In the spring of 1995, the authors of this chapter participated in a conference call with R. Orin Cornett, developer of Cued Speech. On numerous occasions during that call, Cornett reiterated his position that the system he devised, Cued Speech, is bimodal and that speaking is a required element of the system. Thus, when discussion turned to the work of individuals who do not speak while cueing, such as practitioners who transliterate from spoken English to cued English, the premise for an interesting question arose. Specifically, when excluding a defining element (i.e., speech) of Cued Speech, what system are these transliterators employing? As that conversation progressed, Cornett proposed that the term "Cued Speech transliterator"

was a misnomer because cueing transliterators do not use speech, and therefore, are not using Cued Speech, as he defined it, when conveying messages originating with hearing speakers. Cornett noted that transliterators are actually using "Cued Speech with suppressed voice."

In light of the ever growing body of research and literature describing the role of Cued Speech as a "supplement to speech," this was no minor distinction. First, it would be recursive logic to suggest that Cued Speech is supplementary to one of its required elements (i.e., audible speech). Nevertheless, if speech is a definitional element of Cued Speech, then successfully conveying linguistic information in its absence, as in the aforementioned transliterator scenario, suggests that it also is not a functional element. Moreover, it suggests that the salient articulatory features of cueing are less broad than the requisite elements of Cued Speech. Thus, this conversation with Cornett brought to light a fundamental discrepancy: audible speech (and thus, the ability to speak) was a requisite of Cued Speech by definition yet, given the transliterator example, seemed unnecessary as an articulatory element. So, what are the required elements, how can they be isolated and examined, and how are they distinct from being "supplement(s) to speech"? Does Cued Speech function as a truly bimodal system, requiring both audible speech and visible elements as Cornett had hypothesized, or are the visible elements alone—a subset of Cued Speech—the only features required to convey linguistic information? Does speech influence linguistic decision making by or is it extraneous to deaf native cuers when cueing and speaking co-occur? Such questions drive the study addressed in this chapter.

McGurk Paradigm for Examining the Relative Influence of Co-Occurring Visual and Auditory Information

Questions related to the relative roles of auditory and visual information in speech have been examined in hearing individuals via the McGurk paradigm (McGurk & MacDonald, 1976). The McGurk paradigm examines the relative influence of visual and acoustic sources of information on what hearing people perceive when accessing both simultaneously. The McGurk paradigm employs four conditions: (1) Audio-Only (AO), in which participants report what they hear when presented with an audio recording of syllables like /pa/ or /ba/, (2) Visual-Only (VO), in which participants report what they lipread when presented with a face articulating the

same syllables, (3) Audio-Visual Congruent (AVC) condition, in which participants watch a synchronized video recording of a speaker's face articulating the same syllable, for example A/pa/V/pa/, and have to report what they hear, and (4) Audio-Visual Incongruent (AVI), in which participants are presented with an audio recording of syllables matched with a video recording of a different syllable, like A/pa/ matched with V/ga/. When individuals are required to report what they hear in the AVI condition, they typically report hearing the illusory syllable /ta/, which is called a *fusion* of the audio-visual stimuli. In the reverse situation, (i.e., hearing an audio recording of /ka/ while watching a synchronized video recording of a speaker's face articulating /pa/, they typically report hearing /pka/, a percept called a *combination*. Note that in the latter case, the /p/ is *not* in the sound track, and is just suggested by the very salient lip movement of abrupt aperture of the mouth. These illusions are robust, and have been demonstrated in adults and children and in numerous languages (see Colin & Radeau, 2003 for a review).

Purpose of the Study

The purpose of the study was to determine whether the spoken mode of Cued Speech affects the linguistic decisions of deaf native cuers or whether such decisions are products of its visible mode. It was hypothesized that deaf participants exposed to cued allophones, syllables, words, and sentences in both audiovisually consistent and audiovisually inconsistent conditions similar to the AVC and AVI conditions in an adaptation of the

McGurk paradigm would provide responses consistent with information presented in the visible channel regardless of co-occurring information presented in the acoustic channel.

Method

Participants

Twenty-six participants, between the ages of 16 and 32 years, participated in this study, including 13 participants who are deaf and 13 individuals with normal hearing. The hearing individuals served as the control group for this study. All participants reported either having no vision problems or vision corrected to normal with either glasses or contact lenses.

Deaf Participants

Deaf participants, ranging in age from 16 to 32 years (mean age of 20 years), were prelingually deaf, native cuers of American English, including eight females and five males. The term *native* here means that participants had been cueing American English since their early years at school, and for at least half of their lives. Regarding degree of deafness, 10 described their hearing loss as profound, one as severe-to-profound, and two as severe. Regarding onset of deafness, 10 participants indicated that they were deaf at birth, and 3 indicated being deaf prior to 18 months. Regarding early language exposure, 10 participants reported initial exposure to cued English prior to the age of 3 years, two reported initial exposure by 5 years of age, and one reported having been exposed to cued English by the age of 8. Twelve partici-

pants indicated having been exposed to cued English by at least one parent, and one reported initial exposure at school, followed by cueing from at least one parent at home. Ten participants reported being exposed to cued English beginning in preschool, two reported being exposed to cued English starting in first grade, and one participant in the fourth grade.

Hearing Participants

The hearing control group consisted of 13 native speakers of American English, including 7 females, and 6 males ranging in age from 18 to 32 years, who reported having no knowledge of Cued Speech. Hearing participants who began using English in the spoken mode no later than their early years at school and who had used spoken English for more than half of his or her life were also considered *native* for this study. All reported that speaking was the primary mode and English the primary language used by their parents and in school.

Instrumentation

A VHS recording of 32 stimuli, including: 10 isolated allophones, 10 monosyllabic and multisyllabic words, and 12 short sentences (e.g., *Lend me your ears*) was made (Table 3–1). These particular groupings provided a unique opportunity to analyze responses to isolated linguistic symbols (i.e., allophones) as well as to increasingly complex combinations of these symbols (i.e., words and short sentences). All test items were simultaneously congruent in cued and spoken modes. This allowed the mouth to simultaneously contribute to the production of symbols

Table 3–1. Test Items

— CUED — Linguistic Items Presented via the Visible Features of Cuem	Test Item	— SPOKEN — Linguistic Items Presented via the Acoustic Features of Speech
/g/	1	/k/
/p/	2	/m/
/i/	3	/l/
/d/	4	/n/
/u/	5	/ʊ/
/k/	6	/k/
/m/	7	/m/
/l/	8	/l/
/n/	9	/n/
/ʊ/	10	/ʊ/
/trɛnd/	11	/drɛd/
/pɪg/	12	/bik/
/tʌnz/	13	/dʌz/
/drɪp/	14	/trɪm/
/pɛt/	15	/mɛn/
/drɛd/	16	/drɛd/
/bik/	17	/bik/
/dʌz/	18	/dʌz/
/trɪm/	19	/trɪm/
/mɛn/	20	/mɛn/
/ɪt kʊd hæpən/	21	/ɪts ə gʊd hæbɪt/
/hi gʌvɚnd ðʌ kɪŋdəm/	22	/ɪt kʌvɚz ðu hɪltap/
/lɛts bi kərir fokəst/	23	/lɛnd mi yɚ ɪrz foks/
/pɛɪ ʌtɛnʃən/	24	/mɛɪk ʌ dʌndʒən/
/aɪ told yu aɪd kʌm/	25	/aɪ dont tʃu ðæt gʌm/
/aɪ pɛɪd for ɪnʃɚɪns/	26	/aɪ mɛt ə forɪn dʒɚnəlɪst/
/ɪts ə gʊd hæbɪt/	27	/ɪts ə gʊd hæbɪt/
/ɪt kʌvɚz ðu hɪltap/	28	/ɪt kʌvɚz ðu hɪltap/
/lɛnd mi yɚ ɪrz foks/	29	/lɛnd mi yɚ ɪrz foks/
/mɛɪk ʌ dʌndʒən/	30	/mɛɪk ʌ dʌndʒən/
/aɪ dont tʃu ðæt gʌm/	31	/aɪ dont tʃu ðæt gʌm/
/aɪ mɛt ə forɪn dʒɚnəlɪst/	32	/aɪ mɛt ə forɪn dʒɚnəlɪst/

(i.e., visible and acoustic) in both modes, even when those symbols did not match linguistically (e.g., cueing *talk* while speaking *dog*). Thus, the stimuli were selected with the goal of copresenting coherent messages in the cued and spoken modes.

Stimuli were presented using four conditions: (1) with sound, (2) without sound, (3) linguistically associated visible and acoustic values (AC) (e.g., *dog* was spoken while *dog* was cued), and (4) linguistically dissociated visible and acoustic values (DC) which had identical mouthshapes (e.g., *dog* was spoken but *talk* was cued). When choosing DC test items, the authors used only those mouthshape-handshape and mouthshape-hand location pairs that occur when cueing American English. Unlike Alegria's (this volume) test items, all test items were congruent in their respective modes. The stimuli were presented such that the first half were AC items, in which the linguistic value of the cued and spoken stimuli were identical, and the second half were DC items, in which the cued stimuli differed linguistically from the spoken stimuli but had identical *mouthshape* (i.e., nonmanual) images. Test items are presented in the sequence shown in Table 3–1.[1]

Test stimuli were presented by a 35-year-old female, hearing native speaker of American English who simultaneously cued and spoke all AC and DC test items. The presenter had 20 years of experience communicating language via the visual mode via American Sign Language (ASL) as well as Cued American English (CAE), including functioning as a signed language interpreter certified by the Registry of Interpreters for the Deaf, Inc.; as a cued language transliterator certified by the Testing, Evaluation, and Certification Unit, Inc.; as a cued language transliterator and signed language interpreter educator. The presenter made no errors on the Basic Cued Speech Proficiency Rating (Beaupré, 1983), a standardized test that evaluates knowledge and skills with regard to expressive cueing mechanics.

Data Collection

Participants were exposed twice to the same videotaped test items. For their first trial, *deaf* participants were exposed to only the visual (cued) stimuli (the acoustic stimuli were removed by having the volume of the television monitor turned down so that there was no sound). For their first trial, *hearing* participants were exposed to only the acoustic (spoken) stimuli (the picture on the television monitor was dimmed completely so that it provided no visual information). For the second trial, both groups received simultaneously presented acoustic (spoken) and visual (cued) information. For the deaf participants, the volume on the television monitor was adjusted during the second trial such that the sound track of the video recording matched the loudness that the hearing control group would

---

[1]During a prestudy review of the testing material, flaws were noted in cued test items numbered 23 and 25; unintended handshapes and/or hand placements were articulated. This is likely a cognitive manifestation of producing mismatched cued-spoken information; the cuer who presented the test items does not regularly strive to simultaneously generate two different linguistic messages. Although participants were exposed to the flawed test items, the test items are not included in the results and analysis portion of the current study as they do not satisfy the test material parameters.

experience in their acoustic trial. Deaf participants who make use of residual hearing and/or assistive listening devices had the opportunity to make use of the same. For the hearing participants, the television monitor was adjusted during the second trial such that the brightness of the video image matched what the deaf participants had seen. Hearing and deaf participants who make use of eyeglasses or contacts had the opportunity to make use of the same. Thus, all participants were exposed first to their most linguistically accessible mode (i.e., visible for deaf participants, acoustic for hearing participants) for all test items, then to simultaneous visible (cued) and acoustic (spoken) information for all test items.

For both trials, participants were given a blank answer sheet numbered from 1 to 32 and the following written English instructions: "For each item, write down what you understand from the presenter." Figures 3–1 and 3–2 illustrate what participants saw in the DC and AC conditions. The cued allophone seen in the photograph in Figure 3–1 and the spoken allophone [m] are rendered simultaneously. The cued allophone seen in the photograph in Figure 3–2 and the spoken allophone [v] are rendered simultaneously.

Results

Responses of participants were compared for the two trials and were scored as being the same or different. As reflected in Table 3–2, both deaf and hearing participants completed both trials with 100% accuracy. On the surface, the only difference between the deaf and hearing groups was that when co-occurring information differed linguistically (e.g., *dog* and *talk*) between modes, the responses of hearing participants corresponded exclusively with what they *heard*, whereas the responses of deaf participants corresponded exclusively with what they saw. The significance of these results is addressed in the next section.

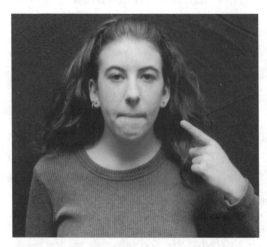

Figure 3–1. Sample DC test item.

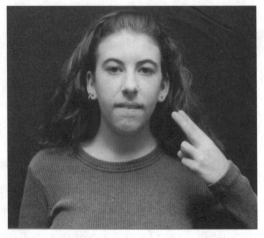

Figure 3–2. Sample AC test item.

Table 3–2. Percentage of Actual Responses Corresponding with Predicted Responses

	Deaf Participants' Predicted Responses	Percentage of Actual Responses Corresponding w/Predicted Responses for Deaf Native Cuers		Test Item	Percentage of Actual Responses Corresponding w/Predicted Responses for Hearing Native Speakers		Hearing Participants' Predicted Responses
		1st Trial (*n* = 13)	2nd Trial (*n* = 13)		1st Trial (*n* = 13)	2nd Trial (*n* = 13)	
DC Test Items	"g"	100	100	1	100	100	"k" "c"
	"p"	100	100	2	100	100	"m"
	"ee" "eee" "ē̄" or "ea"	100	100	3	100	100	"i"
	"d"	100	100	4	100	100	"n"
	any of: "ue" "ooo" "ō̄o"	100	100	5	100	100	any of: "oo" "ŏŏ"
AC Test Items	"k" "c"	100	100	6	100	100	"k" "c"
	"m"	100	100	7	100	100	"m"
	"i"	100	100	8	100	100	"i"
	"n"	100	100	9	100	100	"n"
	any of: "oo" "ŏŏ"	100	100	10	100	100	any of: "oo" "ŏŏ"
DC Test Items	"trend"	100	100	11	100	100	"dread"
	"pig"	100	100	12	100	100	"beak"
	"tons"	100	100	13	100	100	"does"
	"drip"	100	100	14	100	100	"trim"
	"pet"	100	100	15	100	100	"men"
AC Test Items	"dread"	100	100	16	100	100	"dread"
	"beak"	100	100	17	100	100	"beak"
	"does"	100	100	18	100	100	"does"
	"trim"	100	100	19	100	100	"trim"
	"men"	100	100	20	100	100	"men"
DC Test Items	"it could happen"	100	100	21	100	100	"it's a good habit"
	"he governed the kingdom"	100	100	22	100	100	"it covers the hilltop"

continues

Table 3–2. *continued*

Deaf Participants' Predicted Responses	Percentage of Actual Responses Corresponding w/Predicted Responses for Deaf Native Cuers		Test Item	Percentage of Actual Responses Corresponding w/Predicted Responses for Hearing Native Speakers		Hearing Participants' Predicted Responses
	1st Trial (*n* = 13)	2nd Trial (*n* = 13)		1st Trial (*n* = 13)	2nd Trial (*n* = 13)	
DC Test Items *continued* "let's be career focused"	N/A	N/A	23	N/A	N/A	"lend me your ears folks"
"pay attention"	100	100	24	100	100	"make a dungeon"
"I told you I'd come"	N/A	N/A	25	N/A	N/A	"I don't chew that gum"
"I paid for insurance"	100	100	26	100	100	"I met a foreign journalist"
AC Test Items "it's a good habit"	100	100	27	100	100	"it's a good habit"
"it covers the hilltop"	100	100	28	100	100	"it covers the hilltop"
"lend me your ears folks"	100	100	29	100	100	"lend me your ears folks"
"make a dungeon"	100	100	30	100	100	"make a dungeon"
"I don't chew that gum"	100	100	31	100	100	"I don't chew that gum"
"I met a foreign journalist"	100	100	32	100	100	"I met a foreign journalist"

Discussion

Previous studies (such as Chilson, 1985; Clark & Ling, 1976; Kaplan, 1974; Ling & Clark, 1975; Neef, 1979; Nicholls, 1979; Nicholls & Ling, 1982; Nicholls-Musgrove, 1985; Périer, Charlier, Hage, & Alegría, 1987; Quenin, 1992; Ryalls, Auger, & Hage, 1994; Sneed, 1972) have found acoustic information not *functionally* relevant to Cued Speech. The current study supports that finding. However, the significance of the current study is that it is the first to further suggest: (1) that cued information exists independently of spoken information even when the two co-occur and (2) that the speech mode of Cued Speech is inconsequential and even extraneous in terms of linguistic decision-making, at least to the deaf participants in this study. Thus, the findings of this study suggest that the visible elements of Cued Speech (for which the term *cuem*[2] was coined by the authors of this study, see Fleetwood and Metzger, 1998) constitute an autonomous articulatory system. The design of this study is the first to allow for such a finding.

The classic McGurk effect (McGurk & MacDonald, 1976) is the product of incongruent information being sent and received in two channels: acoustic and visible. Where hearing people are concerned, a mismatch between what is heard and what they expect to see (i.e., accompanying mouthshape) creates a sound-articulation incongruency. In light of the deaf participants' responses to the stimuli presented in the current study, it appears that they received no such incongruencies. Thus, although the current study was intended as a modification of the McGurk effect—*linguistic* mismatches between modes were substituted for the classic sound-articulation mismatches—findings suggest that no cross-modal incongruencies were received by the deaf participants. This suggests that

only a study designed with incongruencies wholly within the visible mode would allow for testing of the McGurk affect on deaf subjects (see Chapter 5).

Cueing and speaking comprised the bimodal information *presented* to the deaf cuers in this study. However, findings indicate that information in only one mode (i.e., the visible mode) was *received, perceived,* and *processed.* Therefore, it would be inaccurate to describe deaf native cuers in this study as responding to Cued Speech (a bimodal system) or even to *spoken* English (an acoustic phenomenon) rendered via Cued Speech. Instead, results indicate that deaf native cuers responded exclusively to the *cued English* (a visible phenomenon) presented.

The primary question addressed in this study was whether the speech mode of Cued Speech affects the linguistic decisions made by deaf native cuers. Results of the study indicate that for this group of deaf native cuers it does not. Findings support the idea that both modes comprising Cued Speech can co-exist. However, when strictly referring to features salient to linguistic decisions made by deaf native cuers, results also suggest that it would be inaccurate to use the term Cued Speech, which is by definition a bimodal system. Thus, these data indicate that while Cued Speech can be *presented* bimodally (i.e., in keeping with its definition), only its visible features (i.e., cuem) constitute the

---

[2]Prior to this study, no single term referred at once and exclusively to all of the strictly visible features (i.e., handshape, hand location, and mouthshape) constituting cued allophones. For example, the term "cue" does not, as it refers strictly to the handshapes and hand locations of Cued Speech. The term "Cued Speech" does not, as it refers to both the visible and acoustic components comprising this bimodal system. Thus, where the term "speech" can refer to the production of strictly acoustic allophones, Fleetwood and Metzger (1997, 1998) found the need for a counterpart term. As a result, the authors coined a term that refers exclusively to the visible symbols resulting from the combination of handshape/location (i.e., "cue") and the mouthshape ("m"). The resulting term "cuem" refers strictly to the visible phonologic segments produced while cueing in the same way that the term "speech" can refer strictly to the acoustic phonologic segments produced while speaking.

articulatory system received, perceived, and processed by the deaf native cuers in this study. This finding has implications for both theory and practice.

Implications

Implications for Theory

1. The finding from this study that phonological information about English can be gleaned entirely from visual information explains the observation that deaf children who are consistently exposed to a cued language in natural interaction develop native or native-like competence in a given consonant-vowel language, including home languages of hearing parents or foreign languages studied in school.

2. The example of cued language illustrates that commonly used definitions of terms such as phone (speech sound), phoneme (primary linguistic value), phonics (sound-letter relationship), internal speech recoding (recoding of print to speech sounds for purposes of internal communication) which use "sound" and "speech" in their definitions are at best restrictive, and from the example of deaf cuers, could be described as inaccurate. The distinction between language *modality* and language *structure* prompts the need to re-examine discipline-specific application of research findings. For example, "inner speech" as a construct is not limited to traditional notions of "speech" or "speech perception." Recognizing that deaf native cuers can internalize through an autonomous visual articulatory system the phonological, morphological, and syntactic aspects of traditionally spoken languages has implications for a variety of disciplines, including *psychology* (e.g., language perception, neurofunctional localization of the brain), *linguistics* (e.g., language acquisition and the development of literacy), and *education* (e.g., bilingual and multilingual programming). Related issues in each of these disciplines are ripe areas for further research.

3. Cued Speech carries linguistic information in two modes, visible and acoustic. Yet, the visible component is sufficient for conveying all linguistic elements. Thus, Cued Speech can exist as the bimodal system defined by its inventor and at the same time function as the unimodal system received, perceived, and processed by deaf native cuers.

4. It is inaccurate to describe cueing as "oral." In oral approaches, access to sound is emphasized and place of articulation, manner of articulation, and voicing status are the salient linguistic features of the spoken utterance; while in cueing, the salient linguistic features are handshape, hand placement, and mouth formation (co-occurring with other visible features).

5. In the same way that written language and spoken language are autonomous modes referring to the same linguistic information, cued language and spoken language are autonomous yet related linguistic manifestations. This finding differs from findings of earlier literature, including studies that examine the effect of Cued Speech on deaf children's speech reception (such as Chilson, 1985; Clark & Ling, 1976; Kaplan, 1974; Ling & Clark, 1975; Neef, 1979; Nicholls, 1979; Nicholls & Ling, 1982; Nicholls-Musgrove, 1985; Périer, Charlier, Hage, & Alegría, 1987; Que-

nin, 1992; Sneed, 1972)and those that have focused on how cueing affects deaf children's speech production (including Ryalls, Auger, & Hage, 1994).[3] For a discussion of the fundamental differences between Cued Speech and cued language, see Fleetwood and Metzger, 1998, and Chapter 4 by Koo and Supalla in this volume.

6. The experience of "speechreading" should be qualitatively different for deaf native cuers than it is for deaf noncuers. When presented with the mouth-only version of a familiar cued language, the visible mouth information that remains (in the absence of handshapes and hand placements) might be processed as part of a visibly impoverished cued message rather than as part of an acoustically impoverished spoken one. If so, the terms *speechreading* or *lipreading* would not apply to deaf native cuers as they might to deaf noncuers (see Fleetwood & Metzger, 1998 for further discussion).

Implications for Practice

1. The finding that Cued Speech can function entirely visually, in the absence of either speech or hearing, suggests that that for parents of deaf children and the professionals that work with them, the decision to cue a particular language is not limited by either the hearing acuity of the deaf child or the deaf child's ability to access, perceive, process, or produce the acoustic and articulatory features of speech.

2. For deaf children for whom speech is a goal, one advantage that native cuers of English or other traditionally spoken languages have is that linguistic segmentations (e.g., onset-rime, syllables) provided by cueing parallel those provided by speaking. That segmentation can subsequently serve professionals such as deaf educators, early interventionists, educational audiologists, or speech-language pathologists as a relevant point of reference for associating linguistic knowledge with speech production. Essentially, because the deaf native cuer has already acquired linguistic segments conversationally via exposure to the visible symbols (handshape, hand placement, and mouthshape) of a particular cued language such as English, the professional working with the deaf child can reference those segments when teaching the deaf cuer how to produce the acoustic symbols of the corresponding spoken language. This is one way that acquisition of a cued language might support oral/aural and even auditory/verbal goals.

3. Given that cochlear implants or digital hearing aids do not provide clear and complete acoustic information to deaf individuals, the visible elements of Cued Speech can play an important role in unambiguously specifying linguistic segments where the acoustic information provided by these devices does not. Of the available communication methods (i.e., speechreading, fingerspelling, manually coded sign

---

[3]Common to these studies is their discussion of cued (visual) and spoken (acoustic) information as if: (1) their co-occurrence reflects an inherent relationship between modes, (2) the definitional requisites (e.g., a bimodal system) and functional elements of Cued Speech are one and the same, and (3) Cued Speech represents or presents spoken language (an acoustic phenomenon) rather than cued language (a visual phenomenon).

systems, cueing), cueing is most theoretically supportable, given that it clearly and completely conveys English and other traditionally spoken languages visibly, and can do so in sync with co-occurring spoken messages (see Chapter 12 in this volume).

4. For those instructional programs that seek to provide only visually-accessible languages to deaf children, such as bilingual programs that include ASL and written English (see LaSasso & Lollis, 2003), Cued English, like ASL, is a viable visual linguistic option (see Kyllo, Chapter 10 in this volume for a discussion of bilingualism via ASL-Cued English).

Conclusion

Cornett invented a system to allow deaf children to naturally acquire consonant-vowel languages that have traditionally been spoken. It was his hope that this system could provide a unique option for parents and professionals interested in bilingual (i.e., English-ASL) and monolingual opportunities for deaf children (Cornett, 1991). He envisioned his system as integrated with speech, conceived of speech as being a part of the system, and named the system Cued Speech (Cornett, 1967). Regardless of discrepancies between Cornett's characterization of his system and findings of the current study, a growing body of research provides evidence that Cornett was very successful in his efforts. As numerous chapters in this volume attest, use of the system that he designed does result in deaf children who acquire consonant-vowel languages that have traditionally been spoken (e.g., English, Thai, French). Many native cuers of these languages are also fluent users of natural signed languages such as ASL (see Chapter 9 in this volume).

Cornett apparently did not fully recognize the autonomous nature of the system that he devised, let alone the ramifications of the system on our understanding of language. Although Stokoe (1960) is widely recognized for his well-accepted notion that languages need not be sound/speech-based, Cornett's contribution is the creation of a system that allows traditionally spoken languages to exist in the absence of speech or hearing. The creation of Cued Speech has led to the existence of cued languages and to the development of a new linguistic community (i.e., cueing community) with ties to other sociolinguistic groups (e.g., oral deaf, signing deaf, and hearing communities). The example of cued language provides linguistic evidence that even spoken languages are only traditionally so.

References

Beaupré, W. (1983). *Basic Cued Speech proficiency rating*. Kingston, RI: University of Rhode Island.

Chilson, R. (1985). Effects of Cued Speech instruction on speechreading skills. *Cued Speech Annual, 1,* 60–68.

Clark, B., & Ling, D. (1976). The effects of using Cued Speech: A follow-up study. *Volta Review, 78,* 23–34.

Colin, C., & Radeau, M. (2003). Les illusions McGurk dans la parole: 25 ans de recherches. *L'Année Psychologique, 104,* 497–542.

Cornett, R. O. (1967). Cued Speech. *American Annals of the Deaf, 112,* 3–13.

Cornett. R. O. (1991). A model for ASL/English bilingualism. In E. Lovato, S. Polowe-Aldersley, P. Schragle, V. Armour, & J. Polowe (Eds.), *Profession on parade: Proceed-*

ings of the CAID/CEASD Convention (pp. 33–39). New Orleans, LA: Convention of American Instructors of the Deaf.

Fleetwood, E., & Metzger, M. (1997). *Does Cued Speech entail speech? A comparison of cued and spoken information in terms of distinctive features.* Unpublished manuscript. Washington, DC: Gallaudet University.

Fleetwood, E., & Metzger, M. (1998). *Cued language structure: An analysis of cued American English based on linguistic principles.* Silver Spring, MD: Calliope Press.

Kaplan, H. (1974). The effects of Cued Speech on the speechreading ability of the deaf. *Dissertation Abstracts International, 36,* 645B.

LaSasso, C., & Lollis, J. (2003). Survey of residential and day schools for deaf students in the United States that identify themselves as bilingual-bicultural programs. *Journal of Deaf Studies and Deaf Education, 8,* 79–91.

Ling, D., & Clark, D. (1975). Cued Speech: An evaluative study. *American Annals of the Deaf, 120,* 480–488.

McGurk, H., & MacDonald, J. (1976). Hearing lips and seeing voices. *Nature, 264,* 746–748.

Neef, N. (1979). *An evaluation of Cued Speech training on lipreading performance in deaf persons.* Unpublished doctoral dissertation, Western Michigan University, Kalamazoo.

Nicholls, G. (1979). *Cued Speech and the reception of spoken language.* Unpublished masters thesis. McGill University, Montreal, Canada.

Nicholls, G., & Ling, D. (1982). Cued Speech and the reception of spoken language. *Journal of Speech and Hearing Research, 25,* 262–269.

Nicholls-Musgrove, G. (1985). *Discourse comprehension by hearing-impaired children who use Cued Speech.* Unpublished doctoral dissertation, McGill University, Montreal, Canada.

Périer, O., Charlier, B., Hage, C., & Alegría, J. (1987). Evaluation of the effects of prolonged Cued Speech practice upon the reception of spoken language. In I. G. Taylor (Ed.), *The education of the deaf: Current perspectives* (pp. 616–628). Beckenham, Kent, UK: Croon Helm, Ltd.

Quenin, C. (1992). *Tracking of connected discourse by deaf college students who use Cued Speech.* Unpublished doctoral dissertation, Pennsylvania State University, University Park.

Ryalls, J., Auger, D., & Hage, C. (1994). An acoustic study of the speech skills of profoundly hearing-impaired children who use Cued Speech. *Cued Speech Journal, 5,* 8–18.

Sneed, N. (1972). The effects of training in Cued Speech on syllable lipreading scores of normally hearing subjects. In *Cued speech parent training and follow-up program* (pp. 38–44). Washington, DC: Project Report to Department of Health, Education, and Welfare, U.S. Office of Education.

Stokoe, W. (1960). *Sign language structure.* Silver Spring, MD: Linstok Press.

Chapter 4

PSYCHOLINGUISTIC STUDY OF PHONOLOGICAL PROCESSES IN DEAF ADULT CUERS

Daniel S. Koo and Ted Supalla

Since the introduction of Cued Speech in 1966 (Cornett, 1967), its use as a cross-modal form of communication by hearing parents of deaf children has grown steadily in the United States as well as other countries (Cornett & Daisey, 1992). An entire generation of deaf cuers has grown up with this visual system of manual hand-shapes and nonmanual mouthing, many adapting it for use in daily conversation and interaction with other deaf cuers (see Chapter 9). The purpose of this chapter is to examine the linguistic outcome of life-long experience with cued English, which may be influenced by nativization forces. Andersen's (1983) theoretical model of nativization proposes that language learners go through an internal structuring process in which they initially construct a unique linguistic system (nativization) using presumed innate linguistic abilities and gradually re-adapt their system (dena-tivization) to match the target environment language. When children discover that their tentative linguistic structure conflicts with the environmental language, they adjust their internal hypotheses about language to match the target language. This model has been used to explain certain circumstances where deaf children may deviate in relation to their language environment, leading some investigators to postulate that deaf children are less reliant on denativization and more dependent on their own internal nativization process (Gee & Goodhart, 1985; Gee & Mounty, 1990; Nelson, Loncke, & Camarata, 1993). As deaf native cuers of English presumably have unambiguous visual access to their language environment, will they depend more on their own internal mechanism or undergo a denativization process toward a complete phonological representation of the target language?

Background

Much of the empirical research on Cued Speech has focused on receptive and reading performance of deaf children (i.e., Alegría, Lechat, & Leybaert, 1988; Leybaert, Alegría, Hage, & Charlier, 1998; Nicholls & Ling, 1982) but some early works have used expressive speech as a measure of linguistic performance or competence (i.e., Cornett, 1973; Mohay, 1983; Nash, 1973;) rather than the expressive or receptive use of cued language. Aside from works by Kipila (1985), Metzger (1994a), and Fleetwood and Metzger (1997), little linguistic analysis has been conducted on deaf individuals' use of the cued language system. In a linguistic case study, Kipila (1985) analyzed a deaf child's use of receptive and expressive morphology during a cued interview with a hearing teacher. The subject, 5;4, had been exposed to cued English for 3 years and was able to use certain morphemes with 100% accuracy (i.e., past regular, past irregular, and plural) but not others. In a follow-up study 6 years later, Metzger (1994a) examined the same subject, aged 11;9, and found morphemes previously used correctly by the subject were maintained and the morphemes previously used with less than 100% accuracy were now used with 100% accuracy (i.e., the contractible copula, present progressive, and articles).

Whereas the above studies focused on an individual child cuer, Fleetwood and Metzger (1997) examined the question of whether cued messages are products of a different set of distinctive features than spoken messages; that is, whether cued and spoken information possess the same or different distinctive features that potentially impact the reception, perception, and processing of information occurring in the other channel. Subjects for this study consisted of a control group of 10 hearing native speakers of American English who did not know the cued system and a group of 10 deaf native cuers of American English. Using the McGurk method (McGurk & MacDonald, 1976), Fleetwood and Metzger's (1997) experiment was designed to examine processing of bimodal linguistic stimuli by cohorts with different perceptual abilities for two channels where manual cues (visual channel) and spoken words (auditory channel) are simultaneously coarticulated. The aim was to determine whether: (1) cued information confounds spoken information; (2) spoken information confounds cued information; (3) neither confounds the other, and the integrity of information in each channel is preserved; or (4) the articulation of cued information and the articulation of spoken information are independent processes, even if they co-occur. Stimuli consisted of two exposures to a set of 32 videotaped items of phonemes, words, and sentences in which information was simultaneously spoken and cued to both groups. Half the test material was designed to converge linguistically across mode (i.e., spoken, cued) and the other half was designed to diverge linguistically across mode. One example of a linguistically divergent item is to simultaneously present the cued form of /p/ with the acoustic form of /m/ as the mouthshape for both phonemes are visually similar. The prediction is that deaf people without acoustic input will respond with "p" whereas hearing speakers who do not know cues will respond with "m." As predicted, responses were consistent across groups where simultaneously cued and spoken test material was designed to converge linguistically across mode, and responses differed across groups where simultaneously cued and spoken test material was designed to diverge across mode. As responses were found consistent within groups across all test material, Fleetwood and Metzger (1997) concluded that individually and separately, the cued mode and the spoken mode are each systematic and sufficient for conveying linguistic information. Because hearing speakers and deaf cuers had different responses to linguistically divergent test items, they also concluded that modality-specific attributes, either aural or visual, determine the specific linguistic value of the perceived message. In summary, findings from the Fleetwood and Metzger (1997) study show that coarticulated cued and spoken information results in co-occurring, yet independently functioning, articulatory systems; that is, the distinctive features of speech are not phonetically relevant to receiving, processing, and comprehending cued messages visually. This important point establishes a paradigmatic framework for any linguistic analysis of cued language, including the present study.

To better understand the potential benefit of cueing with and by deaf cohorts who either do not acquire language primarily through audition and/or who do not primarily use speech to communicate language, this chapter explores the effect of lifelong experience with a visual phonological system, namely cued English, which relies on nonmanual mouthshapes and manual cues instead of acoustic features. Specifically, how do deaf native cuers process their acquired knowledge of phonological and morphological rules? What is the psycholinguistic outcome from lifelong experience with cueing? These questions subsequently lead to a set of important inquiries addressed in a series of empirical studies (Koo, 2003): (1) what, if any, phonological properties from English are preserved or modified by deaf native users of cued English and (2) do deaf cuers sufficiently internalize morphophonemic rules from spoken language via cues to be able to generalize to new words? In this chapter, we report the findings of two psycholinguistic studies from the Koo (2003) dissertation: Experiment 1 explores the phonological processes of deaf adults raised with cued English through linguistic analysis of sentence production, and Experiment 2 investigates the morpho-phonological interface in word representations and strategies in deaf adult cuers using a modified morphological experiment. As deaf cuers primarily receive and express cued languages in the visual modality rather than audition, the present study examines deaf adult cuers' use of expressive and linguistic cueing rather than speech. Finally, we interpret the findings within the theoretical framework of the nativization model.

Experiment 1: Linguistic Analysis of Sentence Production

More than 30 years after its conception, the basic elements of cueing as originally developed have not changed; however, in the natural course of dialogue, its users may have altered its physical properties in ways the developer may not have anticipated. For example, Metzger (1994b) found evolutionary changes in expressive phonology of deaf cuers, such as the use of syllabic stress by thrusting the chin and lengthening the duration of hand contact to the appropriate placement, which were not included in Cornett's original system. In Experiment 1, we employed a sentence production task which allowed us to examine the phonological processes that occur in natural cueing production. Specifically, this experiment uses a set of controlled sentence utterances to not only extend Metzger's (1994b) linguistic analysis but also to demonstrate how cueing operates under two distinct phonological rules or systems. On one hand, the phonotactics and phonological rules of English are well preserved in fluent deaf cuers. On the other hand, phonological processes unique to the visuogestural modality impose physical constraints on phonological forms. Whereas Metzger (1994b) identified suprasegmental features from a naturally occurring dialogue between two cueing interlocutors, Experiment 1 describes the phonetic outcome of phonological processes that occur during natural cued language production. One advantage of this sentence recitation task is that it allows us to identify and report linguistic phenomena from several different subjects using controlled linguistic contents.

Method

Four deaf native cuers were asked to read and cue 78 common sentences as naturally as possible. Sentences ranged in length from 4 to 13 words (i.e., "*I will be there tonight*") with some utterances containing embedded clauses or more than one sentence (Appendix 4–A). All items were intentionally kept short and easy to remember so subjects can recite them when facing the camera and avoid a "reading along" intonation. All four subjects were born deaf or became deaf before 14 months of age and attended public educational institutions with cued English transliterators. All had been exposed to cued English before the age of 4 by their hearing parents or educators and reported using the system for more than 18 years. All sub-

jects at the time of testing were between the ages of 22 and 24 years.

Because the manual aspects of cueing occurs at such a rapid pace, we used a JVC GR-DVL 9800 digital camcorder to record utterances of the subjects at 240 fields per second, or four times the standard rate used in most digital camcorders. The use of special high-speed video recording gives us clear images for freeze-frame and slow motion analyses of rapid hand movements in cueing and the ability to track the synchrony between the handshape and mouthshape movements. However, we did not analyze or code their mouth movements because: (1) they resemble the natural mouth movements of typical English speakers, and (2) they are difficult to code considering all the possible manifestations of mouthshapes during normal articulation.

Data Analysis

Data analysis by a deaf native cuer of American English consisted of slow-motion, frame-by-frame analysis of videotaped utterances from four deaf native users of Cued Speech with a particular focus on their phonological processes and assimilations. Several interesting phenomena were revealed from the analysis, which we describe below, including: (1) subjects' production errors and corrections, (2) phonological rules preserved from spoken languages, and (3) phonological processes specific to the manual modality.

Subjects' Production Errors and Corrections

Subjects' production errors and use of repairs are a linguistic phenomenon that lends insight into the psycholinguistic implications of cueing. Occasionally, deaf cuers would restart their words when stumbling on a particularly complex phonemic sequence or when they noticed their handshapes or hand placements were not particularly clear. For instance, one subject initially misproduced the manual forms for the word-final cluster /kts/ in *conflicts*. After cueing the entire word, he realized he had omitted the /k/ handshape in the /kts/ cluster. He then repeated the full form of *conflicts* producing each consonant and vowel clearly on the second attempt. Other mispronunciations have occurred in interword transitions often involving function words. Slow motion analysis showed that one cuer did not clearly cue the function word *a* in the phrase "*was a real.*" Instead of changing from handshape 2 (for /z/ in *was*) to a 5-Ø handshape[1] (for *a*), she produced what looked like handshape 4 with no side-down movement (Figure 1–2 depicts the numbered handshapes). As the preceding handshape 2 and the subsequent handshape 3 do not have thumb extension, rapid coarticulation likely did not allow her to fully extend the thumb for the intervening 5-Ø handshape. After realizing her error, she repeated the entire sentence again with clear 5-Ø handshape and side-down movement for the function word *a*. This example suggests that function words such as *a* or *to* are not given much processing attention, a phenomenon that is also common in spoken languages (i.e., *gonna*). Such evidence of self-monitoring and self-corrections indicate that cuers are at least subconsciously aware of synchronizing their hands with mouthshapes while they cue.

Native cuers, however, are not always aware of their production errors, suggesting that synchronizing their cues with their mouth movements is often an automatic process for them. One example is found in the phrase "*of the year.*" Instead of cueing /θə/ for *the*, the cuer produced what appears to be /jə/ or *yuh* with handshape 8 from *year* replacing the /θ/ even when her mouthshapes clearly indicate "*the year.*" This unconscious "slip of the hand" shows how processing and articulation of manual features can occur independently of mouthshapes. Although such misarticulations rarely occur, they provide evidence for dissociation between mouthshape and manual tiers.

Phonological Rules Preserved in Sentence Recitations

The second phenomenon revealed in the analysis of sentence production of native cuers of American English relates to the cued morpho-phonological processes that are derived from spoken languages, including: English past tense and plural allomorphs, the use of liaisons of phonemes from two adjacent words, and elisions in contractions. First, cuers consistently used the correct English past tense and plural allomorphs when reciting sentences. Allomorphs are defined as phonetic variations of the same morpheme (i.e., /s/, /z/, and /əz/ are allomorphs of the plural English morpheme). Of the 35 possible instances of plural or past tense allomorphs in the sentence list, all four subjects recited the correct allomorph 34 or 35 times. This might seem remarkable since allomorphic forms such as the plural /z/ or past tense /t/ are not indicated in the orthographic text. However, most of the word items in the sentence list contained common morphophonemic alternates for plural /s/ and

---

[1][5-Ø] refers to handshape 5 at the side position to indicate no consonant.

past tense /d/. Therefore, it is not presently clear whether their correct use of allomorphs is due to learning rote rehearsal or generative rules. We explore this further in Experiment 2 described below.

A second indicator of spoken phonological processes used during cueing is the use of liaisons where segments from two adjoining words are tied together such as "*all of*" changing into /ɔ lʌv/. Deaf cuers used this liaison as they blend the word-final /l/ into the subsequent vowel /ʌ/ of the next word and delete the initial 5-Ø handshape paired with /ʌ/. Although the outcome of this liaison /ɔ lʌv/ is ambiguous with "*all love*," deaf cuers would rely on the syntactic context of the phrase to decipher this as "*all of*" in the same manner as hearing speakers. For example, without pragmatic or semantic context, *ladder* and *latter* are nearly indistinguishable on the basis of acoustic properties alone because the /t/ in *latter* can receive voicing attributes from the preceding vowel, giving it the appearance of /d/ (Fleetwood & Metzger, 1998). Cued English, on the other hand, makes a clear and visible distinction between /t/ and /d/ in handshapes 5 and 1, respectively.

A third indicator of spoken phonological processes used during cueing is the use of elisions in contractions such as *you've* or *he'll* where a syllable is deleted from the original phrase. Elisions are commonly used in spoken English and their use is preserved in cued English.

The above phonological processes not only illustrate how spoken English rules are preserved in the manual modality through the uses of cues but also supports Fleetwood and Metzger's (1997) claim that cued languages is sufficiently systematic to operate independent of spoken (or auditory) attributes. As a result, one implication of these cross-modality findings is that accurate representation of the phonology of a spoken language in a new medium can be successfully achieved by individuals who are deaf. A concern among parents and educators has been the integrity of the structure of cued English in faithfully conveying the structure of spoken English to deaf and hard-of-hearing children. Yet, at the same time, cued languages are not limited to phonological influences from spoken language structures.

Phonological Processes Specific to the Visuogestural Modality

The third phenomenon observed in native American cuers' sentence recitations is that of phonological assimilations that operate specifically in the visuogestural modality. By definition, phonological assimilations, or coarticulations, are naturally occurring processes in which the features of one segment change to match that of the preceding or subsequent segment. Traditionally, phonological assimilation is often viewed in terms of speech-related changes but there are also examples in signed languages (Battison, 1978). For instance, the citation form for the sign *father* is articulated at the forehead, but in natural discourse, the locus of the sign may shift based on placement of the preceding or subsequent sign.

Given that cuers use both manual and nonmanual (mouthing) articulators to communicate, cued phonological processes are constrained not only by the above-mentioned rule-governed conditions but also by manually defined (cued) conditions and articulatory constraints unique to the visuogestural modality. Thus, instead of using constraints of voicing assimilation and nasalization found in spoken conditions, the cued condition imposes manually defined constraints on cued phonological processes similar to the articulatory processes and constraints in natural sign languages. In this analysis, we describe three examples of phonological assimilations operating under manual constraints: (1) handshape blends, (2) reductions in movement paths, and (3) locative assimilations.

Using frame-by-frame analysis of cuers' sentence production, one example of handshape blend is revealed in the second syllable of the word *towards*. Starting with the /wɜ˞/ syllable, the handshape 6 for /w/ has vowel placement at the mouth and changes into handshape 1 for /d/ followed by handshape 2 for /z/ while moving outward to the side placement. However, the cuer does not show the handshape 1, an extended index finger, because handshape 6's extended thumb and index finger quickly changes into extended index and middle fingers for handshape 2. As the extended thumb in handshape 6 folds down for the targeted handshape 1, the middle finger for handshape 2 had already begun to unfold in anticipation of /z/ phoneme, bypassing handshape 1 for /d/. This occurs so rapidly that handshape 1 with only an extended index finger is obscured or deleted by the anticipation of the subsequent handshape 2. Accompanying mouthshapes provide evidence for the occurrence of phonemes not clearly seen in manual cues. Because the cuer's mouthshape shows the /d/ phoneme, it appears that the anticipatory process in manual articulation merely obscures the presence of the handshape 1 and not the /d/ phoneme.

This handshape blending phenomenon is best described in the context of its surrounding phonetic environment where the phonetic outcome of the targeted handshape is shaped by the preceding and subsequent handshapes. Fleetwood and Metzger (1998) discussed a similar example, called cued allophone, where a /b/ handshape-mouthshape may be inadvertently inserted in the transition between handshape 3 for /s/ and handshape 1 for /p/ in the phrase "*That's petty.*" However, this phenomenon is not an extra phonemic unit inserted between two words but rather, this allophone is a phonetic byproduct of its physical articulators (Fleetwood & Metzger, 1998). Even though their example of an "inserted" allophone differs slightly from an "underspecified" allophone of /d/ in *towards*, both phonetic outcomes are still physical byproducts of their phonetic environment and transitions.

Phonetic changes in handshapes are not unique to cueing, as handshape blends or deletions have been found in ASL fingerspelling of lexical items (Battison, 1978). Although ASL fingerspelling undergoes additional modifications in hand orientation and movement (Battison, 1978), the manual components of cued English and ASL fingerspelling both utilize a set of complex handshapes changing in rapid succession. This similarity between the two systems suggests they share the same articulatory processes and constraints from the visual-gestural modality. Hand configurations in cueing systems and fingerspelling systems are not only governed by the phonotactic rules of their respective languages but also are constrained by manually defined coarticulatory processes comparable to phonetic forms in spoken languages being influenced by the acoustic properties of neighboring phonemic units.

A second example of coarticulatory assimilation lies in transitional changes in the movement parameter. In a sequence of rapidly changing placements, deaf cuers often will reduce or shorten the paths of their hand movements from one placement to another, which facilitates speed and conversational efficiency. One example starts from the throat placement, moves to the side placement, and ends at one of the three placements: the mouth, chin, or back at the throat placement. Although they show citation forms with full movement paths to each placement, slow motion analyses of their sentence utterances also show cuers taking shorter movement paths within (e.g., *continue*) and across word boundaries (e.g., *man who*). For instance, in a throat-to-side-to-chin sequence, movement path from the throat placement barely brushes the side placement on the way to the chin placement and is subtle enough that the medial placement appears to be dropped. However, the handshape designated for the side placement still appears in the sequence but on a direct path upward from the throat placement so that three handshapes appear in rapid sequence during the transition from throat to chin. A similar reduction pattern is observed in other sequences such as a throat-to-side-to-throat sequence where movement to the side placement is brief and visible enough to assume placement of a handshape at the side placement. It is interesting to note that all observed movement reductions appear in strings where the side placement is interspersed between two nonside placements. Thus far, there is no evidence of movement reductions in other sequences involving only contact placements (i.e., throat-mouth-throat or chin-throat-mouth).

A third example of coarticulation specific to the manual modality is called placement assimilation and is observed in the side placement. Although placement assimilations have been known to occur in ASL signs with body contact (e.g., shifting the contact placement of the sign *father*), cued English utilizes this assimilatory phenomenon only when more than two different handshapes are targeted for the side placement. For example, when cueing the word *explain*, the target form requires three different handshapes for phonemes /k s p/ cued at the side placement before moving back to the chin placement. But instead of changing handshapes *at* the side placement for the consonant cluster, cuers often change their handshapes *while* moving to or away from the side placement. One native cuer quickly changed handshape 5 to handshapes 2 and 3 while his hand was moving out to the side placement. Then, as his hand moved back inward to the chin placement for the onset of a diphthong, handshape 3 changed to handshape 1 to handshape 6 before finally contacting the index finger on the chin placement. During full directional movement from the chin to the side and back to the chin, each handshape was not formed at the same physical placement as the preceding handshape because the handshapes change while the hand moves outward and back. Additional examples of placement assimilation have been observed in word-final consonant clusters (i.e., *asked*), word-initial clusters (i.e., *spring*), and across word boundaries (e.g., *is trying*). This phenomenon is a phonetic byproduct of cuers' goal of fluent language production.

Conclusions from Experiment 1

Findings from Experiment 1 indicate that in the quest for rapid and efficient communication, deaf cuers undergo a dichotomous phonological process gleaned from the two modes. On one hand, the physical expression of manual cueing is influenced by the fact that its users are operating with a different set of articulators. Their manual and nonmanual (i.e., mouthing, facial expression) forms are influenced by physical constraints unique to the visuogestural modality as evident in modifications in movement, handshape, and/or placement. These physical changes are not found in spoken languages and yet they serve to facilitate the production of cued languages. On the other hand, the fundamental structure of cued English is designed to represent the phonology of spoken language and all its phonemic units. This aim is achieved as the sentence production data show that certain phonological rules from spoken languages are preserved in their sentence utterances among deaf cuers (i.e., contractions and allomorphs). Even though cued and spoken phonological processes represent the same abstract phonemic values (and corresponding phonological rules), the two different modes have two entirely different sets of allophonic variations as postulated in Fleetwood and Metzger (1998). In other words, cued English does not use or differentiate allophones of spoken English, such as nasalized vowels or the aspirated and plosive /p/. Conversely, spoken English does not exhibit or distinguish visual-manual allophones found in cued English such as placement or handshape assimilation.

The above linguistic phenomena observed in cuers' sentence production clearly demonstrate how any serious inquiry into the linguistic structure of cueing needs to be conducted independent of the acoustic properties of speech or traditional phonological models of spoken and signed languages, consistent with Fleetwood and Metzger's (1998) claims. A phonological model of cueing is described in depth in Koo (2003). In summary, the above exam-

ples illustrate how the Cued Speech system developed by Cornett (1967) is not a fixed or rigid system but a dynamic one whose phonological information is uniquely influenced by its users operating under a set of articulators and production constraints.

Experiment 2: Affixing Allomorphs to Pseudowords

In Experiment 1, deaf subjects consistently produced the correct allomorph in a sentence recitation task. However, many inflected words in the sentence recitation task were real words containing high frequency word-final segments such as /k/; thus, it remains to be seen whether their performance is a result of rote rehearsal or an implicitly learned system. As a system that extracts the phonology of spoken language and presents them in a different modality involving both hand and mouth articulators, cued English allows us a unique opportunity to investigate the underlying representations and phonological rules learned by deaf users of cued English. In this visuogestural medium, deaf cuers are not required to use the vocal tracts when cueing, and as such are not bound to the same physical constraints of spoken languages. With this in mind, the empirical focus of Experiment 2 was to determine whether deaf people with lifelong experience with cued English faithfully adhere to the same allomorphic rules of spoken English or whether they assume a different internalized system. This is an important question because it addresses the psycholinguistic effects of a cross-modal system that claims to represent the phonology of spoken languages. In the absence of auditory input, will deaf people be able to implicitly learn, through use of cues, the allomorphic rules of English? The learnability of this rule is further compounded by the fact that English orthography does not always reveal the phonetic form. If deaf cuers, without the benefit of auditory input and orthographic information, demonstrate the same use and generalization of allomorphs as hearing speakers, then this validates the structural integrity of cued languages as a cross-modal linguistic system.

English is not a language with heavy use of allomorphs but two well-known sets are the plural (and third person singular) affix (-s) and the past tense affixes (-ed) with each containing three allomorphic variations. The phonetic forms of these allomorphs are constrained by the voicing quality from the preceding segment in what is commonly known as the voice assimilation rule. In other words, an unvoiced word-final segment will influence the suffix to adopt the same phonetic property— an unvoiced allomorphic form. However, when affixing an allomorph to a stem whose word-final segment is identical to the affix, a schwa vowel is inserted between the stem and the suffix (i.e., /z ə z/) because two identical segments appearing in sequence cannot be perceptually discriminated (e.g., roses).

Method

For this experiment, we modified a morphological production study by Berko (1958) who prompted children ages 4 to 7 to produce inflectional allomorphs for pseudowords (i.e., "*wug*"). During the Berko (1958) task, a subject is shown a line drawing of an amorphous figure and asked to complete the sentence when

shown more than one of the figures: "*This is a WUG . . . Now there are two _____.*" The appropriate response is "*Wugs*" with the /z/ phoneme (/wʌgz/). Using novel nonwords that conform to English phonotactic rules in a production task allows us to determine whether subjects mastered the English allomorphic rule without the benefit of previous lexical knowledge or rehearsal. In a pilot study of hearing adults, subjects consistently affixed the plural and past tense suffixes to pseudowords in accordance to the voice assimilation rule (Berko, 1958). In this experiment, deaf cuers were asked to produce either a plural or past tense form of the target word. Each inflection type was further divided into real and pseudowords to test their ability to produce the same allomorph in different contexts. Each of the four experimental conditions (real-past, real-plural, pseudo-past, pseudo-plural) contained three instances of ten different word-final segments for a total of 30 items per condition. These word-final consonants (/n, g, b, d, z, t, k, s, ʃ, tʃ/) were chosen because they elicit all three allomorphic forms for both plural and past tense conditions (see Appendix 4–B for a list). Target word-items were three to four segments in length and presented as (C)CVC always ending in a consonant.

All word-final segments were then further divided into high and low frequency segments based on their frequency distribution in their respective grammatical categories (nouns for plurals and verbs for past tense). Frequency rates of word-final segments for verbs and noun word-forms were obtained from the Celex English database (Baayen, Piepenbrock, & Gulikers, 1995). Target items were placed in sentence frames designed to elicit plural or past tense forms from subjects: "*One (C)CVC, two _____*" and "*He had to*

(C)CVC. So yesterday he _____." As many adult subjects in Berko's (1958) experiment produced the irregular form for pseudowords (e.g., *"bang"* (/bæŋ/) or *"bung"* (/bʌŋ/) for *"bing"* (/bɪŋ/), we included a small number of pseudoword items as extra stimuli designed to elicit irregular forms by using sequences similarly cued as irregular real words. For example, the manual cues for *"thoos"* (/θus/) are produced in the exact same manner as for *"goose"* but only the initial mouthshape differs. In order to ensure subjects have complete mastery of irregular words, twelve irregular real words were added to the experimental stimuli, six for plurals (*goose, foot*, etc.) and another six for past tense (*shoot, fight*, etc.). A total of 132 items used in this experiment was then randomized and divided into two test sessions.

To avoid undue influence from orthographic forms, as in the first experiment described above, all stimuli items were cued on digital videotape by a deaf native cuer and presented to subjects in Quick-Time format on a Powerbook G3. Subjects were instructed to view the stimuli on the laptop and at the end of each item, repeat the entire sentence with uninflected forms and correct responses. A Sony Hi-8 video camcorder situated directly in front of them recorded their responses.

Ten deaf native cuers of English participated in this experiment. All subjects became deaf at birth or before the age of 2 years; had been exposed to cueing from their parents before the age of 5 years; attended mainstreamed public schools; and were either in college or had bachelor's degrees at the time of testing. The average age of 10 deaf cuers at the time of testing was 22.5.

Correct responses are based on the spoken language rule (i.e., /z/ for voiced word-final segments). For word-final segments with fricatives identical to the affixes, subjects must produce a schwa vowel in their affixes (i.e., /əd/ or /əz/), otherwise the item is marked as incorrect. In consideration of various regional dialects and differences in parental input, three alternative forms of the schwa vowel are accepted: /ʌ/, /ɪ/, or /ə/. Also, if subjects gave irregular allomorphs in response to pseudowords or misunderstood the target word and inflected a different word, then their responses were set aside from the scoring and not included in the adjusted score. If, however, subjects do not produce the correct irregular form for real words that require them, it was scored as incorrect and noted for error analysis. Two other deaf cuers not involved as subjects scored their responses and a reliability score of .92 was achieved.

Results

A repeated measures analysis of variance was computed with affixes, word-type, and frequency of word-final segments as within-subject factors. With irregular real words removed from the analysis, main effects of affixes ($F(1, 8) = 21.30$, $p = .002$) and word-type ($F(1, 8) = 21.03$, $p = .002$) were significant. Subjects performed better in plural affixation than past-tense and did better with real words than with pseudowords. Subject errors in the plural condition displayed no particular pattern or trend (see Appendix 4–C for a list). Interaction between affixation and word-type was not significant ($F(1, 8) = .002$, $p = .964$). Table 4–1 shows the adjusted scores from each of the four conditions with real irregular words removed. To the right of adjusted scores for each condition are scores from high and low frequency word-final segments. Main effect for frequency of word-final segments did not approach significance ($F(1, 8) = 1.18, p = .310$).

Since standard deviations were significantly large in both past-tense conditions (.18 and .16), post hoc analysis revealed 10 subjects can be divided into two more homogeneous groups. This group demarcation comes from their performance in the past-tense condition where six subjects scoring higher than .80 in real words are assigned to Group A. Four subjects with real-past tense performance below

.80 are placed in Group B. Figure 4–1 illustrates the difference between Group A and B in past-tense performance but little difference in the plural condition.

Between-subject analysis showed significant group differences ($F(1, 8) = 22.67$, $p = .001$) in the past tense condition but not in the plural condition. Six cuers in Group A indicated mastery of all three past-tense allomorphic forms with average past-tense scores of .92 and .81 in real and pseudowords, respectively—performances that are comparable to the scores of all subjects in the plural condition. The

Table 4–1. Adjusted Scores in Plural and Past Tense Conditions With Scores From High and Low Frequency Word-Final Segments

		Plurals (SD)		Past Tense (SD)	
Real Words	Hi	.94 (.06)	.94	.81 (.18)	.77
	Lo		.86		.74
Pseudowords	Hi	.86 (.06)	.79	.70 (.16)	.68
	Lo		.82		.65

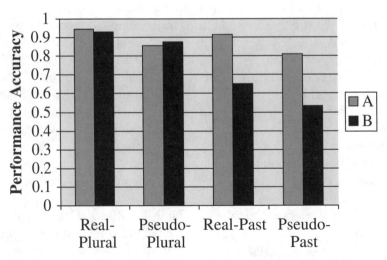

Figure 4–1. Group performance in plural and past tense conditions for real words and pseudowords.

four cuers in Group B averaged .65 for real words and .53 for pseudowords in the past tense condition. After excluding Group B cuers from the data, Group A cuers showed significantly better performance in real words over pseudowords ($F(1, 5) = 307.64$, $p < .05$) but no significant difference between plural and past-tense conditions ($F(1, 5) = 0.895$, $p = .338$). Moreover, Group A cuers still show no frequency effects from word-final segments ($F(1,5) = 1.51$), $p = .273$).

In addition to the difference in performance scores, the type of errors that cuers in Groups A and B make serves as additional motivation for splitting the group into two. Cuers in Group A produced few, seemingly random errors in real and pseudowords whereas Group B cuers showed a strong predisposition toward a particular allomorph (see Appendix 4–D for an overview of errors). For instance, subject 1 did not show a particular bias in his errors incorrectly using /d/ allomorph in 9 of his 16 errors and /t/ allomorph 4 times. The error rate in Group A is relatively small (an average of 7.8%) compared to Group B which not only show higher error rates but often biases toward a particular past-tense form, the /d/ allomorph. For instance, three Group B cuers often affixed the /d/ allomorph to real and pseudowords that required the /t/ allomorph using it in more than 80% of word items. One cuer (subject 7) never used the /t/ allomorph with target words requiring the /t/ form even in real words which suggests she did not have the /t/ allomorph as her past tense form. Although all four cuers in Group B demonstrated the ability to use / d/ forms in appropriate word-final situations, they still made enough overall affixation errors in this and other word-final contexts to justify the demarcation.

Discussion

Overall results in the plural condition indicate that cuers' highest scores were during real words (.94) with 4 out of 10 subjects showing perfect scores. But a substantial drop occurred when cuers affixed plural forms to pseudowords (.86 for pseudoplurals). Even after excluding no-change forms or responses that undergo irregular vowel-changes (i.e., *"plood"* (/plud/) to *"plod"* (/plad/), this decrease in performance reflected affixations that do not follow the constraints of spoken language such as /jɪkəz/ (see Appendix 4–D for a list of plural error responses). Yet, many of these same subjects have used the appropriate rule-oriented allomorphic form with real words (i.e., *"decks"* (/dɛks/). Closer analysis indicated that all subjects employ three phonetic variations of the plural form in real and pseudowords. So what causes a cuer to produce plural allomorphs in pseudowords that do not conform to spoken language constraints? Although most cuers do not show specific error patterns, certain subjects may have a predisposition toward a particular phoneme. For instance, one subject has a tendency to favor the /əz/ allomorph in pseudowords using it in all six of his incorrect responses in the pseudo-plural condition. Despite few idiosyncratic tendencies in the pseudoword condition, all 10 deaf cuers exhibit fairly consistent and rule-oriented use of the three allomorphic forms in all plural conditions.

Overall performance in the past-tense condition was significantly less than the plural condition at .81 for real words and .70 for pseudowords. However, closer examination of subject scores from post-hoc analyses reveal two different types of cuers regarding how they affix past tense forms to word-stems. Table 4–2 shows the

Table 4–2. Individual Subjects' Performance in Past Tense Conditions

	Subject	Real-Past	Pseudo-Past
Group A	1	.81	.67
	2	.89	.79
	3	.89	.76
	4	.94	.86
	5	.97	.83
	6	1.00	.96
	Total	.92	.81
Group B	7	.65	.54
	8	.66	.50
	9	.65	.59
	10	.67	.50
	Total	.65	.53

same grouping of 10 individual subjects into Groups A and B and their past-tense performances.

What is particularly striking about Group B is its frequent use of the /d/ allomorph in *real* words that require the /t/ allomorph. One motivation behind their heavy use of /d/ form may be attributed to the cued input they receive from their parents or other language sources. It is possible that their parents or cueing models did not cue the /t/ form to them, and consequently they were not aware of this form since they do not have the auditory ability to discriminate between /d/ and /t/. A second possibility may be due to the fact that the /d/ allomorph is more commonly used as a past tense form since voiced word-final consonants are high in frequency among verb classes (Baayen et al., 1995) which in turn is further com-

pounded by word-final vowels. As a result, they may have over-estimated the distribution of /d/ to all word-stems even though they are aware of /t/ allomorphs. Another explanation may be attributed to the fact that English has more irregular past-tense words than plural irregulars and this may have an adverse effect on the subjects' ability to confidently generate regular past-tense forms for pseudowords. A fourth possibility may come from the writing system where the "ed" form influences subjects to use the /d/ form. But this orthographic account will have to explain how subjects know when to use the /əd/ form versus the /d/ form.

Although it is possible that cuers in Group B do use the /t/ allomorph in other word-final contexts not included in the stimuli (e.g., /p/), the design of this experiment and the extremely small subject population do not allow ample opportunities to explore a variety of different word-final contexts in depth. Regardless of whether Group B cuers know the /t/ form or not, it is difficult at this point to draw any firm conclusions about their knowledge of past-tense allomorphs without testing their parents, transliterators, or other cueing models. In the future, a morphological judgment test can confirm whether Group B cuers know about the use of /t/ allomorphs in appropriate word-final contexts.

Nonetheless, one of the central aims of this experiment was to see how well deaf subjects affix morphophonological forms in novel situations. Their performance in the pseudoword condition will help identify which of the three possible phonological strategies they use to affix English allomorphs. First, the speech articulatory hypothesis, which predicts deaf cuers will use the same voicing constraint as hearing speakers, is rejected due to the fact that deaf subjects' responses did not conform to the voicing assimilation rule of spoken languages. They made affixations that were in violation of the voicing assimilation rule. Second, the rote rehearsal hypothesis where subjects learn English word affixation through repeated exposure is not well-supported based on the performance of Group A cuers in plural and past tense pseudowords. They could not have memorized the correct allomorph pairing for pseudowords they have never encountered before.

This leaves a third hypothesis—an internalized mechanism where subjects implicitly learned the allomorphic rule and were able to generalize it to novel situations. One example of this hypothesis is the use of frequency rates for word-final segments with high-frequency word-final segments predicting more successful pairings in pseudoword condition than low-frequency segments. However, as the above results show, subjects showed no word-final frequency effect in real or pseudowords. Even when removing Group B cuers from the analysis, the frequency of word-final segments had no significant impact on deaf cuers' ability to attach appropriate allomorphs. Nonetheless, the above-chance performance of Group A cuers in affixing plurals and past-tense forms to pseudowords supports the internalized hypothesis. Even though subjects in Group B generally have only two past-tense forms for real and pseudowords, they did not randomly affix these forms to pseudowords, often using the /əd/ form in voiceless word-final contexts and /d/ in other contexts. So Group B cuers, similar to those in Group A, may be using an internalized mechanism, albeit incorrectly, to affix /əd/ forms in certain word-final contexts and overgeneralize the /d/ allomorph.

Finally, the performance of Group B cuers in plural pseudowords (.81) is comparable to Group A cuers, which lends further support to the internal mechanism hypothesis as a general learning strategy. In terms of Andersen's (1983) nativization model, this internal mechanism would be the driving force behind the nativization-denativization process. Because deaf cuers in Group A demonstrated comparable performance in past and plural pseudowords to hearing speakers, they provide supporting evidence for the nativization-denativization process. Ultimately, this internalized mechanism would have to be sufficiently well-learned through exposure to the model language to be able to account for deaf cuers' ability to affix allomorphs to novel situations in a fairly systematic and rule-consistent fashion.

Irregular Words

Recall that 12 real irregular words were added to the stimuli to determine whether subjects had knowledge of lexicalized irregular forms. As a whole, 10 subjects scored .91 on irregular words, with six subjects showing no errors. The four remaining cuers who gave incorrect regular forms for real irregular words (i.e., "*shooted*" (/ʃutəd/) were equally distributed in Groups A and B. Two cuers made one error and the other two each reported three errors. Table 4–3 lists all the errors subjects made for real irregular words.

Two subjects responded with "*lifes*" (/laɪfs/) as a plural form of *life* and were scored as incorrect because the /z/ allomorph was not used. The other error responses they gave generally followed the spoken language rule. For instance, they inserted a schwa vowel when the word-final segment was identical to the allomorphic form, such as "*gooses*" (/gusəz/) or "*shooted*" (/ʃutəd/). One explanation for their irregular word errors is that subjects were persevering in their task to affix a past tense or plural form to the word-stem and had forgotten that an irregular form exists. Support for this view comes from false starts by other subjects who initially affixed a regular form, but immediately changed their responses to the correct irregular form when they realized a lexicalized word exists.

Several subjects also gave irregular forms to pseudowords. A list of their irregular word responses is shown in Table 4–4 and in Appendixes 4–C and 4–D. Of the 10 subjects, only three subjects (1, 5, and 10) did not give any irregular pseudoforms in the plural and past-tense conditions. The most frequent form of irregular word produced for pseudowords is a vowel change—subjects changed the word-medial vowel in 23 out of the 26 irregular pseudowords they produced. Many vowel changes for plurals are characterized as changing from /u/ or /ɪ/ to /i/ as in "*voob*" (/vub/) to "*veeb*" (/vib/) or "*fleece*" (/flis/) to "*fleeces*" (/flisɪz/). For past tense vowel changes, the most common vowel change is /u/ to /a/, such as "*plood*" (/plud/) to "*plod*" (/plad/) or /ɪ/ to /æ/ such as "*drig*" (/drɪg/) to "drag" (/dræg/). Their pseudoword responses were clearly generalized from vowel changes found in real irregular words. Another type of irregularity in pseudowords occurs when subjects give no-change forms, which are the same pseudoform as the target word (i.e., "*woog*" (/wʊg/) to "*woog*" (/wʊg/). But same-form responses only occurred seven times or in 1.8% of all possible pseudoword responses compared to 4.3% for irregular form responses.

Included in the stimuli were two pseudowords: "*thoos*" (/θus/) and "*woot*" (/wut/) whose cued forms are identical to real irregular words (*goose* and *shoot*), in order to determine whether the similarities in physical forms will elicit irregular pseudoforms. Three subjects did produce the irregular form for "*thoos*" (/θus/) as "*theese*" (/θis/) similar to *goose* and another two gave a no-change form in which they answered with "*thoos*" (/θus/). In addi-

Table 4–3. Subjects' Errors With Real Irregular Words

Plurals	Past Tense
Gooses	Shootud
Livs (2×)	Bleded
Teeths, Toothz	
Mousuz	

Table 4–4. Irregular Word Responses From the Pseudoword Condition

| Plurals | | Past Tense | |
Stimuli	Responses	Stimuli	Responses
Voob	Veeb (2×)	Woot	Shot (3×)
Thoos	Thees (3×)	Drig	Drag (2×)
Flis	Flisn Fleesez	Plood	Plod
Pooz	Peez (2×) Poo	Vesh	Vawd
Nish	Neesh	Frood	Freed
Prib	Preeb	Flot	Flit
Woog	Leeths	Nade	Nid
Stig	Stag		

tion, three subjects gave an irregular real word, *shot*, for "*woot*" (/wut/) as they seemed to misunderstand the target word as being *shoot*. In short, subjects produced irregular pseudowords in isolated incidents with no particular pattern in their selection of irregular responses.

Summary of Experiment 2

The first aim of Experiment 2 was to see how well deaf cuers attach allomorphs to novel situations since it has been shown that they do well with real words. Although subjects as a whole performed well in the plural condition, two groups of cuers were identified on the basis of their performance in the past-tense condition. One group of six cuers demonstrated mastery of both past and plural allomorphic rules even in novel pseudowords. The other group of four subjects generally employed only two past-tense forms—/d/ and /əd/ —in which they showed either inconsis-

tent use or overgeneralization of a single allomorph.

The second aim of Experiment 2 was to determine the processing strategy deaf cuers utilize to make stem-affix pairings. The use of pseudowords in this experiment was designed to determine whether subjects memorized the real words as inflected wholes or used another processing strategy capable of generating the same allomorphs used in spoken language. The results of Experiment 2 refute the rote learning and speech articulatory hypotheses as subjects showed the ability to attach correct and incorrect allomorphs to pseudowords they had never encountered before. The performance from six Group A cuers in past-tense and plural pseudoword conditions and four Group B cuers in plural pseudowords indicate they are able to affix the correct allomorphic form to the appropriate word-final contexts and provide compelling support for a commonly learned mechanism that they used to generalize a rule to novel situations.

Conclusion and Future Directions

This chapter summarizes the findings from two empirical studies of deaf adult users of cued English. Using a sentence recitation task, the first experiment illustrates how linguistic rules from spoken systems and articulatory constraints from manual systems differentially influence the use of cues. As a system designed to manually represent the phonology of spoken language, the evidence from deaf cuers' sentence production data shows highly consistent conformity to the phonotactic rules of English. Yet, as a manual system operating in the visuo-gestural medium, certain phonological processes unique to the visuogestural modality were observed in their sentence utterances. During natural production of sentences, deaf cuers revealed many examples of phonological assimilations previously seen in sign languages such as handshape blends, movement reductions, and placement assimilations. Because cuers operate under this unique phonological dichotomy, a theoretical framework of cue phonology is needed—one that accounts for both their phonological representations and the physical outcome of their phonological processes (Koo, 2003).

Whereas Experiment 1 describes the linguistic behavior of native users of cued English while reciting sentences, Experiment 2 allows us to determine how well deaf cuers internalize English allomorphic rules using an experimental paradigm that elicits the use of plural and past tense forms in novel situations. Results from the plural condition indicate that subjects were able to internalize and generalize the allomorphic rule to pseudowords in a highly consistent fashion despite the fact that this rule typically is neither explicitly taught nor available in the orthography to readers. However, subject performance in the past-tense condition revealed mixed results with consistent and correct use of allomorphic affixations in six subjects and incorrect overgeneralizations in four subjects. In any case, their pesudoword performance shows that cuers cannot rely on rote memory to affix morphemes to novel words nor are they bound to spoken articulatory constraints because they made stem-affix pairings to pseudowords that violate the speech articulatory hypothesis. Instead, the evidence supports an internalized mechanism that cuers use to affix morphemes to novel pseudowords in a highly systematic manner. The six cuers from Group A clearly demonstrated a strong nativization-denativization process in which they adjusted their internal linguistic hypothesis about allomorphs to match that of the English model. They were able to generalize their internal rule to novel situations as demonstrated in the plural and past-tense conditions in Experiment 2. Although the four cuers from Group B went through the same process for plurals, their poor performance in the past-tense pseudoword condition suggests that they did not adjust their internal hypothesis or undergo denativization process vis-à-vis past-tense allomorphs. Without knowing the quality of Group B's cued input from their language models, we cannot draw any conclusions as to whether Group B persisted in using their own linguistic hypotheses in the face of correct or incorrect language modeling. Because deaf cuers do not have auditory access to the spoken language, incorrect or inconsistent cued input will invariably lead the cuer to make incorrect inferences about phonological rules. For instance, Krause (2006) noted that the accuracy of cued words conveyed by cued English transliterators who facilitate communication between deaf and hearing individuals is "substantially less" than 100% and deteriorates as speaking rate increases. Nonetheless, Group B's past-tense performance underscores Andersen's (1983) model as an explanation for the language learner's adaptation the target language by means of nativization but failed to reach denativization.

Future studies will need to look at parental language models, educators, and/or transliterators to determine whether they accurately conveyed the morphophonemic information in their cueing. Moreover, forced-choice recognition tests of past-tense and plural allomorphs can verify whether Group B cuers can correctly distinguish between allomorphic variations but simply do not produce it in a manner consistent with the spoken English rule. Future studies can also explore whether deaf cuers use different allomorphic variations of function words such as *a* in the same manner as hearing speakers. In any case, the findings from this study have not only important educational and psycholinguistic implications for the future of deaf education but theoretical significance in the fields of language acquisition, cross-modal linguistic systems, and general linguistic theory.

References

Alegría, J., Lechat, J., & Leybaert, J. (1988). Role of Cued Speech in the identification of words by the deaf child. *Glossa*, 9, 36–44.

Andersen, R. (1983). *Pidginization and creolization as language acquisition*. Rowley, MA: Newbury House.

Baayen, R., Piepenbrock, R., & Gulikers, L. (1995). The CELEX lexical database (CD-ROM), LDC, University of Pennsylvania, Philadelphia, PA.

Battison, R. (1978). *Lexical borrowing in American Sign Language*. Silver Spring, MD: Linstock Press.

Berko, J. (1958). The child's learning of English morphology. *Word*, 14, 150–177.

Cornett, R. O. (1967). Cued Speech. *American Annals of the Deaf*, 112, 3–13.

Cornett, R. O. (1973). Comments on the Nash case Study. *Sign Language Studies*, 3.

Cornett, R. O., & Daisey, M. (1992). *The Cued Speech resource book for parents of deaf children*. Raleigh, NC: National Cued Speech Association.

Fleetwood, E., & Metzger, M. (1997). *Does Cued Speech entail speech? A comparison of cued and spoken information in terms of distinctive features*. Unpublished manuscript. Washington, DC: Gallaudet University.

Fleetwood, E., & Metzger, M. (1998). *Cued language structure*. Silver Spring, MD: Calliope Press.

Gee, J., & Goodhart, W. (1985). Nativization, linguistic theory, and deaf language acquisition. *Sign Language Studies*, 49, 291–342.

Gee, J., & Mounty, J. (1990). Nativization, variability and style shifting in the sign language development of deaf children of hearing parents. In S. Fischer & P. Siple (Eds.), *Theoretical issues in sign language research Volume 2: Psychology* (pp. 65–84). Chicago, IL: University of Chicago Press.

Kipila, B. (1985). Analysis of an oral language sample from a prelingually deaf child's Cued Speech: A case study. *Cued Speech Annual*, 1, 46–59.

Koo, D. (2003). *On the nature of phonological representations and processing strategies in deaf cuers of English*. Unpublished doctoral dissertation, University of Rochester, Rochester, NY.

Krause, J. (2006). The effect of speaking rate and experience on transliterator accuracy. Paper presented at *Cued Speech 40th Anniversary Convention-Celebrating Language, Literacy and Diversity*, July 22, 2006, Towson, MD.

Leybaert, J., Alegría, J., Hage, C., & Charlier, B. (1998). The effect of exposure to phonetically augmented lipspeech in the prelingual deaf. In R. Campbell, B. Dodd, & D. Burnham (Eds.), *Hearing by eye (Vol. II): Advances in the psychology of speechreading and auditory-visual speech* (pp. 283–301). Hove, UK: Psychology Press.

McGurk, H., & MacDonald, J. (1976). Hearing lips and seeing voices, *Nature, 264* (5588), 746–748.

Metzger, M. (1994a). *First language acquisition in deaf children of hearing parents: Cued English input.* Unpublished manuscript, Georgetown University, Washington, DC.

Metzger, M. (1994b). *Involvement strategies in cued English discourse: Soundless expressive phonology.* Unpublished manuscript, Georgetown University, Washington, DC.

Mohay, H. (1983). The effects of Cued Speech on the language development of three deaf children. *Sign Language Studies, 38,* 25–49.

Nash, J. (1973). Cues or signs: A case study in language acquisition. *Sign Language Studies, 3,* 80–91.

Nelson, K., Loncke, F., & Camarata, S. (1993). Implications of research on deaf and hearing children's language learning. In M. Marschark & D. Clark (Eds.), *Psychological perspectives on deafness* (pp. 123–151). Hillsdale, NJ: Lawrence Erlbaum Associates.

Nicholls, G., & Ling, D. (1982). Cued Speech and the reception of spoken language. *Journal of Speech and Hearing Research, 25,* 262–269.

Appendix 4–A

SENTENCE LIST

1. He was going to talk about his love life.

2. Where are my sunglasses? I thought I left them on the table?

3. Who came in first?

4. Regardless of the outcome, we will still fight on.

5. When the team came in, everyone cheered loudly.

6. I think it is Mr. and Mrs. Smith.

7. The tall, lanky, blond gentleman looks like my dad.

8. He thinks this whole scam stinks.

9. Explain the mess in the kitchen.

10. The young, red-haired woman felt the system was necessary.

11. The North and South had many conflicts before the war.

12. Most of her education was in English.

13. Chicken soup is good for your body.

14. You should try to get more interest on your money.

15. Is it far enough for you?

16. The cafe on Sixth Street looks really good to me.

17. Should we go get more books from the library?

18. She saw his face. But now, she doesn't remember it.

19. This house has historical significance.

20. Are they going to expand the street?

21. Which way did they run? I didn't see them.

22. We came. We saw. We conquered.

23. We live out in the country. We like the peace and quiet there.

24. They went from Washington to New York by air.

25. Strolling down the street, Martha felt something was amiss.

26. We will have to make a major change in the program.

27. John who was robbed is still in a coma.

28. Didn't you see the Super Bowl last year?

29. Columbus was an explorer. And so was Balboa.

30. She thinks it is worth a million dollars.

31. We will be in Washington for six weeks.

32. Mike, our football expert, is not going to the game.

33. If you can't stand the heat, get out of the kitchen.

34. But, he said all of this goes to the Red Cross.

35. She said, "Look, pal. I'm not going to jump into that!"

36. The race starts after the gun goes off.

37. Did you see my new pants?

38. Can you ask the men to raise the bridge?

39. And this is what he said, "I think, therefore I am."

40. The general gave his men the order to attack.

41. He said he was gonna be here tonight.

42. Turn right and go towards town. Then, make a left on Main Street.

43. He said he will give it to you tomorrow.

44. Betty didn't like small nosy children.

45. Mike asked her, "Is it free?"

46. Hollywood, full of glamour, is just like an ordinary town.

47. I feel that the law is above such an action.

48. Are you going to change the will?

49. What year were you born?

50. Go down this road, take a left, and then another left at the intersection.

51. When are you going to finish the painting?

52. They gave Joe, the Rookie of the Year, a ten million dollar contract.

53. You've got to see this movie. It is really good.

54. After dinner, we will retire to the den.

55. Bill earns about 40,000 dollars a year.

56. You've got to keep the can full.

57. Before the war, there were dissenting factions.

58. The man who won the race continues to donate money to our cause.

59. If no one registers, then class will be cancelled.

60. I have a present for you. Go ahead and open it.

61. It was a real pleasure having you here with us.

62. We can have a party at the new community center.

63. Do you know if they found a reason?

64. I could not handle the pressure. The pressure was too much for me.

65. Doctors are not always good listeners.

66. At the meeting, we decided to approve the caucus.

67. She didn't like the British visitors. They were drunk and disrespectful.

68. I saw my old car. One of its doors is broken.

69. I have the money with me. Where should I put it?

70. When are you going to get it?

71. You should ask your father about this issue.

72. We got to the stadium two hours early.

73. Jeff, the foreman, came in to make sure everything was in order.

74. I don't know the face but I sure know the voice.

75. They will move into the old brick house next week.

76. Come in. The swimming pool is warm.

77. Did I break any rules?

78. Have I gotten any money lately?

Appendix 4–B

STIMULI LIST FOR EXPERIMENT 2

Plurals	Frequency	WF Cons	Real Words			Pseudowords		
Voiced-/z/	high	n	fin	pen	brain	frun	doon	plin
	high	d	tide	dad	mood	geed	lud	frood
	low	b	tribe	bib	lab	prib	leeb	voob
	low	g	rug	dog	flag	stig	fug	woog
Unvoiced-/s/	high	t	pet	lot	kite	noot	freet	trit
	high	k	book	deck	leak	veek	jik	smook
Identical-/əz/	low	z	prize	maze	dose	pooz	griz	paze
	high	s	glass	kiss	purse	fes	*thoos	flis
	low	sh	dish	lash	wish	nish	besh	loosh
	low	ch	beach	match	coach	weech	slech	spoch

Past Tense	Frequency	WF Cons	Real Words			Pseudowords		
Voiced-/d/	high	n	fan	plan	train	gan	poon	feen
	high	z	gaze	seize	pose	fize	briz	lerz
	low	b	rob	nab	bribe	reeb	spab	klib
	low	g	wag	beg	brag	pleg	drig	shoog
Unvoiced-/t/	high	s	miss	guess	pass	wis	fras	nis
	high	k	pick	lock	bake	pake	verk	gak
	low	ch	ditch	fetch	punch	heach	wech	klich
	low	sh	fish	rush	wash	doosh	vesh	noosh
Identical-/əd/	high	t	loot	fit	net	*woot	lurt	flot
	high	d	need	pad	kid	merd	nade	plood

Real Irregular Words								
Plural			foot	goose	mouse	life	man	tooth
Past Tense			swim	fight	read	shoot	bite	bleed

* = Planted irregular pseudoword.

Appendix 4–C

SUBJECT ERROR RESPONSES FOR PLURAL CONDITION

Sub ID	Real /s/ (n = 6)	Real /z/ (n = 12)	Real /ez/ (n = 12)	Pseudo /s/ (n = 6)	Pseudo /z/ (n = 12)	Pseudo /ez/ (n = 12)	Subject Error Biases
1			/es/ (3)	/ez/ (3)	/ez/ (3)		/ez-es/ (9 out of 9)
2				/ez/ (1) /z/ (1)		/z/ (2) Irreg (1)	
3				/uz/ (1)	/z/ (4) /s/ (1) Irreg (1)	/z/ (4 out of 7)	/z/ (4 out of 7)
4	/ziz/ (1)	/s/ (4)			/s/ (6) SF (1)	Irreg (1)	/s/ (10 out of 13)
5					/ez/ (1)	SF (2)	
6	/iz/ (1)	/s/ (1)		/eez/ (1)	Irreg (2) /iz/ (1)	Irreg (1) SF (1)	
7				/ez/ (2) /sz/ (1)	/ez/ (4) /s/ (1)	SF (1)	/ez/ (6 out of 9)
8	/iz/ (1)		/z/ (1)		Irreg (1)	Irreg (2) /z/ (1)	
9	/uz/ (1)		/z/ (2)		Irreg (2)	Irreg (3) /is/ (1)	
10			/s/ (1)	/uz/ (1) /gz/ (1)*	/__z/ (1)**	SF (2) /z/ (1)	

SF = same form response; Irreg = irregular pseudoword response. See Table 4–4 for actual form.

*Subject misunderstood /k/ for /g/ but gave the appropriate /z/ form.

**Subject did not produce the word-final /b/ but gave the correct /z/ form.

Appendix 4–D

SUBJECT ERROR RESPONSES FOR PAST-TENSE CONDITION

Sub ID	Real /t/ (n = 12)	/d/ (n = 12)	/ed/ (n = 6)	Pseudo /t/ (n = 12)	/d/ (n = 12)	/ed/ (n = 6)	Subject Error Biases
1	/d/ (4)	/t/ (2)		/d/ (5) /dt/ (1) /ed/ (1)	/t/ (2) /ed/ (1)		/d/ (9 out of 16)
2		/t/ (4) MW (1)			/t/ (2) /ed/ (2) Irreg (1)	/d/ (2)	/t/ (6 out of 12)
3	/d/ (2)	/t/ (2)		/d/ (6)		/d/ (1) Irreg (1)	/d/ (9 out of 13)
4		/t/ (1)	MW (1)	/d/ (1) /id/ (1)	/t/ (1) Irreg (1)	SF (1)	
5	/d/ (1)			/d/ (2)	/t/ (2) /ed/ (1)		
6					/t/ (1)	Irreg (2)	
7	/d/ (12)		MW (2)	/d/ (10) /zd/ (2)		/d/ (1) Irreg (1) SF (1)	/d/ (23 out of 29)
8	/d/ (11)		/d/ (1) MW (1)	/d/ (7) /dt/ (4)	/t/ (1) /dt/ (1)	/d/ (1)	/d/ (20 out of 27)
9	/d/ (10)	MW (1)	/id/ (1) MW (1)	/d/ (11) Irreg (1)		Irreg (2)	/d/ (21 out of 27)
10	/d/ (9)	/t/ (1)	/d/ (2)	/d/ (7), /zd/ (3) /id/ (1) SF (1)	/t/ (1)	/d/ (1) /t/ (1) SF (1)	/d/ (19 out of 28)

SF = same form response; Irreg = irregular pseudoword response. See Table 4–4 for actual form.

MW = misunderstood word: subjects misunderstood the real word and gave an irregular form (i.e., *loot* as *shoot* and responded with *shot*).

Section II

CUED SPEECH FOR PHONOLOGICAL PERCEPTION

Chapter 5

AUDIOVISUAL PHONOLOGY: LIPREADING AND CUED LIPREADING

Jesus Alegria

Introduction

Cued Speech, a system of manual gestures conceived by Orin Cornett (1967), accompanies speech production in real time. The system was designed to provide deaf children an unambiguous and complete phonological message based exclusively on visual information. The delivery of accurate information regarding phonological contrasts via a purely visual input was designed to produce equivalent abstract (phonemic) speech representations in the perceiver's mind. Cornett hypothesized that if phonemic representations could be elaborated on the basis of a visual well-specified input, then linguistic development, as well as all of the cognitive abilities that depend upon such linguistic abilities, would be equivalent in deaf and hearing children. This theory is discussed quite thoroughly in Chapters 1 to 4 of this book.

Cornett's creation has spurred a vast amount of research from scholars in Belgium, France, Spain, Australia, and the United States, and most of the contributions to this volume examine different aspects of that research. This chapter focuses on research conducted by our team related to Cued Speech processing. The primary questions addressed in the two studies reported in this chapter relate to: (1) how mouth movements and hand cues articulate with one another to produce phonemic information and (2) whether there is a difference in cued language between early Cued Speech users and late Cued Speech users.

As discussed in detail by Shull and Crain in Chapter 2 in this volume, a cue is made of two parameters: a manual parameter (i.e., handshape plus hand placement near the mouth) and a nonmanual parameter (i.e., visual information from lipreading). Handshapes combined with mouth movements provide fully specified, unambiguous information about conso-nants, whereas hand placements do the same for vowel information. In Cornett's system, phonemes that are easily distin-guished by lipreading are coded by the same handshape; for example the conso-nants /p/, /d/, and /ʒ/ are coded with handshape 1. Conversely, phonemes that have similar mouthshapes are coded with different handshapes; for example the bilabials /p/, /b/, and /m/ are coded with handshapes 1, 4, and 5, respectively. Consequently, a bilabial lip posture ac-companied by handshape 1 represents the phoneme /p/ without ambiguity. The same rule governs the coding of vocalic phonemes by using hand locations instead of handshapes.

Information provided by the cues and mouth movements is thus comple-mentary. Each time a speaker pronounces a consonant-vowel (CV) syllable, a spe-cific cue (i.e., a particular handshape at a specific location) is produced simultane-ously. Syllabic structures other than CV (e.g., VC, CCV, CVC) are produced with additional specific cues (this will be exam-ined in further detail later). It is important to emphasize that handshapes and hand placements alone are not interpretable as linguistically relevant features. They must be integrated with the visual information provided by lipreading. It is the integrated signal of labial and manual information that points to a single, unambiguous, phonological percept that deaf children could not have achieved from either source alone. Deaf cuers are afforded a reliable visual language in which the gestures (i.e., the combination of mouth movements and manual cues) are entirely specified, both at the syllabic and at the phonemic levels. Each syllable (and each phoneme) corresponds to one (and only one) combi-nation of labial and manual information, and vice versa, a characteristic that makes Cued Speech, or cueing, entirely functional for speech perception.

We will now discuss three aspects of Cued Speech structure that possibly influ-ence the integration between manual cues and lip movements. First, the arbitrary decision to code the vowels by hand loca-tions and the consonants by handshapes seems ecologically valid; that is, the Cued Speech system accounts for the relative duration of consonants and vowels. Specif-ically, vowels have a relatively longer duration than consonants at the acoustic level, which corresponds to the relatively longer time required to pass from one hand location to another. In contrast, con-sonants are relatively shorter events than vowels, and it is possible to move rapidly from one handshape to another. This lin-guistic distinction is more obvious for Cued Speech *production*, but it is probably also relevant for cueing perception (i.e., hand location should be better perceived than handshape in conditions where per-ception is rendered difficult).

A second significant aspect of Cued Speech structure relates to the ability of cueing to transmit information regarding a consonant and a vowel in a single spe-cific cue. This allows a rapid rate of infor-mation transmission, largely compatible with temporal constraints of speech per-ception. Actually, the production of cues seems to slow the speech rate by about 30% (i.e., from 6 syllables per second to 4 syllables per second) (Duchnowski, Braida, Lum, Sexton, Krause, & Banthia, 1998; see Chapter 20). A third significant aspect of Cued Speech relates to the importance of nonmanual information from lipreading. Lipreading is the only component shared by both cued language and spoken language. In the absence of hearing, lipreading makes a strong contribution to linguistic representation for deaf individuals, even if it does not permit normal language development. Dodd (1976) has shown that more that 60% of oral production errors in orally educated deaf individuals result from the ambiguities of lipreading, including: stopping (*tip* for *ship*), suppression of final segments (*ma* for *mat*), and suppression of weak syllables (*nana* for *banana*). Similarly, Leybaert and Alegria (1995) have shown that certain spelling errors are also determined by lipreading properties, such as: devoicing (*pichama* for *pijama*), and suppression of final consonants in syllables (*catable* for *cartable*, *ecalier* for *escalier* (see also Leybaert, 1998).

The role of lipreading in speech perception has been increasingly acknowledged, even for hearing individuals, as the following summary of the research will show. Until the mid 1970s, the theoretical role of lipreading was modest. It was recognized that lipreading improves speech understanding in poor hearing conditions (Binnie, Montgomery, & Jackson, 1974; Erber, 1969; Sumby & Pollack, 1954). Lipread information was supposed to be optional; that is, it could be exploited if the subject felt that it could be useful, and ignored otherwise. Data collected from the mid 1970s onward, however, has shown that when the listener sees the speaker's face, he cannot ignore the lipread information. The visual information accompanying speech production inevitably integrates into an audio-visual compound, which is perceived as a speech sound that can differ from the auditory signal. McGurk and McDonald (1976) showed that seeing a face pronouncing the syllable /ga/ together with a simultaneous auditory stimulus

/ba/ produces a combined percept /da/. If auditory and visual stimuli are inverted, that is, when the visual stimulus presents a bilabial feature such as /ba/ or /pa/, this feature is inevitably included in the subject's perception, which sounds like /bga/ or /bda/. These results have been confirmed by other researchers and their implications for speech perception theories elaborated upon (Burnham, 1998; Green, 1998; Liberman & Mattingly, 1985; Massaro 1987; Schwartz, Abry, Boë, Cathiard, 2002; Summerfield, 1987; see Campbell, Dodd, & Burnham, 1998 for an excellent collection of papers concerning this notion). The main point of these studies is that speech processing in hearing persons is not purely auditory but must be considered as an audiovisual phenomenon.

Furthermore, the processing of lipread information by hearing persons can be demonstrated in prelingual infants. Kuhl and Meltzoff (1982) and McKain, Studdert-Kennedy, Spieker, and Stern (1983) found that 4- to 6-month-old infants, presented with two faces, prefer to look at the face executing the articulatory gesture corresponding to the stimulus simultaneously presented through audition. Finally, using the habituation paradigm, Burnham and Dodd (1996) showed that 4- to 6-month-old infants are susceptible to the McGurk effect. It can be speculated, on this basis, that deaf infants probably possess the ability to process lipread information and that cueing (when integrated with lipreading), if presented during infancy, can preserve the value of lipreading as a natural part of the phonetic transmission system. Some aspects of the data discussed in this chapter, especially the effects of exposure to Cued Speech at an early age, can be considered as evidence in favor of this hypothesis.

Research Related to Cued Speech and Speech Perception

Studies aimed at determining the efficiency of Cued Speech in deaf children have convincingly demonstrated its value. Studies conducted in English, French, and Spanish have shown that the addition of cues to lipreading improves speech reception for deaf children (Alegria, Charlier, & Mattys, 1999; Nicholls & Ling, 1982; Périer, Charlier, Hage & Alegria, 1990; Torres, Moreno-Torres, & Santana, 2006). Nicholls and Ling (1982) found that the speech reception scores of profoundly deaf children taught at school with Cued Speech for at least three years increased from about 30% for both syllables and words in the lipreading alone condition to more than 80% when cues were added. Périer et al. (1990) showed that the advantage to sentence comprehension provided by the addition of cues was greater for children whose parents intensively used Cued Speech to communicate with them at home at an early age than for those children who were exposed to Cued Speech later, and only at school (usually beginning around the age of six years). This differential benefit displayed by the early and late Cued Speech users may be explained in two ways: early Cued Speech users might be more familiar with words presented in Cued Speech, and/or they might have a more efficient phonological processor, which depends of the quality of the mental representations of the phonemes. More recently, Alegria et al. (1999) have shown that early Cued Speech users, compared to peers who began cueing later, displayed a greater improvement related to the addition of cues both for word perception and for pseudoword perception. Because pseudowords were unfamiliar for both groups of subjects, these results support the notion that experience with Cued Speech enhances the efficiency of the processing of phonological information in early users.

Studies concerning linguistic abilities of deaf students involving access and manipulation of precise phonological representations like rhyming, memorizing, as well as reading and spelling, have demonstrated the positive effects of Cued Speech (Campbell & Wright, 1988, Dodd, 1987; Harris & Moreno, 2004; Leybaert & Alegria, 2003; see Chapter 11 in this volume). Exceptionally high performance in those tasks has been observed in early cuers (Charlier & Leybaert, 2000; Colin, Magnan, Ecalle, & Leybaert, 2007). These results constitute strong evidence that cued language permits the elaboration of phonemic representations that can support the same functions that spoken language does, especially as regards reading and spelling.

Our Research Related to the Integration of Lip Movements and Hand Cues

Alegria et al. (1999) investigated how lips and hands combine to produce available phonological information for deaf children by examining the conditions where cues and mouth movements *fail* to combine. They speculated that, in order to provide a phonetically unambiguous message, lips and cues necessarily must be integrated; that is, neither element can be taken into account without considering the other. Alegria et al. (1999) looked for instances in which specific features of Cued Speech create phonological interpretations that are absent in spoken language. One of these instances are situations were syllables do not have the canonical CV structure. In this case, cueing adds additional specific cues (i.e., a handshape produced at a location) to transmit all of the phonemic information. For example, a CCV syllable needs to be articulated using two specific cues: the initial consonant employing the corresponding handshape produced at the side placement, and the canonical specific cue for the remaining CV portion of the syllable (see Figure 2–7 in Chapter 2). The side placement corresponds to the vowels /a, o, ə/ in cued French. In this situation, the syllable /bli/ could mistakenly be perceived /ba-li/ or /bo-li/ in French, though not in English (see Chapter 2 for a discussion of differences among cued languages). Alegria et al. (1999) using bisyllabic items containing four phonemes, found significant differences between canonical structures: CV-CV, and noncanonical structures: V-CCV, V-CVC, and VC-CV, the former being correctly perceived as bisyllabic while the other three were sometimes perceived as trisyllabic. This probably results from the fact that, in French, these CV syllables translate into one specific cue (i.e., a handshape produced at a location) whereas the noncanonical syllabic structures include an extra specific cue, which seems to have been interpreted, at least in some occasions, independently from the labial information. It obviously is necessary to examine, in a detailed manner, the temporal organization of lipread syllables and specific cues. In the same vein, examination of the syllabic structure of mental representations of words in native French-language cuers might be useful. It is possible that for these persons monosyllabic

words like "bras" /bra/ (arm) are represented as if they were bisyllabic: /bə-ra/, and bisyllabic words like "cheval" /ʃe-val/ represented as trisyllabic /ʃe -va-le/.

A second instance where misperceptions arise because manual cues are processed independently from mouth movements are phonemic substitution errors which preserve handshape or location. The syllable /pa/ presented via mouth movements plus cues perceived as /da/ or as /ʒa/ is an example of this type of error, probably resulting from a prioritizing of manual Cued Speech information (i.e., "it is handshape 1"), without taking into account nonmanual lipread information (i.e., "it is bilabial").

Our Research Related to the Effects of Early Versus Late Exposure to Cued Speech on Integration of Labial and Manual Information

To better understand the phenomenon of integration of labial and manual information in Cued Speech, Alegria and Lechat (2005) examined phonemic substitution errors of deaf cuers using a design inspired by the McGurk effect. As previously mentioned, in the classic McGurk and McDonald (1976) study, it was observed that the presentation of synchronized, but noncongruent, lipread and auditory information produced a unique percept: a visual /ga/ coupled with an auditory /ba/ produced a perceptual /da/. This was interpreted as showing that the phonemic features brought by each source of information were combined. The Alegria and Lechat experiment exposed deaf participants to a situation where lips and cues are sometimes incongruent: for example, the mouthed syllable /va/ accompanied by handshape 1 /p/, /d/, and /ʒ/. These two sources of information are incongruous in that the handshape permits the disambiguation of the lipread information in the context of three specific labial features: (1) if lips present the "bilabial feature" then "it is /p/" (instead of /b/ or /m/, which are also bilabials); (2) if lips suggest the "alveolar feature" then "it is /d/" (instead of /t/); and (3) if the lips present the "lips protrusion feature" then "it is /d/" (instead of /tʃ/). The mouthshape needed for /va/ is not one of those concerned by handshape 1, so these two pieces of information are incongruous.

The empirical question addressed by Alegria and Lechat (2005) was: what information from lips and/or cues are taken into account by the participant? If both types of information are considered by participants, what sort of compromise in phonological processing will occur? Findings from previous studies (Erber, 1967; Green & Miller, 1985; Summerfield, 1987) suggest that lipreading gives information about *place of articulation* but no information about *voicing* or *nasality*. Auditory information, however, is rather precise concerning voicing and nasality but is less precise concerning the place of articulation. Moreover, the *place of articulation* feature can be more or less salient. The bilabial feature, for example, is the most salient place of articulation, and if it is present in the stimuli, it is always integrated into the percept (a visual /ba/ plus an auditory /ga/ will produce a /bda/ or /bga/ percept). Models of audiovisual speech perception (Green & Miller, 1998; Massaro, 1987; Summerfield, 1987) try to conceptualize the notion of specificity and salience of each source of information. In the Alegria and Lechat (2005) experiment,

it was hypothesized that because phonemes like /r/ and /k/ produce less salient visual features than /v/ and /f/ do, they are more likely to allow cues to determine the perceptual response. Similarly, the vocalic context can modify the salience of consonants. So, the /v/ is probably easier to perceive in a /va/ context than in a /vo/ context. Montgomery, Walden, and Prosek (1987) have shown that the consonantal context affects the lipreading of vowels. Consonants bearing highly visible features, like bilabials and labiodentals, might reduce vowel intelligibility, while vowels with highly visible features tend to decrease the perception of consonants (Owens & Blazek, 1985).

In the Alegria and Lechat (2005) experiment, when manual cues were congruent with mouthshapes, cueing substantially improved performance compared with pure lipreading conditions. These findings confirm results of previous studies (Alegria et al., 1999; Nicholls & Ling, 1982). Interestingly, the positive effects were also greater in children exposed to cueing at home prior to the age of 2 years (the "early group") compared to children exposed later and only at school (the "later group"). These findings support the notion that deaf children do possess a processor responsible for extracting phonological information from lipread input and, when present, from cued language. When manual cues and mouth movements gave incongruent information, the global frequency of errors increased. It is important to specify that errors were evaluated relative to the lipreading condition, that is to say, without cues. This suggests that cues cannot be ignored when they are present, even though they are incongruent with mouth movements. There is no reason to suppose that congruent manual cues contribute to speech perception while incongruent manual cues are ignored. It is reasonable to consider that the mechanisms involved in both cases function automatically.

Alegria and Lechat (2005) were interested in examining the presence of "Cued Speech errors" defined, for example, as erroneously responding /d/ or /ʒ/ for /p/ when the labial /va/ is presented with the incongruent handshape 1 (see Figure 1–2 in Chapter 1). The presence of Cued Speech errors would constitute strong evidence in favor of the notion that manual cues are processed even if they are incongruent with the lipread information. Stated differently, these errors indicate that participants "overread" the phonetic information delivered by the hands. This interpretation is tenable only if the amount of Cued Speech errors is larger when incongruent labial-manual information is presented than when only labial information is presented (lipreading alone condition). The results did show a significant increase of Cued Speech errors when incongruent labial-manual cues were presented, relative to the lipreading alone condition. Importantly, almost all (94%) of the errors on consonants collected in the "early" group were Cued Speech errors (i.e., erroneously responding /d/ or /ʒ/ for /p/ when the labial /va/ is presented with the incongruent handshape 1). The corresponding percentage of errors in the "late" group was only 37%. For vowels, the results were even clearer (100% and 15%, respectively).

The visibility factor (i.e., the salience of phonetic features in lipreading) in the Alegria and Lechat study, played the expected role for the "early" but not in the "late" group. The "early" group experienced more cueing errors for posterior (i.e., less visible) consonants than for anterior (i.e., more visible) consonants (83% and 75%, respectively of the errors observed

were cueing errors). Similarly, when consonants were presented in an unfavorable vocalic context, the proportion of cueing errors was greater than in favorable contexts (i.e., 87% and 70%, respectively). These results indicate that the susceptibility of lipread information to be "invaded" by manual cues depends on the lipread information's salience, at least in the "early" group. The more that mouth movements provide reliable phonological information, the smaller the influence of the manual cues. The contrast observed between "early" and "late" deaf children strongly suggests that the "early" group made a more careful analysis of the information presented by mouth movements than did the "late" group.

A final and important point concerns the choice of response made by the "early" and the "late" groups. For example, when handshape 1 was presented in an incongruent lipread context, the participant could "see" /p/, /d/, or /ʒ/. Regarding consonants, the results show that the participants routinely chose the less marked alternative from the point of view of lipreading (i.e., /d/). Similarly, with handshape 4 (corresponding to /b, n, w/), the most frequent choice was /n/. The speech processing system thus seems to operate on the assumption that "if the target had been /p/ or /ʒ/ this should be seen on the lips. When /p/ or /ʒ/ are not seen on the lips, they could be excluded so the decision then is "it must be /d/." The same processes lead to choosing /n/ from among /b, n, w/, given that /b/ and /w/ present more salient phonetic features of lipreading. A similar mechanism has been proposed to explain some aspects of the classic McGurk effect. For example, an auditory /ba/ combined with a lipread /ga/ never produces the response /ba/. Such a response is incompatible with lipread information which unambiguously shows that the input does not possess the bilabial feature. The response /da/ is a compromise between the two sources of information.

Conclusion

The evidence available from other studies (Alegria et al., 1999; Nicholls & Ling, 1982; Périer et al., 1990; Torres et al., 2006) clearly shows that the manual components (i.e., handshape and hand placement) of Cued Speech combined with lipreading allows deaf children to perceive phonological contrasts. The more specific question addressed in this chapter regards the manner in which lipreading and manual components of Cued Speech combine. Two models are compatible with the data reviewed in this chapter:

1. Both sources of phonological information (i.e., nonmanual information from lipreading and manual information) are hierarchically processed, the former giving the core phonological information, and the latter intervening optionally. That is, cues are taken into account when necessary to resolve lipreading ambiguities. According to this model, the contribution of Cued Speech to speech processing takes place at a later, postperceptual stage.
2. The speech processing device automatically integrates all of the available visually based phonological information, including the manual information and nonmanual information from lipreading. The functioning of this device might be similar to the audiovisual speech processing device postulated in hearing individuals (Green, 1998; Massaro, 1987; Schwartz, Abry, Boe, &

Cathiard, 2002; Summerfield, 1987; Summerfield & McGrath, 1984). Phonemes are defined as abstract units allowing the distinction between different morphemes, so that lipreading with cues may logically elaborate phonemic contrasts. This formulation implies that the phonological processing device can combine exotic signals (e.g., manual cues) with natural phonological information available from lipreading (and residual hearing, if available). Fowler and Deckle (1991) have shown that auditory and labial information perceived by a finger touching the lips combine to produce McGurk-like effects. Additional evidence (Breeuwer & Plomp, 1986; Green & Miller, 1985; Rosen, Fourcin, & Moore, 1981) demonstrating that nonspeech auditory signals also combine with lipreading to produce genuine phonetic percepts is also relevant in this context.

Which model is more representative of the manner in which lipreading and Cued Speech combine to form a single percept? The answer likely lies somewhere between these two models. Regarding the conceptualization of how nonmanual visual information from lipreading combines with manual cues, an important direction for future research should be to better understand the exact nature of this integration, either as a *conscious*, postperceptual mechanism or as an *automatic*, compulsory one. Further, this alternative must be considered in light of the "early exposure" versus "late exposure" contrast, because its resolution could depend on the age of exposure to Cued Speech. The results of Alegria and Lechat (2005) show important differences between the groups, but these differences are all compatible with the notion that the "early" group of children is more efficient exploiting both manual cues and lipreading than the "late" group. The difference might simply be a difference of degree and not of nature. The results reported by Leybaert and D'Hondt (2003) also could be relevant in the present context. They have explored the hemispheric specialization of Cued Speech processing as a function of earliness of exposure to Cued Speech. Their results clearly show that early exposed cuers, but not late cuers, process Cued Speech in the left hemisphere. This might be considered as a difference between these groups of children at a qualitative level, not simply at a quantitative one.

It is important to highlight some aspects of the data examined in this chapter that might have practical consequences for the education of deaf children. The notion that speech is multimodal and that it includes a natural visual dimension (i.e., lipreading) which permits an artificial visual signal (i.e., Cued Speech) to elaborate a phonological signal has important consequences. This means that the manual cues of Cued Speech are not merely an artifact aimed at helping deaf children to distinguish between words, but rather, they become a genuine part of speech processing and speech representation. The conditions necessary for Cued Speech to reach this perceptual and cognitive status are related to the age of exposure to it. The empirical evidence reviewed is not totally conclusive regarding the notion that early exposure is a condition sine qua non for the integration of cues in phonological processing at a perceptual automatic level. As a matter of fact, experimental studies show that deaf children exposed to Cued Speech later in their life also exploit cues to improve perception, although to a lesser extent than children exposed earlier. The present analysis suggests that when the decision to adopt an oral education has been made, intervention should take place as early as possible so that the deaf child can be exposed to a complete and unambiguous phonological model.

References

Alegria, J., Charlier, B., & Mattys, S. (1999). Phonological processing of lipread and Cued-Speech information in the deaf. *European Journal of Cognitive Psychology, 11*, 451–472.

Alegria, J., & Lechat, J. (2005). Phonological processing in deaf children: When lipreading and cues are incongruent. *Journal of Deaf Studies and Deaf Education, 10*, 122–133.

Binnie, C., Montgomery, A., & Jackson, P. (1974). Auditory and visual contributions to the perception of consonants. *Journal of Speech and Hearing Research, 17*, 619–630.

Breeuwer, M., & Plomp, R. (1986). Speechreading supplemented with auditorily presented speech parameters. *Journal of the Acoustical Society of America, 79*, 481–499.

Burnham, D. (1998). Language specificity in the development of auditory-visual speech perception. In R. Campbell, B. Dodd, & D. Burnham (Eds.), *Hearing by eye (Vol II): Advances in the psychology of speechreading and auditory-visual speech* (pp. 27–60). Sussex, UK: Psychology Press.

Burnham, D., & Dodd, B. (1996). Auditory-visual speech perception as a direct process: The McGurk effect in infants and across languages. In D. Stork & M. Hennecke (Eds.), *Speechreading by humans and machines* (pp. 103–114). Berlin: Springer-Verlag.

Campbell, R., Dodd, B., & Burnham, D. (1998). *Hearing by eye (Vol. II.): Advances in the psychology of speechreading and auditory-visual speech.* Sussex, UK: Psychology Press.

Campbell, R., & Wright, H. (1988). Deafness, spelling and rhyme: How spelling supports written word and picture rhyming skills in deaf subjects. *Quarterly Journal of Experimental Psychology, 40A*, 771–788.

Charlier, B., & Leybaert, J. (2000). The rhyming skills of deaf children educated with phonetically augmented speechreading. *Quarterly Journal of Experimental Psychology, 53A*, 349–375.

Colin, S., Magnan, A., Ecalle, J., & Leybaert, J. (2007). A longitudinal study of the development of reading in deaf children: Effect of Cued Speech. *Journal of Child Psychology and Psychiatry, 48*, 139–146.

Cornett, R. O. (1967). Cued Speech. *American Annals of the Deaf, 112*, 3–13.

Dodd, B. (1976). The phonological system of deaf children. *Journal of Speech and Hearing Disorders, 41*, 185–198.

Dodd, B. (1987). Lipreading, phonological coding and deafness. In B. Dodd & R. Campbell (Eds.), *Hearing by eye: The psychology of lipreading* (pp. 177–189). London, UK: Lawrence Erlbaum.

Duchnowski, P., Braida, L., Lum, D., Sexton, M., Krause, J.,& Banthia, J. (1998). Automatic generation of Cued Speech for the deaf: status and outlook. In D. Burnham, J. Roberts-Ribes, & E. Vatikiotis-Bateson (Eds.), *International Conference on Auditory-Visual Speech Processing* (pp. 161–166). Terrigal, Australia, December 4–7, 1998.

Erber, N. (1969). Interaction of audition and vision in the recognition of oral speech stimuli. *Journal of Speech and Hearing Research, 12*, 423–424.

Fowler, C., & Deckle, D. (1991). Listening with eye and hand: Cross-modal contributions to speech perception. *Journal of Experimental Psychology: Human Perception and Performance, 17*, 816–828.

Green, K. (1998). The use of auditory and visual information during phonetic processing: implications for theories of speech perception. In R. Campbell, B. Dodd, & D. Burham (Eds.), *Hearing by eye (Vol II): Advances in the psychology of speechreading and auditory-visual speech* (pp. 3–26). London, UK: Psychology Press.

Green, K., & Miller, J. (1985). On the role of visual rate information in phonetic perception. *Perception and Psychophysics, 38*, 269–276.

Harris, M., & Moreno, C. (2004). Deaf children's use of phonological coding: Evidence from reading, spelling, and working memory. *Journal of Deaf Studies and Deaf Education, 9*, 253–268.

Kuhl, P., & Meltzoff, A. (1982). The bimodal perception of speech in infancy. *Science, 218*, 1138–1141.

Leybaert, J. (1998). Phonological representations in deaf children: The importance of early linguistic experience. *Scandinavian Journal of Psychology, 39*, 169–173.

Leybaert, J., & Alegria, J. (1995). Spelling development in hearing and deaf children: evidence for use of morpho-phonological regularities in French. *Reading and Writing, 7*, 89–109.

Leybaert, J., & Alegria, J. (2003). The role of Cued Speech in language development of deaf children. In M. Marschark & P. Spencer (Eds.), *Handbook of deaf studies, language, and education* (pp. 261–274). New York, NY: Oxford University Press.

Leybaert, J., & D'Hondt, M. (2003). Neurolinguistic development in deaf children: The effect of early language experience. *International Journal of Audiology, 42*(Suppl 1), S34–S40.

Liberman, A., & Mattingly, I. (1985). The motor theory of speech perception revised. *Cognition, 21*, 1–36.

Massaro, D. (1987). Speech perception by ear and by eye. In B. Dodd & R. Campbell (Eds.), *Hearing by eye: The psychology of lipreading*. London, UK: Lawrence Erlbaum.

McGurk, H., & MacDonald, J. (1976). Hearing lips and seeing voices. *Nature, 264*, 746–748.

McKain, K., Studdert-Kennedy, M., Spieker, S., & Stern, D. (1983). Infant intermodal speech perception is a left hemisphere function. *Science, 219*, 1347–1349.

Montgomery, A., Walden, B., & Prosek, R. (1987). Effects of consonantal context on vowel lipreading. *Journal of Speech and Hearing Research, 30*, 50–59.

Nicholls, G., & Ling, D. (1982). Cued speech and the reception of spoken language.

Journal of Speech and Hearing Research, 25, 262–269.

Owens, E., & Blazek, B. (1985). Visemes observed by hearing-impaired and normal-hearing adults viewers. *Journal of Speech and Hearing Research, 28,* 381–393.

Périer, O., Charlier, B., Hage, C., & Alegria, J. (1990). Evaluation of the effects of prolonged Cued Speech practice upon the reception of spoken language. *Cued Speech Journal, 4,* 47–59.

Rosen, S., Fourcin, A., & Moore, B. (1981). Voice pitch as an aid to lip-reading. *Nature, 291,* 150–152.

Schwartz, J., Abry, C., Boë, L., & Cathiard, M. (2002). Phonology in a theory of perception-for-action-control. In J. Durand & B. Laks (Eds), *Phonology: From phonetics to cognition* (pp. 255–280). Oxford, UK: Oxford University Press.

Sumby, W., & Pollack, I. (1954). Visual contributions to speech visibility in noise. *Journal of the Acoustic Society of America, 26,* 212–215.

Summerfield, Q. (1987). Some preliminaries to a comprehensive account of audio-visual speech perception. In B. Dodd & R. Campbell (Eds.), *Hearing by eye: The psychology of lipreading* (pp. 3–51). London, UK: Lawrence Erlbaum Associates.

Summerfield, Q., & McGrath, M. (1984). Detection and resolution of audio-visual incompatibility in the perception of vowels. *Quarterly Journal of Experimental Psychology, 36A,* 51–74.

Torres, S., Moreno-Torres, I., & Santana, R. (2006). Quantitative and qualitative evaluation of linguistic input support to a prelingually deaf child with Cued Speech: A case study. *Journal of Deaf Studies and Deaf Education, 11,* 438–448.

Chapter 6

CUED SPEECH FOR ENHANCING SPEECH PERCEPTION OF INDIVIDUALS WITH COCHLEAR IMPLANTS

Jacqueline Leybaert, Cécile Colin, and Catherine Hage

Introduction

This book documents how deaf children who have been provided with Cued Speech successfully use language representations in major cognitive activities like reading, spelling, remembering, and rhyming without auditory input. The main source of improvement in these cognitive skills is the advantage provided by Cued Speech for speech perception, which leads to the natural acquisition of English and other traditionally spoken languages.

In one of the first studies addressing the issue of spoken language perception, Nicholls and Ling (1982) studied a group of Australian profoundly deaf children educated with Cued Speech at school for at least 3 years. They found that speech reception scores of these children increased from about 30% for both syllables and words in the lipreading condition to more than 80% in the lipreading + cues condition. They emphasized that the children's average scores in the lipreading + cues condition were within the range of normal hearing listeners' reception scores of similar material from audition.

Périer, Charlier, Hage, and Alegria (1988) studied the advantage provided by the addition of cues to French sentence comprehension. They found an increase from 39% correct responses in the lipreading condition to 72% in the lipreading + cues condition for a group of children exposed early to Cued Speech, and from 37 to 53% for those who were exposed to Cued Speech later and only at school, suggesting a variability related to experience in perceiving and discriminating the phonetic structure of Cued Speech.

Now that most children born profoundly deaf are fitted with a cochlear implant during the early language learning years (Spencer & Marschark, 2003), the need for using Cued Speech might be less apparent. Improvement in children's hearing via cochlear implants is impacting strategies of perception of oral language (Geers, 2006). That is, with auditory training, many children with cochlear implants may understand speech sufficiently without having to look at the speaker. However, even for normally hearing people, speech detection and intelligibility are influenced by a speaker's face. From the seminal work of Sumby & Pollak (1954), it is known that visual speech information dramatically enhances the identification of speech when the auditory information is degraded by noise. Auditory and visual modalities are complementary in the transmission of phonetic features. Although *voicing* and *manner of articulation* are quite resistant to noise, *place of articulation* is not. Information about place of articulation, in contrast, is transmitted well via the visual modality (Summerfield, 1987). This multimodal nature of speech reception has been shown through the well-known and commonly cited McGurk effect (McGurk & MacDonald, 1976).

Another compelling reason for considering the multimodal nature of speech reception through a cochlear implant and the benefit of visual integration in speech perception is the fact that the signal delivered by the cochlear implant remains imprecise and incomplete. Recent advances in psychoacoustic research have clarified the role of two types of temporal information in speech perception: (1) frequency information and (2) temporal fine structure.

The auditory system performs a limited-resolution spectral analysis of sounds using an array of overlapping "auditory filters" with center frequencies spanning from 50 to 15,000 Hz. The output of each filter is like a bandpass-filtered version of the sound, which contains two forms of information: fluctuations in the envelope (the relatively slow variations in amplitude over time) and fluctuations in the temporal fine structure (the rapid oscillations with rate close to the center of the frequency of the band). The temporal fine structure is often described as a "carrier," whereas the envelope is described as "an amplitude modulator applied to the carrier." (Lorenzi, Gilbert, Carn, Garnier, & Moore, 2006)

Currently, cochlear implants typically use 16 to 22 electrodes placed along the tonotopic axis of the cochlea, each electrode being designed to provoke a frequency-specific neural activation; however, within each region of stimulated neurons, the temporal fine structure of neural response is quite different from that occurring in a normal cochlea (Shannon, 2007). Modern cochlear implants provide good information about the slow variations in amplitude of the envelope; however, they are poor at transmitting frequency information and information about temporal fine structure (Glasberg & Moore, 1986; Grosgeorges, 2005; Lorenzi et al., 2006).

The lack of temporal fine structure in cochlear implants has consequences on the perception of phonetic features, on degradation of speech perception by noise, and on the perception of musical pitch. At the phonetic level, place of articulation, and voicing are mostly impaired, whereas the transmission of manner is well-preserved. Consequently, individuals with a cochlear implant confound minimal word pairs that differ only by place of articulation, such as *buck/duck* (Giraud, Price, Graham, Truy, & Frackowiak, 2001), which creates confusions in acquisition of meanings by children. Due to the fragility of the transmission of phonetic features, speech perception through a cochlear implant is dramatically impaired in noisy listening environments (Fu & Nogaki, 2004; Lorenzi et al., 2006). Individuals with a cochlear implant also have difficulties in perceiving musical information related to pitch, whereas the information about rhythm is relatively well preserved (Fearn & Wolfe, 2000; Frère & Leybaert, 2007). These problems currently are being addressed by the companies that develop cochlear implant technology, and will certainly be reduced in the future (see for example http://www.phys.unsw.edu.au/jw/Cochlear.html). Until that time, however, these problems might best be addressed via visual support.

Given these limitations of cochlear implants, it is reasonable to believe that speechreading and manual cues of Cued Speech remain of valuable use for speech perception by children with a cochlear implant who are in the process of language development. In the following sections, we will discuss research related to the positive effect of visual speech information on language perception at the level of: (1) phonemic syllables; (2) word and pseudoword identification, and (3) morphosyntactical development.

Integration of Auditory and Speechread Information on the Phonetic Perception of Syllables

Deaf children fitted with a cochlear implant have been found to perform better on speech recognition tasks when visual information is available conjointly with the auditory information rather than when only the auditory information is available (Lachs, Pisoni, & Kirk, 2001; Rouger, Lagleyre, Fraysse, Deneve, Deguine, & Barone, 2007). Given their limited auditory experience, individuals with a cochlear implant might rely *more* on speechreading than normally hearing children (Clarke, 2003; Rouger et al., 2007).

If audiovisual integration depends mainly on the balance between the weight devoted to the processing of auditory and visual information, it is likely that the way the cortex integrates auditory and visual signals is different in children with a cochlear implant than it is in normally hearing children. A critical variable in the development of audiovisual integration might be the precocity of implantation. Auditory speech perception scores after implantation are better when children have been fitted before the age of 3, and even 2 years old (Baumgartner, Pok, Egelierler, Franz, Gstoettner, & Hamzavi, 2002; Snik, Makhdoum, Vermeulen, Brokx, & van den Broeck, 1997; Svirsky, Teoh, & Neuburger, 2004; Tyler, Fryauf-Bertschy, Kelsay, Gantz, Woodworth, & Parkinson, 1997). Early implantation would allow auditory networks to maintain more of their initial functionality. Children fitted early with a cochlear implant could more readily exploit the phonetic relations between auditory and visual signals, and thus develop audiovisual processing mechanisms earlier and more efficiently.

Researchers interested in audiovisual integration in children with a cochlear implant have used the McGurk paradigm (McGurk & Mac Donald, 1976). A typical McGurk experiment consists of four conditions: Audio Only (AO), Visual Only (VO), Audio Visual Congruent (AVC), and Audio Visual Incongruent (AVI). In the AO condition, participants have to report what they hear when presented with an audio recording of syllables like /pa/ or /ba/. In the VO condition, they have to report what they lipread when presented with a face articulating the same syllables. In the AVC condition, participants watch a synchronized video recording of a speaker's face articulating the same syllable, for example A/pa/ V/pa/, and have to report what they hear. In the AVI condition, they are presented with an audio recording of syllables matched with a video recording of a different syllable, like A/pa/ matched with V/ka/. When required to report what they hear, they typically report hearing the illusory syllable /ta/, which is called a *fusion*. In the reverse situation (i.e., hearing an audio recording of /ka/ while watching a synchronized video recording of a speaker's face articulating /pa/), they typically report hearing /pka/, a percept called a *combination*. Note that in the latter case the /p/ is *not* in the sound track, and is just suggested by the very salient lip movement of abrupt aperture of the mouth. These illusions are robust, and have been demonstrated in adults and children and in numerous languages (see Colin & Radeau, 2003 for a review).

Schorr, Fox, van Wassenhove, and Knudsen (2005) were the first researchers to report the outcomes of a McGurk experiment with children who have a cochlear implant as participants. They tested 35 children (mean age: 5.85 years) who were deaf from birth and had used their cochlear implant for at least 1 year, and they compared them to normally hearing children matched for chronologic age. In the AVI condition A/pa/ V/ka/, of the 35 children with normal hearing, 57% (n = 20) showed "consistent fusions" /ta/ on seven or more of the 10 trials. The remaining children who showed less consistent fusions, responded /pa/, which indicates that their speech perception was dominated by the auditory processing. The situation was rather different for the children with a cochlear implant. Five of the 35 children were removed from further analyses because they responded with the syllable /ta/ on congruent A/ka/ V/ka/. Out of the 30 remaining children, only 6 showed consistent fusions on the incongruent trials. The 24 remaining children gave fewer than 6 fusion responses on the 10 trials, meaning that they integrated poorly or inconsistently. They predominantly reported /ka/ (i.e., the visual component of the incongruent stimulus), indicating that their speech perception was dominated by the visual stimulus under bimodal conditions. The likelihood of strong audiovisual integration is shaped by experience with bimodal spoken language during early life. Although the six children who made consistent fusions all received their implant before the age of 30 months (representing only 38% of the "early fitted" population), none of the children fitted after the age of 30 months exhibited consistent audiovisual fusions.

In our own research program with the McGurk paradigm (Colin, Deltenre, Radeau, & Leybaert, 2007; Colin, Leybaert, et al., 2008; Leybaert & Colin, 2008), we also have been interested in determining whether children fitted early with a cochlear implant (i.e., before 3 years of age) display more combinations and fusions percepts than children fitted later with a cochlear implant. Our McGurk experiment consisted of the four syllables /pi/, /ki/, /bi/, and /gi/, presented in four conditions described above: AO, VO, AVC, and AVI. Voiced /bi/ and /gi/ and voiceless /pi/ and /ki/ were presented in separate blocks of stimuli. Children reported what they heard (or lipread) by showing one of four written syllables, for example, PI, KI, TI, PKI for the voiceless blocs, and BI, GI, DI, BGI for the voiced ones.

We began with a single-case study. The participant, referred to here as N was an 8-year-old girl, diagnosed as profoundly deaf at 18 months, and fitted with a Nucleus 22 electrodes cochlear implant at 3 years of age. Her parents used the French version of Cued Speech (Langage Parlé Complété) intensively. Her language development was good both at the lexical and morphosyntactical levels. Her score at the standardized test for morphosyntax L'ECOSSE (Lecoq, 1996) was between the 25th to 50th percentile for children of the same chronologic age. She demonstrated effective use of the cochlear implant; indeed, she was able to handle a conversation at the phone with an unknown person.

The performance of N for voiceless consonants is reported in Table 6–1 (for a detailed account of her results, and a comparison with those of 20 normally hearing children of the same grade-level, see Leybaert & Colin, 2008).

Inspection of Table 6–1 reveals several interesting findings: First, speech recognition though AO was good for the bilabial /pi/, while the palatal /ki/ was often misperceived and categorized as the dental /ti/. The same tendency was observed in the VO condition. All congruent audiovisual stimuli were correctly perceived. The improvement was particularly impressive for A/ki/ V/ki/, which was recognized at 100% when audio and visual information were redundant, while this syllable was not perceived accurately either in AO or in VO conditions. On the incongruent audiovisual stimuli however, N did not report *any* auditory response. When auditory and visual information were in conflict, her speech perception was dominated by the visual stimulus and she seemed to "hear what she saw." It is difficult to consider the large number of /ti/ responses to the stimulus A/pi/ V /ki/ as classical audiovisual fusions because she already gave /ti/ responses in the VO and in the AO conditions (see Table 6–1). The surprising pattern of visual dominance in N could be interpreted either as a consequence of her relatively late fitting with the cochlear implant, or of intensive exposure to Cued Speech.

In order to test the first interpretation, we compared two groups of children with cochlear implants. One group of 10 participants had been fitted early (i.e., between 1 year 10 months to three years). They ranged in age from 4 years 11 months to 14 years 10 months. The second group of 14 participants had been fitted late (i.e., between 3 years 11 months to 16 years 10 months). They ranged in age from 5 to 25 years. All children had been exposed to the Langage Parlé Complété (French version of Cued Speech) to various degrees. They all participated in the same experiment McGurk experiment as the child N. They responded either by designating the written syllables or by repeating what they perceived (this was

Table 6–1. Percentage of Designations of the Written Syllables PI, KI, TI, and PKI as a Function of the Target Syllables Presented AO, VO, AVC, and AVI conditions for the Child N

Audio Only	AO/pi/	AO/ki/
Pi	91.7	
Ki	–	58.3
Pki	–	
Ti	8.3	41.7
Visual Only	**VO/pi/**	**VO/ki/**
Pi	75	–
Ki	–	17
Pki	25	–
Ti	–	83.3
Audio Visual Congruent	**A/pi/V/pi/**	**A/ki/V/ki/**
Pi	100	–
Ki	–	100
Pki	–	–
Ti	–	–
Audio Visual Incongruent	**A/pi/V/ki/**	**A/ki/V/pi/**
Pi	–	100
Ki	8	–
Pki	–	–
Ti	92	–

of course the case for nonreaders, and also for some of the older participants). The results for the voiceless consonants /pi/ and /ki/ are presented for the AO, VO, and AVI conditions in Table 6–2.

Three aspects of the results are striking. First, the percentage of auditory responses was always much lower in the AVI condition than in the AO condition, showing a strong influence of the visual information on speech perception: 18% /pi/ responses for A/pi/ V/ki/ in the early group, compared to 65% /pi/ responses to A/pi/ for the same group in the AO condition. Second, and even more striking, is the fact that the percent of visual

Table 6–2. Percentage of PI, KI, PKI, and TI Responses to the Target Syllables Presented in AO, VO, AVC and AVI Conditions for Deaf Children Fitted Early (*n* = 10) or Late (*n* = 14) with a CI

	Early Fitted Participants		Late Fitted Participants	
Audio Only	**AO/pi/**	**AO/ki/**	**AO/pi/**	**AO/ki/**
Pi	65	19	60	20
Ki	12	54	10	45
Pki	11	9	9	10
Ti	10	17	20	23
Visual Only	**VO/pi/**	**VO/ki/**	**VO/pi/**	**VO/ki/**
Pi	71	20	72	13
Ki	6	36	6	45
Pki	13	15	17	13
Ti	8	27	3	26
Audio Visual Incongruent	**A/pi/V/ki/**	**A/ki/V/pi/**	**A/pi/V/ki/**	**A/ki/V/pi/**
Pi	18	77	12	77
Ki	30	8	38	7
Pki	17	8	9	11
Ti	30	5	40	5

responses to bimodal incongruent stimuli was nearly the same as the percent of correct visual responses in VO condition. Compare, for example, the 77% /pi/ responses to A/ki/ V/pi/ in the early group to the 71% /pi/ responses to VO /pi/ in the same group. Third, no significant difference appeared between the pattern of responses given by the early and the late groups (although the early group seems to be a little better than the late group at the AO condition, and the late group a little better than the early group in the VO condition).

In order to test the effect of exposure to Cued Speech, Colin et al. (2008) administered the same experiment to a group of deaf children fitted with a cochlear implant, who had not been exposed to Cued Speech. These children showed the same reliance on speechreading as the Cued Speech-users when the visual syllable did not correspond with the auditory syllable.

Taken as a whole, these findings suggest that when faced with conflicting audiovisual stimuli, children fitted with a cochlear implant seem to rely mostly on *visual* speech information. Their auditory speech skills, which appear to be moderate in the AO condition, may be too fragile to resist when they are put into competition with visual processing. It must be noted that the McGurk experiment mimics fairly well the watching of a dubbed film on television; that is, the auditory information is not congruent with the information they can read on the lips. Given that many of the children have confidence in what they read on the lips, without perceiving the sound, it means that they should have problems watching dubbed films. Many of the participants reported this was the case.

Children with cochlear implants rely more on speechreading than normally hearing children for different reasons. First, they may assign more weight to the visual speech information because the auditory information is degraded. This is evident in the case of normally hearing participants who must recognize stimuli consisting of spectrally reduced speech (SRS). The information about place of articulation is only partially transmitted in SRS, and normally hearing participants show larger McGurk fusion effects with SRS than with normal speech (Berthommier, 2001; Grant, Tufts, & Greenberg, 2007). The parallel between perception of SRS by normally hearing adults and perception of speech by children with a cochlear implant is that, in both cases, the speech information conveyed by the high frequencies, which is important to perceive the place of articulation, is *degraded*. Therefore, it is not surprising that children with a cochlear implant who have only partial access to place of articulation information through the auditory channel rely more on speechreading to process place of articulation. When auditory and visual information are put into conflict, their perception of speech is *captured* by visual information.

Second, the visual predominance of cochlear implant users might also be explained in terms of reorganization of neural resources in the case of deafness followed by cochlear implantation. Early deprivation of auditory information, as in congenital hearing impairment, can lead to a reorganization of neural resources, with a potentially larger involvement of auditory cortex in the processing of visual stimuli (Neville, Schmidt, & Kutas, 1983; Neville & Lawson, 1987). It has been found that the auditory cortex of deaf persons, once reorganized by cross-modal plasticity after years of deafness, can no longer respond to signals from a cochlear implant (Champoux, Lepore, Gagné & Théoret, 2009; Doucet, Bergeron, Lassonde, Ferron, Lepore, 2006; Lee et al., 2001). Children and adults implanted at later ages are at a relative disadvantage compared to children implanted early, because the auditory cortex has already been appropriated by the visual modality. As Shannon (2007) notes, the auditory system of children implanted at early ages competes for cortical real estate whereas late implantation may be unable to dislodge existing cortical "squatters." The results of Schorr et al. (2005) showing that children implanted later than 30 months of age fail to integrate visual cues with the auditory cues, is compatible with this view.

In summary, speech perception through a cochlear implant presents some important differences compared to speech perception in normally hearing individuals. Children with cochlear implants rely *more* on *visual* speech information, probably because this information is more reliable than the auditory information, particularly in noisy environments. From the available research, there is no reason to discourage children with a cochlear implant from employing speechreading or using the visible manual cues of Cued Speech in addition to the auditory information available via the cochlear implant. Rather, research suggests that they need *both* for optimum speech perception.

Word and Pseudoword Identification in Children with Cochlear Implants

Recently, a number of researchers have found that deaf people with a cochlear implant not only have better speechreading abilities, but that they also show a better combination of the visual signal with the degraded auditory signal for word perception than hearing individuals are able to do (Rouger et al., 2007). Shannon (2007) interestingly suggests that cochlear implant listeners are able to compensate for the loss of fine temporal information with exploitation of visual cues. Should that be the case, one would expect that adding visual cues of Cued Speech (i.e., mouth-shapes and handshapes) might improve the reception of lexical and nonlexical information by children who are cochlear implant users.

Some researchers have expressed the opposite prediction, specifically that the processing of the manual information, either in manually coded English (MCE) systems or Cued Speech, could *compete* for limited resources in auditory-visual tasks. For example, when a child with a cochlear implant is administered an auditory memory task that is conveyed via an MCE sign system such as Signing Exact English (Gustason, Zawolkow, & Pfetzing, 1993) or Cued Speech, the child is confronted with manual signs or cues that must be interpreted simultaneously with the audi-

tory information. This task involves paying attention to both the hand(s) of the speaker in addition to the lips on the speaker's face (Burkholder & Pisoni, 2006, p. 352).

Nouelle (2005) designed an experiment aimed at testing how well cochlear implantees, who were exposed to Cued Speech, could repeat aloud words and pseudowords presented in six different conditions: Visual Alone (VO), Audio Alone (AO), V (Visual) + Cues (V + C), Audio Visual (AV), AV + Cues (AV + C), AV + Noise (AV + N). The noise consisted of children's conversations recorded in a playground. The stimuli presented in the six conditions were matched in terms of the number of syllables, number of consonant clusters and number of final consonants with low visibility (examples are the words *enfant* and *oiseau* matched with the pseudowords *eufant* and *ouzeu*). The stimuli from the six conditions were randomly mixed, so that participants were in a situation with high uncertainty about the modality in which the next stimulus would be presented. Nineteen children (aged 4 years 10 months to 12 years; mean age 8;8 years) participated in the experiment (see also Leybaert et al., 2007). The proportion of correct repetition for words and pseudowords in VO and V + C (Table 6–3) suggest that the performance was enhanced when cues were present in addition to speechreading, indicating that children could make an efficient use of the cues. The proportion of correct responses was on average 89.5% in word repetition in V + C condition (with 11 participants reaching 90% and above) but only 52.0% for pseudoword repetition (ranging from 17% to 82.4%). It would appear that children use their lexical knowledge to repeat words presented via Cued Speech; however, when lexical knowledge was not

Table 6–3. Mean Percent Correct Repetitions for Words and Pseudowords Presented in Lipreading (VO) or Lipreading + Cues (VO + C)

Participant	Words: VO	Words: VO + C	Pseudowords: VO	Pseudowords: VO + C
1	50	95	12	35
2	55	95	18	65
3	45	90	29	60
4	40	95	18	65
5	55	95	41	47
6	55	95	35	77
7	65	85	18	60
8	20	95	5,9	47
9	55	100	12	77
10	65	95	24	35
11	55	95	24	71
12	30	85	0	53
13	60	75	0	35
14	50	90	41	35
15	50	95	24	41
16	40	90	18	29
17	50	85	18	65
18	40	50	0	18
19	60	95	29	82
Mean	**49,47**	**89,47**	**19,31**	**52,47**
SD	**11,53**	**11,17**	**12,59**	**18,49**

available, in the case of pseudowords, their performance decreased.

Table 6–4 gives the proportion of words and pseudowords correctly repeated for the AO, AV, AV + C conditions for each of the 19 participants. For word identification, the performance in the AO condition was above 75% of correct responses for half of the participants; for pseudoword identification, only two participants reached a score higher than 75%. For words, the addition of speechreading and of the hand cues facilitated performance for every participant, except for one who was already 90% in the AO condition. Performance increased more in the AV condition for those participants performing very poorly in the AO condition. In the AV + C condition, performance was 100% for 16 participants, and 95% for the three

Table 6–4. Mean Percent Correct Repetitions for Words and Pseudowords Presented in Auditory (audiovisual + cues [AV + C])

Participant	Words: AO	Words: AV	Words: AV + C	Pseudo-words: AO	Pseudo-words: AV	Pseudo-words: AV + C
1	75	85	100	71	60	88
2	70	90	100	77	88	100
3	75	95	100	53	77	100
4	80	100	100	71	71	82
5	85	95	100	71	71	82
6	80	100	100	82	94	100
7	40	75	100	24	71	88
8	90	85	95	60	71	94
9	80	100	100	71	60	100
10	10	80	100	18	29	77
11	65	90	100	65	65	82
12	35	55	95	35	47	82
13	80	95	100	71	88	88
14	50	75	100	53	60	77
15	60	75	100	29	71	100
16	70	95	100	35	47	77
17	60	90	100	47	60	77
18	70	80	95	35	60	60
19	75	95	100	47	77	88
Mean	**65,79**	**87,11**	**99,21**	**53,42**	**66,68**	**86,42**
SD	**19,88**	**11,58**	**1,87**	**19,60**	**15,60**	**10,85**

others. For pseudowords, the performance was systematically lower in the AO, AV, and AV + C than for the word repetition. The addition of speechreading to AO, and addition of hand cues to AV increased the correct repetition of pseudowords: in the AV + C condition, the mean correct performance was 86.4%, and 4 subjects achieved 100% correct responses (all subjects showed an improvement).

The following conclusions can be drawn from these data: First, AV information might be sufficient enough to recognize *familiar words*, but AV might not contain enough information in order to repeat pseudowords, which could be considered as potentially *novel words*. If this is true, it means that at least some deaf children could be at risk for delayed vocabulary development if they are forced to rely solely on auditory and speechread information. Second, the processing of manual cues from Cued Speech improves word repetition, but plays an even greater role in the processing of pseudowords (from 67% to 86% on average), seeming to provide support for the improved input via Cued Speech for children's acquisition of new words.

Contrary to Burkholder and Pisoni's (2006) concern, the cues from Cued Speech seem to be well integrated in the processing of audiovisual information; however, children with a cochlear implant do not seem to fully exploit the possibilities of Cued Speech, as indicated by the fact that the correct repetition of pseudowords presented in V + C was only 52% on average (one pseudoword of two was correctly repeated). Although there are no data about where the children's eyes are fixated when attending to a person producing cued language, we may, a priori, think that the perceiver does not need to fixate directly on the talker's lips or hands but could be looking at other parts of the face or even somewhat away from the face, as already demonstrated for speechreading by hearing listeners (Smeele, Massaro, Cohen, & Sittig, 1998). Transliterators frequently complain that children with a cochlear implant do not look to them enough in classroom situations (personal communication, Marthouret, May 2007).

To conclude, it seems that the provision of manual cues from Cued Speech to the auditory and speechread signal enhances word, and even more *pseudoword*, repetition, thereby enhancing the condition for acquiring lexical representations for new words. The important role of "reading the cues" in children's perception of the articulatory movements related to new words may be related to *phonemic* and *attentional* factors. For example, the cues combined

with the lip gestures afford the opportunity of perceiving all phonemes without any ambiguity. In terms of the attention factor, we know that the lip movement anticipates itself the emission of sound (Schwartz, Berthommier, & Savariaux, 2004), and the manual gesture anticipates the opening of the lips (see Chapter 19 in this volume). If a child sees the manual cue configuration corresponding to /p, d, ʒ/ near the cheekbone, he implicitly *knows* that the auditory consonant will be one of these three and could use speechreading to finally remove the remaining ambiguity. For example, /du/ and /gu/ have the same lipread image; however, if the hand is making the /p, d, ʒ/ configuration near the chin, the child will be able to maximize the processing of the following speechread (an alveodental with lips protrusion) and the auditory information (a voiced plosive consonant).

The Effect of Cued Speech Experience on the Development of Morphosyntax

Nouelle's (2005) results, together with other results reviewed elsewhere (see Hage & Leybaert, 2006), lead one to think that children with a cochlear implant whose parents use Cued Speech will develop more precise phonological representations than children who do not use Cued Speech. Consider the hypothetical case of a young deaf child, aged 24 months, fitted with a cochlear implant at 18 months, who converses with parents in a noisy context (e.g., a family dinner). "Are you sick?" asks the mother speaking and cueing to their child. The auditory input received by this child in this noisy situation would probably be too incomplete to allow the child to perceive the words, and thus, the meaning of the question. In contrast, the manual Cued Speech gestures used by the mother attract the child's attention to the communicative intention of the mother. If the child is able to decode the manual cues combined with the lip movements corresponding to *sick*, and the interrogative expression of his mother, the child might be able to associate the auditory stimulus /sɪk/ with a meaning because of the manual coding. Therefore, using Cued Speech may help parents and their deaf child to build up episodes of joint attention in which the first lexical representations, the beginning of morphosyntax and of sociocognitive development, are well anchored.

Data supporting the view that Cued Speech enhances speech perception have been reported by Le Normand (2003), who assessed 50 French-speaking children at 6, 12, 18, 24, and 36 months after cochlear implantation. The children had received a cochlear implant between 21 and 78 months of age. In addition to the socioeconomic status of the families and gender, the mode of communication used with the children was found to be predictive of language production. In addition, children who used Cued Speech produced a higher number of content words and function words than did those educated with other modes of communication, including oral, sign language, signed French.

In a recent study, Szagun (2004) showed that children with a cochlear implant made morphosyntactic errors of gender and omissions of articles. Szagun argued that "due to their hearing impairment, these children frequently miss unstressed pronominal articles in incoming speech (which) would lead to a reduced

frequency of actually processed article input" (p. 26), and that "the difficulties hearing-impaired children experience in constructing a case and gender system are due to processing limitations. While such processing limitations may have their root in a perceptual deficit, they may become a linguistic cognitive deficit during the children's developmental history" (p. 27).

Hawes (2004) speculated that the use of Cued Speech might help to overcome this "perceptual deficit" in children with a cochlear implant by transmitting *complete* information about these unstressed elements of language and might help to avoid the development of a "cognitive deficit" during the child's developmental history of language. Hawes (2004) investigated the effect of Cued Speech exposure upon the development of grammatical gender in French-speaking children fitted with a cochlear implant. She compared the linguistic development of five children of approximately the same age, same school level, and equivalent durations of cochlear implant stimulation, but who differed in the mode of communication to which they were exposed (Table 6–5). Two of them (C and L) were orally educated by their parents, one (D) was exposed to Cued Speech, but relies more on audition and does not attend much to the lips and to the cues, whereas R and O were exposed intensively to Cued Speech by their parents and rely on auditory, visual, and manual cues.

These children were given three language tests. The first was L'ECOSSE (Lecoq, 1996), a French adaptation of the Test for Reception of Grammar (TROG) (Bishop, 1989). L'ECOSSE is designed to investigate morphosyntactic development of hearing children. It contains 72 items testing a wide range of linguistic constructions, including: affirmatives, negatives,

Table 6–5. Characteristics of the 5 Children

Name of the child	R	C	D	L	O
Age in months	81	78	80	87	86
Age at fitting	37	32	30	50	31
Duration of stimulation	44	46	50	37	45
Grade level	1st	KG	1st	1st	1st
CAP	7	5	6	6	7
Mode of communication	O + CS	O	O	O	O + CS

Note. CAP = Category of auditory performance; Scale from 1 to 7 (7 = child understands telephone conversation); mode of communication: O = oral; CS = Cued Speech.

passives, and embedded relatives. On each trial, a sentence is spoken with the cues to the child and the child has to choose, among four pictures, the one corresponding to the sentence. In a second test, children were given eight pictures and asked to tell a story in response to the question "what happened?" They were also given the book "Frog, Where Are You?" and asked to comment about each picture of that book (see Le Normand, 2003). Their productions were transcribed in the Childes database (MacWhinney, 2000). Table 6–6 presents the results from the five children on the L'Ecosse test of morphosyntax.

The children R and O, who had been exposed intensively to Cued Speech, achieved scores on the L'Ecosse test that were within the normal distribution of scores for their age level. In the semi-spontaneous talks, they use closed-class words at a level corresponding to their age (not illustrated here). The child D, who was relying more on her auditory capacities, and who did not seem to take benefit from the cues, had difficulties with complex sentences on the L'Ecosse test (e.g., relatives, double negations) but she used closed-class words in her spontaneous talking. The children, C and L, who

were educated orally, displayed significant language delay on the L'Ecosse test as well as in their spontaneous use of closed-class words.

Finally, the five children with cochlear implants were given a gender generation test (the Bicron test), derived from that designed by Hage (1994), consisting of 24 trials. In each trial, two pictures of the same imaginary animal were presented to the child while saying, "Here are two bicrons." One of the two characters is then hidden, and the child is asked, "What remains?" The child is expected to answer "le (the) bicron" or "un (one) bicron." The appeal of this test is that some phonological endings like "-on" are statistically associated with the masculine gender, others (like "-ette") with the feminine gender, and others are not associated with a particular gender. This test thus examines whether children have established co-occurrences between the suffixes and the grammatical gender, which, in French, are expressed by articles ("le," "un" versus "la," "une"). A control group of 32 hearing children aged 5 years 6 months in average was also given the Bicron test. These children made between one and six errors (Table 6–7).

Table 6–6. Results Obtained by the 5 Children at L'Ecosse Test and Corresponding Ages of Grammatical Development

Name	R	C	D	L	O
Percentile obtained at L'Ecosse test	P25–P50	<P 10	<<P 10	<<P 10	P 25
Age of grammatical development (in months)	72–77	48–53	54–59	54–59	72–77

Table 6–7. Number of Hearing Kindergarteners Who Made 1, 2, 3, . . . Errors on the Bicron Test

Number of Errors	1	2	3	4	5	6
Number of Children	10	12	5	2	0	0

The distribution of errors for our five children with a cochlear implant at the Bicron test was the following: R: 4 errors, C: 13 errors, D: 3 errors, L: 10 errors, and O: 2 errors. To sum up, the children R, D, and O were clearly within the distribution of errors of hearing children, whereas C and L were outside this distribution, meaning that they made a number of gender errors which cannot be found in the distribution of normally hearing children. Age at implantation is not sufficient to explain the variability in the development of morphosyntax of these five children. Access to the language input seems a critical variable. Children who benefitted from the combination of Cued Speech and a cochlear implant (i.e., R and O) seem to have undergone a normal development of morphosyntax. Child D, who exploited her auditory capacities effectively, has developed a good morphosyntax of gender, but made more errors in the complex sentences of the L'Ecosse test. Finally, the children L and C, who only rely on auditory information delivered through the cochlear implant do not seem to have extracted the regularities between phonology and morphology. They also displayed important delays to the L'Ecosse test and in spontaneous production of closed-class words. Thus, exposure to Cued Speech seems to help deaf children master delicate aspects of morphosyntax.

Conclusions

Data collected in the 1980s and 1990s demonstrated that the use of Cued Speech can be a powerful tool for language development and subsequent formal reading achievement by profoundly deaf children equipped with hearing aids. Cued Speech enhances speech perception through the visual modality, the acquisition of vocabulary and morphosyntax, and metalinguistic development, as well as the acquisition of reading and spelling (see Chapter 11 in this volume). More recent data seem to indicate that children who received cochlear implants benefit from prior exposure to Cued Speech; however, use of Cued Speech before implantation is likely to become increasingly more rare. Indeed, most children are now fitted with a cochlear implant around the age of one year. During the first months or years of cochlear implant use, speech perception of an implanted child remains imperfect. Oral comprehension does not develop exclusively through the auditory channel but necessitates audiovisual integration. Therefore, the addition of Cued Speech to the signal delivered by the cochlear implant might help deaf children in identifying new words. Children fitted early with a cochlear implant, thus, would benefit from multimodal input during the development of phonological representations, which would serve as the platform from which subsequent phonological awareness, reading, and spelling acquisition could be launched (see Chapter 11 in this volume).

The use of Cued Speech by children with a cochlear implant is not an automatic solution to language development of deaf children. Children may not reliably look at a speaker's lips and hands, and they may tend to rely on auditory information alone. Some parents may lose their motivation to cue, feel discouraged, or simply abandon coding with the hands. Therefore, it would be important for educators and related service providers to regularly assess whether cueing remains necessary, and under what circumstances after implantation. It is likely that after some period of auditory (re)habilitation, children fitted with a cochlear implant would be capable of learning new words by auditory means and reading alone. Continued attention, nonetheless, should be devoted to the development of delicate, but vital, aspects of language, such as morphosyntax. This domain of language

acquisition is particularly important and sensitive to a lack of precise input, as Szagun's (2004) data show. The capacity to develop morphosyntax easily in response to a well-specified input also tends to diminish with age, although the limits of a precise "sensitive period" cannot be fixed at the present time (Szagun, 2001).

References

Baumgartner, W., Pok, S., Egelierler, B., Franz, P., Gstoettner, W., & Hamzavi, J. (2002). The role of age in pediatric cochlear implantation. *International Journal of Pediatric Otorhinolaryngology, 62*, 223–228.

Berthommier, F. (2001). Audiovisual recognition of spectrally reduced speech. *Proceedings of the International Conference on Auditory-Visual Speech Processing* (pp. 183–189). Aalborg, Denmark.

Bishop, D. V. M. (1989) *Test for receptive grammar.* Manchester, UK: Age and Cognitive Performance Research Center, University of Manchester.

Burkholder, R., & Pisoni, D. (2006). Working memory capacity, verbal rehearsal speed, and scanning in deaf children with cochlear implants. In P. Spencer & M. Marschark (Eds.), *Advances in the spoken language development of deaf and hard-of-hearing children* (pp. 328–359). New York, NY: Oxford University Press.

Champoux, F., Lepore, F., Gagné, J.-P., & Théoret, H. (2009). Visual stimuli can impair auditory processing in cochlear implant users. *Neuropsychologia, 47*, 17–22.

Clarke, G. (2003). Cochlear implants in children: Safety as well as speech and language. *International Journal of Pediatric Otorhinolaryngology, 67*, S7–S20.

Colin, C., Deltenre, P., Radeau, M., & Leybaert, J. (2007). La perception audiovisuelle de la parole chez l'enfant muni d'un implant cochléaire: Première données. In L. Collet, C. Corbé, M. Doly, M. Imbert, & Y. Christen,

Percevoir & Protéger: Collection Neurosciences sensorielles et cognitives (pp. 193–207). Marseilles, France: Editions Solal.

Colin, C., Leybaert, J., Charlier, B., Mansbach, A.-L., Ligny, C., Mancilla, V., & Deltenre, P. (2008). Apport de la modalité visuelle dans la perception de la parole. *Les Cahiers de l'Audition, 21,* 42–50.

Colin, C., & Radeau, M. (2003). Les illusions McGurk dans la parole: 25 ans de recherches. *L'Année Psychologique, 104,* 497–542.

Doucet, M., Bergeron, F., Lassonde, M., Ferron, P., & Lepore, F. (2006). Cross-modal reorganization and speech perception in cochlear implant users. *Brain, 129,* 3376–3383.

Fearn, R., & Wolfe, J. (2000). The relative importance of rate and place: Experiments using pitch scaling techniques with cochlear implantees. *Annals of Otology, Rhinology, and Laryngology, 109,* 51–53.

Frère, C., & Leybaert, J. (2007, September). *Perception de la musique par les enfants sourds munis d'un implant cochléaire.* Poster presented at the meeting Music and Emotion, Brussels.

Fu, Q., & Nogaki, G. (2004; 2006 ds txt). Noise susceptibility of cochlear implant users: The role of spectral resolution and smearing. *Journal of the Association for Research in Otorhinolaryngology, 6,* 19–27.

Geers, A. (2006). Spoken language in children with cochlear implants. In P. Spencer & M. Marschark (Eds.), *Advances in the spoken language development of deaf and hard-of-hearing children* (pp. 244–270). New York, NY: Oxford University Press.

Giraud, A., Price, C., Graham, J., Truy, E., & Frackowiak, R. (2001). Cross-modal plasticity underpins language recovery after cochlear implantation. *Neuron, 30,* 657–663.

Glasberg, B., & Moore, B. (1986). Auditory filter shapes in subjects with unilateral and bilateral cochlear impairments. *Journal of the Acoustical Society of America, 79,* 1020–1033.

Grant, K., Tufts, J., & Greenberg, S. (2007). Integration efficiency for speech perception within and across sensory modalities by normal-hearing and hearing-impaired individuals, *Journal of the Acoustical the Society of America, 121,* 1164–1176.

Grosgeorges, A. (2005). *L'analyse des scènes auditives et reconnaissance de la parole,* Unpublished doctoral dissertation, Institut de la communication parlée (ICP/INPG), Université Stendhal, CNRS.

Gustason, G., Zawolkow, E., & Pfetzing, D. (1993). *Signing Exact English.* Los Alamitos, CA: Modern Signs Press.

Hage, C. (1994). *Développement de certains aspects de la morpho-syntaxe chez l'enfant atteint de surdité profonde: Rôle du Langage Parlé Complété.* Unpublished doctoral dissertation, Université libre de Bruxelles.

Hage, C., & Leybaert, J. (2006). The effect of Cued Speech on the development of spoken language. In P. Spencer & M. Marschark (Eds.), *Advances in the spoken language development of deaf and hard-of-hearing children* (pp. 193–211). New York, NY: Oxford University Press.

Hawes, V. (2004). Développement de la morphosyntaxe chez 5 enfants sourds porteurs d'un implant: Complémentarité des informations auditives et visuelles. *Mémoire non publié de licenciée en logopédie.* Université libre de Bruxelles.

Lachs, L., Pisoni, D., & Kirk, K. (2001). Use of audiovisual information in speech perception by prelingually deaf children with cochlear implants: A first report. *Ear and Hearing, 22,* 236–251.

Lecoq, P. (1996). *Epreuve de Compréhension Syntaxico-Sémantique.* Villeneuve d'Ascq, France: Presses universitaires du Septentrion.

Lee, D., Lee J., Oh, S., Kim, S., Kim, J., Chung, J., . . . Kim, C. (2001). Cross-modal plasticity and cochlear implants. *Nature, 409,* 149–150.

Le Normand, M-T. (2003). Acquisition du lexique chez l'enfant implanté. *Liaison LPC, 40,* 97–110.

Leybaert, J., & Colin, C. (2008). Perception multimodale de la parole dans le développement normal et atypique: Premières données. In M. Kail, M. Fayol, & M. Hickmann (Eds.), *Apprentissage des langues premières et secondes* (pp. 529–547). Paris, France: CNRS Editions.

Leybaert, J., Colin, C., Willems, P., Colin, S., Nouelle, M., Schepers, F., . . . Ligny, C. (2007). Implant cochléaire, plasticité cérébrale, et développement du langage. In J. Lopez (Ed.), *Audition et langage* (pp. 13–67). Paris, France: Presses Universitaires de Vincennes.

Lorenzi, C., Gilbert, G., Carn, H., Garnier, S., & Moore, B. (2006). Speech perception problems of the hearing impaired reflect inability to use temporal fine structure. *Proceedings of the National Academy of Sciences, 103,* 18866–18869.

MacWhinney, B. (2000). The *CHILDES Project: Tools for analyzing talk.* Mahwah, NJ: Lawrence Erlbaum Associates.

McGurk, H., & MacDonald, J. (1976). Hearing lips and seeing voices. *Nature, 264,* 746–748.

Neville, H., & Lawson, D. (1987). Attention to central and peripheral visual space in a movement-detection task: An event-related potential and behavioural study. II. Congenitally deaf adults. *Brain Research, 405,* 268–283.

Neville, H., Schmidt, A., & Kutas, M. (1983). Altered visual-evoked potentials in congenitally deaf adults. *Brain Research, 266,* 127–132.

Nicholls, G., & Ling, D. (1982). Cued Speech and the reception of spoken language. *Journal of Speech and Hearing Research, 25,* 262–269.

Nouelle, M. (2005). La perception de mots et de pseudo-mots dans le bruit chez l'enfant sourd porteur d'un implant cochléaire: Impact du LPC. *Mémoire de licence en logopédie, non publié.* Université libre de Bruxelles, Université catholique de Louvain.

Périer, O., Charlier, B., Hage, C., & Alegria, J. (1988). Evaluation of the effects of prolonged Cued Speech practice upon the reception of spoken language. In I. G. Taylor (Ed.), *The education of the deaf: Current perspectives* (Vol. I, pp. 47–59). London, UK: Croom Helm.

Rouger, J., Lagleyre, S., Fraysse, B., Deneve, S., Deguine, O., & Barone, P. (2007). Evidence that cochlear-implanted deaf patients are bet-ter multisensory integrators. *Proceedings of National Academy of Sciences, 104,* 7295–7300.

Schorr, E., Fox, N., van Wassenhove, V., & Knudsen, E. (2005). Auditory-visual fusion in speech perception in children with cochlear implants. *Proceedings of National Academy of Sciences, 102,* 18748–18750.

Schwartz, J., Berthommier, F., & Savariaux, C. (2004) Seeing to hear better: Evidence for early audiovisual interactions in speech identification. *Cognition, 93,* B69–B78.

Shannon, R. (2007). Understanding hearing through deafness. *Proceedings of National Academy of Sciences, 104,* 6883–6884.

Smeele, P., Massaro, D., Cohen, M., & Sittig, A. (1998). Laterality in visual speech perception. *Journal of Experimental Psychology: Human Perception and Performance, 24,* 1232–1242.

Snik, A., Makhdoum, M., Vermeulen, A., Brokx, J. P., & van den Broeck, P. (1997). The relation between age at the time of cochlear implantation and long-term speech perception abilities ion congenitally deaf subjects. *International Journal of Pediatric Otorhinolaryngology, 41,* 121–131.

Spencer, P., & Marschark, M. (2003). Cochlear implants: Issues and implications. In M. Marschark & P. Spencer (Eds.), *Oxford handbook of deaf studies, language, and education.* Oxford, UK: Oxford University Press.

Sumby, W., & Pollack, I. (1954). Visual contribution to speech intelligibility in noise. *Journal of Acoustical Society of America, 26,* 212–215.

Summerfield, Q. (1987). Some preliminaries to a comprehensive account of audiovisual speech perception. In B. Dodd & R. Campbell (Eds.), *Hearing by eye: The psychology of lipreading* (pp. 3–51). London, UK: Erlbaum.

Svirsky, M., Teoh, S., & Neuburger, H. (2004). Development of language and speech perception in congenitally, profoundly deaf children as a function of age at cochlear implantation. *Audiology and Neuro-otology, 9,* 224–233.

Szagun, G. (2001). Language acquisition in young German-speaking children with cochlear implants: Individual differences and implications for conceptions of a "sensitive phase." *Audiology and Neuro-otology,* *6,* 288–298.

Szagun, G. (2004). Learning by ear: On the acquisition of case and gender marking by German-speaking children with normal hearing and with cochlear implants. *Journal of Child Language, 31,* 1–30.

Tyler, R., Fryauf-Bertschy, H., Kelsay, D., Gantz, B., Woodworth, G., & Parkinson, A. (1997). Speech perception by prelingually deaf children using cochlear implants. *Otoryngology-Head and Neck Surgery, 117,* 180–187.

Section III

CUEING FOR NATURAL LANGUAGE ACQUISITION

Chapter 7

EARLY LINGUISTIC INPUT RECEIVED BY A DEAF CHILD EXPOSED TO LA PALABRA COMPLEMENTADA DURING THE PRELINGUISTIC PERIOD

Ignacio Moreno-Torres and Santiago Torres-Monreal

Language Development of Deaf Children

Hearing children of hearing parents have contact with oral language before birth (Bijeljac-Babic, Bertoncini, & Mehler, 1993; Christophe, Mehler, & Sebastian-Gallés, 2001; Mehler, Jusczyk, Lambertz, Halsted, Bertoncini, & Amiel-Tison, 1988; Nazzi, Bertoncini, & Mehler, 1998; Peña et al., 2003). Then, during their first months of life, they receive the necessary oral input to acquire language. In the first years of life, and until the child has acquired language, most adults and older children tend to communicate with the infant using a specific register that has been called *motherese*, *baby talk*, or simply *child-directed speech*. Among other features (Anula,

1998), motherese involves a lower speech tempo, clearer articulation and higher pitch, simpler sentence structure, repetitions, and a reduced lexicon.

As some cultures do not use motherese (Heath, 1983), we may assume that although motherese might facilitate language acquisition (Kuhl, 2000), it is not *necessary* for language acquisition. However, some amount of linguistic input *is* absolutely necessary. Typical language acquisition offers positive evidence: children learn the language that they receive. Negative evidence comes from language delays in children who receive no input (Goldin-Meadow, 2003) or poor input, as is often the case of children who are deaf with hearing parents, who comprise 95% of the deaf population (Mitchell & Karchmer, 2004). Compared with the hearing infant, the infant who is deaf receives less input and of a degraded quality. Due to this poor input, children who are deaf typically accumulate a delay in language acquisition. The delay tends to increase with time, at least until some augmentative or compensatory measures are adopted, including: (1) technical devices, such as cochlear implants, (2) an early intervention speech and language rehabilitation program, and/or (3) home-based use of an augmentative communication system, such as Cued Speech or Manually Coded English (MCE). After the adoption of these measures, a concerted effort must be made by parents and other caregivers to provide linguistic input before critical periods have passed (Locke, 1997).

An important variable during the critical language learning period is parent motivation (Spencer, 2004). The importance of family motivation is evident when we consider what typically happens once the aforementioned measures have been adopted, and assuming the infant is under two years of age. As regards assistive listening devices, they are fitted and checked by specialist doctors who will examine the child on only a few occasions. Language rehabilitation programs are carried out by language educators who might work at most five hours a week with the child. Finally, the use of an augmentative communication system requires parents to participate actively and to use it throughout the day with the child. For this reason, it is important that parents understand the importance and implications of their decision regarding which communication system to use.

The Need to Support Oral Language

During the last 15 years, we have seen important health, educational, and tech-nological changes that have motivated a resurgence of interest in oral approaches. Neonatal universal screening has made it possible to detect deafness in the early stages of life, resulting in the implementation of programs at a very early age. Furthermore, the use of cochlear implants has expanded greatly in many countries. Cochlear implants have been shown to provide important benefits for *speech perception* (e.g., Blamey, Sarant, et al., 2001), *production* (e.g., Blamey, Barry, et al., 2001; Horga & Liker, 2006), *linguistic development* (e.g., Connor, 2006), and *intelligibility* (Descourtieux, Groh, Rusterholtz, Simoulin, & Busquet, 1999).

Despite the important technological advances related especially to cochlear implants (summarized in Chapter 6), it is important to note that many children fitted with cochlear implants do not reach normal linguistic levels. For instance, Szagun (2001) studied a group of children who received a cochlear implant before the age of 4 years and found that 55% of the children in her study remained at the stage of two-word utterances even after three years of language development with the implants. Some researchers have observed very specific grammatical deficits in deaf children fitted with cochlear implants. For instance, Svirsky, Lynne, Ying, Lento, and Leonard (2002) compared the use of grammatical bound morphemes (such as the –s for plural in *boys*) and free grammatical morphemes (such as the copulative verb *is*) in hearing and deaf children. They found that hearing children made more errors with free verbal morphemes, while deaf children made more errors with number bound morphemes. Szagun (2004) compared the errors made by deaf children fitted with a cochlear implant with the errors made by hearing children with the same mean length of utterance

(MLU). In hearing children, errors of case predominated, while in deaf children, most common errors were gender and article omission. Note that these errors appear in the simplest syntactic structures, such as the combination of a determinant and a noun. As these structures are needed to build almost any other syntactic structure, it is easy to see that the effects of this deficit will negatively affect almost any complex structure. Both Svirsky and colleagues, and Szagun suggest that the limitations of hearing children might be related to differences in perceptual saliency, that is, children make more errors with particles which are difficult to perceive, such as articles or bound morphemes.

It should be noted that not all researchers have confirmed the perceptual saliency hypothesis. In a recent study of the acquisition of the phoneme system in Cantonese, Barry, Blamey, and Fletcher (2006) examined the linguistic, articulatory, and perceptual factors determining the rate and order of vowel acquisition. Factors associated with articulatory difficulty were shown to explain the composition of preimplant vowel inventories. Subsequent to receiving an implant, all children demonstrated a steady and systematic expansion in the size of their vowel inventories, though the rate of acquisition varied between individuals. The order of vowel acquisition was affected by a combination of linguistic and articulatory factors. More research is needed to explain why children fitted with a cochlear implant show such grammatical deficits as observed by Szagun, and Svirsky and colleagues.

In summary, educational and technologic advances have placed deaf children in a much better position than their predecessors to acquire oral language, but this position is still not comparable to that of normally hearing children (see Chapter 6). As Blamey, Barry, et al. (2001) note, only 22 electrodes do the work of thousands of hair cells, which reduces the amount of information for acoustic structure that can be transmitted to the auditory cortex for further processing. In this context, an important question for parents, educators, and researchers is this: how can we support oral language development after implantation?

Communication Modes to Support Oral Language

Communication modes used in oral-language based interaction with deaf children have been dichotomized into oral communication (OC) approaches and total communication (TC) approaches (Geers, 2005). As Geers notes, proponents of OC approaches maintain that dependence on speech and audition is critical for achieving maximum auditory benefit from any sensory aid. Proponents of the TC approach maintain that the deaf child benefits most when some form of signing accompanies speech.

Oral communication approaches differ from one another in their emphasis on the auditory and visual channels for the reception of spoken language, ranging from Cued Speech (only visual) to the auditory-verbal approach, in which lipreading is discouraged. Given that there are a number of oral communication approaches (see Beattie, 2006 for a review), and that our objective here is to analyze the benefits of Cued Speech, we divide oral communication approaches into Cued Speech (CS) and non-Cued Speech (NCS) oral approaches.

Some researchers have studied the benefits of different approaches (CS, NCS, and TC) when used with cochlear implants. Leybaert, Colin, and Hage (Chapter 6 in this volume) found that the use of Cued Speech in combination with a cochlear implant improves *speech perception* (Descourtieux, 2003), speech *intelligibility* (Cochard, 2003; Vieu, Mondain, Blanchard, Sillon, Reuillard-Artières, & Tobey, 1998), and *linguistic development* (Le Normand, 2003). All of these results suggest that children can benefit from a multimodal (visual/auditive) phonological input.

Some studies have compared TC and NCS approaches in deaf children fitted with a cochlear implant (see Geers, 2005 for a review). For instance, Connor, Hieber, Arts, and Zwolan (2000) studied 147 children (1–10 years) placed in TC and OC settings. TC programs were defined as programs that used some form of signing in addition to spoken language. OC programs were defined as programs that used spoken language without the reliance on signing. The authors found an advantage in vocabulary for TC children. However, other researchers (e.g., Moog, 2002) have observed that oral approaches can be very effective in terms of children reaching levels closely approximate to those of hearing age mates. More research is needed to evaluate the benefits of each educational approach, especially in the case of Cued Speech.

It is important to note that the lack of experimental data regarding educational approaches might reflect a loss of interest in the field. It can be speculated that the impressive success of cochlear implants has had the effect of minimizing the importance of communication support, both in families and in researchers. As for families, the authors have had the opportunity to observe, both in Spain and in the United States, that once a child has been implanted, the family tends to stop using augmentative communication systems.

As for research, Schauwers, Gillis, Daemers, Beukelaer, and Govaerts (2004), describe a girl implanted bilaterally (at 5 and 15 months respectively). The authors do not mention the communication mode used to support oral language communication at all, suggesting to us that the researchers do not view this variable to be critical.

As there are few experimental data about the three approaches (CS, NCS, and TC) when used with a cochlear implant, it is useful to examine how each approach enriches the linguistic input provided by the cochlear implant. Note that we will not describe all the features of each system. Instead, we concentrate on the linguistic nature of the input provided by each approach. Given the key role of phonology for language acquisition (Leybaert, 1998), we pay special attention to phonology. The hearing child develops phonology mainly with oral input received primarily through the ears. The aim of the cochlear implant is to emulate this process; however, to the extent that the cochlear implant is not providing clear phonological information, the deaf child cannot be expected to acquire all the phonemes or the child might acquire them too slowly. Different strategies are used by each approach (NCS, CS, and TC) to enhance phonological information provided by the cochlear implant.

NCS Approaches

Generally speaking, NCS approaches stimulate the child to concentrate on the sound production, but they do not provide a comparable phonological input alternative to that provided by speech. Note that use of prosodic visual input, as in Verbotonal (Guberina & Asp, 1981), or even lipreading if present, are not at all equivalent-to-phonological input. Thus, for a child fitted with a cochlear implant and educated in a NCS setting, the only phonological input is that provided by the cochlear implant. As this input is incomplete, one might ask whether the NCS approaches produce any direct benefit in terms of the linguistic input received by the child.

Cued Speech Approach

Cued Speech offers an appealing alternative to NCS approaches by providing a full visual representation of the phonemic input (Cornet, 1967). Cued Speech is an oral-based system comprised of a limited series of handshapes used together with the lipreading of normal speech. See Chapter 2 for a detailed description of Cued Speech. Cued Speech was created by Cornett (1967) with the aim of offering a possible solution to oral communication between deaf children and their parents, mainly in the early years. Children exposed to Cued Speech have been found to develop phonological abilities comparable to hearing peers (Santana, 1999; Santana, Torres, & García, 2003). See Chapters 11 to 14 in this volume for summaries of research related to phonological abilities of deaf students from Cued Speech backgrounds. Thus, Cued Speech is an ideal complement to cochlear implants in that Cued Speech visually conveys to the child the phonological information that cannot be perceived or distinguished auditorily via the cochlear implant alone. The task of the cochlear implant is to link acoustic cues to phonemes, while the task of Cued Speech in the collaboration is to link visual cues with phonemes.

TC Approach

TC systems combine spoken language syntax with sign vocabulary. The signs in TC approaches are borrowed from signed languages such as ASL; and thus are an alternative lexicon to the spoken language lexicon. The use of signs can have an impact on the development of symbolic processing, but they do not collaborate directly in the development of phonology. Thus, if a child fitted with a cochlear implant is educated in a TC setting, development of phonology would depend mostly on the input received from the cochlear implant. Lipreading, available in TC approaches, provides some phonetic input; however, several studies have shown that lipreading by itself is insufficient for speech perception (Charlier, Hage, Alegría, & Périer, 1990; Nicholls & Ling, 1982; Villalba, Fernández, & Ross, 1996), which typically is not enough to develop a complete, accurate phonology.

In short, both NCS and TC systems are limited in terms of optimizing the incomplete phonetic input of the cochlear implant. The main advantage of Cued Speech is precisely that it collaborates with the cochlear implant in the development of phonological representations which serve as the foundation for morphological, syntactic, and semantic aspects of English, Spanish, or any other spoken language.

Potential Difficulties for Early Use of Cued Speech by Hearing Parents

In order to make an efficient use of Cued Speech, parents must overcome certain potential obstacles (Torres, Moreno-Torres, & Santana, 2006). First, parents must learn Cued Speech in a short period of time. Second, they must use it to communicate efficiently. Learning Cued Speech is relatively simple, compared to learning MCE sign systems because: (1) little memory is required to learn the handshapes and placements needed to produce a closed set of phonemes; (2) there is no need to learn new grammatical rules because Cued Speech uses the rules of spoken language; and for the same reasons, (3) there is no need to learn a new vocabulary as is needed in TC approaches (see Chapter 12 for a comparison of Cued Speech and MCE sign systems). In general, after 1 to 3 months' practice, parents are able to begin using Cued Speech with their children (Torres, Moreno-Torres, & Santana, 2006).

There are three potential obstacles for parents becoming efficient Cued Speech communicators: first, it may be difficult for parents initially to use Cued Speech all of the time until they become accustomed to it; however, in our experience, it is probable that they will get used to it after some weeks or months of practice. A second potential obstacle relates to the fact that Cued Speech is a manual communication system in which the hands must also be used for other activities, such as object manipulation and gesturing. It seems inevitable that the adult cuer will leave a part of the oral production uncued. We have found, however, due to the characteristic redundancy of oral language input, this should not be a problem. A third potential obstacle for effective communication via Cued Speech is the need for visual contact. The deaf child who uses a visual communication mode cannot look at an object while it is being described. For this reason the child will have to look sequentially (Gallaway, 1998; Harris, 2000; Mohay, 2000). Here, we find an important difference with hearing children, who may look at an object while it is described (Tomasello & Farrar, 1986). It has been observed (Swisher, 1992) that native sign-ing deaf mothers maximize visual contact with different strategies (i.e., changing the position of objects, placing signs in the visual field, waiting for attention, etc.). We have observed that cueing mothers use similar strategies when cueing to their deaf child.

In brief, despite Cued Speech being a relatively easy system to learn, intensive use of Cued Speech requires a certain amount of effort by the parents who will need to adapt themselves to the visual communication channel, and will have to learn new strategies to maximize interaction with their children. In addition, the presence of a cochlear implant might have a negative effect on visual contact; that is, as the deaf child may receive input without actually looking at the subject in question, the child might not pay as much attention as she or he would if the only input were visual.

Our Research Related to Language Input

Until recently, most of the research related to Cued Speech has examined the positive effects of Cued Speech on different aspects of language perception and production, and on reading (see Chapters 11 and 12 for summaries of that research). Comparisons of cueing children with other groups of deaf children show that generally speaking, children exposed to Cued Speech have good language and reading levels. An implication of these results is that children exposed to Cued Speech must have received adequate linguistic input; however, no researchers before our team (Torres, Moreno-Torres, & Santana, 2006) had examined in detail the nature of the linguistic input that deaf children receive via Cued Speech. Our research focuses on determining why Cued Speech appears to work so well.

Our methodology differs from previous Cued Speech research. For instance, research by Alegría and colleagues from the Université Libre de Bruxelles (Alegría, Charlier, & Mattys, 1995; Leybaert & Alegria, 2003) have used test-based experimental methodologies. Tests have the advantage of allowing researchers to control different variables and study specific effects. Certain phenomena, however, involve too many variables, and it is not easy to control all of them in the laboratory. This is the case of interactions of a mother with her prelinguistic child. For this reason, our research on linguistic input has used a corpus-based methodology. The subjects are videotaped in their natural context, and then the interactions are transcribed. In order to analyze the interactions, the productions (e.g., oral words, cues, gestures) and several other details of research interest are explicitly identified using a standard coding norm (MacWhinney, 2000). Videos are recorded on a weekly or monthly basis, depending on the objectives of the research. The videos are 30 minutes in length. The full coding scheme and other general criteria are described in Moreno-Torres and Torres (2005). Part of the material produced by the authors can be downloaded from the Child Language Data Exchange System (CHILDES) Project Database (http://childes.psy.cmu.edu/).

Using this methodology, we have examined several questions related to the linguistic input received by children exposed to Cued Speech. In one line of research (Torres et al., 2006), we examined the quantity and the linguistic quality of the input received through Cued Speech.

We compared the production of two adults (a mother and a speech-language therapist), in their interaction with a deaf girl. We assumed that in order for the mother to provide her daughter with rich input, her cued production should be as similar as possible to her own oral production, and also to that of the therapist. The next section of this chapter summarizes the major findings from this study. Another line of research (Moreno-Torres, Torres, & Santana, 2006) explored the impact of Cued Speech on other forms of input. We compared data from the mother-child dyad in the previous study with data from a mother-child dyad that employs a NCS approach. The comparison between these two dyads offered interesting data regarding the amount of oral input and gestures produced by each mother. The final section summarizes some results of this study.

Cued Input in the Prelinguistic Period

In our first study, we examined the nature of the input received by a deaf child exposed to Cued Speech in the final part of her prelinguistic period (18–25 months). Our primary hypothesis was that parents who use Cued Speech are able to provide a significant amount of linguistically rich input. The subject of this study started a Cued Speech-based rehabilitation program, referred to as Oral Cued Model (MOC; see http://www.uma.es/moc) when she was 14 months and 15 days. The child was fitted with a cochlear implant when she was 17 months old. In all, we examined 15 sessions recorded at home, and 15 sessions recorded in the lab. The last four sessions

(Figure 7–1) of this study coincide with a lexical burst (i.e., a sudden increase in the number of words produced by a child), which suggests that the input provided in these 30 weeks was enough to initiate the language acquisition process.

Quantity of the Input

Data were obtained for the following five variables: *oral input, cued input, cued ratio, attended input,* and *attended ratio. Oral input* refers to word tokens produced orally by adults; *cued input* represents the number of oral tokens that were cued; *cued ratio* represents the proportion of oral tokens that were cued; *attended input* refers to the number of oral tokens that were cued by the adults and attended by the deaf child; and *attended ratio* represents the proportion of oral words that were cued by the adult and attended by the child. The number of *word tokens* refers to the total number of words produced. The number of *word types* refers to the number of different words produced.

Mean oral input was above 1,300 word tokens per session for the therapist, and above 1,000 for the mother; both adults cued more than 60% of their oral input; the girl attended more than 55% of the oral tokens (i.e., more than 86% of total cued tokens) produced by the adults (Table 7–1). Differences between the therapist and mother were significant for oral input ($U = 52$, $p = .011$, Mann-Whitney U-test) and attended ratio ($U = 49$, $p = .008$), but not for cued ratio ($U = 70$, $p = .078$); that is, the therapist and mother cued the same proportion of words.

Throughout all 15 sessions with each adult there was an important progression in the attended input both for the therapist and the mother. Linear regression analysis (Figure 7–2) showed that this progression was significant both for the therapist ($\beta_{session} = 46$; $p < .001$) and the mother ($\beta_{session} = 27$; $p < .001$). Since progression is significant in both adults, it might indicate a change in the girl. The more her attentional capacity increases, the more the adults communicate.

Analysis of attended ratio showed a progression in the therapist ($\beta_{session} = .52$;

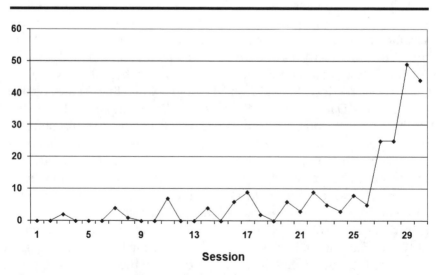

Figure 7–1. Lexical production of B (18–25 months).

Table 7–1. Input Quantity of Therapist (*n* = 15) and Mother (*n* = 15)

Speaker	Word Production			Standard Deviation		
	Oral	Cued	Cued + Att	Oral	Cued	Cued + Att
THE	1,370.8	.62	.6	280.1	.1	.09
MOT	1,086.9	.64	.55	241.0	.09	.07
	$p = .011*$	$p = .078$	$p = .008*$			

Source: From Torres, S., Moreno-Torres, I., and Santana, R. (2006). Quantitative and qualitative evaluation of linguistic input support to a prelingually deaf child with Cued Speech: A case study. *Journal of Deaf Studies and Deaf Education, 11,* 438–448. Reprinted with permission.

*Statistically significant.

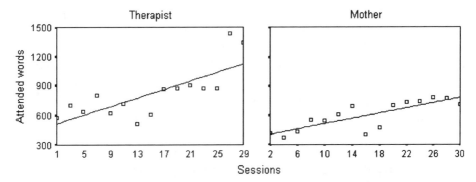

Figure 7–2. Attended input per adults. From Torres, S., Moreno-Torres, I., and Santana, R. (2006). Quantitative and qualitative evaluation of linguistic input support to a prelingually deaf child with Cued Speech: A case study. *Journal of Deaf Studies and Deaf Education, 11,* 438–448. Reprinted with permission.

$p < .047$), but not in the mother ($\beta_{session} = .39$; $p < .145$). These results suggest that as time passed, the mother did not seem to adapt her strategies to augment the child's attention.

Grammatical Quality and Lexical Variety

To determine input quality, Torres and colleagues examined the mean length of utterance (MLU) of oral and cued input, as well as the frequency of major word classes (lexical, grammatical, and pragmatic words). MLU traditionally has been used to reflect syntactic complexity of children's language (Brown, 1973) and child-directed adult language (Snow, 1995). In this study, MLU was used to compare the syntactic complexity of oral input versus cued input. Note that if speakers leave part of the utterances uncued, oral MLU should be higher than MLU for cued production. Note also that a common feature of motherese register is low MLU. In order to obtain reliable MLU values, utterances were divided according to strict criteria. Every full sentence was coded as an independent utterance. Linguistic expressions which do not have a syntactic function in a sentence (i.e., pragmatic markers, interjections, salutations, and any word produced alone) were also coded as independent utterances. MLU was obtained both for oral input and for cued input (Table 7–2).

MLU values were always lower for oral input than for cued input. This difference was significant both for the therapist (t (14) = –2.287, p = .038) and for the mother (t (14) = –3.617, p = .003). This finding might be caused by two linguistic properties of cued input. On the one hand, speakers often tended to leave pragmatic expressions uncued. As these expressions are generally one word utterances, oral MLU tends to decrease. On the other hand, speakers tended to cue every word in each utterance, which tends to increase cued MLU. It is worth noting that no significant differences were found between the mother and therapist either for oral MLU (U = 84, p = .250) or for cued MLU (U = 88, p = .310). Such results suggest a considerable similarity between the mother and the therapist in terms of the syntactic complexity of their input.

In order to analyze the frequency of word classes, the 100 most frequently cued words of each adult were examined. Each word was classified according to its primary linguistic function: pragmatic, grammatical, or lexical. Torres et al. omitted words that admitted double classification such as *vale* (which in Spanish can stand for *O.K.* or for the lexical *to cost*). Words used to guide linguistic interaction or to express emotions were classified as pragmatic: interjection (*ah, oh,* etc.), discourse markers (*a ver,* let's see), and attention-getters (the girl's name, the imperative form *mira* look, etc.) which are common in interaction with deaf children (Gallaway & Woll, 1994). Deictic words such as *aquí* (here) and *allí* (there) were also included in the pragmatic group, as they were very often used with POINT gestures, and play a central role in guiding the child to the appropriate objects. Grammatical words included pronouns, articles, determiners, prepositions, conjunctions, and auxiliary and copulative verbs.

Analysis of the 100 most frequent words showed that the pragmatic group represented 32% of the therapist's production, and 34% of the mother's produc-

Table 7–2. Global Input Quality of Therapist and Mother

Speaker	MLU		% Cued		
	Oral	Cued	Pragmatic	Lexical	Grammatical
THE	1.6	2.31	.41	.65	.63
MOT	1.49	2.12	.35	.62	.69

Source: From Torres, S., Moreno-Torres, I., and Santana, R. (2006). Quantitative and qualitative evaluation of linguistic input support to a prelingually deaf child with Cued Speech: A case study. *Journal of Deaf Studies and Deaf Education, 11,* 438–448. Reprinted with permission.

tion. The rest were lexical or grammatical words. As Table 7–2 shows, words classified as pragmatic were not cued as often as grammatical or lexical ones. Noncueing pragmatic and deictic expressions can be related to the nature of these expressions, often produced to express emotions and used with natural gestures. This was the case with deictic *aquí* (here) and attention-getter *mira* (look), which were often produced with a POINT gesture. The low percentage of cueing pragmatic expressions summed to their high frequency also may explain the low MLU values obtained for uncued production.

In order to examine the lexical variety of the input received by the child, the authors obtained the number of types (different words) and tokens (total number of words) attended by the child. The total number of word tokens produced by the therapist in her 15 sessions was the largest for the two adults (20,562, $M = 1,371$ per session, $SD = 280.09$ vs. 16,304, $M = 1,087$ per session, $SD = 240.97$). The therapist's number of word types, however, was the smallest (1,281 vs. 1,511). This difference may be related to the fact that the therapist always interacted with the girl in the same context, while the mother interacted in varied functional contexts (playing, eating, etc.). The percentage of attended tokens with respect to oral tokens ranged between 55% to 60%. But the percentage of attended types rose to 83% for both adults, which shows that B was receiving a varied lexicon.

Quality of the Cued Speech Input for the Deaf Child

As we noted in the introduction, in order for Cued Speech to be effective, some potential obstacles must be overcome: (1) the parents must achieve a good command of Cued Speech; (2) parents and therapists must cue a large proportion of their oral input; and 3) the child must pay attention to the adults. Our data show that the mother's command of Cued Speech was equivalent to that of the therapist. Both adults cued the same proportion of oral words. Both show the same MLU for oral and cued input. Both use a similar proportion of lexical, grammatical, and pragmatic expressions, each group being cued to the same proportion. The main difference between the adults refers to the number of words produced per session, which is significantly higher in the therapist. It is important to note at this point that the mother had been using Cued Speech for only two months prior to the start of the project, whereas the therapist had 10 years' experience. In this context, results confirm that Cued Speech is not a barrier to effective communication, as a mother with little experience may learn Cued Speech very quickly. Our data also show that cued production is *linguistically rich*. Specifically, the proportion of cued tokens was 65% for the therapist and 62% for the mother. The quality of the input is confirmed lexically and grammatically. Adults cued 83% of the oral word types, which shows that the input is lexically rich. As for grammatical input, adults cued more grammatical tokens (63% for the therapist and 69% for the mother) than pragmatic expressions (41% for the therapist and 35% for the mother). This difference between grammatical and pragmatic words, and the fact that the MLU of Cued Speech input was significantly higher than the MLU of oral production for both adults, suggests that the input is grammatically rich. Finally, the results show that the child attended to a very high proportion of the input produced by the adults. Results also show that the adults often used attention-getters and the strategy of utterance repetition. Altogether, these results confirm the hypothesis that adults who use Cued Speech are able to provide a significant amount of linguistically rich input.

Effects of Cued Speech on Oral Production and Use of Natural Gestures

In a second line of research, we explored the potential influence of Cued Speech on adult-child communication. On one hand, we examined whether Cued Speech might have a negative impact on other forms of input (i.e., oral production and natural gestures). On the other hand, we explored whether Cued Speech had a positive impact on early symbol processing, which is an essential area of language development.

Regarding the impact on input, it could be speculated that oral production might be reduced because parents must make a greater effort to communicate with cues than would be needed without cueing. Also, use of Cued Speech might have a negative impact on gesture production, as they are both manual (Mohay, 1990). Regarding symbol processing, it has been suggested that natural gestures and manually coded English (MCE) signs may be helpful in promoting symbol processing (Szagun, 2001). However, Hage, and Leybaert (2006) note that Cued Speech might also be used to promote symbol processing. We explored this possibility.

In order to study the potential advantages and disadvantages of Cued Speech, we compared the input and production of the girl in the study summarized above with another girl with similar characteristics, except for the communication mode (Moreno-Torres, Torres, & Santana, 2006). The second girl participating in these studies was educated under a NCS setting, with no help from visual input (i.e., no signs). The two girls were very similar for other important variables: level of deafness, age of deafness (birth), age at cochlear implant programming (NCS: 15 months; CS: 17 months). Neither family had a history of deafness. Both girls had an older sibling (NCS: sister 7 years older; CS: brother 18 months older). Both families were very much involved in the language development of the girls. In both cases the mothers were the girls' main communication partner.

Our initial objective was to analyze the subjects for one year, in 13 sessions; however, when the NCS subject was 23 months old (after 7 sessions), her parents decided to start a Cued Speech rehabilitation program because they felt that their daughter was developing slowly compared with other children of her age. For that reason, only seven sessions were used to compare the dyads. However, the NCS parents provided two further videotapes. In the last of these two sessions, the mother used Cued Speech for the first time. This last session was analyzed separately.

Given that there were some differences in the duration of the videos, the results were normalized assuming the same duration in all files. For this reason there are some differences between quantity results in this section and those in the previous section. Criteria to identify gestures followed Butcher and Goldin-Meadow (2000). These authors classify gestures as iconic, deictic, conventional, and ritual. Only the first three types were included in the calculations.

Oral and Gesture Input

Oral and gestural input produced by adults was examined. We hypothesized that both adults would provide similar oral input, but differences might be found in manual input. If our hypotheses were confirmed, differences in the girls' language production should be related to nonoral input (Cued Speech and/or natural gestures). Examination of the quantity of oral input of both mothers confirmed that there were not significant differences (i.e., both mothers produced approximately the same number of words per session). Throughout the 7 sessions, there was an important progression in the number of words produced, which was statistically significant for both mothers (NCS: $\beta_{session}$ = 149.8; p = .017; CS: $\beta_{session}$ = 77.6; p = .042).

In order to detect grammatical differences, MLU was calculated. For both mothers, MLU was very low (Table 7–3), as expected for a motherese register (Anula, 1998). The difference between the mothers' MLU was statistically significant; however, from a linguistic point of view, the differences might reflect individual differences, as the difference between child directed language MLU and adult directed language MLU was similar in both mothers. Throughout the seven sessions, the MLU of the NCS mother increased significantly ($\beta_{session}$ = .08; p = .002), whereas the MLU for the CS mother remained stable ($\beta_{session}$ = .01; p = .736). In order to have a more precise idea of the use of grammatical particles, a selection of the 100 most frequent words used by each mother was classified in three groups (lexical, grammatical, and pragmatic). As shown in Figure 7–3, both mothers used each group with similar frequencies.

In order to detect differences in lexical variation, the number of types (different words) and tokens (total words) produced by each mother was calculated. As noted above, the total number of tokens was higher in the NCS mother (11,907) than in the CS mother (10,605). However, the number of types was higher in the CS mother (978) than in the NCS mother (767). This result might indicate that the CS mother had a richer vocabulary, but there were no reasons to believe that the effect is caused by the use of Cued Speech.

Examination of gesture production (Figure 7–4) showed that the NCS mother produced significantly more gestures than the CS mother (M_{NCS} = 107.7; M_{CS} = 65.5; Mann-Whitney U = 1.0; z = -3.003; p = .003).

Table 7–3. Word Tokens and MLU of the Mothers

Speaker	Words		MLU	
	M	SD	M	SD
NCS	1701.1	383.1	2.331	0.19
CS	1515.3	217.0	1.903	0.16
			p = .002*	

*Statistically significant.

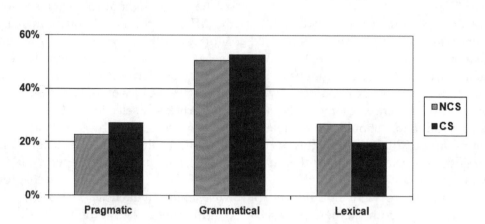

Figure 7–3. Word groups used by NCS and CS mothers.

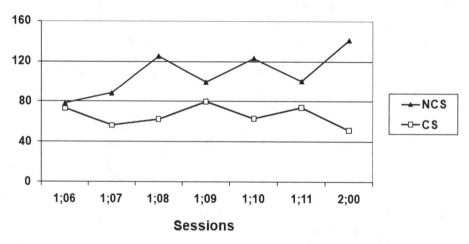

Figure 7–4. Number of gestures per session produced by the mothers.

Gesture production by the NCS mother increased throughout the 7 sessions ($\beta_{session}$ = 7.5; p = .067), although variation does not reach statistic significance. Gesture production in the CS mother remained stable ($\beta_{session}$ = 1.0; p = .645). The ratio of gestures per 100 oral words was 6.3 for the NCS mother and 4.4 for the CS mother, showing that despite the differences and variations, both mothers produced most input orally.

For both mothers, deictic gestures were the most common ones (M_{NCS} = 70.3%; M_{CS} = 56.6%), while iconic gestures represented only 15.5% in the NCS mother and 13.3% in the CS mother. Given that iconic gestures might promote symbol processing, the full list of these gestures was obtained for both mothers. The NCS mother produced 117 iconic gestures, whereas the CS mother produced 61. The major difference in gesture production appears in the gestures used to describe actions. The NCS mother produced 57 gestures of this type, while the CS mother produced only 19. An important subgroup of iconic gestures in both mothers was animal gestures. Overall, the CS mother produced 28 animal gestures for 13 different animals. The NCS mother produced 27 gestures for 19 different animals. In both cases the gestures were understandable only in context.

Use of Cued Speech as a Lexical Visual Augmentative System

In a study currently in progress, we are exploring the possibility that Cued Speech can be used as a lexical visual augmentative system. The study examines the use of a set of 69 onomatopoeias (see http://www.uma.es/moc). Standard onomatopoeias are commonly used to name animals in baby-talk in many languages (i.e., the name for dog in Spanish is /guau/, for cat /miau/). Torres and colleagues have extended this list to include a large portion of Spanish syllables. As most of these onomatopoeias are monosyllabic, each one is cued with a unique complement (i.e., a unique combination of *handshape + hand position + lip shape*). This feature makes this set of onomatopoeias fairly similar to many signs used in total communication.

Examination of how often the adults used this set of complements showed that both CS adults used them intensively (20 per session for the mother, and 50 for the CS therapist). Examination of the last video recorded by the NCS mother—two

months after Cued Speech rehabilitation —showed that the only words she was cueing were onomatopoeias. Note that she had been instructed to cue all words, but instead she seemed to have memorized this closed set. It is also important to note that use of these tokens does not necessarily involve phonological processing. However, the possibility is there for the child to process them phonologically or lexically. In sum, results show that Cued Speech can be used to provide a rich symbolic input (and not only a rich phonological input).

Oral and Gesture Output

The first symbols produced by children are *natural gestures* (Caselli & Volterra, 1990; Volterra, Caselli, Capirci, & Pizzuto, 2005). In hearing children, gestures appear before words, but soon the amount of oral production surpasses gesture production both in the number of types and in the combination of more than one symbol. Capirci, Iverson, Pizzuto, and Volterra (1996) studied oral and gesture production in a group of hearing children 16 to 20 months of age and found that while the number of gestures remained stable, oral production exceeded gesture production in 91.6% of the children. Such results contrast with those observed in deaf children. Mohay (1990) studied two deaf children of hearing parents 20 to 30 months of age. In both children, gesture production remained the main communication mode. Furthermore, the increase in gesture production is more important, which makes it unclear whether oral production will ever exceed gesture production. Goldin-Meadow (2003) observed that children with no oral input continue using gestures as their main communicative means, creating a gesture lexicon and a gesture grammar. Such results show that when linguistic input is poor, children tend to communicate with gestures. Results obtained by Moreno-Torres et al. (2006) suggest that whereas the CS girl follows a pattern similar to that of hearing children, the pattern of the NCS girl might follow a different trend (Figure 7–5).

In the first three sessions, both girls used almost no words and between 8 and 21 gestures. In the next sessions their communication trends differ considerably. The number of gestures in the NCS girl increases significantly ($\beta_{session}$ = 8.3; p = .014), whereas the number in the CS girl remains stable ($\beta_{session}$ =.53; p = .711). In the last two sessions the NCS girl produced less than five words, whereas the CS girl produced 28 in the last session alone.

Deictic gestures were the most common ones in both girls; they represented just over 60% in each girl. In the NCS girl, iconic gestures represented 34%, whereas in the CS girl they represented 13.2% of the total number of gestures. These results suggest that the NCS girl might be starting to use a gesture vocabulary which was not present in the CS girl. The most important features of the trend observed in the NCS girl were confirmed in a session taped when she was 25 months old. In that session she produced only 10 words and again a large number of gestures.

In sum, patterns of language acquisition are fairly different in each girl. Although the CS girl follows the pattern observed in hearing children, the NCS girl shows a marked tendency to communicate with gestures. A possible explanation is that the NCS girl probably has the need to communicate, but her command of oral language is not enough to express herself; thus, she relies on gestures. This can be a consequence of poor input suggesting that the input received by the cochlear implant and the help of the NCS rehabilitation program was insufficient in this case.

Using Cues as Signs

In order to know whether Cued Speech was promoting symbolic processing, we examined the CS girl's first productions in a selection of sessions of the period 18 to 30 months. In this part of the corpus, the girl cued expressively on 39 occasions. Most of the cues (70%) were incorrect. In

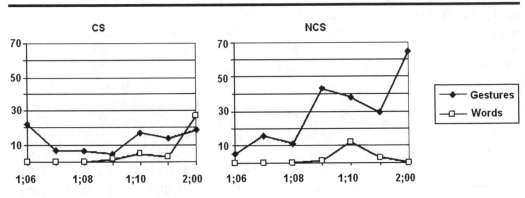

Figure 7–5. First gestures and words.

most cases, the girl produced the right position, or the right shape, but not both parameters at the same time. Also, in most cases (82%) the girl did not produce the correct syllable orally (i.e., the third parameter.) On all 39 occasions, she cued onomatopoeias. As noted above, given that these units are one-syllable words, therefore produced by a single manual complement, it is possible that the girl was not using phonology. She well could be producing unparseable units.

We also examined the video in which the NCS mother started to use Cued Speech. As noted above, in this video the mother hardly ever uses Cued Speech (4% of her oral production). All of her cued words are monosyllabic onomatopoeias. Examination of the NCS girl showed that she was using Cued Speech expressively. In fact she produces as many as 20 cued productions (50% of her oral production was cued). Also in this case, many cues are wrong in position or shape. However, the important point in this context is that the girl only uses Cued Speech actively with these onomatopoeias, which suggests that she might not be using phonology. These results suggest that Cued Speech can help children to produce their first words, even in the absence of good articulation.

Effects of Cued Speech: Some Conclusions

Despite the limited data that have been analyzed, the results summarized in this section offer new details about the differences in the input provided by adults depending on the communication mode used (CS versus NCS) and some advantages of Cued Speech. To date, our research has focused on getting answers to the following questions:

- Does the use of Cued Speech negatively affect the input produced orally by the adults?
- Does Cued Speech reduce the symbolic input received by the prelinguistic child?
- Does Cued Speech block a tendency toward gesture communication?
- Can Cued Speech promote symbolic processing?

In the case study reported in Torres et al. (2006), the adults' oral production is fairly similar both quantitatively and qualitatively. Quantitatively, both adults produced a similar number of words. Qualitatively, both adults used similar ratios of lexical and grammatical words, and their MLUs are similar in both cases. Furthermore, both adults showed some typical features of motherese: simple syntactic structures (confirmed by low MLU), and repetitions both of words and full sentences. Therefore, at least in this case, Cued Speech had *no* negative impact on the linguistic input produced by the parents.

Examination of gesture input showed that there were some differences between the mothers, the most important being that the NCS mother used significantly more gestures than the CS mother. It is possible, or even natural, that Cued Speech will reduce gesture input, as both are manual modes. However, our data show that Cued Speech and gestures are *not* incompatible. Moreover, as the CS mother uses Cued Speech to transmit symbols (especially onomatopoeias), the amount of symbolic visual input received by the CS child is by far more important than the one received by the NCS girl.

Examination of the word-gesture pattern showed important differences between the two girls. Although the NCS girl tended to communicate with gestures and significantly reduced her oral production, the CS girl showed her first lexical burst. It is important to be cautious with this result. Just two months after this last session, the NCS girl also showed a lexical burst. Cued Speech was used in 50% of the tokens produced. It is difficult to determine what caused this change in the girl. Several variables might have promoted the lexical burst. First, the mother became more relaxed when she started to use a different communication mode; second, Cued Speech may have helped the girl to produce her first symbols. Finally, it is possible that the girl's productions are recognizable now that she uses Cued Speech (i.e., previously they were too unintelligible to be understood). The final question relates to the children's first productions. Examination of the first symbols in both girls suggested that children used Cued Speech to produce their first symbols, possibly before they could have full phonological representations.

Conclusions

This chapter has summarized the research carried out by the MOC group on input received by children exposed to Cued Speech at an early age. Despite the scarce data available, results are promising regarding Cued Speech. Our study shows that parents can become competent cuers in a relatively short period of time (three months in our case study). With Cued Speech, adults can make a large part of the oral input visible. Use of Cued Speech does not negatively affect oral input, and Cued Speech can be used to encode full symbols. Results also suggest that use of Cued Speech might have a positive impact

on the adult-child interaction, with oral language being the main communicative mode as opposed to natural gestures. Finally, the results show that children may use Cued Speech to encode lexical symbols, as is done with MCE signs, in the prelinguistic period. This result shows that benefits of Cued Speech go farther than in its capacity to encode phonological input.

More research is needed in this area before we can explain why Cued Speech works and how we can best use it, not only with children who are deaf, but also, as reflected in Chapter 16, with other groups of children showing delay in language acquisition. For instance, it might be interesting to know which type of input best promotes language acquisition in the prelinguistic period. Another area of research is visual contact, and more specifically the best strategies to gain the children's attention. Finally, it is important to know more about the sensitive or critical periods for Cued Speech exposure. At least two questions need an answer here: (1) when can parents stop using Cued Speech without negatively affecting language acquisition and (2) how intensively should Cued Speech be used? Research related to linguistic input should help parents, early educators, and others in making the most of Cued Speech.

References

Alegría, J., Charlier, B., & Mattys, S. (1995). The role of lipreading and Cued Speech in the processing of phonological information in deaf children. *European Journal of Cognitive Psychology, 11*, 123–146.

Anula, A. (1998). *El abecé de la psicolingüística [Basic concepts of psycholinguistics]*. Madrid, Spain: Arco libros.

Barry, J. G., Blamey, P. J., & Fletcher, J. (2006). Factors affecting the acquisition of vowel phonemes by pre-linguistically deafened cochlear implant users learning Cantonese. *Clinical Linguistics & Phonetics, 20,* 761–780.

Beattie, R. (2006). The oral methods and spoken language acquisition. In P. Spencer & M. Marschark (Eds.), *Advances in the spoken language development of deaf and hard of hearing children* (pp. 103–135). New York, NY: Oxford University Press.

Bijeljac-Babic, R., Bertoncini, J., & Mehler, J. (1993). How do four-day-old infants categorize multisyllabic utterances? *Developmental Psychology, 29,* 711–723.

Blamey, P., Barry, J., Bow, C., Sarant, J., Paatsch, L., & Wales, R. (2001). The development of speech production following cochlear implantation. *Clinical Linguistics and Phonetics, 15,* 363–383.

Blamey, P., Sarant, J., Paatsch, L., Barry, J., Bow, C., Wales, R., . . . Tooher, R. (2001). Relationships among speech perception, production, language, hearing loss, and age in children with impaired hearing. *Journal of Speech, Language, and Hearing Research, 44,* 264–285.

Brown R. (1973). *A first language.* Cambridge, MA: Harvard University Press.

Butcher, C., & Goldin-Meadow, S. (2000). Gesture and the transition from one- to two-word speech: When hand and mouth come together. In D. McNeill (Ed.), *Language and gesture* (pp. 235–257). Cambridge, MA: Cambridge University Press.

Capirci, O., Iverson, J., Pizzuto, E., & Volterra, V. (1996). Gestures and words during the transition to two-word speech. *Journal of Child Language, 23,* 645– 673.

Caselli, M., & Volterra, V. (1990). From communication to language in hearing and Deaf Children. In C. Erting & V. Volterra (Eds.), *From gesture to language in hearing and deaf children* (pp. 263–277). Berlin, Germany: Springer.

Charlier, B., Hage, C., Alegría, J., & Périer, O. (1990). Evaluation d'une pratique prolongée du LPC sur la compréhension de la parole par l'enfant atteint de déficience auditive [Evaluation of the effects of prolonged cued cpeech practice upon the reception of oral language in deaf children]. *Glossa, 22,* 28–39.

Christophe, A., Mehler, J., & Sebastián-Gallés, N. (2001). Perception of prosodic boundary correlates by newborn infants. *Infancy, 2,* 385–394.

Cochard, N. (2003). Impact du LPC sur l'évolution des enfants implantés [Impact of Cued Speech on the development of implanted children]. *Actes des Journeés d'études Nantes, 40,* 65–77.

Connor, C. (2006). Examining the communication skills of a young cochlear implant pioneer. *Journal of Deaf Studies and Deaf Education, 11,* 449–460.

Connor, C., Hieber, S., Arts, H., & Zwolan, T. (2000). Speech, vocabulary, and the education of children using cochlear implants: Oral or total communication? *Journal of Speech, Language and Hearing Research, 43,* 1185–1204.

Cornett, R. O. (1967). Cued Speech. *American Annals of the Deaf, 112,* 3–13.

Descourtieux, C. (2003). Seize ans d'expérience pratique à CODALI: Evaluation-evolutions [Sixteen years of practical experience at CODALI: Evaluation-evolutions]. *Actes des Journées d'études Nantes, 40,* 77–88.

Descourtieux, V., Groh, A., Rusterholtz, I., Simoulin, D., & Busquet, D. (1999). Cued Speech in the stimulation of communication: An advantage in cochlear implantation. *International Journal of Pediatric Otorhinolaryngology, 47,* 205–207.

Gallaway, C. (1998). Early interaction. In A. Weisel (Ed.), *Insights into deaf education. Current theory and practice* (pp. 49–67). Tel Aviv, Israel: Academic Press of the School of Education, Tel Aviv University.

Gallaway, C., & Woll, B. (1994). Interaction and childhood deafness. In C. Gallaway & B. Richards (Eds.), *Input and interaction in language acquisition* (pp. 197–208). Cambridge, MA: Cambridge University Press.

Geers, A. (2005). Spoken language in children with cochlear implants. In P. Spencer & M. Marschark (Eds.), *Advances in the spoken language development of deaf and hard of hearing children* (pp. 244–270). Cary, NC: Oxford University Press.

Goldin-Meadow, S. (2003). *The resilience of language.* New York, NY: Psychology Press.

Guberina. P., & Asp, C. (1981). *The verbotonal method for rehabilitation people with communication problems.* New York, NY: Ed. World Rehabilitation Fund.

Hage, C., & Leybaert, J. (2006). The effects of Cued Speech on the development of spoken language. In P. Spencer & M. Marschark (Ed.), *Advances in the spoken language development of Deaf and hard of hearing children* (pp. 193–211). New York, NY: Oxford University Press.

Harris, M. (2000). Social interaction and early language development in deaf children. *Deafness and Education International, 2,* 1–11.

Heath, S. (1983). *Ways with words: Language, life, and work in communities and classrooms.* New York, NY: Cambridge University Press.

Horga, D., & Liker, M. (2006). Voice and pronunciation of cochlear implant speakers. *Clinical Linguistics & Phonetics, 20,* 211–217.

Kuhl, P. (2000). A new view of language acquisition. *Proceedings of the National Academy of Sciences, 97,* 11850–11857.

Le Normand, M. (2003). Acquisition du lexique chez l'enfant implanté [Acquisition of lexicon in implanted children]. *Actes des Journe'es d'études Nantes, 40,* 97–108.

Leybaert, J. (1998). Phonological representations in deaf children: The importance of early linguistic experience. *Scandinavian Journal of Psychology, 39,* 169–173.

Leybaert, J., & Alegría, J. (2003). The role of Cued Speech in language development of deaf children. In M. Marschark & P. Spencer (Eds.), *Oxford handbook of deaf studies, language, and education* (pp. 261–274). Oxford, UK: Oxford University Press.

Locke, J. (1997). A theory of neurolinguistic development. *Brain & Language, 58,* 265–326.

MacWhinney, B. (2000). *The CHILDES project: Tools for analyzing talk.* Mahwah, NJ: Lawrence Erlbaum Associates.

Mehler, J., Jusczyk, P., Lambertz, G., Halsted, N., Bertoncini, J., & Amiel-Tison, C. (1988). A precursor of language acquisition in young infants. *Cognition, 29,* 143–178.

Mitchell, R., & Karchmer, M. (2004). Chasing the mythical ten percent: Parental hearing status of deaf and hard of hearing students in the United States. *Sign Language Studies, 4,* 138–163.

Mohay, H. (1990). The interaction of gesture and speech in the language development of two profoundly deaf children. In C. Erting & V. Volterra (Eds.), *From gesture to language in hearing and deaf children* (pp. 187–204). Berlin, Germany: Springer.

Mohay, H. (2000). Language in sight: Mothers' trategies for making language visually accessible to deaf children. In P. Spencer, C. Erting, & M. Marschark (Eds.), *The deaf child in the family and at school* (pp. 151–166). Mahwah, NJ: Erlbaum.

Moog, J. (2002). Changing expectations for children with cochlear implants. *Annals of Otology, Rhinology, and Laryngology, 111,* 138–142.

Moreno-Torres, I., & Torres, S. (2005). *MOCHAT: Sistema de trascripción CHAT adaptado al MOC* [CHAT system adapted to Complemented Oral Model]. Retrieved April 29, 2008, from http://www.uma.es/moc/CorpusBl/mochat.pdf

Moreno-Torres, I, Torres, S., & Santana, R. (2006). Efectos de LPC en la interacción diádica adulto-oyente niño-sordo: Gestos espontáneos [Effects of Cued Speech in dyadic hearing adult-deaf child interaction: Spontaneous gestures]. In E. Mendoza & G. Carballo (Coords.), *25 Congreso Internacional de AELFA* (pp. 457–472). Granada, Spain: University of Granada.

Nazzi, T., Bertoncini, J., & Mehler, J. (1998). Language discrimination by newborns. Towards an understanding of the role of rhythm. *Journal of Experimental Psychology: Human Perception and Performance, 24,* 1–11.

Nicholls, G., & Ling, D. (1982). Cued Speech and the reception of spoken language. *Journal of Speech and Hearing Research, 25,* 262–269.

Peña, M., Maki, A., Kovaãiç, D., Dehaene-Lambertz, G., Koizumi, H., Bouquet, F., & Mehler, J. (2003). Sounds and silence: An optical topography study of language recognition at birth. *Proceedings of the National Academy of Science, 100,* 11702–11705.

Santana, R. (1999). *Papel de La Palabra Complementada en el desarrollo y uso de las representaciones fonológicas en el sordo* [The role of Cued Speech on the development and use of deaf's phonological representations]. Las Palmas de Gran Canaria, Spain: University of Las Palmas de Gran Canaria.

Santana, R., Torres, S., & García, J. (2003). The role of Cued Speech in the development of Spanish prepositions. *American Annals of the Deaf, 148,* 323–332.

Schauwers, K., Gillis, S., Daemers, K., De Beukelaer, C., & Govaerts, P. (2004). The onset of babbling and the audiologic outcome. *Otology & Neurotology, 25,* 263–270.

Snow, C. (1995). Issues in the study of input: fine tuning, universality, individual and developmental differences, and necessary causes. In P. Fletcher & B. MacWhinney (Eds.), *Handbook of child language* (pp. 180–193). Oxford, UK: Blackwell Reference.

Spencer, P. (2004). Individual differences in language performance after cochlear implantation at one to three years of age: Child, family, and linguistic factors. *Journal of Deaf Studies and Deaf Education, 9,* 396–412.

Svirsky, M., Lynne, M., Ying, E., Lento, C., & Leonard, L. (2002). Grammatical morphologic development in paediatric cochlear implant users may be affected by the perceptual prominence of the relevant markers. *Annals of Otology, Rhinology & Laryngology, 111,* 109–112.

Swisher, M. (1992). The role of parents in developing visual turn-taking in their young deaf children. *American Annals of the Deaf, 137,* 92–100.

Szagun, G. (2001). Language acquisition in young German-speaking children with cochlear implants: Individual differences and implications for conceptions of a "sensitive phase." *Audiology & Neurotology, 6,* 288–297.

Szagun, G. (2004). Learning by ear: On the acquisition of case and gender marking by German-speaking children with normal hearing and with cochlear implants. *Journal of Child Language, 31,* 1–30.

Tomasello, M., & Farrar, M. (1986). Joint attention and early language. *Child Development, 57,* 1454–1463.

Torres, S., Moreno-Torres, I., & Santana, R. (2006). Quantitative and qualitative evaluation of linguistic input support to a prelingually deaf child with Cued Speech: A case study. *Journal of Deaf Studies and Deaf Education, 11,* 438–448.

Vieu, A., Mondain, M., Blanchard, K., Sillon, M., Reuillard-Artières, F., Tobey, E. (1998). Influence of communication mode on speech intelligibility and syntactic structure of sentences in profoundly hearing impaired French children implanted between 5 and 9 years of age. *International Journal of Pediatric Otorhinolaryngology, 44,* 15–22.

Villalba, A., Fernández, J. A., & Ross, V. (1996). Instrumentos de valoración de la percepción del habla [Instruments to evaluate speech perception]. *Asociación Española de Educadores de Sordos* [Spanish association of teachers of the deaf], *45,* 4–10

Volterra, V., Caselli, M., Capirci, O., & Pizzuto, E. (2005). Gesture and the emergence and development of language. In M. Tomasello & D. Slobin (Eds.), *Beyond nature-nurture. Essays in honor of Elizabeth Bates* (pp. 3–40). Hillsdale, NJ: Lawrence Erlbaum Associates.

Chapter 8

EARLY LANGUAGE DEVELOPMENT OF DEAF TWINS OF DEAF PARENTS WHO ARE NATIVE CUERS OF ENGLISH

Kelly Lamar Crain

Introduction

Language Development of Hearing Children

The language development of normally developing hearing children born to hearing speakers of English is well documented, and forms the basis of entire textbooks used in the field of speech-language pathology (cf. Berko-Gleason, 2004; Hulit-Howard, 2002; Owens, 2001). It is generally held that hearing children of hearing parents progress through early communication and language milestones in a highly predictable manner. That is, children typically develop different cries and other vocal behaviors by 1 month of age, develop visual attention around 2 to 3 months, begin cooing and babbling by 3 to 4 months, use social gestures and respond to spoken words by 9 months, and say their first real word by 12 months of age. By 15 months, the typical hearing child will demonstrate a spoken vocabulary of 4 to 6 words, which grows rapidly to 20 words or larger by 18 months, at which point he or she can produce two-word utterances. By 2 years of age, the child has an expressive vocabulary of 200 to 300 words, which grows to 900 words or more by the age of 3 years, at which point he or she can produce a wide variety of sentence structures (Owens, 2001).

Language Development of Deaf Children

The language development of deaf children has been less extensively studied and documented. Available research reports provide some information; however, regarding deaf children's development of signed language and of spoken language, although information regarding the language development of deaf children raised with Cued Speech is extremely limited.

The availability of research on the development of signed languages in deaf children is not yet sufficient to suggest a clear pattern of signed language development (Marschark, Schick, & Spencer, 2006). Existing studies of the signed language development of deaf children, however, suggest that deaf children of deaf signing parents naturally acquire signed languages in a fashion and at a rate comparable to hearing children's acquisition of spoken languages from hearing parents (Newport & Meier, 1985; Schlesinger & Meadow, 1972), including similarities in the emergence of first words/first signs (Anderson & Reilly, 2002; McIntire, 1977).

Studies tracking the *development* of spoken language over time in deaf children are not found in the literature. Studies related to the spoken language *abilities* of preschool or school-age deaf children, however, are available, and focus on the relationships among speech perception, speech production, and language ability (Blamey et al., 2001; Paatsch, Blamey, Sarant, & Bow, 2006), the development of phonological awareness (James, Rajput, Brown, Sirimanna, Brinton, & Goswami, 2005; Spencer & Tomblin, 2008); and the attainment of spoken language milestones (Mayne, Yoshinaga-Itano, & Sedey, 2000; Mayne, Yoshinaga-Itano, Sedey, & Carey, 2000; Sarant, Holt, Dowell, Rickards, &

Blamey, 2009). Collectively, these data point to delays in the areas of receptive (language comprehension) and expressive (phonology, morphology, vocabulary, and syntax) language experienced by deaf children acquiring spoken language through oral-aural means.

To date, there has been no published longitudinal research documenting the language development of children raised with Cued Speech. However, Kipila (1985) conducted a case study of the expressive and receptive cueing of a 5-year-old deaf child and found many age-appropriate morphological structures used by the child with 100% accuracy. In a follow-up study with the same child, Metzger (1994) found that the child produced at 100% accuracy morphological structures previously found to be inconsistent. The findings from these two studies of one child, taken together, suggest a developmental trajectory of language acquisition similar to that of hearing children.

Prelinguistic Communication in Deaf Children

During the prelinguistic period of communication, precursors to conversations between parents and children develop, such as: eye gaze and visual attention, babbling, perlocutionary and illocutionary intent, gesturing, and turn-taking. Turn-taking and babbling begin as imitations and allow for early interactions which form a base for communication to evolve into language (Stine & Bohannon, 1983). Visual attention includes the child's ability to focus on objects and people, track movement, and maintain eye contact. Perlocutionary intent refers to behaviors (typically between 2 to 9 months) that appear to be unintentional and unrelated to the communication of others, such as reflexive crying and physical exploration. Illocutionary intent develops from perlocution (Bates, Camaioni, & Volterra, 1979) and includes the child's earliest attempts to request (e.g., stretching hands to be picked up). During this period, the development of foundational behaviors in the child are dependent on the mother's (or father's) ability to recognize and respond to the child's intentions (Harding, 1983).

Studies of the earliest communication behaviors of deaf infants of deaf and hearing parents have focused on the areas of eye-gaze and visual attention (Spencer, 2000; Swisher, 1992; Waxman & Spencer, 1997) perlocutionary and illocutionary intent (Bates, Camaioni, & Volterra, 1979; Dromi, 2003; Lichtert, 2003), and babbling (Petitto & Marentette, 1991).

Studies of eye-gaze and visual attention in deaf infants have found that these infants develop regular patterns of visual fixation and following (e.g., looking at mother vs. looking at another object) by the age of 6 months (Koester, Traci, Brooks, Karkowski, & Smith-Gray, 2004). Differences were found between deaf infants of deaf mothers and deaf infants of hearing mothers, with deaf infants of deaf mothers establishing the to-and-from-mother pattern sooner than the deaf infants of hearing mothers. Differences have also been found between hearing and deaf mothers regarding their use of attention related strategies with their 9- to 18-month-old infants, particularly in regard to strategies directing the child's visual attention to language (Meadow-Orlans & Spencer, 1996; Waxman & Spencer, 1997).

Studies of perlocution and illocution in deaf infants have found reliable use of proto-imperatives, in which an infant appears to wish to bring something to the attention of an adult (e.g., gesturing the function of a common object, shifting eye gaze between an adult and a desired object) by 8 months (Dromi, 2003) and proto-declaratives, in which an infant appears to wish to influence or manipulate an adult's behavior (e.g., pointing to an unattainable object while vocalizing and shifting eye gaze between the object and an adult) by 18 months (Lichtert, 2003). Expected age ranges for a hearing infant's progression through these overlapping developmental stages vary (Bates, 1979), making comparisons difficult. However, the available research suggests a similar developmental trajectory for deaf infants.

Studies of babbling in deaf infants focus either on *vocal* babbling or *manual* babbling. It is commonly held that deaf infants begin vocal babbling at the same time as hearing infants do (as a form of vocal play) and cease babbling to the extent that speech sounds not heard are not reinforced (see Oller, 2000 for a discussion of deaf infant vocalizations). Regarding babbling in the manual mode, Petitto and Marentette (1991) found that infant babbling is not a speech-dependent maturational phenomenon; rather, it is also observed in the manual mode by both hearing and deaf babies. Over multiple observations with deaf infants of ASL-native deaf parents and hearing infants of speaking, nonsigning hearing parents, Petitto and Marentette observed that the deaf infants produced significantly more manual babbling behaviors than did the hearing infants, and produced a reduced subset of phonetic units found in ASL. They suggest that deaf infants in signing environments demonstrate visual tracking behaviors and differential attention to faces and hands similar to the way that hearing infants differentially attend to speech and environmental sounds, and deaf infants focus on the hands of signers in their environment and begin to mimic handshapes that eventually will be used in the child's expressive signing (Petitto & Marentette, 1991). What is still not known, and what the present study can begin to inform, is whether the manual babbling in the visual mode is *modality*-specific (i.e., signing only) or whether it develops in response to any visible manual behaviors to which linguistic meaning can be attached (e.g., signing, cueing).

The Effect of Parental Hearing Status on the Early Language Development of Infants and Toddlers Who Are Deaf

Many studies of the early language development of deaf children have compared parenting behavior of mothers who are deaf who sign to their children to parenting behavior of mothers who are hearing. These studies have found that: (1) signing deaf mothers provide less stressful, more natural early communication for their deaf infants than do hearing mothers of deaf infants (Jamieson, 1995; Pipp-Siegel, Sedey, & Yoshinaga-Itano, 2002; Swisher, 1992; Waxman & Spencer, 1997); (2) deaf mothers of deaf infants are more sensitive to their babies' early visual needs and attention than are hearing mothers of deaf children (Meadow-Orlans, 1997; Spencer & Meadow-Orlans, 1996); and (3) the degree of maternal sensitivity and interaction correlates to child language gains (Pressman, Pipp-Siegal, Yoshinaga-Itano, & Deas, 1999).

Findings from studies comparing early language interactions with deaf infants and toddlers of signing deaf parents with hearing parents highlight the importance of early, natural language-rich interactions between deaf infants and

their primary caregivers in the attainment of early communication and language development milestones. Studies to date, however, have been limited to *signing* deaf parents and have not included Cued Speech or *cueing* deaf parents in their comparisons. The present case of deaf parents who cue their home language (i.e., English) to their deaf children might further clarify whether the salient feature of a deaf parent's early interactions with a deaf infant is: (1) immediate and fluent *signing* by a deaf parent, or (2) immediate and fluent *visually accessible language* by a deaf parent.

Early Language Acquisition and Subsequent Literacy Development

The link between early oral language ability and subsequent literacy achievement for hearing children is widely understood and well-documented (cf. Chall, 1983; Katz, Shankweiler, & Liberman, 1981; Kemper & Vernooy, 1993; Mann, Shankweiler, & Smith, 1984; Weaver, 1994). Generally, hearing children acquire phonological, morphological, and syntactic rules of their home language naturally, without formal instruction, prior to formal reading instruction in that language, and subsequently apply those language abilities to the tasks of decoding, rehearsal, and reading comprehension.

Less is known about the link between early oral language ability and subsequent literacy achievement for deaf children, although Perfetti and Sandak (2000) argue that the link between spoken languages and reading achievement is applicable to the case of deaf readers, as evident by demonstrated phonological awareness in deaf readers, and its association with higher levels of reading skill in those populations.

Although the research literature related to oral language and literacy for deaf children is limited, relationships between and among early oral language, phonological awareness, and reading comprehension in deaf children from oral backgrounds have been documented (Desjardin, Ambrose, & Eisenberg, 2009; Harris & Beech, 1998).

Very little is known about the link between early signed language ability and subsequent English literacy achievement for deaf children. Strong and Prinz (1998) reported an association between higher levels of American Sign Language (ASL) skills and higher English literacy skills (as evidenced by measures of vocabulary, syntax, and written narrative) among deaf students ranging in age from 8 to 15 years although, unfortunately, the study did not include a measure of reading comprehension. Despite a lack of empirical data, considerable theoretical support for the connection between signed language ability and subsequent literacy achievement can be found in the literature (cf. Chamberlain & Mayberry, 2000; Grushkin, 1998; Padden & Ramsey, 2000; Wilbur, 2000). As Leybaert, Colin, and LaSasso note in Chapter 11, this phenomenon may relate, in part, to children of signing deaf parents coming to formal reading instruction with more general world knowledge, which they have acquired in their linguistic interactions with parents prior to reading instruction. Furthermore, as LaSasso and Crain note in Chapter 12, deaf children who have fewer questions about the content of the materials they are reading can focus on the vocabulary, syntactic structures, and decoding of print.

Much of the literature regarding the connection between exposure to Cued Speech and subsequent literacy achievement in deaf children comes from work conducted in the French language by Leybaert and her colleagues (Alegria, Dejean, Capouillez, & Leybaert, 1990; Alegria, Lechat, & Leybaert, 1990; Leybaert, 1993; Leybaert & Alegria, 1993, 1995; Leybaert, Alegria, Hage, & Charlier, 1998; Leybaert & Charlier, 1996; Perier, Charlier, Hage, & Alegria, 1987), which document phonological awareness, spelling, decoding, and reading measures of deaf children exposed to Cued Speech commensurate to hearing peers and superior to deaf children educated orally or with sign communication. Wandel (1989) matched groups of deaf elementary school students by communication mode (Oral, TC, Cued Speech) and compared them to a hearing control group matched for age, gender, and cognitive ability. Results revealed no significant difference in reading achievement between the hearing control group and the Cued Speech group. Crain and LaSasso (Chapter 14) compared the generative rhyming abilities and measured reading comprehension of 10- to 14-year-old deaf readers from Cued Speech and oral English-language backgrounds to that of a hearing control group. They found that although the oral group had higher levels of hearing and better speech intelligibility than the cueing group, the cueing group demonstrated higher levels of phonological awareness and higher measured reading comprehension. To date, no studies have been published suggesting a developmental course between the early language development of deaf cuers of English and subsequent literacy development and reading achievement.

Purpose of the Study

The purpose of study described in this chapter was to document the early language and preliteracy development of two (twin) prelingually, profoundly deaf children born to profoundly deaf native cuers of English. Specifically, the study described sought to determine whether: (1) these deaf children of deaf cueing parents would progress through early stages of visual attention, perlocutionary and illocutionary intent, and manual (i.e., cue) babbling in a manner similar to those observed in deaf children of deaf signing parents; (2) the cued language development milestones documented in these deaf children would resemble the language milestones of hearing children acquiring spoken English from hearing parents; (3) the deaf cueing parents would demonstrate the same early parenting and communication behaviors observed in deaf signing parents and thought to benefit early communication and language development of deaf children; (4) whether the contribution of Cued Speech to the language acquisition of these deaf children would be evident as a purely visual phenomenon, or as a visual component of an audiovisual phenomenon; and (5) whether these children, exposed to cueing from birth by native cuers of English, would demonstrate early literacy and prereading behaviors by the age of 3 years.

Method

Participants

Participants include twin prelingually, profoundly deaf girls who were 10 months of age at the beginning of the study and 36 months at the conclusion, and their deaf parents, who are native cuers of English. The infants and their parents are described separately.

The parents are both deaf native cuers of English, aged in their 30s. The mother was born with a profound bilateral hearing loss, diagnosed at 18 months, and was raised with Cued Speech as the primary mode of communication starting at the age of 30 months. The father was born with a profound bilateral hearing loss, diagnosed at 24 months, and was raised with Cued Speech as the primary mode of communication starting at the age of 42 months.

The infants were born at 34 weeks gestation, and were referred for audiologic testing through universal newborn hearing screening prior to release from the hospital. The first twin, who will be referred to as Emily, was later diagnosed as having a severe-to-profound bilateral hearing loss. The second twin, who will be referred to as Laura, was diagnosed with a severe bilateral hearing loss. No other complications were reported. At the onset of the study, the twins were 10 months of age. Both girls were fitted with bilateral BTE hearing aids at the age of 4 months. Parents report consistent use of hearing aids from 4 to 6 months, after which the children would continually remove the hearing aids. Hearing aid use was inconsistent and minimal from 6 months until cochlear implantation at 18 months. The twins were implanted at 18 months of age, and the implants were activated 1 month later. Parents report consistent use of the cochlear implants, with the children rarely removing the magnetic component following implantation and activation, and very rarely since.

Instruments

Instruments developed or adapted for use in this study included: a parent interview protocol related to beliefs and perceptions of the importance of early amplification, cochlear implantation, communication, language, and socialization of deaf children raised with Cued Speech; a checklist of prelinguistic gestures (adapted from Camaioni, Caselli, Volterra, & Luchenti, 1992); a protocol for the assessment of prelinguistic intentional communication (adapted from Casby & Cumpata, 1986); and a speech intelligibility measure modeled after the NTID Speech Intelligibility Rating Scale. Published instruments used in this study included: The MacArthur Bates Communicative Development Inventories (Fenson et al., 1993) and the Goldman-Fristoe Test of Articulation, 2nd edition (American Guidance Service, 2000).

Interview Protocol

The interview protocol used in this study focused on parents' beliefs and attitudes about communication, language, amplification, and implantation of children who are deaf and hard of hearing. The interview protocol contained questions relating to the following themes: choice of Cued Speech for self; communication ability of self and family; communication strategies; quality of peer relationships; quality/nature of family relationships; school experiences; self-identity; choice of Cued Speech for children; and amplification and implantation.

Checklist of Prelinguistic Gestures

The checklist of prelinguistic gestures used in this study is an adaptation by Dromi (2003) of a checklist originated by Camaioni et al. (1992). The checklist consists of 15 prelinguistic referential gestures that infants frequently produce prior to the onset of speech (or, in the case of deaf infants, any combination of speech, signs, or cues). Gestures appearing on the checklist include: *stretching hands to be picked up*, *shakes head for no, nods head for yes*, and *gives and takes objects*. For each gesture on the checklist, the parent is asked to indicate whether and/or how reliably the gesture is produced, by marking *never*, *sometimes*, or *always*. Additionally, the researcher makes direct observations of these gestural behaviors as they are elicited in natural contexts.

Protocol for the Assessment of Prelinguistic Intentional Communication

The protocol for the assessment of prelinguistic intentional communication used in this study was the same as that described by Lichtert (2003), which itself was adapted from one originated by Casby and Cumpata (1986). The protocol used in this study consists of Lichtert's 10 tasks intended to elicit proto-imperative behaviors from the infants. In each task, the infant is presented with a problem that cannot be solved independently. The infant's communicative behaviors are recorded and rated for complexity.

Speech Intelligibility Rating Scale

The speech intelligibility measure used in this study was adapted from the NTID Speech Intelligibility Rating Scale (Subtelny, 1977). Judgments are made regarding five features of speech: pitch register and control; prosody; respiratory control; resonance; and vocal tension. A Likert-like 5-point scale is employed, to rate an individual's speech from 1 (speech is unintelligible) to 5 (speech is completely intelligible).

MacArthur Bates Communicative Development Inventory

The MacArthur-Bates Communicative Development Inventories (CDIs) are a pair of widely used assessment instruments by which parents can report the communicative skills of their infants and toddlers by filling in ovals corresponding to words the child understands and/or produces. Using these parent reports, the inventories assess early language skills of children between the ages of 8 and 30 months. The CDI/Words and Gestures inventory is for use with infants between the ages of 8 and 16 months. The inventory's gestures section contains a list of 63 gestures for communication, play, imitation of parents and other adults. The inventory's words section contains a 28-item list of phrases and a 396-item list of words, and is used to assess both comprehension and production of words and phrases. The CDI/Words and Sentences inventory is for use with infants between the ages of 16 and 30 months. This inventory's word section contains a list of 680 words. The second part of the inventory is used to document the toddler's use of possessives, plurals, and tenses, as well as the development of complex sentences.

Goldman-Fristoe Test of Articulation, 2nd Edition (GFTA-2)

The GFTA-2 is a tool for the systematic measurement of articulation for individuals ranging in age from 2 to 21 years. Examinees respond verbally to picture plates and verbal cues from the examiner with single-word answers that demonstrate common speech sounds. For example, the examinee will see a drawing of a duck and will be asked by the examiner,

"What is this?" to which the examinee will be expected to say, "A duck," thereby producing the targets /d/ and /k/. The test is intended to measure speech articulation and categorize types of misarticulation. As such, the GFTA-2 was not formally administered; the stimulus plates were chosen for their ability to readily elicit all cued consonants and vowels in a short period of time.

Data Collection and Analysis

From the age of 10 months to 36 months, the children and their parents were visited in their home every 3 to 4 months by the author, who is a skilled cuer with a background in the language development of deaf children, and/or the research assistant who is a fluent cuer with a background in linguistics and experience working with young children and families. The duration of visits ranged from 60 to 120 minutes. During these visits, the researchers videotaped the twins and at least one parent in natural activities (e.g., play/exploration, book sharing, feeding), videotaped structured activities related to prelinguistic intentional communication, and/or interviewed one or both parents regarding their attitudes and beliefs about the role of Cued Speech in communication and language, and/or the receptive and expressive language of their children.

Videotapes and documents were analyzed to document the infants' prelinguistic, vocal, gestural, and cued expressive and receptive behaviors, and the parents' spoken and cued language input and modeling. Through analyses of interviews, observations, and language samples, communication and language milestones have been documented, and certain domains or themes have emerged from the data.

Results

Parents

Parental hearing loss is based on self-report. The mother reported being born with a profound bilateral hearing loss, diagnosed at 18 months. The father reported being born with a profound bilateral hearing loss, diagnosed at 24 months. Both parents reported being exposed to Cued Speech in early childhood, and their own parents learned to cue well and cued consistently at home. Each was the only deaf member of his or her family, and each experienced some of the isolation and frustrations common to deaf individuals from hearing families (e.g., missing incidental conversations, not always being able to visually track group discussions). Both reported, however, generally feeling included in family discussions and activities, and credited the ability of all family members to communicate in a single common language.

Both parents reported feeling successful and self-confident, and content with their identity as deaf individuals and cuers. Both attended public schools, excelled academically, and received regular high school diplomas. Both went on to receive bachelor and master's degrees from state or private colleges, accessing the services of Cued Language Transliterators (CLT).

The mother grew up as the only deaf cuer in her area, and was fully mainstreamed during her school years. She reported having a small number of close friends, all hearing. The father grew up in an area with several cueing families (i.e., hearing parents with deaf children), who joined together to create a Cued Speech program in the local schools, which already had programs for oral or signing deaf children. The father, therefore went to school with a mix of hearing and deaf peers, and enjoyed varying levels of access to communication with those peers.

The mother reported that both she and the father assumed the possibility of having deaf children, but were somewhat surprised at the initial diagnosis, as they were the only deaf member of their respective families, and neither of them had undergone genetic testing to determine the odds of having a deaf child. Both parents reported initially feeling overwhelmed with scheduling appointments (e.g., pediatrician, audiologist, early intervention specialist) and making decisions, but the mother indicated feeling fortunate that she had her own experiences with deafness to reassure her and lessen her stress. She also reported feeling immediately relieved at knowing she could communicate visually with her children as soon as she realized they were deaf.

Regarding the question of how the children would communicate expressively, the mother reported recognizing an important difference between her (and the father's) childhood experience and that of her own children. Both reported having been cued to by their hearing parents, and generally speaking (with or without cues) in response. In the case of deaf parents, the mother recognized, it would be important for the children to cue expressively sooner and more often than in the typical case of deaf children raised by hearing parents. The parents both stated their belief that the children, provided sufficient communication modeling, would naturally copy what they see, and could also be reminded to cue, if and when necessary.

The mother and father reported placing a high value on their children's access to auditory information, not only for access to environmental sounds, but also for speech and spoken language development and ease of spoken communication with hearing individuals. The mother reported that the children were fitted with hearing aids at 4 months. Both parents reported great difficulty keeping the hearing aids on the children (the father described it as, "a constant battle with a most worthy opponent"). This, along with the children's degree of deafness and promising advances in cochlear implantation, led to the decision to implant the children. The parents reported having made the decision with the goal in mind of the children having the greatest access possible to all sensory experiences and forms of communication.

Both parents are fluent receptive and expressive cuers. Their cueing skills were not assessed for this study, however, both reported extensive experience receiving language input via cues (from direct communication and through transliterators). The mother is a certified Cued Speech instructor, a designation which requires passing an expressive Cued Speech assessment, and both parents were judged by certified Cued Speech instructors and transliterators to be technically accurate and highly intelligible cuers.

The parents' speech intelligibility was judged by three professionals in aural rehabilitation (the author, a speech-language pathologist and an educational audiologist) with extensive experience with speech perception and production of deaf individuals. Raters viewed a videotape of each parent reading the Rainbow Passage (Fairbanks, 1960) aloud, first without cues, and again with cues. Using a 5-point scale modeled on the NTID Speech Intelligibility Rating Scale (Subtelny, 1977), each professional independently rated each parent's speech intelligibility, noting speech characteristics that contributed to the overall score. After independently rating each parent's speech, the raters met to discuss their ratings and reach consensus. The mother's speech was rated as a 3 in the audio-only condition (speech is difficult to understand; however, the gist of the conversation can be understood) with slight improvement in the audiovisual condition. Her speech was described as "somewhat intelligible," and was characterized as hypernasal and slightly above normal pitch, with limited variability in loudness, pitch, and stressing patterns within or between words. The father's speech was rated at 4 (speech is intelligible, with the exception of a few words or phrases) in both the audio-only and audio-visual conditions. His speech was described as "mostly intelligible," and was characterized as slightly de-nasal, with slightly more variability in loudness, pitch, and stressing patterns within and between words.

Both parents were observed using voice while cueing to the children. The mother reported always voicing while cueing, with the expressed purpose of stimulating the auditory channel during hearing aid use, as well as after cochlear implantation. The father also reported voicing while cueing for the same purpose, with the exception of occasional "experiments" of voice-off cueing to determine whether the children understood cues independently of speech. This will be discussed further in findings related to the children's receptive language.

At the beginning of data collection and continuing throughout, both parents were observed to consistently employ attention strategies commonly reported and assumed to be intuitive among deaf parents of deaf children (Meadow-Orlans

& Steinberg, 2004; Spencer, 1993; Waxman & Spencer, 1997). Specifically, the parents were observed to: (1) exaggerate cueing space to gain or maintain attention, (2) wave the hand or a held object (e.g., toy) briefly, (3) gently tap a part of the child's body (e.g., arm or leg), (4) produce the manual portion of cues away from the face and into the child's field of vision and return to cueing at the face upon regaining attention, and (5) wait for the child to move attention from a jointly held object back to the parent before resuming cueing.

Visual attention and redirecting behaviors were seen to gradually decrease over time, as the children responded more readily to vocal prompts as received through the cochlear implant. Initially, according to parent report, visual attention strategies were almost always accompanied by vocalization. With the children demonstrating increasingly reliable responses to vocal attention and redirecting prompts by the age of 22 months (4 months post-implant), use of visual strategies along with vocal prompts decreased. By the age of 25 months, the parents reported (and were observed) using voice to gain attention (even from separate rooms), followed by cued and spoken messages after visual contact was made.

Children

Prelinguistic Behaviors

Children typically begin to communicate expressively before they demonstrate the first signs of expressive language (Hulit & Howard, 2002). The use of prelinguistic behaviors by the twins in this study was documented, starting at the age of 10 months, to establish a baseline of communication from which early language use could be assumed to develop. Of particular interest were the development and use of visual attention, prelinguistic gestures, prelinguistic intentional communication, vocalization, and cue babbling.

Eye Gaze and Visual Attention. According to parental reports, both children progressed through the early stages of visual attention and purposeful eye contact and engagement typically seen in hearing and deaf infants (Adamson, 1995; Swisher, 1992). Specifically, by the age of 4 months, the children were reported to maintain eye contact with the parent holding them. By the age of 5 months, they were reported to shift eye contact between the parent holding them and the parent not holding them cueing to them. By the age of 6 months, they were reported to alert to visual stimuli, move their eyes and turn their heads to orient themselves, attend to objects and features of objects, and track the movement of objects in the visual field. By the age of 10 months, they were reported to consistently shift attention from a parent to an object referred to by the parent (by pointing or head shift) and back to the parent.

Regarding visual attention to cues, the parents reported that by 6 months, the children demonstrated increased visual attention to a "speaking" face accompanied by a cueing hand, as compared to a "speaking" face with no cues. At this point, the parents reported, the children's eye gaze could be seen to shift between face and hand as frequently as every 1 to 2 seconds.

At the beginning of data collection (at 10 months of age), both infants were observed by the author to engage in joint visual attention with the mother and with the father. During both unstructured interactive play sessions and the activities designed to elicit prelinguistic gestures and proto-imperatives, the children were observed to maintain visual attention with an animated face or with a cueing adult for a number of seconds before looking at/reaching for an object or other person, or looking around the room. They were observed to attempt to visually track a cued conversation between two adults and among three adults. Cued conversations among four adults did occur, but visual tracking at this rate was not apparent.

Prelinguistic Gestures. The children's use of prelinguistic gestures was documented by the author at 10 months, 12 months, and again at 25 months, using a checklist of prelinguistic gestures adapted by Dromi (2003) from one originally described by Camaioni et al. (1992). At 10 months, the mother was asked to recall the age at which each child had begun to use a gesture reliably (i.e., intentionally for the same purpose). The parents were asked to make note of the emergence and consistent use of gestures not yet demonstrated by the age of 10 months, for reference at future visits from the author. Two gestures not reported by the parents or observed by the author were: *shakes index finger to scold*, and *moves hands/arms for "going" or "moving."* Gestures not included on the checklist but reported by the parents and observed by the author were: *pointing at an object for "I want that," pointing in a direction for "I want to go there,"* and *pointing at the palm of the hand for "I want more," or "I want it again."* Results from these checklists indicate that the children developed ways to communicate needs and desires prior to uttering their first words. Table 8–1 provides a composite of results (10, 12, and 25 months) for each child.

Prelinguistic Intentional Communication. The children's use of proto-imperative communicative intentions was documented using an elicitation task adapted by Lichtert (2003) from one originally created by Casby and Cumpata (1986). In this elicitation task, the child sits on the parent's lap, and is presented with a problem she cannot solve independently (e.g., a favorite toy with an important part missing). The child's use of proto-imperatives (i.e., prelinguistic "demands") is documented, and scored from 0 (no response; no communicative behavior toward adult) to 4 (use of conventional linguistic form; true word, phrase, etc.). An average score is taken from the 10 elicitations.

The first attempt to document the children's proto-imperative use, at 10 months, was unsuccessful, as both children appeared more interested in the adults (i.e., the author, the research assistant, the mother) than the objects selected for the task. The task was repeated at 17 months. Emily's responses ranged from 0 to 3, with an average score of 1.9. Laura's responses ranged from 1 to 4, with an average score of 2.1. These results compare favorably with the average response score of 1.6 at 18 months as reported by Lichtert (2003). The task was repeated again at 25 months. Emily's responses ranged from 1 to 4, with an average score of 3.3. Laura's responses ranged from 3 to 4, with an average score of 3.2. These results compare quite favorably with the average response score of 1.9 at 24 months as reported by Lichtert. Results from these elicitation tasks indicate that both children progressed from simple gestures to indicate wants and needs to more sophisticated means of communication, including the use of proto-words and first words well within expected time lines. Table 8–2 provides composite scores for the two tasks.

Table 8–1. Composite Results for Checklist of Prelinguistic Gestures

Gesture	Emily		Laura	
	Age Observed	Context	Age Observed	Context
Stretches hands to be picked up	8 months	Parent stands up	9 months	Parent stands up
Bye-bye	10 months	Adult waves good-bye	9 months	Adult waves good-bye
Shows objects	8 months	Toys, food	7 months	Toys, food
Claps hands	8 months	Enjoying activity	7 months	Enjoying activity
Shakes head for "no"	10 months	Refusing food	9 months	Refusing food; protesting interruption
Gives and takes objects	11 months	Toys, food	11 months	Toys, food
Stretches hands to sides for "all gone"	11 months	Food: all gone Activity: all done	13 months	Food: all gone Toy: gone Activity: all done
Nods head for "yes"	10 months	Do you want more?	11 months	Do you want more?
Shakes index finger to scold	N/A		N/A	
Moves lips for "food is tasty"	9 months		8 months	
Moves hands for "that was wrong"	19 months	Points to sister	19 months	Points to sister
Combs hair	12 months	Play	14 months	Play
Puts fingers to lips for "shh–quiet"	24 months	Baby/doll is sleeping	24 months	Baby/doll is sleeping
Pretends to use phone	25 months	Toy cell phone	25 months	Toy cell phone
Moves hands backward or forward for "going" or "moving"	N/A		N/A	
Other: flexes body	6 months	To be picked up	5 months	To be picked up
Other: point at object/food	12 months	"I want that."	12 months	"I want that."
Other: point in a direction	14 months	"I want to go there."	14 months	"I want to go there."
Other: point at palm of hand	12 months	"I want more/ I want it again."	12 months	"I want more/ I want it again."

Table 8–2. Composite Results for Proto-Imperative Elicitation Task

Stimulus	Response Score			
	Emily		Laura	
	17 mos	25 mos	17 mos	25 mos
Give child a wind-up toy that runs down	2	3	2	3
Give child a bottle of play bubbles that she cannot open	2	4	2	4
Place toy in a clear plastic container and give to child	0	2	1	2
Hit play drum with a stick, then give child drum only	2	3	2	3
Hit pegs on toy workbench with hammer, then give child workbench only	2	3	2	3
Show child doll and bottle, then give child doll only	3	4	2	4
Hold a favorite book* just out of child's reach	3	4	3	3
Show child stacking rings, then give child only one ring	2	3	3	4
Place candy in a clear plastic bag, hold just out of child's reach	2	3	2	3
Give child an empty glass and present juice just out of reach	1	4	2	3
Average Response Score	**1.9**	**3.3**	**2.1**	**3.2**

*book replaced toy per mother's suggestion.

Response Scores: 0 = No response; no communication behavior toward adult. Looks at or reaches for object only; 1 = Gestural or pointing response toward object and adult. Deictic gaze. Looks at or reaches for object and looks at adult; 2 = Gestural or pointing response toward object or adult, plus vocalization. Gestures or points toward object and vocalizes. Gestures or points toward adult and vocalizes; 3 = Verbalization toward adult or object (may be accompanied by gesture). Use of "proto-words"; 4 = Use of conventional linguistic form. True word, phrase, and so forth.

Vocalization. Parents reported that the children's vocalizations were minimal prior to implantation at the age of 18 months. Hearing aid use from 3 months to 18 months was inconsistent, although vocalization was noted to increase during times of hearing aid use. Vocalizations also increased with the onset of expressive cueing (at 11 months). These vocalizations initially did not constitute speech production, but did appear to be intentionally used as an accompaniment to cues, most often as a match between cued syllables and spoken syllables (i.e., one vocal burst for one placement, two vocal bursts for two placements or a repeated placement).

At the beginning of data collection, the children were observed by the author to squeal (often in response to a pleasurable activity or offering, and occasionally with no apparent stimulus) and cry. At 17 months, during a time when the children wore hearing aids (i.e., before removing both hearing aids at the same time), vocalizations were noted by the author, including an elongated or repeated neutral vowel, and a repeated approximation of /ma/ (the elongated neutral vowel interrupted by the repeated closing of the jaw). At 25 months (6 months postimplant activation), the children were observed to vocalize for the majority of the home visit (approximately 2 hours), except when eating, drinking, concentrating, or watching an adult cue. By 36 months, the children were observed to use vocal speech with and without cues.

Cue Babbling. Cue babbling, as its name suggests, refers to the emergence of approximations of cued handshapes and placements on the part of the child. Parents reported that at 8 months the children began raising one arm (either arm, but only one) to the side of the face when observing an adult cueing. By the beginning of data collection (at 10 months), both girls were observed to do this, and to alternately extend and retract all fingers (as though grasping). When the adult stopped cueing, the child's imitative behavior stopped. This starting and stopping was repeated several times to rule out coincidence. By 11 months, the girls had ceased the purely imitative behavior, and used the cueing posture only during their own conversational turns. At the same time (11 months) the girls first used a correctly formed handshape at a correct placement to express meaning, moving them from the babbling stage to the protoword stage of language development.

Receptive Language Development

Comprehension of Cued/Spoken Language. Children develop receptive language (i.e., the ability to understand what is said to them) months before they utter their first true word (Hulit & Howard, 2002). Children demonstrate their comprehension of language through appropriate responses to what is said, either by vocalization (e.g., squealing), gesture (e.g., pointing), or gross motor action (e.g., reaching up, pushing away). It is impossible to accurately measure a child's receptive language in terms of number of words understood (Benedict, 1979), though observations can be made. Of particular interest to this study was the ways in which these children demonstrated their comprehension of cued/spoken vocabulary, phrases, and directions, both before and after cochlear implantation.

The parents reported that, by 3 months, the children maintained visual attention, and responded to objects differently than to the parents' faces. By 6 months, the children attended to the face and cueing hand for longer periods (on the order of seconds), and attended to the face longer if the cueing hand was present. At 9 months, the mother reported, Emily first responded to the question, "Where's Daddy?" a few moments after he had left the room, by looking around and settling on the doorway. By 10 months, both children were observed by the author to respond behaviorally to many "Where is . . . " questions, and began playing games of routine, such as peek-a-boo and hand-clapping.

At 17 months (2 months before implant activation), the children were observed by the author to respond appropriately to a number of "Where is . . . " questions, such as "Where's Daddy?" "Where's Mommy?" and "Where's Laura?" They were observed to respond differentially to a number of "Go get . . . " commands, such as "Go get Elmo" versus "Go get Blue" (two different stuffed animals) and "Go get a ball" versus "Go get a book."

By 19 months (around the time of implant activation), the mother reported that they consistently responded to "Come here," "Give [name] a kiss," "Give [name] a hug," and "Nice touch" without accompanying gestures. The mother reported that Laura first began playing "the nose game," in which she would appropriately respond to "Where is . . . " questions regarding a number of body parts (e.g., nose, eyes, ears, hair, belly button) and the words *your* and "Mommy's." By this time, both children were observed by the author to respond appropriately to "Say hello to . . . " and "Say good-bye to . . . " by repeating the phrase without the word *say*.

At 25 months (6 months after implant activation), both children were observed by the author to respond appropriately (e.g., gesturally, behaviorally, or speech/cues) to a wide variety of animals and animal sounds (e.g., who says "moo," what does the sheep say?), colors (e.g., what color is a banana? find your pink socks), and one- and two-step directions (e.g., "Give mommy the broom"; "Give Daddy a kiss and come here"). They were observed by the author to recognize the names of many individual toys and objects by name (e.g., purse and bag; pen, pencil, and crayon; binoculars and glasses).

At 36 months, the children were observed by the author to correctly answer questions of "Who" (e.g., Who will we see tomorrow? Response: Aunt Barbara), "Where" (e.g., Where does Alan live? Response: Montreal), "What" (e.g., What is Daddy doing? Response: Reading), and "Which one" (e.g., Which basket is it in? Response: That one).

Comprehension of Cues. Of particular interest to the author was whether the children continued, after cochlear implantation, to comprehend cued messages without accompanying speech. To determine whether this was the case, the author intentionally cued voice off for portions of each visit, starting at 22 months (3 months postimplant activation). Additionally, the father reported and demonstrated "cueing comprehension" activities of his own.

At 22 months, at the beginning of the visit, the author asked each child a series of "Who is . . . " and "Where is . . . " questions, regarding people and objects, respectively. All questions were posed via cueing, voice off, and included both "Who am I?" and "What's my name?" and "What's that?" and "What's that called?" Both children responded to all questions correctly.

At 28 months, the author engaged the children in a play session with a tube of 12 small canisters of Play-Doh, each a different color or shade. During this play session, the author did not voice, and the children's utterances varied (i.e., voice and cues, cues only, voice only). The author asked a series of questions to determine that the children knew the colors (e.g., What color is this one? Which one is pink? May I have the orange one?). The author taught the children *light* and *dark*, to distinguish between two canisters of blue Play-Doh (the mother reported that the children had not used the words *light* and *dark* in reference to colors). The children responded appropriately to the author's statements, such as, "Let's make a ball. Can you make a snake? Don't mix them together. What did you make?" At the end of the play session, the author pointed to the light blue asked Laura to tell the research assistant which color it was. Laura hesitated, and the research assistant cued with voice, "What color is it?" Laura cued *with voice*, "It's light blue."

Also at 28 months, the father reported to the author during an interview having wondered about the children's cueing reception, and provided a brief demonstration. He sat with Emily in the living room and asked her, voice off, "Where's your elbow?" Emily pointed to her elbow. He then cued, without gesture or break of eye contact, "Where's your Elmo?" Emily looked around the room, and pointed down the stairs (the play room). The father cued, "Right, go get it." A few minutes later, he successfully repeated the task with Laura, asking her first about her Elmo, and then her elbow. The father indicated that he took the children's ability to discern these two otherwise visually identical messages as evidence that they could receive and comprehend cued messages without accompanying speech.

At 32 months, the father demonstrated a "game" he had invented for the children. After gaining Emily's attention, he cued to her without voicing or moving his mouth (i.e., only the manual cue handshapes and placements), "Sit down." Emily sat down, at which the father cued "Good job," again without voice or mouth movements. He then asked her, "What color is your shirt?" to which Emily replied, "Red." He asked her, "What kind of shirt is it?" to which she replied, "It's a football shirt" (a football jersey). He then cued, still without voice or mouth movements, "Go get Laura," at which point Emily left the room yelling her sister's name. The "game" was repeated with Laura, with similar results. Laura was asked, "What is your name?" (Laura.) "Where is Kelly?" (Right there.) and "Do you like applesauce?" (Yes, applesauce!)

These examples indicate that the children continued to focus on the visual aspects of communication, including both the mouth movements associated with cueing, and the manual cues specifically, after the development of listening skills and speech/spoken language observed postcochlear implantation.

Expressive Language Development

Phonology. No attempt was made to document the children's speech production and articulation independent of their cued phonological development. The normal speech development of hearing children includes approximations and misarticulations up to the age of 8 years (Sander, 1972), and the wide variability in speech intelligibility and articulation among deaf children make such judgments difficult at best. Observations are made regarding the children's speech sounds and spoken phonemes when they help to illustrate their overall (cued or spoken) phonological development.

Parents reported that the first handshape emerged for each child at 11 months: handshape 5 for Emily and handshape 1 for Laura (which also emerged for Emily). Almost immediately thereafter, each of these handshapes was paired with a cueing placement: both girls cued handshape 5 at the chin (creating the first phoneme of Emily's name) and handshape 1 at the chin (poo). Soon after, according to parental report, Laura began using handshape 6 at the side placement and, immediately after that, at the side-forward placement (creating the first syllable of her own name). For Laura, handshapes emerged in the following order: 1, 6, 5, 2, 4, 3, 7, and 8, with handshape 8 beginning to emerge by 36 months. For Emily, handshapes emerged in the following order: 5, 1, 6, 2, 4, 7, 3, and 8. According to parent report, handshapes emerged largely intact. Handshape 5 emerged as an approximation (fingers separated when they should be together), but quickly self-corrected. At the same time the children began using handshape 6, a non-handshape emerged, wherein the middle finger, index finger, and thumb were all extended. This non-handshape was used interchangeably with handshape 5 before being extinguished with the emergence of handshapes 2 and 4.

The first cueing placement (chin) emerged with the first handshape. Side-forward placement emerged next, followed closely by side-down placement. Mouth placement emerged by 18 months, and throat placement by 22 months. As opposed to handshapes, which emerged largely intact, cueing placements were initially gross approximations of their location. Side placement occurred in a fairly large area to the child's side, and side-forward and side-down placements were produced with greatly exaggerated movements. Mouth placement was observed to occur anywhere from the side of the mouth to the middle of the cheek. Chin placement emerged largely intact, whereas throat placement was observed to occur anywhere from the throat to the middle of the chest. By 36 months, these placements were observed to be closer to their targets, but not yet technically accurate.

Starting at 14 months, two clear trends were observed by the author regarding the emergence of cues and the relationship between cued and spoken segments. The first trend regarded manual cues preceding spoken speech sounds. When attempting to "say" a new word, (the word *pony* will be used as a real example) both children produced the first cued syllable (handshape and placement combination), while vocalizing the vowel or vowels (i.e., handshape 1 at side-forward while vocalizing /o/ /i/). In the next approximation (in the same observation or later), the second cued syllable would appear, followed by the same vocalization (i.e., handshape 1 at side-forward while vocalizing /o/ and handshape 4 at mouth while vocalizing /i/). Finally, the word was cued and spo-

ken completely. This was observed a number of times, with words such as: pony, daddy, nana, Elmo, baby, and diaper. By 32 months, many correctly integrated two- and three-syllable words were observed, such as: mommy, daddy, table, paper, apple, dinner, and sorry. The second trend regarded spoken speech sounds preceding manual cues. When attempting to "say" a word with a consonant cluster (e.g., grass, blue, milk, slide, fast), the children were observed to pronounce the word to include both sounds in the cluster (giving credit for developmentally appropriate articulation and the effects of hearing loss on speech production), while cueing only the first handshape if the cluster appeared at the beginning of the word, and cueing only the last handshape if the cluster appeared at the end of the word. In this way, *grass* was spoken, and *gas* was cued. Similarly, *fast* was spoken, and *fat* was cued. By 32 months, many correctly integrated cued/spoken consonant clusters were observed in such words as: *twinkle, blue, green, brown, black, please, fix,* and *draw.*

At 25 months, when the children were able to express themselves in sentences, they were observed by the author to produce cues in conjunction with vocalizations for syllables, but without mouth movements or intelligible speech. Words observed to be cued and spoken correctly in isolation were cued without speech or mouth movements during this time. By 28 months, the children were observed to coordinate manual cues and speech production in sentences.

The children's phonological inventory was investigated by the author at age 36 months, using the plates (stimuli) from the Goldman-Fristoe-2 Test of Articulation (GFTA-2) (American Guidance Service, 2002). Due to visual and auditory distractions, and in keeping with the attention span of 3-year-olds, each child completed half of the GFTA-2 plates at a time, alternating from one child to the other. Both children voiced and cued most responses, and were asked by the author or by the mother to provide manual cues when they provided a response via speech alone.

Emily spontaneously produced all individual consonant cues except handshape 7 for /dʒ/ and handshape 8 for /tʃ/ and /ŋ/. In cases where handshape 8 was required for /tʃ/, she produced handshape 5, which is the neutral open handshape. In cases where handshape 8 was required for /ŋ/, she produced handshape 2. Handshapes 8 and 2 are similar, except that in handshape 8 the two fingers are separated, while in handshape 2 they are together. Emily did not produce handshape 8 when provided a model. Provided a model of a word requiring handshape 7 (e.g., jumping) and asked to repeat, she produced handshape 2. Handshapes 7 and 2 look alike, except for the thumb being extended in handshape 7, but not in handshape 2.

Laura spontaneously produced all individual consonant cues except handshape 7 for /g/ and /dʒ/, handshape 8 for /tʃ/ and /ŋ/. In all cases where handshape 8 was required, she produced handshape 5, which is the neutral open handshape. Provided a model and asked to repeat, she produced handshape 7 for /g/, but produced handshape 1 instead of handshape 7 for /dʒ/. Laura provided a combination of cues and speech in her responses. Most of the time, the cues and speech sounds were produced together. At times, a response was only spoken, and Laura was asked to cue the response. Other times, her speech was unintelligible or she produced the articulation errors expected of a child her age, but the cues

were correct, indicating the phonemes contained in the words. In one instance, the word *gorilla*, neither the cue nor the speech sound were produced (spontaneously or after modeling) for the initial /g/. In this case, handshape 5 was used, and the speech sound was omitted, producing a cued and spoken response of –*orilla*. It should be noted that *gorilla* is not a stimulus item in the GFTA-2; this was Laura's initial response to the stimulus for *monkey*. Laura exhibited inconsistent use of handshapes 2 and 3 for /z/ and /s/. She was observed to use handshape 2 for /z/ correctly and handshape 3 for /s/ correctly, but she also used handshape 3 at the end of plurals and possessives requiring /z/, which would require handshape 2. It was not clear from her cueing or from her speech whether she was aware of this distinction.

A final aspect of cued phonology observed in the children's expressive cueing relates to the use of liaisons (see Chapter 2 in this volume for a discussion of liaisons in cued languages). Liaisons in the children's cueing were observed starting at 28 months, in the recitation of learned songs and rhymes. An example is found in "the clean-up song" (*clean-up, clean-up; everybody, everywhere . . .*) in which both children were observed to cue the /n/ of *clean* with the side-down placement /ʌ/ for *up* (klee–nup). Another example is found in a favorite game of "waking up" Sesame Street characters in a toy, in which both children were observed to cue the /k/ of *wake* with the side-down placement /ʌ/ for *up* (way–kup). Another example is found in Laura's cueing/singing of "Twinkle, Twinkle, Little Star," in which she cues the final /d/ of *diamond* with the throat placement /ɪ/ for *in* (diamon–din). These examples, and other observed instances, suggest that these children, much like hearing children with speech (Gombert, 1992), learn to cue large phonological segments prior to gaining an understanding of word boundaries.

Vocabulary. The parents reported that both children expressed their first word at 11 months and that by 13 months, the children had an expressive vocabulary of approximately 8 words, including: *Emily, Laura, mommy, daddy, moo, poo-poo, up,* and *uh-oh.* At 23 months, the mother completed the MacArthur-Bates Communicative Development Inventory (CDI): Words and Gestures, and the children's expressive vocabulary was estimated at 130 words. At 36 months, the author and the mother completed the MacArthur-Bates Communicative Development Inventory (CDI): Words and Sentences, and based on the items presented in the inventory, the children's expressive vocabulary was estimated at 625 words. An accurate count or estimate was not possible, due to the children's use of a large number of synonyms (e.g., couch/sofa, large/big/huge, pretty/beautiful), and additional words in a number of semantic categories not accounted for in the CDI, including: actions (e.g., crawling, flying, marching), objects (e.g., battery, binoculars, string, tutu), people (e.g., artist, ballerina, player), and proper nouns (e.g., brand name grocery items, cities, store names).

Morphology, Mean Length of Utterance, and Syntax. Following Brown's (1973) rules for counting morphemes, the mean length of utterance (MLU) was calculated for each child at 25 months, 30 months, and 36 months. Each time the middle 50 utterances in the language sample attributed to each child were used. Also, in keeping with Brown's guidelines for stages of language and sentence types, the children's developing syntax was documented. At 25 months, Emily's MLU was calculated as 2.4 with utterances ranging from 1 to 3 words, an example being, "That not me." Laura's MLU was calculated at 2.1 with utterances ranging from 1 to 3 words, an example being, "In, mommy, please." Also at 25 months, examples of Brown's Stage I *operations of reference* were documented, in which both children created 2 to 3 word sentences for the purposes of: (1) nomination, as in, "That mommy"; (2) recurrence, as in, "More water" and "More water please"; (3) negation for denial, as in, "No hit Laura" (I didn't hit Laura); (4) negation for rejection, as in, "No peach"; and (5) negation for nonexistence, as in, "Baby all gone." Examples of Brown's Stage I *semantic relations* were documented, in which both children created 2 to 3 word sentences to express: (1) agent + action, as in, "Emily hit Laura!"; (2) action + object, as in, "Feed baby"; (3) agent + object, as in, "Mommy school"; (4) action + locative, as in, "We go park"; (5) entity + locative, as in, "Pony there"; (f) possessor + possession, as in, "Laura baby," "Emily purse," and "Daddy key"; (g) entity + attribute, as in, "Baby sleepy"; and (h) demonstrative + entity, as in, "That one."

This language sample included examples of most of Brown's (1973) 14 morphemes, including: present progressive; in, on (and other prepositions); regular pluralization; and regular and irregular past tense. This suggests that by 25 months both girls had progressed through Brown's Stage I, with an approximate age range of 12 to 26 months, and had entered Stage II, with an approximate age range of 27 to 30 months (Brown, 1973).

At 30 months, Emily's MLU was calculated at 3.2 with utterances ranging from 2 to 6 words, an example being, "Can you draw a Barney here?" Laura's MLU was calculated at 2.9 with utterances ranging from 1 to 5 words, an example being, "Kelly, I hurt my toe." This language sample included a number of sentence forms, such as declaratives (e.g., "I need more paper"), negatives (e.g., "That not Baby Bop"), and interrogatives (e.g., "Who that?"). This language sample also included such structures as irregular past tense (e.g., "Laura hit me!") and use of articles (e.g., *a*, *an*, *the*). This suggests that by 30 months, both children had entered Brown's Stage III, with an approximate age range of 31 to 34 months. It should be noted that Mother reported "an explosion of language" between 27 and 30 months, in which both parents observed a marked increase in vocabulary and sentence length.

At 36 months, Emily's MLU was calculated at 4.1 with utterances ranging from 2 to 10 words, an example being, "We will go to [city] to see Grandma and Grandpa." Laura's MLU was calculated at 3.8 with utterances ranging from 2 to 8 words, an example being, "Can we go to the really really really big park?" This language sample included a variety of sentence forms and functions, including articles, regular past tense, conjunctions, and joined clauses (e.g., if, when, so, because), suggesting that by 36 months, both girls had entered Brown's Stage V, with an approximate age range of 41 to 46 months.

By 36 months, all of Brown's 14 morphemes were observed as emerging or mastered, with the girls generally initiating use of a new morpheme at roughly the same time, and with Emily generally mastering its use 4 to 6 weeks before Laura. At the 36-month mark, the most recent morpheme to be mastered was the regular 3rd person –s, which Emily mastered at 34 months and Laura at 35 months. Also at this point, the contractible and uncontractible copula and the contractible auxiliary (included in Brown's Stage V, with an approximate age range of 41 to 46 months) had emerged in both girls, but had not yet reached mastery.

Pragmatics and Metalinguistic Awareness. The children were reported and observed to use language for a variety of intentions and purposes. Beginning with proto-imperatives and continuing with more sophisticated language forms, they were observed to use language to state/report/complain, deny/refuse/protest, and request/inquire.

By the age of 32 months, they were also reported and observed to use language to aid in pretend play, to play jokes, and to manipulate their parents. As an example of using language to play jokes, the father reported that, at the age of 31 months, the children had come to understand that they could hear things that neither of their parents could. At this point, they began a game in which they would run into a room and cue, "Daddy, baby crying, [points upstairs] waa-waa!" The father would go upstairs to check on the baby, and the girls, knowing this to be untrue, would run, giggling, in the opposite direction. The behavior was reportedly extinguished in a short period of time. The use of language to manipulate a situation is clearly illustrated in the following exchange, observed at 32 months:

Mother: *[first, middle, and last name], what did mommy say about jumping on the bed?!*

Laura: *Laura not jumping; Laura marching* [laughs]

Mother: *You know what I mean.*

The children's metalinguistic awareness (i.e., awareness of their use of language and that of other's) was reported on by the parents and observed by the author through the children's comprehension of the difference between speaking and cueing, their ability to "code switch" depending on the expressive communication of another, and their recognition of differences in people's use of language.

By 28 months, the children were observed by the author to respond appropriately to requests to: cue a word/phrase which they had recently spoken only; say a word/phrase without cues; and cue "quietly, without saying anything." The parents reported that by 25 months, the children had begun cueing and speaking in response to individuals who cued expressively, and speaking only to individuals who did not cue expressively. This "code switching" was observed by the author at 28 months during a play session, when the author intentionally did not cue his statements and the research assistant cued all of her statements. Both children responded to the author with speech only, and responded to the research assistant either with speech only, or with speech and cues. Perhaps the most interesting example of metalinguistic awareness observed during this study centers on the recognition of other people's specific word choices, demonstrated by Emily at the age of 36 months in the following exchange.

[the mother and author are sitting together, discussing observations]

[Emily approaches, reaches for the mother]

Mother: *Do you want up on the sofa with mommy?*

[Emily does not respond; tries to climb]

Mother: *Do you want on the sofa, yes or no?*

Emily: *Mommy says, sofa; Daddy says couch.*

Author: *What did she just say?*

Mother: *She came up with that yesterday; it was new to me.*

Early Literacy

Behaviors supportive of early literacy development were observed at the beginning of data collection (10 months) and during every subsequent visit. Observations were made regarding: book sharing, cued response to pictures in books, learning rhymes and songs, drawing and scribbling, letter naming, and early sight word learning.

Book Sharing. The parents reported exposing the children to books as soon as the children were able to sit up, around 6 months. The exact nature of this book sharing changed over time, regarding visual access to cues, visual attention, and child responses.

At the beginning of data collection (10 months), the father was observed to sit cross-legged on the floor with a child in his lap facing forward, and a picture book (with or without text) facing the child. The father cued the text on the page and/or what was seen, often pointing to an image on the page. The father cued with his hand in front of the child, between the child and the book. Instead of using his own cueing placements, he produced the manual cue handshapes at the child's mouth, chin, throat, and side placements.

At 12 months, the children were observed to locate a favorite book and bring it to the father. The father cued, "Do you want to read? Do you want to read a book?" At this point, the father sat cross-legged on the floor, and the child crawled into his lap. During this book sharing, the father again cued "on the child." The child's visual attention (eye gaze and head position) shifted from one position when the father cued in front of the book to a second position when the father pointed into the book. The child was observed to point to an object relating to the word cued, then turn her head around and up toward the father. The father cued in his own space (e.g., "Yes! The baby chick!").

By 17 months (2 months before implant activation), the children had favorite books, and had names for them (e.g., "Goo Goo," referring to an expression repeated in the book). At this point, either child was observed to shift attention between the father and the book, point to objects cued by the father, and repeat the cues.

At 25 months (6 months after implant activation), the children were observed to request books be read two or three times at a sitting. The child sat in the father's lap, with the father continuing to cue in the child's visual field. The child was observed to point to an object or area of text in advance of the father cueing that part.

At 32 months (13 months after implant activation), the children were observed to engage in books sharing together with the father, sitting in chairs to either side. The children pointed to the objects or areas of text in the book and cued (with speech) what they pointed to. They were observed to argue over who should turn the page, and whether it was "time" to do so.

Cued Response to Pictures in Books.
Also at 32 months, the children were observed to interact with books independently. Each time, the child selected a book, oriented it correctly, opened the book toward the beginning, and turned one or more pages at a time. On each page, the child pointed to one or more objects and named them (with or without cues). This behavior was observed both when the child knew an adult was watching, and when the child appeared to be unattended.

Learning Rhymes and Songs. At 28 months, the children were observed to sing (with cues) songs for routines, such as *The Clean-Up Song*, and *The Nighty-Night Song*. By 32 months, both children were observed singing (with cues) *The Barney Song* in its entirety (*I love you, you love me, we're a happy family . . .*). Emily was observed singing *Twinkle, Twinkle, Little Star* in its entirety (*. . . up above the world so high . . .*), and Laura was observed singing *The ABC Song* in its entirety (*. . . now I know my ABC's, next time won't you sing with me?*).

Drawing and Scribbling. At 28 months, the children were observed by the author to repeatedly draw pictures of their favorite dinosaur characters, Barney and Baby Bop. The children drew a picture, and the mother asked, "What did you draw?" The child responded (either Barney or Baby Bop), and the mother cued, "I'll write [name] underneath, right here." At 32 months, the children were observed to draw a character with one color of crayon, and "write" beneath the drawing with another color. Also at 32 months, the children sat at a table with the author and "drew" shapes. The children's consistent use of the verbs *draw* and *write* were noted (e.g., "I'll draw a circle; Mister Kelly, draw a star; Kelly, write Laura."). At 36 months, Laura was first observed to "write" letters. Specifically, upon completing a drawing of Barney, she asked the author to write the dinosaur's name beneath. The author wrote each letter, stopping to cue the name of the letter before writing the next. Laura then "wrote" beneath the author's writing three separate scribbles, calling them B, E, and Y, respectively.

Early Sight Word Learning. At 36 months, the children were observed to match (inconsistently) printed words to their spoken referents. Specifically, seated at a table with the mother (holding baby brother) and the author, the children took turns writing words with the author. Laura asked the author to write words for shapes she had attempted to draw (i.e., circle, heart, moon, star). Emily asked the author to write the names of people present (i.e., Daddy, Emily, Kelly, Laura, Matthew, Mommy). The author wrote names, making note of the first letter and the sound/cue it makes. Both children quickly matched printed names to cued/spoken names. After 5 minutes of "play," all written names were consistently identified, except for *Mommy* and *Matthew*, as the most salient feature (i.e., first letter) was the same, both have double consonants, and the two words are similar in length.

Conclusion

Results from this study add to our understanding of the language development of children who are deaf, as well as specifically our understanding of how children who are deaf develop traditionally spoken language visually. These results also shed light on the role of Cued Speech in the receptive and expressive language of cueing deaf adults and children. Finally, results from this study provide insight to the role of early language exposure in the preliteracy achievement of very young deaf children.

Results from this study support the position that language acquisition is a generally irrepressible phenomenon, provided a child has early, clear, and complete access to the phoneme stream of the language and opportunities to interact with fluent models of that language (see Chapter 12). Just as hearing children acquire spoken languages from hearing parents and signing deaf children acquire signed languages from signing deaf parents, the cueing deaf children in this study were observed acquiring cued language from cueing deaf parents.

Results from this study also support the position of LaSasso and Metzger (1998) that early exposure to Cued English and opportunities to interact with fluent English language models allows children who are deaf to acquire English naturally, in the same ways and at the same rate as hearing peers. Findings from the study reported here provide evidence that prelingually, profoundly deaf children *can*, with clear, complete access to the continuous phoneme stream of English, achieve English language development milestones within the ranges expected of children of hearing parents. These milestones include prelinguistic and early English language milestones observed both prior to cochlear implantation as well as receptive and expressive language milestones observed after implant activation. The children in this study exhibited eye gaze and joint attention behaviors and prelinguistic intentional communication comparable to that expected of hearing infants. They developed a large receptive vocabulary prior to uttering their first words at approximately 11 months, in keeping with hearing norms. They gained morphemes along with varied grammatical sentence structures along expected trajectories for hearing peers. They developed rich and varied receptive and expressive vocabularies and syntactically complex sentence structures. In terms of the mechanics of expressive cueing, they progressed through stages of: hand/finger movements in response to adult cueing; cue babbling; early words cued as single movements; cued approximations; fully cued words; partially cued sentences; and fully cued sentences. As this is the first study to document this progression of expressive cueing behavior in deaf infants, comparisons cannot be made.

Results of this study also add to our understanding of the role of the manual mode used by deaf parents related to infant babbling in the manual mode. Prior to this study, the term "manual mode" was taken to mean signing only. Both of the cueing children in this study as infants progressed through stages of "cue babbling" on a time line that appears to mirror "sign babbling" observed in deaf infants of signing deaf parents (Petitto & Marentette, 1991). Previous data related to deaf infants of signing deaf mothers coupled with data reported here related to cueing deaf infants, suggests a universal tendency of deaf infants to seek visual stimuli, mimic and practice visible gestures, and selectively keep those which eventually will be used to express meaning, regardless of whether the language is a signed language or a traditionally spoken language that is cued.

Results of this study also add to our understanding of the respective contributions of *parental deafness* versus language access in the early development of deaf children. The same behaviors long observed in signing deaf mothers (e.g., responding to the child's eye movements, anticipating and labeling the child's gestures, communicating within the child's visual field) were observed in the cueing deaf parents in this study. These behaviors have been linked to early bonding and language acquisition (Koester, Traci, Brooks, Karkowski, & Smith-Gray, 2004). This finding of intuitive responses to the deaf child's visual needs and immediate exposure to visual language input with these deaf cueing parents suggests that such advantages that have been typically associated with early exposure to *signing by deaf parents* (Loots & Devisé, 2003) might better be more accurately attributed to deaf parents' intuition and visually convey and model their language clearly and completely rather than the nature of the language (i.e., signed or traditionally spoken).

Results of this study also add to our understanding of the nature of Cued Speech and its role in the cued and spoken language development of deaf children. First, the cueing deaf parents in this study, like hearing parents of hearing children and signing deaf parents in other studies (Loots, Devisé, & Jacquet, 2005; Newport & Meier, 1985; Schlesinger & Meadow, 1972) served as effective language models for their children, and in this case, served as effective models of English, a language that is traditionally spoken, to children who could not hear speech. From birth through 18 months, when hearing aid use by the girls in this study was minimal and inconsistent, the girls reached normal language milestones. Even before the girls' cochlear implantation, the manual, facial, and prosodic components of cueing provided all of the linguistic information of English visually that the girls needed to acquire the English language naturally. This finding supports the finding of Metzger and Fleetwood (Chapter 3) that cueing *can* function as a purely visual means of language transmission. It also supports the view that deaf children, like hearing peers are able to acquire English and other traditionally spoken languages naturally as long as they have early, clear, and complete access to the continuous phoneme stream of the language and consistent, fluent language models (LaSasso & Metzger, 1998).

A second insight about Cued Speech obtained in this study is that Cued Speech can serve as a real-time audio-visual bridge for cued and spoken language development of children who are deaf during the period of cochlear implant activation and the children's learning to construct meaning from the novel acoustic signal. This is in keeping with the discussion by Aparicio, Peigneux, Charlier, and Leybaert (Chapter 24) regarding the multimodal nature of speech and spoken language reception. Immediately following cochlear implant activation, cueing provided a bridge between phonology that is *seen* and phonology that is *heard*. The girls in this study, after their cochlear implants were activated, were quickly able to pair the "new and strange" acoustic signal from the implant with the "already known" handshapes and placements of familiar words and phrases. This is in contrast to a child with limited visual input (i.e., speechreading) prior to implantation, who must attempt to simultaneously acclimate to new acoustic signals and discover the existence of the phonemes represented therein.

A third insight about Cued Speech obtained in this study was its value for augmenting or supplementing the degraded acoustic signal supplied by a cochlear implant (Fu & Shannon, 2000). As the girls in this study learned to make sense of the auditory information avail-able to them via the cochlear implant, and they learned new spoken words and phrases, Cued Speech was observed to provide visual support and clarification for continued spoken language development. As the children simultaneously developed expressive cueing and speaking abilities, cueing was observed to provide an additional means through which words could be perceived and/or expressed; words could be acquired first as cued phenomena and then added to the spoken lexicon, or vice versa.

A fourth insight about Cued Speech gained from this study relates to its effectiveness for parents who are deaf. The parents in this study, despite differences in speech intelligibility, were observed to provide clear and complete visual representation of spoken language via the visible manual and facial aspects of cueing, decreasing their children's dependence on speech intelligibility to understand a cued English message.

Results of this study also provide insight into the role of Cued Speech in the development of literacy in young deaf children. Early language ability is closely linked to later literacy achievement for deaf children (Desjardin, Ambrose, & Eisenberg, 2009; Strong & Prinz, 1998) and hearing children (Bryant, MacLean, Bradley, & Crossland, 1989). Given that written language is based on spoken language and encoded in an alphabetic script (Musselman, 2000; Perfetti & Sandak, 2000), it stands to reason that a deaf child's early experience with a spoken language could only serve to support that child's acquisition of the written form, more so than explicitly learning the language when learning to read (Mayer & Akamatsu, 1999).

Reading comprehension can be viewed as a process that goes forward or breaks down as a result of reader's questions; that is, comprehension breaks down if readers have too many or no questions about what they are reading (Smith, 2006). In this view, three types of questions that a deaf reader might have relate to *language*, *content*, and *code* (LaSasso, 1994). A reader's questions about language might relate to vocabulary, syntax, figurative language in the text. Questions about content relate to the reader's background knowledge and experiences brought to the reading task. Questions about code refer to the reader's knowledge of the letters and punctuation used to form printed words and sentences, and how these relate to the spoken form of the language. Refer to Chapter 12 by LaSasso and Crain for examples of readers' questions.

Cued Speech, as exhibited in the findings of study reported in this chapter, is a powerful tool for implicitly and simultaneously exposing a deaf child to the language (vocabulary, syntax, figurative expressions), content (labels and explanations for experiences), and code (the continuous phoneme stream) necessary to later successfully and independently decode and comprehend text.

Perhaps most importantly, the parents in this study were observed to cue all conversations and interactions in the children's presence, providing labels for people, objects, and ideas. In return, the parents expected (and received) age-appropriate expressive language from the children. These parents, like parents of hearing children, were observed to consistently lead their children in nursery rhymes and sing-song games, practicing rote language in the same way that hearing parents and children do. Through this exchange of language, the parents and children were able to build shared experiences and memories, adding to the children's schema and background knowledge. At all times

during the observations, the allowable sequences of phonemes used to construct every word in the English language were being supplied by the parents in a completely visual manner and practiced by the children every day. Toward the end of data collection (at 36 months of age), the deaf toddlers were observed to isolate phonemes (e.g., /m/) and recognize and call by name printed letters (e.g., "It's an *m*."). They were observed to recognize their first sight words, memorized not only by the letter shapes they contained, but by the letters and their initial sounds. This is the beginning of the development of the critically important alphabetic principle, and decoding. Although questions about code represent only one potential barrier to reading comprehension, as documented in this chapter, the language experience and comprehension that these prelingually, profoundly deaf children will need to bring to the task of early reading are already in place.

Epilogue

One year after the end of data collection, eight days after the girls' fourth birthday, the girls were administered the Test of Early Reading Assessment, Third Edition (TERA-3) by a qualified teacher of students who are deaf. The TERA-3 (Reid, Hresko, & Hammill, 2001) assesses the mastery of early developing reading skills in hearing children between ages 3.5 to 8.5 years. The TERA-3 has three subtests: (1) alphabet knowledge and phonics, (2) conventions of print (e.g., how to hold a book, text is read left to right and top to bottom), and (3) construction of meaning (i.e., comprehension) of symbols and words. The test requires 30 minutes to administer and

Table 8–3. TERA-3 Hearing Age Equivalents Expressed in Years-Months

	Alphabet Knowledge	Conventions of Print	Comprehension of Symbols and Print
Emily	5-5	4-3	4-9
Laura	6-4	4-9	5-4

yields standard scores, percentile ranks, and normal curve equivalents. A version of the test for children who are deaf or hard of hearing exists,[1] but the decision was made to test the girls with the hearing version of the TERA-3 and compare their performance with hearing norms. The test was administered to each girl individually, via cued American English.

As reflected in Table 8–3, both girls scored above the age levels expected of their hearing peers in all three measures of early reading ability. These results corroborate the observations and parent reports collected during the 26 months of data collection.

References

Adamson, L. (1995). *Communication development during infancy.* Madison, WI: Brown and Benchmark.

Alegria, J., Dejean, K., Capouillez, J., & Leybaert, J. (1990). Role played by Cued Speech in the identification of written words encountered for the first time by deaf children. *Cued Speech Journal, 4,* 4–9.

Alegria, J., Lechat, J., & Leybaert, J. (1990). Role of Cued Speech in the identification of words in the deaf child: Theory and preliminary data. *Cued Speech Journal, 4,* 10–23.

American Guidance Service (2000). *The Goldman-Fristoe Test of Articulation* (2nd ed.). Circle Pines, MN: Author.

Anderson, D., & Reilly, J. (2002). The MacArthur Communicative Development Inventory: Normative data for American Sign Language. *Journal of Deaf Studies and Deaf Education, 7,* 83–106.

Bates, E. (1979). *The emergence of symbols: Cognition and communication in infancy.* New York, NY: Academic Press.

Bates, E., Camaioni, L., & Volterra, V. (1979). The acquisition of performatives prior to speech. In E. Ochs & B. Schieffelin (Eds.), *Developmental pragmatics* (pp. 111–113). New York, NY: Academic Press.

Benedict, H. (1979). Early lexical development: Comprehension and production. *Journal of Child Language, 6,* 183–200.

Berko-Gleason, J. (2004). *The development of language* (6th ed.). New York, NY: Allyn & Bacon.

Blamey, P., Sarant, J., Paatsch, L., Barry, J., Bow, C., Wales, R., . . . Tooher, R. (2001). Relationships among speech perception, production, language, hearing loss, and age in children with impaired hearing. *Journal of Speech, Language, and Hearing Research, 44,* 264–285.

---

[1]The TERA–D/HH test is an individually administered test of reading designed for children with moderate to profound sensory hearing loss (i.e., ranging from 41 to beyond 91 decibels, corrected). The test was standardized on a national sample of more than 1,000 students who were deaf or hard of hearing from 20 states. Normative data are given for every 6-month interval from 3-0 through 13-11.

Brown, R. (1973). *A first language: The early stages.* Cambridge, MA: Harvard University Press.

Bryant, P. E., Bradley, L., Maclean, M., & Crossland, J. (1989). Nursery rhymes, phonological skills and reading. *Journal of Child Language, 16*(2), 407–428.

Camaioni, L., Caselli, M. C., Volterra, V., & Luchenti, S. (1992). Questionario sullo sviluppo comunicativo e linguistico nel 2° anno di vita [A questionnaire for the assessment of communication and language in the second year of life]. Manuale, Firenze: OS.

Casby, M., & Cumpata, J. (1986). A protocol for the assesment of prelinguistic intentional communication. *Journal of Communication Disorders, 19*, 251–260.

Chall, J. (1983). *Stages of reading development.* New York, NY: McGraw-Hill.

Chamberlain, C., & Mayberry, R. (2000). Theorizing about the relation between American Sign Language and reading. In C. Chamberlain, J. Morford, & R. Mayberry (Eds.), *Language acquisition by eye* (pp. 221–260). Hillsdale, NJ: Lawrence Erlbaum Associates.

Desjardin, J., Ambrose, S., & Eisenberg, L. (2009). Literacy skills in children with cochlear implants: The importance of early oral language and joint storybook reading. *Journal of Deaf Studies and Deaf Education, 14*, 22–43.

Dromi, E. (2003). Assessment of prelinguistic behaviors in deaf children: Parents as collaborators. *Journal of Deaf Studies and Deaf Education, 8*, 367–382.

Fairbanks, G. (1960). *Voice and articulation drillbook* (2nd ed.). New York, NY: Harper & Row.

Fenson, L., Dale, P., Reznick, J., Thal, D., Bates, E., Hartung, J., . . . Reilly, J. (1993). *The MacArthur Bates Communicative Development Inventories User's Guide and Technical Manual.* Baltimore, MD: Paul H. Brooks.

Fu, Q., & Shannon, R. (2000). Effect of stimulation rate on phoneme recognition in cochlear implants. *Journal of the Acoustical Society of America, 107*, 589–597.

Gombert, J. (1992). *Metalinguistic development.* London, UK: Harvester Wheatsheaf.

Grushkin, D. (1998). Why shouldn't Sam read? Toward a new paradigm for literacy and the deaf. *Journal of Deaf Studies and Deaf Education, 3*, 179–201.

Harding, C. (1983). Setting the stage for language acquisition: Communication development in the first year. In R. Golinkoff (Ed.), *The transition from prelinguistic to linguistic communication* (pp. 93–113). Hillsdale, NJ: Lawrence Erlbaum Associates.

Harris, M., & Beech, J. (1998). Implicit phonological awareness and early reading development in prelingually deaf children. *Journal of Deaf Studies and Deaf Education, 3*, 205–216.

Hulit, L., & Howard, M. (2002). *Born to talk: An introduction to speech and language Development* (3rd ed.). New York, NY: Allyn & Bacon.

James, D., Rajput, K., Brown, T., Sirimanna, T., Brinton, J., & Goswami, U. (2005). Phonological awareness in deaf children who use cochlear implants. *Journal of Speech, Language, and Hearing Research, 48*, 1511–1528.

Jamieson, J. (1995). Interaction between mothers and children who are deaf. *Journal of Early Intervention, 19*, 108–117.

Katz, R., Shankweiler, D., & Liberman, I. (1981). Memory for item order and phonetic recoding in the beginning reader. *Journal of Exceptional Child Psychology, 32*, 474–484.

Kemp, M. (1998). Why is learning American Sign Language a challenge? *American Annals of the Deaf, 143*, 255–259.

Kemper, R., & Vernooy, A. (1993). Metalinguistic awareness in first graders: A qualitative perspective. *Journal of Psycholinguistic Research, 22*, 41–57.

Kipila, E. (1985). Analysis of an oral language sample from a prelingually deaf child's Cued Speech: A case study. *Cued Speech Annual, 1*, 46–59.

Koester, L., Brooks, L., & Traci, M. (2000). Tactile contact by deaf and hearing mothers during face-to-face interactions with their infants. *Journal of Deaf Studies and Deaf Education, 5*, 127–139.

Koester, L., Traci, M., Brooks, L., Karkowski, A., & Smith-Gray, S. (2004). Mother-infant behaviors at 6 and 9 months: A microanalytic view. In K. Meadow-Orlans, P. Spencer, & L. Koester (Eds.), *The world of deaf infants: A longitudinal study* (pp. 40–56). New York, NY: Oxford University Press.

LaSasso, C. (1994). Reading comprehension of deaf readers: The impact of too few or too many questions. *American Annals of the Deaf, 138*, 435–441.

LaSasso, C., Crain, K., & Leybaert, J. (2003). Rhyme generation in deaf students: The effect of exposure to Cued Speech. *Journal of Deaf Studies and Deaf Education, 8*, 250–270.

LaSasso, C., & Metzger, M. (1998). An alternate route for preparing deaf children for BiBi programs: The home language as L1 and Cued Speech for conveying traditionally-spoken languages. *Journal of Deaf Studies and Deaf Education, 3*, 265–289.

Leybaert, J. (1993). Reading in the deaf: The role of phonological codes. In M. Marschark & M. Clark (Eds.), *Psychological perspectives on deafness* (pp. 269–309). Hillsdale, NJ: Lawrence Erlbaum Associates.

Leybaert, J., & Alegria, J. (1993). Is word processing involuntary in deaf children? *British Journal of Developmental Psychology, 11*, 1–29.

Leybaert, J., & Alegria, J. (1995). Spelling development in hearing and deaf children: Evidence for use of morpho-phonological regularities in French. *Reading and Writing, 7*, 89–109.

Leybaert, J., Alegría, J., Hage, C., & Charlier, B. (1998). The effect of exposure to phonetically augmented lipspeech in the prelingual deaf. In R. Campbell, B. Dodd, & D. Burnham (Eds.), *Hearing by eye (Vol.II): Advances in the psychology of speechreading and auditory-visual speech* (pp. 283–301). Hove, England: Psychology Press.

Leybaert, J., & Charlier, B. (1996). Visual speech in the head: The effect of Cued Speech on rhyming, remembering, and spelling. *Journal of Deaf Studies and Deaf Education, 1*, 234–248.

Lichtert, G. (2003). Assessing intentional communication in deaf toddlers. *Journal of Deaf Studies and Deaf Education, 8*, 43–56.

Loots, G., & Devisé, I. (2003). The use of visual-tactile communication strategies by deaf and hearing fathers and mothers of deaf infants. *Journal of Deaf Studies and Deaf Education, 8*, 31–42.

Loots, G., Devisé, I., & Jacquet, W. (2005). The impact of visual communication on the intersubjective development of early parent-child interaction with 18- to 24-month old deaf toddlers. *Journal of Deaf Studies and Deaf Education, 10*, 357–375.

Mann, V., Shankweiler, D., & Smith, S. (1984). The association between comprehension of spoken sentences and early reading ability: The role of phonetic representations. *Journal of Child Language, 11*, 627–643.

Marschark, M., Schick, B., & Spencer, P. (2006). Understanding sign language development of deaf children. In B. Schick, M. Marschark, & P. Spencer (Eds.), *Advances in the sign language development of deaf children* (pp. 3–19). New York, NY: Oxford University Press.

Mayer, C., & Akamatsu, C. (1999). Bilingual-bicultural models of literacy education for deaf students: Considering the claims. *Journal of Deaf Studies and Deaf Education, 4*, 1–8.

Mayne, A., Yoshinaga-Itano, C., & Sedey, A. (2000). Receptive vocabulary development of infants and toddlers who are deaf or hard of hearing. *Volta Review, 100*, 29–52.

Mayne, A., Yoshinaga-Itano, C., Sedey, A., & Carey, A. (2000). Expressive vocabulary development of infants and toddlers who are deaf or hard of hearing. *Volta Review, 100*, 1–28.

McIntire, M. (1977). The acquisition of American Sign Language hand configurations. *Sign Language Studies, 16*, 247–266.

Meadow-Orlans, K. (1997). Effects of mother and infant hearing status on interactions at twelve and eighteen months. *Journal of Deaf Studies and Deaf Education, 2*, 26–36.

Metzger, M. (1994). *Involvement strategies in cued English discourse: Soundless expressive phonology.* Unpublished manuscript: Georgetown University, Washington, DC.

Musselman, C. (2000). How do children who can't hear learn to read an alphabetic script? A review of the literature on reading and deafness. *Journal of Deaf Studies and Deaf Education, 5,* 9–31.

Newport, E., & Meier, R. (1985). Acquisition of American Sign Language. In D. Slobin (Ed.), *The crosslinguistic study of language acquisition* (pp. 881–938). Hillsdale, NJ: Lawrence Erlbaum Associates.

Oller, K. (2000). *The emergence of the speech capacity.* Hillsdale, NJ: Lawrence Erlbaum Associates.

Owens, R. (2001). *Language development: An introduction* (5th ed.). New York, NY: Allyn & Bacon.

Paatsch, L., Blamey, P., Sarant, J., & Bow, C. (2006). The effects of speech production and vocabulary training on different components of spoken language performance. *Journal of Deaf Studies and Deaf Education, 11,* 39–55.

Padden, C., & Ramsey, C. (2000). American Sign Language and reading ability in deaf children. In C. Chamberlain, J. Morford, & R. Mayberry (Eds.), *Language acquisition by eye* (pp. 165–189). Hillsdale, NJ: Lawrence Erlbaum Associates.

Perier, O., Charlier, B., Hage, C., & Alegria, J. (1987). Evaluation of the effects of prolonged Cued Speech practice upon the reception of spoken language. In I. G. Taylor (Ed.), *The education of the deaf: Current perspectives* (pp. 616–628). Kent, UK: Crom Helm Ltd.

Perfetti, C., & Sandak, R. (2000). Reading optimally builds on spoken language: Implications for deaf readers. *Journal of Deaf Studies and Deaf Education, 5,* 32–50.

Pettito, L., & Marentette, P. (1991). Babbling in the manual mode: Evidence for the ontogeny of language. *Science, 251,* 1493–1496.

Pipp-Siegel, S., Sedey, A., & Yoshinaga-Itano, C. (2002). Predictors of parental stress in mothers of young children with hearing loss. *Journal of Deaf Studies and Deaf Education, 7,* 1–17.

Pressman, L., Pipp-Siegal, S., Yoshinaga-Itano, C., & Deas, A. (1999). Maternal sensitivity predicts language gain in preschool children who are deaf and hard of hearing. *Journal of Deaf Studies and Deaf Education, 4,* 294–304.

Reid, D., Hresko, W., & Hammill, D. (2001). *Test of Early Reading Achievement* (3rd ed.). Austin, TX: Pro-Ed.

Sander, E. (1972). When are speech sounds learned? *Journal of Speech and Hearing Disorders, 37,* 54–63.

Sarant, J., Holt, C., Dowell, R., Rickards, F., & Blamey, P. (2009). Spoken language development in oral preschool children with permanent childhood deafness. *Journal of Deaf Studies and Deaf Education, 14,* 205–217.

Schlesinger, H., & Meadow, K. (1972). *Sound and sign: Childhood deafness and mental health.* Berkeley, CA: University of California Press.

Smith, F. (2006). *Reading without nonsense* (4th ed.). New York, NY: Teachers College Press.

Spencer, L., & Tomblin, B. (2009). Evaluating phonological processing skills in children with prelingual deafness who use cochlear implants. *Journal of Deaf Studies and Deaf Education, 14,* 1–21.

Spencer, P. (1993). The expressive communication of hearing mothers and deaf infants. *American Annals of the Deaf, 138,* 275–283.

Spencer, P. (2000). Looking without listening: Is audition a prerequisite for normal development of visual attention during infancy? *Journal of Deaf Studies and Deaf Education, 5,* 291–302.

Spencer, P., & Meadow-Orlans, K. (1996). Play, language, and maternal responsiveness: A longitudinal study of deaf and hearing infants. *Child Development, 67,* 3176–3191.

Stine, E., & Bohannon, J. (1983). Imitation, interactions, and acquisition. *Journal of Child Language, 10,* 589–604.

Strong, M., & Prinz, M. (1997). A study of the relationship between American Sign Language and English literacy. *Journal of Deaf Studies and Deaf Education, 2,* 37–46.

Subtelny, J. (1977). Assessment of speech with implications for training. In F. Bess (Ed.), *Childhood deafness: Causation, assessment, and management* (pp. 183–194). New York, NY: Grune & Stratton.

Swisher, V. (1992). The role of parents in developing visual turn-taking in their young deaf children. *American Annals of the Deaf, 137,* 92–100.

Wandel, J. (1989). *Use of internal speech in reading by hearing and hearing-impaired students in oral, total communication and Cued Speech programs.* Unpublished doctoral dissertation, Teachers College, Columbia University, New York, NY.

Waxman, R., & Spencer, P. (1997). What mothers do to support infant visual attention: Sensitivities to age and hearing status. *Journal of Deaf Studies and Deaf Education, 2,* 104–114.

Weaver, C. (1994). *Reading process and practice: From sociopsycholinguistics to whole language.* Portsmouth, NH: Heinemann.

Wilbur, R. (2000). The use of ASL to support the development of English and literacy. *Journal of Deaf Studies and Deaf Education, 5,* 81–104.

Wilbur, R., Montanelli, A., & Quigley, S. (1975). Pronominalization in the language of deaf students. *Journal of Speech and Hearing Research, 19,* 120–140.

Chapter 9

EXPERIENCES AND PERCEPTIONS OF CUEING DEAF ADULTS IN THE UNITED STATES

Kelly Lamar Crain and Carol J. LaSasso

The Literature Related to Cultural Identity, Psychosocial Adjustment and Self-Esteem of Individuals Who Are Deaf

Much has been written about cultural identity, psychosocial adjustment and self-esteem of individuals who are deaf from oral and signing backgrounds over the past 25 years; however, very little has been written about individuals from Cued Speech backgrounds. Our knowledge of the cultural identity, psychosocial adjustment, and self-esteem of children, adolescents, and adults who are deaf from oral and signing backgrounds comes primarily from research and autobiographic literature.

Research Literature

A recent review of the published research literature related to self-esteem, psychosocial adjustment, and/or cultural identify of children, adolescents, and adults who are deaf revealed 19 studies from 1982 to 2007. Table 9–1 summarizes those studies, including: the various research protocols (e.g., questionnaires, interviews, psychosocial scales) employed, the aspect of self-esteem, psychosocial adjustment, or cultural identity assessed, numbers of participants in the study, ages and communication backgrounds, and whether the study explored home and/or school variables.

Participants in previous reports came from either oral and/or signing backgrounds. Specifically, five of the 19 studies examined participants from oral backgrounds

Table 9–1. Summary of Studies of Self-Esteem, Psychosocial Adjustment or Cultural Identity of Deaf Children, Adolescents, or Adults

Authors (year)	Method	Identity, Self-Concept, or Self-Esteem	No. of D/HH Subjects	Ages	Degree of Deafness	Oral, MCE, ASL,	Home, School, or Both
Bat-Chava & Deignan (2001)	Interview; Parent Reporting	Peer relationships	25	Child	Profound/ Cochlear Implant	Oral	Both
Brunnberge et al. (2007)	Questionnaire	Mental health and school adjustment	149	Adolescent	Mild-Moderate	Oral	Both
Crowe (2003)	Scales	Self-esteem	152	Adult	Not reported	Sign	School
Hintermair (2007)	Questionnaire	Self-esteem and contentedness	629	Adult	Severe-profound	Oral and Sign	N/A
Israelite et al. (2002)	Qualitative Questionnaire Interviews	Hard-of-hearing identity	7	Child	Moderate to Profound	Oral	School
Jambor & Elliot (2005)	Questionnaire	Self-esteem and doping strategies	78	Adult	Self-report Moderate to Profound	Oral and Sign	Both
Kent (2003)	Questionnaire	Hard-of-hearing identity	52	Adolescent	Not reported	Oral	School
Koelle & Convey (1982)	Scale	Self-concept, locus of control, and academic achievement	90	Adolescent	Not reported	Unclear: signing assumed (residential)	School
Leigh (1999)	Questionnaire	Self-perception and personal development	34	Adult	Not reported	Oral	Both

Authors (year)	Method	Identity, Self-Concept, or Self-Esteem	No. of D/HH Subjects	Ages	Degree of Deafness	Oral, MCE, ASL,	Home, School, or Both
Lukomski (2007)	Self-reporting Scale	Perceptions of socioemotional adjustment	205	Adult	Not reported	Oral and Sign	Both
Most (2007)	Self-report Questionnaire; Scale	Loneliness and sense of coherence	19	Adolescent	Severe to Profound	Oral and Sign	School
Musselman et al. (1996)	Scale	Social adjustment and degree of mainstreaming	72	Adolescent	Severe to Profound	Oral and Sign	School
Musselman & Akamatsu (1999)	Language samples	Interpersonal Communication skills	67	Adolescent	Unclear Avg. 101 dB	Oral and Sign	School
Nikolaraizi & Hadjikakou (2006)	Interview	Deaf vs. hearing identity	25	Adult	Not documented; 70 dB+ assumed	Oral and Sign	Both
Polat (2003)	Reporting Scale	Psychosocial adjustment	1,097	Child, Adolescent	Not reported	Oral and Sign	Both
van Gurp (2001)	Questionnaire	Self-concept	90	Adolescent	Moderate-Profound	Oral and Sign	School
Wallis et al.	Reporting scales	"Mode match"	57	Adolescent	Profound	Oral, Sign,	Both

continues

Table 9–1. *continued*

Authors (year)	Method	Identity, Self-Concept, or Self-Esteem	No. of D/HH Subjects	Ages	Degree of Deafness	Oral, MCE, ASL,	Home, School, or Both
Weisel & Kamara (2005)	Questionnaire	Attachment and self-esteem	38	Adult	Not reported	As child: unknown As adult: Oral or Signs	N/A
Yachnik (1986)	Questionnaire	Self-esteem and parental hearing status	56	Adult report on adolescence	Severe to Profound	Oral and Sign	Both

(Bat-Chava & Deignan, 2001; Brunnberg, Boström, & Berglund, 2008; Israelite, Ower, & Goldstein, 2002; Kent, 2003; Leigh, 1999), two examined participants from signing backgrounds (Crowe, 2003; Koelle & Convey, 1982), and 12 examined both oral and signing participants (Hintermair, 2007; Jambor & Elliot, 2005; Lukomski, 2007; Most, 2007; Musselman & Akamatsu, 1999; Musselman, Mootilal, & MacKay, 1996; Nikolaraizi & Hadjikakou, 2006; Polat, 2003; Wallis, Musselman, & MacKay, 2004; van Gurp, 2001; Weisel & Kamara, 2005; Yachnik, 1986). Research protocols varied, including: questionnaires, interviews, psychosocial scales, or parental reports. Of the 19 studies, 12 examined self-esteem and social adjustment of children and adolescents who are deaf (Bat-Chava & Deignan, 2001; Brunnberg et al., 2008; Israelite et al., 2002; Kent, 2003; Koelle & Convey, 1982; Most, 2007; Musselman & Akamatsu, 1999; Musselman et al., 1996; Polat, 2003; van Gurp, 2001; Wallis et al., 2004; Yachnik, 1986) and seven examined self-esteem of adults (Crowe, 2003; Hintermair, 2007; Jambor & Elliot, 2005; Leigh, 1999; Lukomski, 2007; Nikolaraizi & Hadjikakou, 2006; Weisel & Kamara, 2005). The study reported here is the first of its kind, in that it focuses on adult deaf *cuers'* self-esteem, psychosocial adjustment, and cultural identity.

Autobiographic Literature

Autobiographies (cf, Bragg, 1989; Chorost, 2005; Jacobs, 1989; Kisor, 1990; Swiller, 2007) are another source of information about cultural identity, psychosocial adjustment, and communication and language experiences of individuals who are deaf. In comparison to adults from oral or signing backgrounds, however, very little is known about per-

ceptions of cueing deaf adults regarding their language, communication, psychosocial adjustment, and cultural experiences.

Prior to the study reported in this chapter, the only information specific to cuers' psychosocial adjustment, self-esteem, and cultural identity comes from publications of the National Cued Speech Association (NCSA). Cornett and Daisey (2001) included a chapter of stories and narratives from 4 to 21-year-old deaf cuers, which described their views about growing up deaf in the United States and how Cued Speech impacted their lives. Many of these were in the form of letters written by the young people to Cornett over a period of several years. In *Letters from Cue Adults* (NCSA, 2002) 12 of those youngsters, as adults, wrote again to Cornett, providing updates on their lives and educational pursuits. These narratives provide *some* insight into the language, communication, culture, academic achievement, and self-concept of young cuers, but they lack the independent voice of adults who are able to reflect and report freely on their experiences with parents/guardians, teachers, and other professionals. Arguably, letters written by minors, perhaps on the urging of parents, to a man known to be "the father of Cued Speech," are at risk of being singularly positive about Cued Speech, perhaps from a sense of gratitude.

Currently, the first generation of native cuers of American English in the United States has reached adulthood; these individuals have graduated or are graduating from college or graduate school, and are beginning families of their own. These young adults provide a unique opportunity for researchers interested in the perceptions of native cuers of English regarding their satisfaction with parents' choice of Cued Speech, feelings of belonging or isolation in the family and with peers as a child or adult, current communication methods (including Cued Speech and sign communication), and whether they currently consider themselves members of the Deaf and hearing communities.

Purpose of the Study

The purpose of the study described in this chapter was to add to the knowledge base related to deaf adults' self-esteem, psychosocial adjustment, and cultural identity by adding reports of the experiences and perceptions of deaf adults who were raised with Cued Speech. Questions in the study were derived from numerous conversations the authors have had over the past decade with deaf children, parents, school administrators, college educators of professionals who will work with deaf children, educational policy makers, signed language interpreters, and Cued Speech transliterators, and were subjected to member check (Mertens, 1998) when reviewed for relevance, bias, and clarity by a deaf adult cuer.

Method

Survey methods were selected for this study. Historically, survey and interview methods have been common in deaf education, with such studies being conducted either via live administration, through postal mail, or via facsimile (fax) transmission. Such surveys have been conducted to collect data from: *social or school programs* and *agencies serving children and/or adults who are deaf or hard of hearing* (Cawthon, 2006; Israelite & Hammermeister, 1986; LaSasso & Lollis, 2003); *professionals serving this population in education or related services*

(Esp, 2001; Freebody & Power, 2001; Kelly, Lang, & Pagliaro, 2003; Marlatt, 2001; Polich, 2001); and *deaf and hard of hearing children or adults themselves* (Akamatsu, Mayer, & Farrelly, 2006; Angelides & Aravi, 2006; Kent, 2003; Richardson, Long, & Woodley, 2004; Richardson, MacLeod-Gallinger, McKee, & Long, 2000; Scherer & McKee, 1993). Regarding deaf adults' perceptions and experiences, Punch, Hyde, and Power (2007) recently reported results of a study designed to determine career and workplace experiences of Australian University graduates who are deaf or hard of hearing. Increasingly, *online* survey methodology is being employed by researchers interested in learning about experiences of deaf or hard of hearing individuals. For example, Porter and Edirippulige (2007) recently reported results from an online survey designed to learn about the experiences of parents of deaf children seeking hearing loss information on the internet.

Researchers electing survey methods have available to them web-based services available to subscribing institutions for creating, administering, and analyzing surveys, among other applications. For example, Porter and Edirippulige used the commercial software program Questionpro (http://www.questionpro.com) that is designed for online surveys.

Survey methods were selected for the present study for several reasons. First, surveys are convenient because participants can respond from the location, at the time, and in the amount of time most convenient for them. Second, surveys are an efficient method for collecting information from respondents in various parts of the country. Third, in contrast to interviews, data collected from questionnaires (electronically, in this case) do not require transcription, as respondents either check boxes or type open-ended responses that can later be analyzed verbatim.

The questionnaire used in this study consisted of 95 questions, 78 of which utilized a forced-choice format and provided responses from which respondents could choose the most appropriate answer(s) among those supplied. Seventeen questions were open-ended and invited respondents to enter responses in their own words. Questions requiring a single choice response were followed by radio buttons that forced respondents to select a single option for the question. Other forced-choice questions allowed respondents to choose all applicable responses. Radio buttons or check boxes marked "other" were followed by text boxes, allowing respondents to qualify such responses. Open-ended questions, allowing respondents to construct responses, were followed by text boxes, and did not include a word limit or suggested response length.

Recruitment of participants consisted of posting an electronic flier on Web sites of local Cued Speech associations as well as the National Cued Speech Association (NCSA). A branch of NCSA, Cued Speech Discovery, disseminates information about Cued Speech and cued language and maintains email lists of NCSA members and nonmembers seeking information or wishing to be informed of Cued Speech-related events and opportunities, and disseminates a quarterly newsletter in paper and digital (.pdf) formats. In the recruitment flier, individuals who identified themselves as being: (1) 18 years of age or older and (2) a deaf cuer, were invited to follow URL links to the survey, located on a secured network. A total of 32 individuals accessed the survey. Upon viewing the Web site flier or opening and reading the listserv E-mail, participants read the description of the study, their rights as research participants as required by the University of South Florida Institutional Review Board for the Protection of Human Subjects (IRB), and the known costs/benefits associated with participation. Participants were informed that, by clicking on the "access survey" link, they were giving their informed consent to participate.

The survey instrument was an online survey, hosted by Flashlight Online (http://www.tltgroup.org/flashlightP .htm), a Web-based service available to subscribing institutions for creating, administering, and analyzing surveys, among other applications. It was developed in 1992 at Washington State University, which still hosts and supports the system. Participant responses are provided online, and investigators conduct simple analyses of data directly from the system or download raw data into separate statistical analysis software.

Data collected were tabulated and displayed via the Flashlight Online tool (http://www.tltgroup.org/Flashlight/flash lightonline.htm), which preserves participants' confidentiality. Responses to forced-choice questions were displayed as simple counts for the different possible choices that could be selected. These were converted to percentages by the researcher. Responses to open-ended questions were listed verbatim in the data file in order of response, and then were categorized thematically, based on the central idea expressed.

Results

Participants

The participant group consisted of 32 individuals, of whom 22 are female. They ranged in age from 18 to 42 years, with a mean age of approximately 26 years and a mode of 22 years. Of the 32 respondents, in response to a question about the extent of hearing loss according to the most recent audiogram, 66% ($n = 21$) reported a profound hearing loss; 28% ($n = 9$) reported severe-to-profound loss; 3% ($n = 1$), reported moderate loss; and 3% ($n = 1$) reported mild loss. Of the 32 responses, 47% ($n = 15$) reported growing up in the Northeast or Mid-Atlantic regions of the country; 16% ($n = 5$) in the Southeast; 19% ($n = 6$) in the Midwest; 16% ($n = 5$) in the West or Southwest; and 3% ($n = 1$) reported growing up outside of the United States. No respondents reported having grown up in the Northwest region of the country.

Analyses of Forced-Choice Responses

Data reported in this section are grouped according to categories of questions regarding: (1) parental choice of Cued Speech, (2) age of exposure to communication, including Cued Speech, (3) early family environment, including: who cued to the deaf child in the family, how the deaf child communicated expressively to family members, and how involved the cueing deaf child felt in family activities, (4) relationships and communication with deaf and hearing peers and classmates, (5) school placements, experiences, and academics, (6) experiences with teachers, transliterators, and related services, and (7) communication in adulthood.

Parental Choice of Cued Speech

Given the paucity of Cued Speech information and services available to parents, compared to those established for oral or signed communication with deaf children (Gallaudet Research Institute, 2005), it was deemed important to understand how cueing deaf adults' parents learned about Cued Speech as a viable option for communication and language, and the reason(s) they chose it.

When Cueing Parents Learned About Cued Speech. When asked how their parents or guardians learned about Cued Speech as a communication option, cueing deaf adults indicated a number of potential referral sources (more than one option could be checked). Of the 32 respondents, 50% ($n = 16$) indicated either "other cueing members of the community" or "word of mouth"; 31% ($n = 10$) indicated "speech-language pathologist," and 22% ($n = 7$) indicated "audiologist." Although "pediatrician" was presented as a possible response, none of the participants selected this option. This suggests that at the time parents were making communication choices, there were gaps in the knowledge base among professionals in related fields. Research is needed to determine whether the same gaps in the knowledge base of professionals working with deaf children exists today.

Reasons Parents Chose Cued Speech. Cueing deaf adults were asked to indicate why they believe their parents chose Cued Speech as the primary means of communication (more than one option could be selected). Of the 32 responses, 78% ($n = 25$) reported: "So I would have access to my home language"; 44% ($n = 14$) responded: "There was a lot of theoretical/research support behind it"; 31% ($n = 10$) responded: "Because it was easier to learn than signing."

Age of Exposure to Cued Speech

Of the 32 respondents, 81% reported learning to cue before the age of 5 years, with 50% ($n = 16$) learning to cue before age 2, and 31% ($n = 10$) learning to cue between

3 to 4 years. In response to a question asking how they communicated before Cued Speech, 25% (*n* = 8) indicated that they had no means of communication prior to Cued Speech; 41%, (*n* = 13) responded they were "oral"; 16% (*n* = 5) responded they used "Signed English"; and 19% (*n* = 6) replied "ASL."

Early Family Environment

A series of questions in this survey related to: (1) which family members cued to the deaf child in the family, (2) how the deaf child communicated expressively to family members, and (3) how involved the cueing deaf child felt in family activities.

Cueing Family Members. In response to a question asking who in the family cued to them, 100% of respondents reported that their mother cued to them; 81% reported that their father cued to them; and 69% (*n* = 22) indicated that both parents cued expressively to them when they were children. Of the 32 responses, 78% (*n* = 25) reported that their mother cued fluently and 35% (*n* = 9) of the 26 respondents whose fathers cued reported that their fathers cued fluently. Respondents' judgments of their parents' cueing abilities are displayed in Table 9–2.

Of the 32 respondents, 91% (*n* = 29) reported having at least one sibling; of those 29, 51% (*n* = 15) reported at least one older sibling; 69% (*n* = 20) reported having at least one younger sibling; 6% (*n* = 2) reported having at least one sibling of the same age; 9% (*n* = 3) reported having no siblings; and 62% (*n* = 18) indicated having at least one sibling who cued. Of those 18 respondents with cueing siblings, 61% (*n* = 11) reported having at least one sibling who "cued fluently"; 22% (*n* = 4) had

Table 9–2. Participants' Judgments of Parental Cueing Abilities (*n* = 32)

Cueing Ability	Mother	Father
Fluently	78%	28%
Above average	13%	16%
Average	9%	13%
Poorly	0%	19%
Very poorly	0%	6%
Did not cue	0%	19%

at least one sibling who "cued above average"; 28% (*n* = 5) had at least one sibling who "cued poorly," and 33% (*n* = 6) had at least one sibling who "cued very poorly." Of the 32 respondents, 34% (*n* = 11) indicated that they cued with extended family members. Of those 11, 27% (*n* = 3) indicated cueing with grandparents, 64% (*n* = 7) with aunts and/or uncles, and 45% (*n* = 5) with cousins.

Cueing Deaf Adults' Expressive Communication with Family. Respondents were asked how, growing up, they communicated expressively with their families, and were asked to select all applicable choices. The most common responses, provided by 84% (*n* = 27) of the 32 responses was "speaking without cueing." The second most common response, provided by 66% (*n* = 21) was "cueing with voice." Table 9–3 reflects complete responses.

Of the 32 respondents, 78% (*n* = 25) reported that they knew when they began cueing. Of those 25, 68% (*n* = 17) reported cueing expressively with family members beginning before the age of 5; and 32% (*n* = 8) reported after the age of 5, with one of those reporting not having cued expressively with family until after the age of 12 (Table 9–4).

Table 9–3. Participants' Expressive Communication Modalities with Family (*n* = 32)

Communication	Percentage
Speaking without cueing	84%
Cueing with voice	66%
Cueing without voice	19%
Signing	9%
Signing with voice	6%
Other	0%

Table 9–4. When Participants Began Cueing Expressively with Family Members (*n* = 32)

Age	Percentage
0–2 years	22%
3–5 years	31%
6–11 years	22%
12–14 years	3%
15–18 years	0%
After age 18	0%
Unknown	22%

Three-fourths (*n* = 24) of the 32 respondents reported cueing expressively with family members at least some of the time, while 25% (*n* = 8) reported never cueing expressively with family. Of the 24 who reported cueing expressively, 29% (*n* = 7) indicated that they "always" cued expressively, 17% (*n* = 4) indicated "often," and 53% (*n* = 13) indicated "sometimes."

Cuers' Perceptions of Inclusion in Family Activities. In response to a ques-tion about whether they always, some-times, or never felt involved with family members growing up, 69% (*n* = 22) of the 32 respondents reported "always"; 28% (*n* = 9) reported "sometimes"; and one reported "never" feeling involved. When asked if they always, often, sometimes, or never felt included in family activities and conversations, 72% (*n* = 23) reported feeling "always" or "often"; whereas one respon-dent reported "seldom" feeling included.

Cuers' Relationships and Communication with Deaf and Hearing Peers and Classmates

A common question raised by those who are unfamiliar with Cued Speech is whether deaf children from Cued Speech back-grounds feel socially isolated. Therefore, a number of questions in this survey addressed peer relationships growing up, in and out of the classroom setting. All (100%) respondents reported developing close friendships growing up. Of the 32 respondents, 66% (*n* = 21) indicated hav-ing "many" close friends growing up, whereas 34% (*n* = 11) reported "a few." When asked to indicate all of the ways in which they communicated with childhood friends, 88% (*n* = 28) responded "orally," 75% (*n* = 24) responded: "cueing with voice," and 47% (*n* = 15) responded "ASL or Signed English." Complete responses are displayed in Table 9–5.

Of the 32 respondents, 69% (*n* = 22) reported having many hearing friends and 38% (*n* = 12) reported having many deaf or hard-of-hearing friends; 16% (*n* = 5) reported having no deaf or hard-of-hearing friends growing up, while only one respondent reported having no hear-ing friends; 78% (*n* = 25) reported having childhood friends who learned how to cue. Of those, 28% (*n* = 7) reported that only

Table 9–5. Participants' Means of Communicating with Childhood Friends (*n* = 32)

Communication	Percentage
Oral	88%
Cueing with voice	75%
Cueing without voice	44%
ASL/signed English	47%
Signed English + speech	34%
Other	16%

their deaf/hard-of-hearing friends cued, 36% (*n* = 9) reported that only their hearing friends cued, and 36% (*n* = 9) reported that both hearing and deaf/hard-of-hearing friends had learned how to cue. In response to the question, "Did you cue at home, at school, or both," approximately 88% (*n* = 28) indicated "both," 7% (*n* = 2) indicated "at home only," and none reported cueing only at school.

Similarly, all respondents (100%) reported having hearing classmates during their K–12 school years. Regarding their level of interaction with hearing classmates, 53% (*n* = 17) reported "always" doing so; 19% (*n* = 6) reported "often" doing so; and 28% (*n* = 9) reported "sometimes" interacting with hearing classmates. None indicated "never" interacting with hearing classmates. Of the 59% (*n* = 19) respondents who reported also having deaf or hard of hearing classmates, 53% (*n* = 10) reported "often" interacting with these classmates; 25% (*n* = 8) reported "sometimes" doing so; and only one respondent indicated "never" interacting with deaf or hard of hearing classmates. When asked specifically whether they interacted more with hearing classmates

or with deaf or hard of hearing classmates, 37% (*n* = 7) of those respondents who went to school with both indicated that they interacted more with *hearing* classmates; while 21% (*n* = 4) reported having interacted more with *deaf or hard of hearing* classmates. The remaining 42% (*n* = 8) reported having interacted with deaf and hearing classmates in equal measure.

All respondents (100%) reported having hearing classmates with whom they communicated directly (as opposed to communicating via a cued language transliterator or other facilitator) at least some of the time. As reflected in Figure 9–1, 53% (*n* = 17) reported hearing classmates "always" communicating with them directly; 19% (*n* = 6) reported that hearing classmates "often" did so; whereas the remaining 28% (*n* = 9) reported that their hearing classmates "sometimes" communicated with them directly. When asked how their hearing classmates communicated with them (a question to which respondents could choose more than one response option), 94% (*n* = 30) reported using oral communication, 34% (*n* = 11) reported using a combination of cueing and oral communication; 28% (*n* = 9) reported using some form of sign communication (either ASL or a form of MCE); 44% (*n* = 14) reported using either written or electronic text-based means; and 6% (*n* = 2) reported using some other means of communicating.

Respondents were asked whether they wish they had more interaction with either hearing classmates or with deaf or hard of hearing classmates. Thirty-four percent (*n* = 11) of the 32 respondents reported that they wish they had more interactions with classmates who were deaf or hard of hearing; 32% (*n* = 10) reported that they did not wish for this; and the remaining 34% (*n* = 11) reported

Communication with Hearing Classmates

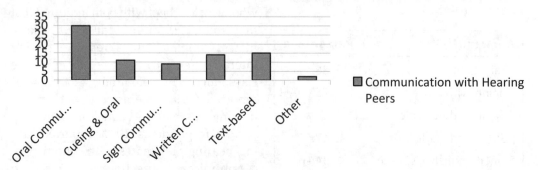

Figure 9–1. Participants' communication methods with hearing classmates.

feeling neutral on the subject, not having a strong desire either way. Thirty-seven percent (n = 12) reported that they wish they had more interactions with hearing classmates; while 19% (n = 6) reported that this was not a wish; and the remaining 44% (n = 14) reported feeling neutral on the subject.

Cuers' School Placements, Experiences, and Academics

A series of questions addressed the types of school placements in which cuers were educated, their experiences with and perceptions of those placements, as well as certain academic experiences. When asked to report the types of school placements they experienced from preschool through high school (a question to which respondents could choose more than one response option), 94% (n = 30) reported having been fully mainstreamed; 19% (n = 6) reported partial mainstreaming; 13% (n = 4) reported being taught in a special education classroom (self-contained); and 6% (n = 2) reported having been home schooled at least part of the time between preschool and 12th grade.

Respondents were asked at which points in their K–12 school years they attended self-contained classes (a question to which respondents could choose more than one response option). Fifty-nine percent (n = 19) of the 32 respondents indicated that they did not attend self-contained classes during the elementary years. Of those 13 respondents who reported having attended self-contained classes during this period, 92% (n = 12) reported having attended such classes during the early elementary years (grades K–2); 62% (n = 8) during the late elementary years (grades 3-5); and 31% (n = 4) during the middle school years (grades 6-8). One respondent indicated having attended self-contained classes at some point during the high school years (grades 9-12). Respondents were also asked at which points in their school years they attended mainstream classes (also a question to which respondents could choose more than one response option). None of the 32 respondents reported having never attended mainstream classes. Eighty-one percent (n = 26) reported having attended mainstream classes in the early elementary years; 91% (n = 29) reported having attended such classes during the late elementary years; and all respondents (100%) reported having attended mainstream classes during their middle school and high school years. Figure 9–2 shows the dichotomy regarding self-contained placements in early elementary years and mainstream placements in middle school and high school.

Respondents were asked a series of questions concerning whether they found school difficult, and which subjects they found particularly easy or particularly difficult. None of the 32 respondents reported that "all" or "many" subjects in school were difficult for them; 19% (*n* = 6) reported that they found "all" subjects in school "easy"; 38% (*n* = 12) reported having found "most" subjects "easy," and the remaining 44% (*n* = 14) found school to be of "average" difficulty, with an equal amount of easy and difficult subjects.

When asked to report their perceptions of the difficulty of subjects in elementary school, 97% (*n* = 31) reported having found

English language arts "easy." Figure 9–3 provides a graph detailing respondents' perceptions of easy and difficult school subjects.

Regarding when and how they learned to read, 78% (*n* = 25) of the 32 respondents reported having learned to read in early childhood (ages 3–5) and 19% (*n* = 6) reported having learned during elementary school. One respondent reported not knowing when she or he had learned to read. Regarding from whom they had learned to read (a question to which respondents could choose more than one response option), 81% (*n* = 26) reported learning to read from their parents; 53% (*n* = 17) reported learning from their regular education teachers; 28% (*n* = 9) reported learning from their special education teacher; 28% (*n* = 9) also reported learning from their speech-language pathologist; and 13% (*n* = 4) reported "other." Nineteen percent (*n* = 6) reported having no idea from whom they learned to read.

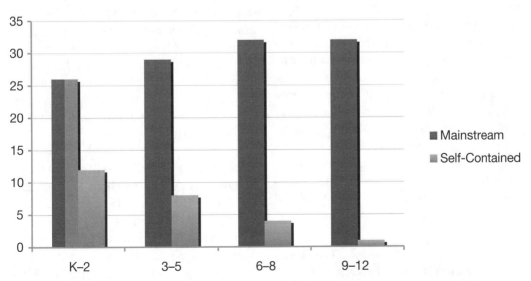

Figure 9–2. Participants' attendance of mainstream and self-contained classes.

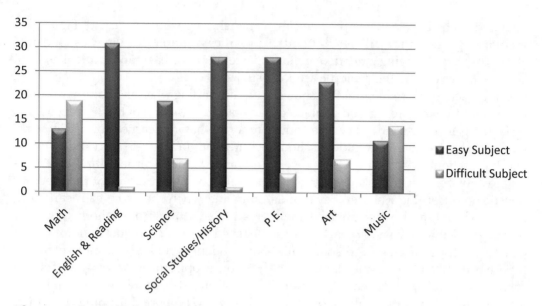

Figure 9–3. Participants' perceptions of easy and difficult school subjects.

Cuers' Experiences with Teachers, Transliterators, and Related Services

In addition to teachers who can and do communicate directly with them (orally, via signs, or with Cued Speech), students who are deaf or hard of hearing can experience a range of other services provided to ensure access to instruction (e.g., interpreters, cued language transliterators, note takers). In order to understand the services afforded to deaf students who cue, and how those services change over time, respondents were asked a series of questions relating to their experiences with teachers and transliterators during their K–12 school years, and to their experiences with transliterators and related services during their college years.

Experiences with K–12 Teachers and Transliterators. Respondents were asked to indicate during which grade lev-

els they were taught by teachers who cued for themselves, and during which grade levels they received instruction facilitated by a cued language transliterator. Respondents could choose any or all response options for each question (a response for each applicable grade level), and could respond in the affirmative to the same grade level for both questions (i.e., indicating having had a cueing teacher and a transliterator during the same school year). Figure 9–4 shows a clear trend away from cueing teachers and toward cued language transliterators from kindergarten toward the 12th grade.

Experiences with Transliterators and Related Services in High School and College. Respondents were asked to indicate which services they accessed in order to receive instruction and curricular content (a question to which respondents could choose more than one response option) in high school and in college. The

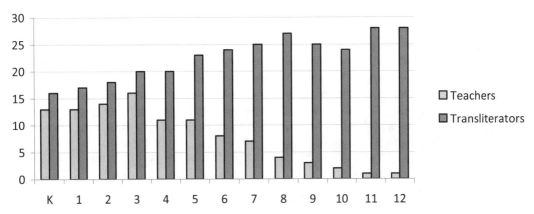

Figure 9–4. Participants' experience with cueing teachers and transliterators by grade.

most common response pertaining to middle school/high school was "cued language transliterator," selected by 91% (*n* = 29) of respondents. Of the 32 respondents, 19% (*n* = 6) reported using the services of a sign interpreter at some point in middle school or high school. The choices "cued language transliterator" and "notetaker" were the most common pertaining to college, with each being selected by 65% (*n* = 20) of respondents who indicated having attended college (one respondent indicated having not yet entered college at the time of the survey). Figure 9–5 shows respondents' use of cued language transliterators, notetakers, and other related services during middle/high school and college.

Respondents were also asked about their choice of college, and whether the availability of cued language transliterators or interpreters factored into their application and decision-making process. Of the 31 respondents indicating that they had attended or were currently attending college, 58% (*n* = 18) indicated that their choice of a school was based at least in part on the availability of transliterator

services. The availability of sign interpreter services was indicated as a factor by 32% (*n* = 10) respondents.

Communication in Adulthood

A series of questions in this survey addressed how cuers of American English communicate with others as adults. Of the 32 respondents, 88% (*n* = 28) reported that they still cue expressively in adulthood. Of those 28, 86% (*n* = 24) rate their current expressive cueing abilities as "very good"; and 14% (*n* = 4) rate themselves as "average." All 32 respondents reported that they still cue-read (i.e., understand the expressive cueing of others), with 94% (*n* = 30) rating their cue reading abilities as "very good," and 6% (*n* = 2) as "average."

Of the 32 respondents, 88% (*n* = 28) reported having learned to sign, with 59% reporting that they considered themselves members of the Deaf community. Respondents who indicated having learned to sign were asked to indicate why they had done so (more than one reason could be given). Of the 28, 75% (*n* = 21) indicated they wanted to "communicate with friends

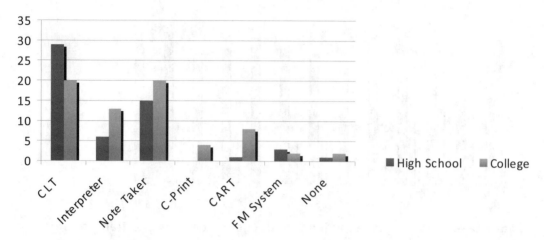

Figure 9–5. Participants' use of communication accommodation services in high school and college.

they already had," 61% ($n = 17$) indicated wanting "to make new friends," 61% wanting to join the signing Deaf community, and 57% indicating they wanted to become bilingual.

Regrets About Cueing

In response to a question asking whether they were glad they were raised cueing, 94% ($n = 30$) of the 32 respondents indicated "yes"; 6% ($n = 2$) indicated "sometimes"; and none responded "no." In response to a question about whether they had any regrets about growing up as a cuer, 81% ($n = 26$) reported having no regrets. In response to a question about whether they believe they incurred any social costs by being a "cue kid," 50% of the 32 respondents ($n = 16$) indicated that they do not believe they incurred any social costs by being a "cue kid"; 13% ($n = 4$) believe they did incur a social cost; and the remaining 37% ($n = 12$) believe that they "sometimes" incurred such a cost. Open-ended responses clarifying respondents' regrets or

perceived social costs of growing up with Cued Speech are discussed in the following section.

Responses to Open-Ended Questions

Results in this section are organized according to cueing deaf adults' responses to open-ended questions regarding: (1) regrets about growing up with Cued Speech; (2) their experiences in and perceptions of mainstream and self-contained educational placements; (3) the respective roles of Cued Speech, speech/speechreading, signing, and reading/writing/texting in their adult lives; (4) their identification with or involvement in the Deaf community; (5) the lasting impact of early exposure to Cued Speech; and (6) what it means to be "a cuer." Due to space constraints, not all responses are included here for every question. When a response represented a unique perspective, it was included. When multiple responses represented the same perspective, contained similar wording, or could otherwise be grouped thematically, one or more responses are presented as representative. In cases of multiple responses, attempts were made to include a variety of response lengths.

Regrets

In response to the forced-choice question about whether cueing deaf adults had any regrets about growing up as a cue kid, 19% indicated that they had some regrets. Respondents provided specific examples of situations in which they felt a sense of not belonging to a particular group or subgroup. For example: (1) "I wish I had been more involved in the deaf community. I also believe that I was in the hearing community for so long that I thought I wasn't welcome or meant to be in a deaf community," and (2) "I grew up almost exclusively in a cuer or hearing environment. I had very little interaction with the signing community. As a result, I share little commonality with the other grown cue kids who both cue and sign. To a certain extent, I feel like an outsider from that particular community."

Half (*n* = 16) of the cueing deaf adults responded in the affirmative to the forced-choice question about whether they incurred a social cost to being raised a "cueing kid." Open-ended responses revealed perceptions related to being deaf in a hearing environment (e.g., speechreading, speech intelligibility, missing spoken information, feeling isolated). Two clear themes emerged: (1) a sense of being "between worlds," and (2) a sense of being misunderstood or mischaracterized by other individuals or groups. The following responses are illustrative of those reflecting respondents' feelings of being caught between hearing and deaf "worlds:" (1) "Always

being left out of both hearing and deaf cultures and always having to have special attention (special accommodations in class, sporting events, etc.) and when you're a teen girl, you just want to blend in, not be front and center," (2) "Being in the middle of the deaf and hearing worlds," (3) "I don't feel like I belong in the Deaf Community at all times," and (4) "I was kind of in between worlds, but I feel like Cued Speech has given me the ability to move between the two worlds. I was able to learn sign language, so I can communicate with members of the deaf community, and I can talk with my hearing friends."

Responses suggesting that respondents felt misunderstood or mischaracterized by noncueing individuals or groups included: (1) "I didn't know any sign at the time and everyone considered me intolerant," (2) "I was judged by the ASL community sometimes simply because I knew how to both cue and sign," (3) "People would assume that I couldn't hear. Or that I was closed-minded because I wasn't fluent in ASL. Also, I was made fun of in school for being deaf and knowing Cued Speech. They would imitate the interpreter as if it was a bad thing."

One respondent questioned the assumption that the "social cost" is directly related to being a cuer or to being deaf:

I responded "no" to this question because I wasn't socially hurt by being a cue kid, but I'm aware that my social opportunities were likely limited because I am deaf. Even though I said "no," I've always felt that the social question wasn't very fair. Social experiences depend so much on more than just communication modality. Students who are shy or introverted are more likely to have problems interacting socially, whether or not they are deaf or hearing (communication mode not-withstanding). And then there's the issue of being a "cue kid" . . . Sometimes it's not about being a cuer, it's just about being deaf. I do know one student who was a deaf cuer in my high school who did not have many deaf or hearing friends and that just had a lot to do with his personality and attitudes. He gave off the attitude that he was smarter/better than the other deaf students (who signed) and he never wanted to learn to sign, so of course they didn't want to socialize with him. And he had a similar attitude with hearing peers—don't get me wrong, he was very smart, but his ego hurt him socially. So, in a nutshell, the social issue is much more than just about being a "cue kid." It has to do with deafness, attitude, personality, as well as the opportunities for socializing in the area where the kid is living.

Experiences in and Perceptions of Educational Placements

Respondents provided a variety of comments regarding their perceptions of benefits and costs associated with mainstreaming and partial mainstreaming (self-contained classes and mainstream experiences in the same school). Comments can best be grouped according to perceived: (1) educational and socialization benefits of mainstreaming; (2) support provided by partial mainstreaming; and (3) costs associated with having been educated in a mainstream or partial mainstream setting, as opposed to a school or program specifically for deaf students.

Perceived Educational Benefits of Mainstreaming. The following comments provided by respondents typify the sense that they received an education comparable to hearing peers that they would not have received in a self-contained setting or special school: (1) "I feel that by not being segregated into a special classroom, I was able to compete against the best in school (rather than the "best" in a small subpopulation)," (2) "I feel like I gained a normal education comparable to hearing children as I was fully mainstreamed in school. I was able to do this with the help of a Cued Speech transliterator," (3) "I had access to the full curriculum and simply went along with the high standards expected from all schools," and (4) "I was challenged and was able to meet my full potential. My reading and writing skills were not hindered in this setting."

Perceived Social Benefits of Mainstreaming. Respondents provided numerous comments regarding the socialization opportunities afforded them by their mainstream education. Comments typical of this sentiment included: (1) "I felt more integrated into society," (2) "Mainstreaming gave me the social skills necessary for life outside the deaf community. By developing my lipreading skills, learning social 'norms' and gaining exposure to a variety of cultures (not just deaf), I better integrate into the world around me," (3) "Full socialization with hearing peers," (4) "I was able to interact with the hearing world much more effectively, and use the experience learned from said interaction to grow as a human being, rather than feeling limited by my hearing loss. You learn from all different types of interactions—you learn from mistakes, and you learn to think and consider how you can change as a person to react and behave better in different situations," and (5) "Better adaptation skills and social skills for later on in life."

Perceived Supports Received in Partial Mainstreaming. Respondents also provided comments regarding their perception of benefits to receiving an education in a partial mainstream setting (one in which students experience both self-contained classes and mainstream experiences). Comments representative of those provided include the following: (1) "The presence of an ASL/Cued Speech program at the school meant that I had the support services (speech therapy, resource specialist, transliterators, etc.) necessary, as well as the companionship of deaf peers (although I tended to be friends with hearing people more than deaf people)," and (2) "I was with my hearing peers, but got help when I needed it."

Perceived Costs Associated with Mainstreaming. Responses to the question of whether the respondents believe they "missed out" on anything by being educated in a mainstream or partial mainstream (as opposed to another) setting can be grouped into three categories: (1) comments indicating respondents not feeling as though they missed out on anything; (2) comments relating to a sense of having missed out on opportunities to interact with signing deaf peers; and (3) comments relating to a sense of having missed out on certain aspects of communication access. Seven respondents simply typed the word "nothing" as a response to this question. Four other, similar, comments included: (1) "I don't think I missed out on anything at all," (2) "I did not lose out on anything. I received the best education possible," (3) "I never felt that I lost out on anything in regard to using Cued Speech," and (4) "From full inclusion, I really didn't lose anything."

Some comments indicated that some respondents feel that by being educated in a mainstream setting, they missed out on opportunities to interact with signing deaf peers. Typical comments indicative of this sentiment included: (1) I hadn't really thought about it before. I suppose it would be not learning sign language and meeting other deaf individuals (and actually be able to communicate with them)," (2) "Socialization like deaf schools have," (3) "I lost out on the opportunity to be in the deaf community," (4) "Sometimes I felt stigmatized by being the only deaf kid," and (5) "More insight into the deaf world."

Role of Cued Speech in Cuers' Lives

Respondents detailed a variety of ways that Cued Speech plays a role in their adult lives. In addition to mentions of cueing with other deaf cuers, responses centered around two main themes: (1) access to spoken language in the absence of assistive devices, and (2) access to education. The following comments are particularly representative of those regarding Cued Speech and assistive technologies: (1) "My family cues to me only if I cannot follow them orally for a reason (tired, not wearing hearing aid, too far away, etc.)" and (2) "It helps me communicate with my family when I don't have my cochlear implant on. For example when I'm at the beach, pool, late at night when I have taken my implant off."

The following comments focus on how Cued Speech impacted their education: (1) "I continue to use it as my preferred mode of communication in the classroom (graduate school) as well as at research conferences," (2) "I have CSTs [Cued Speech transliterators] for some of my college classes. It allows me to access knowledge and information in my college courses and to communicate with my family," (3) "I would request a cuer for a Ph.D. class so that I could access the language used in a particular field and grow in knowledge and vocabulary," (4) "I use CLTs [cued language transliterators] now in graduate school. They're a blessing! No CART [computer assisted real-time translation] or ASL terp [interpreter] could replace them."

Many respondents wrote about what they perceive to be the "power" of Cued Speech, as highlighted by the following statement: "It is because of Cued Speech that I'm able to get a good start to my adult life. It has shaped my social skills with hearing people so powerfully, as well as my mind, that I will be able to function in the environment of one of the nation's most elite universities. One thing I appreciate about Cued Speech so much is that it has enriched my imagination by allowing me to detect linguistic subtleties that make English—as well as Spanish— a beautiful medium for art as well as communication."

Role of Speech/Speechreading in Cuers' Lives

Two themes emerged related to responses to the question: "What role, if any, does speech/speechreading play in your life as an adult?" One theme related to speech/speechreading playing a significant, primary role in adulthood. A second theme related to lesser, more situational roles for oral communication. The following responses indicate that speech and speechreading play a very important role currently in their lives: (1) "Huge. I'd say probably 99% of the time I have to speechread, except when I'm at deaf happy-hour gatherings," (2) "Speech and speechreading play a huge role as I often interact with

hearing people who do not know any form of visual communication," (3) "Speech/speechreading plays an important role in my life. Being able to hear with my hearing aids and having the ability to speechread is pretty much the only mode of communication I use today," and (4) "Speech and speechreading play a MAJOR role— that's how I communicate at work and in my daily life."

The following responses reflect specific, situational uses for speech/speechreading related to brief and/or casual exchanges with hearing noncuers: (1) "I order my lattes with [speech/speechreading]. Chat with my hearing family with them. Otherwise, speech and lipreading play minimal roles," and (2) "To be able to communicate when I go shopping, etc." One respondent described speechreading as a visual backup strategy for oral communication with hearing noncuers: "Yes. I get lazy with my implant, even though I do well with it . . . so I read people's lips when I'm tired."

Role of Signing in Cuers' Lives

Responses to the question, "What role, if any, does signing play in your life?" varied considerably, but centered on six themes: (1) signing plays a major role in daily life; (2) signing serves to help in social situations; (3) signing serves to broaden one's communication or language abilities; (4) signing allows for communication in family relationships; (5) signing allows for artistic expression; and (6) signing plays no role or a very minimal one. Selected comments representative of these six themes are provided in the following paragraphs.

Signing Plays a Major Role in Daily Life. Certain comments provided by respondents indicated that signing plays a major role in their daily lives as adults. Such comments include: (1) "I use it to communicate with my friends, students, and on the job, (2) "I'm in a deaf sorority, so I sign every day with them as well as with my teammates, classmates, and professors," (3) "I am a Gallaudet student so I use signing daily now to communicate," (4) "Quite a fair amount. I started picking up signs as early as age 5 or 6 and am now teaching ASL at a local community college," and (5) "I teach in a deaf school (ASL) and typically use sign language in every social environment."

Signing Helps in Social Situations. Certain comments provided by respondents indicated that signing, while not playing a major role in their daily lives as adults, does help in certain social situations. Such comments include: (1) "Mostly social, I don't use it for anything else, " (2) "I use it to communicate with my ASL-only friends," (3) "Socialization," (4) "I only use ASL with deaf peers," and (5) "More friends and learned another language."

Signing Broadens Communication or Language Abilities. Comments provided by certain respondents indicated that signing has helped them to broaden their communication and language abilities in adulthood. Such comments include: (1) "Signing played a role of learning another language to communicate with other deaf people that have grown up with it," (2) "Signing has become one of the many languages I know," (3) "Signing allows me to communicate with a wider range of deaf/hh people," (4) "I use it when communicating with other signers," and (5) "[Signing helps] communication with other deaf people."

Signing Helps in Family and Relationships. Comments provided by other respondents indicated that they use sign communication in family and romantic relationships forged in adulthood. Comments include: (1) "I sign with my husband," (2) "My home language with my deaf partner and daughter is ASL; my social language is ASL," and (3) "My girlfriend is a signer, and that's pretty much how we communicate."

Signing Is a Vehicle for Artistic Expression. Comments provided by still other respondents indicated that they view signing as a vehicle for artistic expression. Such comments include: (1) "I enjoy the visual arts of it. I think Sign Language is beautiful and very expressive. That is what Cued Speech lacks, but Cued Speech makes up for it by teaching me how to speak and write proper English," and (2) "I use it for deaf theatre, and I use it to express myself creatively. I love reciting poems and signing them at the same time in front of hearing audiences . . . they become quite awed by the language's beauty."

Signing Plays No Role or Only a Minimal Role. Comments provided by certain respondents, however, indicated that sign communication plays a minimal role, or no role at all, in their adult lives. Such comments include: (1) "It doesn't really play a role, other than my feeble efforts to communicate with signers," (2) "It's not an important part of my life," (3) "Very little. I use it as a fallback mode of communication with my deaf peers if they don't know Cued Speech. I'm not fluent, and have no desire to develop fluency in signing," (4) "I do not sign, so it does not have a role in my life," (5) "Very minimal. I know a few basic signs, but that's it," and (6) "Just a tool to communicate with deaf people if necessary."

Role of Reading, Writing, and Texting

All of the respondents (100%) responded either "yes" or "sometimes" to the forced-choice question, "Do you like to read?" In response to the question, "What role, if any, does reading, writing, and texting play in your life?" respondents were unanimous regarding the importance of these literacy-dependent activities. Adjectives to describe the role of reading, writing, and texting included "big," "huge," "massive," and "vital." Themes that emerged from responses of cueing deaf adults centered on the role of reading, writing, and texting for: (1) enjoyment; (2) communication; (3) learning and self-improvement; and (4) professional activity. Selected comments representative of these four themes are presented in the following paragraphs.

Reading and Writing for Enjoyment. Comments provided by certain respondents indicated a love of reading and writing for pleasure. Such comments include: (1) "Reading and writing IS my life. I do it every day: for homework, for communication with my friends, for pleasure. I make regular trips to the bookstore to buy a variety of books to peruse and enjoy," (2) "Reading is huge. I have a love for literature and only wish I had more time to read for the sheer pleasure of it," and (3) "I read voraciously."

Reading and Writing as Forms of Communication. Comments provided by other respondents indicated use of reading and writing as a means of communicating with deaf or hearing individuals.

Such comments include: (1) "Text messaging is the primary way I communicate with friends and family when we need to get a message to each other quickly. If it's not urgent, we just use e-mail then," (2) "Good grief . . . reading and writing basically make up my entire life. I don't know where I would be without them. Texting is wonderful as well . . . I use it to communicate with both hearing and deaf friends to make plans and learn about how they are doing," and (3) "a HUGE role. I use both every single day."

Reading and Writing for Learning and Self-Improvement. Comments provided by other respondents indicated a view that reading and writing are vehicles to self-improvement and learning. Such comments include: (1) "They're a big part of my life as they're what I do in college," (2) "I love reading, and wish I had more time to read. I tend to write a lot of technical stuff for my research," (3) "Pretty much everything, I'm going to college and it lets me keep up in my classes as well as keep in touch with my mom while I'm out of state," and (4) "Without reading or writing, I would not be where I am. As it is, I have an excellent command of the English language, syntax, and idiom in prose, poem, and song."

Reading and Writing as Professional Activities. Comments provided by still other respondents speak to the role of reading and writing as an integral part of the work experience. Such comments include: (1) "A huge part. Writing for work, communication. Same thing for reading. Texting plays a part mostly for emergency use," (2) "I'm an English teacher, English student, and English lover. Reading and writing are like air. Texting is water, I guess (smile)," and (3) "As a professional in a highly technical field, the attention to detail is very important. So e-mails, along with written notes/reports/markups, really help convey what is needed. Texting is my main mode of communication with others, along with emails/relay via [cellular device]/computer."

Cueing Deaf Adults and the Deaf Community

As discussed previously, nearly three-fifths (59%) of respondents indicated that they currently consider themselves members of the Deaf community, whereas the other 41% indicated that they do not. Cueing deaf adults were asked to respond to one of two follow-up questions: "If yes, when and how did you become involved?" or "If not, why not?" The following responses relate to respondents becoming involved with the Deaf community in high school, either at mainstream programs or at a school for the deaf: (1) "Well, that depends on your definition of community membership. I'll be liberal with the definition and say that it was when I started interacting with deaf peers/friends outside of school. That would be high school for me, I think, when I joined a community theatre company that included deaf and hearing high school students," (2) "The minute I was born deaf. More seriously or culturally: when I transferred to a deaf school my senior year of high school," and (3) "I always went to school with other deaf people, and some were signers. I wanted to learn sign language so I could become friends with them. I took ASL as a foreign language my freshman year and sophomore year of high school, and became immersed in the culture. I would sit at lunch with all the other deaf kids and pick up even more ASL from them. Today, I am fluent."

Other respondents indicated that they became members of the Deaf community during college. Two respondents mentioned Gallaudet University specifically, and it is possible that others are referring to Gallaudet as well. The following four responses are representative: (1) "It was about midway through college that I started becoming involved in deaf-affiliated organizations. I realized that it was an easy way for me to expand my leadership experience as well as improve my communication skills." (2) "I became more involved in college at Gallaudet," (3) "College— learned sign and was able to communicate with other deaf people," and (4) "When I went to Gallaudet." Still other respondents did not indicate a time period, but felt they had become members of the deaf community through participation with deaf organizations or attendance at deaf activities/events. For example: (1) "I just started going to deaf events," (2) "I'm involved with a local coalition and a deaf church," and (3) "When I learned how to sign and become more involved in the deaf community activities." One participant's response was short and simple, but sums up many of the previous responses: "As soon as I picked up ASL, I simply blended in."

Responses to the question, "If you did not join the Deaf community, why not?" seem to defy categorization. One respondent equated the Deaf community with signing: "No, because I'm not a Signer." A second respondent specifically mentioned feeling excluded by the Deaf community, either for being a cuer or for having a cochlear implant:

> I was told a criterion of being involved in the Deaf Community when I was younger, by a very ASL person that being involved with Cued Speech

somehow (even if you also know how to sign) automatically excluded you from the Deaf Community. I knew a lot of anti-cuers and anti-CI [cochlear implant] people and it shaped my opinion of the Deaf Community to a point that I was a little bit negative of it. However, later years and talking to people, I do understand the reason why the Deaf Community exists and now look upon it with great affinity.

A third respondent mentioned negative feelings and/or perceived maltreatment from members of the Deaf community: "The deaf culture, where I came from, was very cruel to my parents and often told me negative things about my mother and quite frankly, you don't insult someone's parents." A fourth participant's response seems to equate membership in the Deaf community with being limited in certain ways: "Growing up, my mom always instilled in me that even though I was hearing impaired, I was not to limit myself. So, from the time she was told my diagnosis, she pushed me to exceed my limits early for the better." A fifth respondent mentioned different subgroups within the Deaf community, separating those with whom she or he enjoys being associated from those with whom she or he does not: "While I hang out with deaf native signers from time to time, I do not enjoy being associated with certain people in the community (such as ASL interpreters and first generation signers) who tend to push deaf "militancy" topics. Ironically enough, it's the second and third generation signers that I enjoy hanging out with the most because they tend to be the most open minded and accepting of who I am. They may be the kind of person who refuses to get an implant, but they think it's great that I have one."

Lasting Impact of Cued Speech

Responses to the question, "What is the impact of Cued Speech on your life today?" indicate that respondents believe that exposure to Cued Speech in childhood has had lasting impact. The most common themes that emerged in their responses concerned: (1) communication and language abilities, (2) literacy, (3) academics, and (4) self-confidence.

Communication and Language Abilities. A common belief expressed among cueing deaf adults regarding the lasting impact of Cued Speech on their lives concerns their communication, and/or language abilities. For example: (1) "My native English skills are on par with (or better than) my hearing friends," (2) "It has given me the ability to speak well and fluently. My speech pathologists were able to access sounds that I never knew existed by actually associating the sounds to cueing. All of my speech pathologists knew how to cue and they were able to communicate in a much more positive and helpful way," (3) "Without it my English wouldn't be as good, I wouldn't have been able to learn Spanish, I wouldn't have been able to compete with my hearing peers and that was important to me, and now I am equal in almost every way to my hearing peers," and (4) "Without my early cueing experiences, I would not have the good communication skills that I have now."

Literacy. Another common perception expressed by respondents relates to the impact of Cued Speech on their access to and development of literacy. Respondents mention their abilities in reading and writing, their love of literature. One respondent mentioned the link between his or her speaking of English and reading of English, typing, "I learned how to speak and read in English very well." Other respondents mention their abilities in reading and writing, and/or their love of literature. The following comments provided by four respondents are representative of such statements: (1) "Without cued English, I wouldn't be literate," (2) "I believe it had an impact on my reading skills," (3) Yes, it made a huge impact because it gave me the literacy I could have not received in any other way," and (4) "DEFINITELY! English became something I love. I am a writer, I love writing poetry, short stories, I've even written a play, which I produced in high school. I read complex novels. I love Shakespeare. I am also an actress, and can read the subtext of the characters onstage. Without words, I feel I would be lost."

Academics. Respondents mentioned the impact of Cued Speech on their access to and/or successes with education. Representative of those comments are: (1) "I can definitely say that it has had a positive impact on my academics and ability to succeed academically," and (2) "I feel I got a good education and a social life due to Cued Speech."

Confidence. One particularly interesting theme that emerged from respondents' reflections on the lasting impact of Cued Speech regards a sense of confidence in cueing deaf adults in this study. Respondents mentioned a sense of confidence interacting with people: (1) "My vocabulary went up and my confidence in interacting with a variety of people has gone up as well," and (2)

If it weren't for my parents teaching me cued speech at such an early age,

I wouldn't have taken honors classes and wouldn't have gone to a wonderful high school. My future would be very different. This way, I can meet several people, both deaf and hearing, and make new friends.

Respondents mentioned a sense of confidence in their abilities and potential in life, and the effect that has had on their motivation: "It made me realize that I had to work hard my entire life to get to where I wanted to be. I could not slack off. Learning to cue at an early age really increased my reading ability and ability to absorb information, and dream of larger things," (2) "I had such unbridled access to language, I don't possess the same hesitation about being meta-lingual that other people seem to have. Learning French was, to my surprise, fun and easy," and (3) "For pretty much the same reasons as most other native Cuers who are still active in the cueing community—I don't feel any limitations as I would have had if I just signed. I feel I can do almost anything."

Reflections on Being a Cuer

Responses to the final open-ended response item on this questionnaire, "What does it mean to you to be a cuer?" could be grouped into four themes, suggesting that one's self-concept as a cuer might be determined in part by: (1) access to language and/or languages; (2) communication abilities; or (3) literacy. A fourth theme that emerged represents an opposite perspective, that being a cuer is not a defining characteristic at all.

Access to Language(s). Respondents wrote of their access to the English language and their ability to learn spoken languages and dialects. Statements representative of this view include: (1) "I'm quite proud of being a cuer, knowing that I was exposed to a system that gave me access to language before I had access to hearing," (2) "To be able to use my natural language (English) and to be proud of what I've done with cueing," (3) "As a cuer, I feel I have the ability to speak any spoken languages as well as sound. Simply that I used Cued Speech to access the spoken language and learned a great deal about phonology. I also learned accents as a result," (4) "I'm a person who's been cueing since I was a wee lassie and prefer to access English through [Cued Speech]," and (5) "Being a cuer means ACCESSIBILITY! I have access to language, which is so crucial. I was able to learn English, and coincidentally, English became one of my favorite subjects in school. I was always placed in classes above grade level, thanks to Cued Speech. I also was able to take Hebrew and Spanish . . . which is exactly why Cued Speech means accessibility. I can learn languages other than ASL as well."

Communication Abilities.   A second theme regarding self-concept as a cuer regards communication abilities and knowledge of Cued Speech as one communication modality, separate from or in addition to speech and signs: (1) "It means that I am fortunate to know Cued Speech. It means that I am able to have better communication with the hearing people than most other deaf people," (2) "Just someone that knows how to use cued speech. I also feel somewhat empowered that I know all three modes of communication; cued speech, ASL, oralism," (3) "Being a cuer makes me feel unique from the ASL group. I feel that I am able to communicate and be a part of the hearing world," and (4) "I feel that it has given me access to good speech skills because my speech pathologists were

able to work with my cueing and speech in order to identify/learn certain sounds that I was not able to recognize before."

Literacy.   A third theme among responses centers on the identity of a cuer as a highly literate person, as highlighted in the following examples: (1) "It means a lot. I used to not want to be a cuer, but I'm glad I am one. I can speak very well and clearly because of cued speech, also I write very well," (2) "Someone who is very literate and can function in the hearing world with few accommodations," (3) "I am able to read Dostoevsky novels with no problems due to Cued Speech," (4) "Cueing has allowed me to discover my talents, which, ironically, are literature comprehension and writing," and (5) "I'm not sure, but I do know that it has helped me become a very literate person."

Being a Cuer Is a Non-Issue.   A final theme, perhaps contrary to the others, centers on the belief that being a cuer is a non-issue, and that deaf individuals need not be labeled based on communication mode(s): (1) "Nothing. I identify myself as a normal deaf person. I don't identify myself as a cuer or a signer, etc." and (2)

> I don't think about it. For me, I don't think of myself as a 'cuer.' That's a small part of who I am. I have always taken issue with members of the deaf, signing community who take pride in being a d/Deaf signer and use that to define their personal identities. I think that limits them, and insulates them from the larger world around us. They use that as a buffer, as a comfort blanket, in my personal opinion. I don't want that, nor do I need to be known as a cuer when I have so much more in me.

Discussion

Major findings discussed in this section are grouped as: (1) self-esteem and cultural identify of cueing deaf adults in this study, (2) early childhood family and peer experiences that may have influenced self-esteem and culturally identity of the cueing deaf respondents, (3) educational experiences and achievement of deaf cuers; and (4) the lasting effect of Cued Speech in the lives of cueing deaf adults in this study.

Self-Esteem and Cultural Identity of Cueing Deaf Adults

Findings from this study reveal that cueing deaf adults who participated in this study identify themselves as being academically successful, socially connected, and linguistically and communicatively flexible. They attribute their self-esteem and psychosocial adjustment to Cued Speech, regardless of whether they currently use Cued Speech at all or most of the time.

Cueing Deaf Adults as Readers

Virtually all cueing deaf adults in this study report ease and a strong affinity for reading and writing (some to the point of considering it part of their identity), and report extensive daily use of text-based communication for recreation, social, academic, and professional purposes. This finding relates closely to another finding in this study, that is, in response to an open-ended question asking "What it means to be a cuer," many responses indicated it means being a highly literate person. This finding is important, given findings from studies showing that the development of reading is challenging for most deaf individuals, with the average high school graduate reading at a third to fourth-grade reading level (Traxler, 2000).

Cueing Deaf Adults as Flexible Communicators

Responses from cueing deaf adults in this study collectively suggest that they tend to be highly flexible communicators and language users, able to use expressive cueing and cue reading, speech and speech-reading, expressive and receptive signing, reading/writing/texting, or combinations thereof as the situation dictates. This is an interesting finding given that often, individuals who are deaf are classified as "oral," "signers," or "cuers," with an unstated assumption that they use a single communication method. Most respondents reported considering themselves to be very good cue readers, even those who do not find themselves in cueing situations often, which suggests that these cuers truly internalized Cued Speech at an early age, and that even without practice, it is natural and automatic. The role of expressive and receptive cueing in the lives of cueing deaf adults in this study ranges from that of a tool for communicating either in noisy environments or when hearing aids/cochlear implants are off or not functioning properly, to communication and conversation with other deaf or hearing cuers, to a means of gaining academic information via CLTs. Cuers appear to be very good speechreaders, and report using this skill often in social, academic, and work environments. Given that speechreading is integral to receptive cueing, it is not surprising that cuers would rely on this when communicating with hearing individuals who do not cue or sign, nor is it surprising that they would use this communication strategy to a great extent.

The majority (88%) of cueing deaf adults in this survey reported gaining some level of sign proficiency by the time they reached adulthood. Given the large number of deaf adults who use signs to communicate, whether manually coded English sign systems, Pidgin Sign English, or American Sign Language (ASL), it is not surprising that cuers would learn to sign in order to access this larger population. Respondents in this study who now sign report skill levels ranging from survival signer to fluent ASL user. Some report almost exclusive use of ASL in adulthood, to the point of marrying ASL native signers, teaching in ASL school environments, and/or becoming ASL instructors. Other cuers report that they have not learned to sign and for them, signing plays a minimal role in their lives as adults.

Cueing Deaf Adults as Members of the Deaf and Hearing Communities

Results of this study suggest that these cueing deaf adults fit into two of the four acculturation categories discussed by Hintermair (2007); specifically, they appear to identify as either hearing acculturated or biculturally acculturated, as opposed to entirely deaf acculturated, or marginally acculturated. All of these cueing deaf adults report growing up in hearing families and attending mainstream school programs, and many statements provided by cueing deaf adults indicate their tendency toward and ease with their hearing communities. Although some cueing deaf adults report negative experiences regarding the Deaf community and do not feel as though they have much in common with its members, nearly three-fifths (59%) of respondents

look on Deaf Culture with affinity and consider themselves to be members of the Deaf community, in addition to their membership in their hearing community.

Respondents who consider themselves members of the Deaf community (in addition to the hearing community) generally report having entered it in high school, in college, or by attending Deaf-specific events. Interestingly, many statements provided by respondents in this study seem to suggest a view that learning to sign is, unto itself, an avenue for entrance into the Deaf community.

Childhood Experience and Perceptions Related to Communication and Inclusion

Previous studies of early childhood experiences of deaf adults from oral or signing backgrounds and adolescents have reported feelings of isolation within families and/or peer groups (Bodner-Johnson, 2003; Kent, 2003; Most, 2007; Weisel & Kamara, 2005). Cueing deaf adults in this study overwhelmingly report that they did not consider themselves isolated, either in their families or in their peer groups, which is in sharp contrast to Bodner-Johnson's (2003) conclusion that:

> Regardless of the communication mode chosen by their hearing parents, the deaf [adult] students interviewed indicated that they were not able to participate fully in the in the language used in their homes . . . Without a shared language, conversation or reciprocal dialogue among family members is a challenging, often frustrating task. (pp. 8–9)

Family

A series of questions in this survey addressed which members of cueing deaf adults' families were able to cue to the deaf child, how well they cued, and the extent to which family members were able to communicate with one another. These questions were included because access to communication determines the extent to which a child is involved in his or her family (Epstein, Coates, Salinas, Sanders, & Simon, 1997) and deaf children of hearing parents are at particular risk of diminished communication access (Yoshinaga-Itano, Sedey, Coulter, & Mehl, 1998).

The vast majority (81%) of cueing deaf adults in this study reported that they were first exposed to Cued Speech before the age of 5 years, with 69% having two parents who cued to them, 62% with at least one sibling who cued to them, and 34% reported extended family members cued to them. This finding, coupled with findings related to self-esteem support findings from studies showing an advantage academically of children who receive Cued Speech at home and school compared to those exposed to Cued Speech only at school, suggests that the same advantage may exist in terms of psychosocial adjustment for deaf children who are exposed to Cued Speech at home. Further research is needed to test this hypothesis, however.

The majority (72%) of cueing deaf adults in this study report that they always felt included in family activities and conversations when they were growing up. This finding may be attributable to the ease with which Cued Speech can be learned by parents and the short time required for parents to a provide rich linguistic environment (Torres, Moreno-Torres, & Santana, 2006) so that the deaf child, like hearing peers, can acquire English and other tra-ditionally spoken languages naturally, in preparation for formal reading instruction and academic achievement. It can be assumed that the access to immediate family members via Cued Speech experienced by the cueing deaf adults in this study as young children is one factor in respondents feeling included in family events and conversations. It remains unclear, however, whether feelings of family involvement are related to the number or type of family members who cued.

Peers

All of respondents in this study reported having close friendships growing up, and seem equally likely to develop friendships with hearing or deaf children. Seventy-eight percent reported that their friends learned to cue. These findings are important, as they suggest that children raised with Cued Speech do not necessarily feel more or less socially isolated than other deaf children. This also speaks to the communicative flexibility of these cuers.

Educational Experiences and Achievement of Deaf Cuers

All but one respondent to this survey indicated having attended college, with the single exception indicating that she or he had not yet enrolled at the point of responding to the survey. Moreover, given the degree to which these individuals accessed transliterators, interpreters, and computer-assisted real-time translation (CART) services for access to instruction (100% using cued language transliterators or interpreters in college classes), it can be assumed that these individuals attended "mainstream" colleges and universities, as opposed to those established specifically for deaf students (i.e., Gallaudet University or the National Technical Institute for the Deaf).

Trends in the data clearly indicate a "typical" educational experience for deaf cueing children in the United States; more often than not, they have fairly equal chances of participating in a self-contained class with a cueing teacher or entering school in the mainstream with a cued language transliterator. By the late elementary years, they become more likely to access most of their curricular instruction as facilitated by CLTs. By middle school, a cueing teacher is a rarity in the experience of these students, and by high school, they are fully integrated into regular education classrooms, with cued language transliterators or other accommodations to ensure access to communication.

The deaf cuers responding to this survey do not appear to have struggled in their mainstream education alongside their hearing classmates. Indeed, 57% of respondents reported that most or all of their subjects in school were easy, with the other 43% reporting an equal amount of easy and difficult subjects. The finding that 97% of respondents found English language arts "easy" is not surprising, given that the majority (78%) of respondents learned to read in early childhood, most often from their parents at home.

The tendency of deaf adult cuers to be "highly flexible communicators" seems to take root in their early family and social experiences, as well as their experiences with hearing (and for some, hearing and deaf) classmates. The deaf cueing individuals responding to this survey report being equally likely to interact with hearing or deaf peers, and report a wide variety of communication methods, including oral communication, cueing, and signing.

The Lasting Impact of Cued Speech

Virtually all cueing deaf adults in this study indicated that they believe exposure to Cued Speech in childhood has had lasting impact on their lives, especially in terms of communication and language abilities, literacy and academics, and self-confidence. Few respondents articulated regrets at having been raised with Cued Speech. Comments about costs associated with being a cuer focused either on feeling "between two worlds," with the cuer either feeling caught between the hearing and deaf "worlds," or the cueing and signing deaf "worlds," or wishing to have been socialized with signing deaf children and/or exposed to sign communication earlier in life. Other frustrations articulated by respondents seem to relate more to being a deaf person in a largely hearing environment than with being a cuer per se, such as feeling different or singled out.

Conclusion

Cueing deaf adults in this study demonstrate a high level of self-esteem and self-confidence, which they credit to their parents' choice of Cued Speech, their early childhood experiences of feeling included in family activities and conversations and in peer groups, and positive feelings of competence and success in school. Virtually all report a strong affinity for and skill in reading and writing. Most respondents report that they continue to think of themselves as cuers, but see cueing now as only one of the many communication options at their disposal for access to hearing and deaf speakers and signers, and they adapt their communication modality as needed to social, academic, and professional settings. This is an interesting finding given that often, individuals who are deaf are classified as "oral," "signers," or "cuers," with an unstated assumption that they use a single communication method. The vast majority of cueing deaf adults in this study report that they function comfortably in both the hearing and deaf worlds with 88% reporting that they have learned to sign, and nearly 60% reporting that they consider themselves to be members of the Deaf community. This last finding supports the rich diversity and ever evolving nature of American Deaf culture and dispels the myth that deaf children from Cued Speech backgrounds are isolated socially.

References

Akamatsu, C., Mayer, C., & Farrelly, S. (2006). An investigation of two-way text messaging use with deaf students at the secondary level. *Journal of Deaf Studies and Deaf Education, 11,* 120–131.

Angelides, P., & Aravi, C. (2006). A comparative perspective on the experiences of deaf and hard of hearing individuals as students at mainstream and special schools. *American Annals of the Deaf, 151,* 476–487.

Bat-Chava, Y., & Deignan, E. (2001). Peer relationships of children with cochlear implants. *Journal of Deaf Studies and Deaf Education, 6,* 186–199.

Bodner-Johnson, B. (2003). The deaf child in the family. In B. Bodner-Johnson & M. Sass-Lehrer (Eds.), *The young deaf or hard of hearing child: A family centered approach to early education* (pp. 3–33). Baltimore, MD: Brookes.

Bragg, B. (1989). *Lessons in laughter.* Washington, DC: Gallaudet University Press.

Brunnberg, E., Boström, M., & Berglund, M. (2008). Self-rated mental health, school adjustment, and substance use in hard-of-hearing adolescents. *Journal of Deaf Studies and Deaf Education, 13,* 324–335.

Cawthon, S. (2006). National survey of accommodations and alternate assessments for students who are deaf or hard of hearing in the United States. *Journal of Deaf Studies and Deaf Education, 11,* 337–359.

Chorost, M. (2005). *Rebuilt: How becoming part-computer made me more human.* New York, NY: Houghton-Mifflin.

Cornett, R. O. (1967). Cued Speech. *American Annals of the Deaf, 112,* 3–13.

Cornett, R. O., & Daisey, M. (2001). *The Cued Speech resource book for parents of deaf children.* Cleveland, OH: National Cued Speech Association.

Crowe, T. (2003). Self-esteem scores among deaf college students: An examination of gender and parents' hearing status and signing ability. *Journal of Deaf Studies and Deaf Education, 8,* 199–206.

Epstein, J., Coates, L., Salinas, K., Sanders, M., & Simon, B. (1997). *School, family, and community partnerships: Your handbook for action.* Thousand Oaks, CA: Corwin Press.

Esp, J. (2001). A national survey of social work services in schools for the deaf. *American Annals of the Deaf, 146,* 320–327.

Freebody, P., & Power, D. (2001). Interviewing deaf adults in post-secondary educational settings: Stories, cultures, and life histories. *Journal of Deaf Studies and Deaf Education, 6,* 130–142.

Gallaudet Research Institute. (2005). *2004–2005 Annual Survey of Deaf and Hard of Hearing Children and Youth.* Washington, DC: Gallaudet University.

Hage, C., & Leybaert, J. (2006). The effect of Cued Speech on the development of spoken language. In P. Spencer & M. Marschark (Eds.), *Advances in the spoken language development of deaf and hard of hearing students* (pp. 193–211). New York, NY: Oxford University Press.

Hintermair, M. (2008). Self-esteem and satisfaction with life of deaf and hard-of-hearing people: A resource-oriented approach to identity work. *Journal of Deaf Studies and Deaf Education, 13,* 124–146.

Israelite, N., & Hammermeister, F. (1986). A survey of teacher preparation programs in education of the hearing impaired. *American Annals of the Deaf, 131,* 232–237.

Israelite, N., Ower, J., & Goldstein, G. (2002). Hard-of-hearing adolescents and identity construction: Influences of school experiences, peers, and teachers. *Journal of Deaf Studies and Deaf Education, 7,* 134–148.

Jacobs, L. (1989). *A deaf adult speaks out* (3rd ed.). Washington, DC: Gallaudet University Press.

Jambor, E., & Elliot, M. (2005). Self-esteem and coping strategies among deaf students. *Journal of Deaf Studies and Deaf Education, 10,* 63–81.

Kelly, R., Lang, H., & Pagliaro, C. (2003). Mathematics word problem solving for deaf students: A survey of practices in grades 6–12. *Journal of Deaf Studies and Deaf Education, 8,* 104–119.

Kent, B. (2003). Identity issues for hard of hearing adolescents aged 11, 13, and 15 in mainstream settings. *Journal of Deaf Studies and Deaf Education, 8,* 315–324.

Kisor, H. (1990). *What's that pig outdoors? A memoir of deafness.* New York, NY: Penguin Books.

Koelle, W., & Convey, J. (1982). The prediction of the achievement of deaf adolescents from self-concept and locus of control measures. *American Annals of the Deaf, 12,* 769–779.

LaSasso, C., & Lollis, J. (2003). Survey of residential and day schools for deaf students in the United States that identify themselves as bilingual-bicultural programs. *Journal of Deaf Studies and Deaf Education, 8,* 79–91.

LaSasso, C., & Metzger, M. (1998). An alternate route for preparing deaf children for Bi-Bi programs: The home language as L1 and Cued Speech for conveying traditionally-spoken languages. *Journal of Deaf Studies and Deaf Education, 3,* 265–289.

Leigh, I. (1999). Inclusive education and personal development. *Journal of Deaf Studies and Deaf Education, 4,* 236–245.

Lukomski, J. (2007). Deaf college students' perceptions of their social-emotional adjustment. *Journal of Deaf Studies and Deaf Education, 12,* 486–494.

Marlatt, E. (2001). Measuring practical knowledge among prospective and current teachers of deaf and hard of hearing students. *American Annals of the Deaf, 146,* 331–347.

Mertens, D. (1998). *Research methods in education and psychology: Integrating diversity with quantitative and qualitative approaches.* Thousand Oaks, CA: Sage Publications.

Most, T. (2007). Speech intelligibility, loneliness, and sense of coherence among deaf and hard-of-hearing children in individual inclusion and group inclusion. *Journal of Deaf Studies and Deaf Education, 12,* 495–503.

Musselman, C., & Akamatsu, C. (1999). Interpersonal communication skills of deaf adolescents and their relationship to communication history. *Journal of Deaf Studies and Deaf Education, 4,* 305–320.

Musselman, C., Mootilal, A., & MacKay, S. (1996). The social adjustment of deaf adolescents in segregated, partially integrated, and mainstreamed settings. *Journal of Deaf Studies and Deaf Education, 1,* 52–63.

National Cued Speech Association (2002). *Letters from cue adults.* Cleveland, OH: NCSA.

Nikolaraizi, M., & Hadjikakou, K. (2006). The role of educational experiences in the development of deaf identity. *Journal of Deaf Studies and Deaf Education, 11,* 477–492.

Polat, F. (2003). Factors affecting psychosocial adjustment of deaf students. *Journal of Deaf Studies and Deaf Education, 8,* 325–339.

Polich, L. (2001). Education of the deaf in Nicaragua. *Journal of Deaf Studies and Deaf Education, 6,* 315–326.

Porter, A., & Edirippulige, S. (2007). Parents of deaf children seeking hearing-loss related information on the internet: The Australian experience. *Journal of Deaf Studies and Deaf Education, 12,* 518–529.

Punch, R., Hyde, M., & Power, D. (2007). Career and workplace experiences of Australian graduates who are deaf or hard of hearing. *Journal of Deaf Studies and Deaf Education, 12,* 504–517.

Richardson J., Long, G., & Woodley, A. (2004). Students with an undisclosed hearing loss: A challenge for academic access, progress, and success? *Journal of Deaf Studies and Deaf Education, 9,* 427–441.

Richardson, J., MacLeod-Gallinger, J., McKee, B., & Long, G. (2000). Approaches to studying in deaf and hearing students in higher education. *Journal of Deaf Studies and Deaf Education, 2,* 156–173.

Scherer, M., & McKee, B. (1993). *The views of adult deaf learners and institutions serving deaf learners regarding distance learning cooperative arrangements with NTID/RIT: The results of two surveys.* U.S. Department of Education. Retrieved August 2, 2007, from http://www.eric.ed.gov/ERICDocs/data/ericdocs2sql/content_storage_01/0000019b/80/16/26/0b.pdf

Swiller, J. (2007). *The unheard.* New York, NY: Henry Holt and Company.

Torres, S., Moreno-Torres, I., & Santana, R. (2006). Quantitative and qualitative evaluation of linguistic input support to a prelingually deaf child with Cued Speech: A case study. *Journal of Deaf Studies and Deaf Education, 11,* 438–448.

Traxler, C. (2000). The Stanford Achievement Test, 9th edition: National norming and performance standards for deaf and hard of hearing students. *Journal of Deaf Studies and Deaf Education, 5,* 337–348.

Van Gurp, S. (2001). Self-concept of deaf secondary school students in different educational settings. *Journal of Deaf Studies and Deaf Education, 6,* 54–69.

Wallis, D., Musselman, C., & MacKay, S. (2004). Hearing mothers and their deaf children: The relationship between early, ongoing mode match and subsequent mental health functioning in adolescence. *Journal of Deaf Studies and Deaf Education, 9,* 1–14.

Weisel, A., & Kamara, A. (2005). Attachment and individuation of deaf/hard-of-hearing and hearing young adults. *Journal of Deaf Studies and Deaf Education, 10,* 51–62.

Yachnik, M. (1986). Self-esteem in deaf adolescents. *American Annals of the Deaf, 131,* 305–310.

Yoshinaga-Itano, C., Sedey, A., Coulter, D., & Mehl, A. (1998). The language of early- and later-identified children with hearing loss. *Pediatrics, 102,* 1161–1171.

Chapter 10

A BILINGUAL (ASL AND CUED AMERICAN ENGLISH) PROGRAM FOR DEAF AND HARD OF HEARING STUDENTS: THEORY TO PRACTICE[1]

Kitri Larson Kyllo

Preceding chapters in this volume clearly establish the linguistic merits of cued American English (CAE) as a visual and linguistically complete medium to convey the language of English, incorporating the visually discrete features of Cued Speech (handshape, hand placement, mouthshape) with prosodic information from nonmanual features, such as head-thrust and brow movement, to convey the linguistic features of American English (Fleetwood & Metzger, 1998a, 1998b). This chapter describes a public school program's application of CAE in the school setting in terms of language acquisition and educational considerations, and provides results in language and achievement of its students over the past decade.

As discussed in Chapter 11 of this volume, the role of phonemic awareness in the early decoding and reading achievement of hearing and deaf children[2] has

---

[1]Portions of this chapter are reprinted in part from, "Phonemic Awareness Through Cued American English," originally published in *Odyssey*, Vol. 5(1). Copyright © 2003, Laurent Clerc National Deaf Education Center. Used with permission.
[2]Deaf and hard of hearing students are referred to as deaf students in this chapter.

been investigated and well-documented. Generally, children (deaf or hearing) with sufficient access to the phoneme stream of a consonant-vowel (C-V) language can develop the ability to parse segments of that language into phonological units and phonemes and can, in turn, learn to apply that ability to decoding the printed form of that language.

Access to Phonology for Deaf Children

As discussed in several chapters of this volume, a shift has been made in our understanding of phonology and the various means of representing phonemes (e.g., acoustically, visually, tactile-kinesthetically). It is now better understood that phonemes are not speech sounds, but are abstract linguistic contrasts that can be represented visually (e.g., via Cued Speech) as well as acoustically (i.e., via speech). Readers immersed in English via CAE can learn to read using *phonemic* strategies and need not rely on a sight-word approach as their main strategy. They have learned the alphabetic code/phoneme correlation be-tween the printed letter and the English phoneme, and can apply phonemic de-coding strategies in an interactive manner with their internalized knowledge of the English language to decode the words on the page.

As discussed in Chapter 12 of this volume, among the typical means of conveying English visually to individuals who are deaf (i.e., speech, fingerspelling, manually-coded English [MCE], Cued Speech), only Cued Speech is capable of doing so clearly and completely and at all levels of language, including the phonological level. This early visual access to phonology aids not only in phonological awareness and phonics decoding, but in the development of more sophisticated language structures, also critical for fluent and independent reading (see Chapter 11).

With the continuing improvements in hearing aid technology and the advent of cochlear implants, it is more important than ever to remember that these devices aim to increase the quantity or quality of acoustic input to a deaf child, but limitations still exist as to their efficacy in all situations.

Natural Acquisition and Language Mastery

Children who are deaf have historically been exposed to English vocabulary, syntax, and figurative language through *direct or formal* teaching efforts during their school years, whereby print has been used in an attempt to make the precise English words and word endings clear. For prelingual, profoundly deaf students exposed to American Sign Language (ASL) or MCE sign systems, reading tends to be a process of trying to match sight words (i.e., words recognized instantly after multiple exposures) with signs in their sign vocabulary. This sight-word approach is used to unravel the words on the page that represent a language of which these learners typically only have minimum or partial knowledge. These learners are being expected to learn to read English and to learn the language of English simultaneously.

In contrast, deaf children who are immersed in English via cued English tend to acquire English vocabulary, syntax, morphology, and idioms naturally through meaningful interactions with cuers. These words and structures are not formally taught through direct instruction, but rather are acquired through conversations with people who cue to them. Their internalized knowledge of English phonology, syntax, morphology, vocabulary, and figurative language allows them to decode and anticipate/predict words as they read. Children exposed early to cued English are not learning the language of English while they learn to read; rather, they are learning to read a language they already know (as hearing children do) using phonemic decoding and linguistic closure strategies (as hearing children do) (Doenges, 2003).

Intermediate School District 917 Program for Deaf and Hard of Hearing Learners

Program Description

The Intermediate School District 917 Program for Deaf and Hard of Hearing Learners (ISD 917), a regional bilingual program in the Minneapolis/St. Paul metropolitan area, develops English phonemic awareness and literacy through language instruction and immersion in spoken/cued American English. Access to American Sign Language (ASL) and CAE is provided through exposure to each language in different activities or settings. The determination of the language(s) of instruction occurs through the process of developing the child's Individualized Education Plan. The program believes that the use of CAE in an immersion model: (1) provides the most visually complete access to the language of English in conversation, (2) allows for the develop-

ment of phonemic awareness and decoding skills, and (3) results in high literacy levels in learners who are deaf. (For more information regarding the program's immersion model, view the segment *Signs of Literacy* featuring the District 917 Deaf and Hard of Hearing Program in the *PBS Reading Rockets: Launching Young Readers* episode, *A Chance to Read*, http://www.readingrockets.org/shows/launching/chance. © 2007. WETA-TV.) The program also believes that immersion in ASL can be critical to the development and social/emotional well-being of many learners who are deaf/hard of hearing.

A central tenet of the ISD 917 program is the belief that advanced proficiency in a language, whether it is ASL, English, or another traditionally spoken language, requires internal mastery of that language. Program administrators and staff believe internalization and mastery of a target language occurs most effectively and efficiently through natural communication and discourse via *immersion* in that language, and not through translation or language-via-print-only methodologies typical of other bilingual education programs for deaf students (LaSasso & Lollis, 2003). Professionals in the field of deaf education appear largely in agreement on the need and requirement for immersion in ASL to acquire internal mastery of that language. The perspectives in deaf education about the means of acquiring internal mastery of English, a traditionally spoken C-V language, however, vary significantly. The program's practice of using Cued Speech to convey English is grounded in the belief that it enables deaf children to acquire an internalized mastery of English at the phonological level necessary to acquire the phonemic awareness skills required to develop: (1) the ability to *decode* the printed form of English for reading and (2) the ability to *encode* the internalized language accurately into the written form of English for writing.

The program also values complete and early access to a learner's home language, that is, the *native language* of the parents, whether that language is ASL, or a traditionally spoken language, such as English, that is conveyed visually using the system of Cued Speech. Program professionals work with parents to promote an understanding of the barriers to language accessibility for deaf children. They assist parents in developing communication skills to provide complete, unambiguous access to language in the home setting in addition to the school setting. Program staff believe that deaf learners can become bilingual in ASL and English when provided: (1) access to adult language models fluent in ASL and models fluent in cued or cued/spoken American English, (2) *immersion* in both ASL and English via CAE, and (3) maximized language learning opportunities through both school and parent participation and commitment to unambiguous language immersion in all settings (Intermediate District 917, 1997; Doenges & Kyllo, 2001).

Determination of Language(s) of Instruction

The program aims for bilingual access to English and ASL and the development of proficiency in those languages to the extent determined by a learner's parents and educational team. It does not presume, however, that all language-of-instruction needs are the same and are to be delivered in a uniform manner for each of its learners. The program recognizes the parents' right to be a critical decision-maker regarding the language(s) of instruction to be used with their child in the school setting. The program aims to achieve unambiguous access to, and immersion in, the languages of both ASL and English in all settings where each has been determined to be used as the language of instruction. Some learners in the program have either ASL or spoken and cued English solely as their language of instruction throughout their school day. Many learners, however, have exposure to both languages in their school day, the ratio of exposure being determined through the learner's Individualized Education Plan (IEP) process.

The mission of the program is to provide comprehensive services to prepare students to become confident, successful, literate, and independent life-long learners. Unequivocally, there is a distinct, driving mission in the program to assist learners in achieving English literacy and communication proficiency on par with their hearing peers. In order to have deaf learners ready to meet the reading and writing demands already present by kindergarten, the program strives for intense exposure to English during the preschool years. For those learners for whom ASL has been deemed a critical vehicle for learning and communication, the program assists in the achievement of proficiency in that language to the maximum extent possible. The program also seeks to maximize the spoken English and auditory skills of its learners through auditory/oral strategies to the maximum extent possible given learners' abilities.

Delivery of Language(s) and Instruction

Many learners served in the program acquire English proficiency and literacy solely through immersion in English via cued/spoken English. Other learners, however, benefit in their acquisition of English skills from the communication bridge afforded through the use of sign communication. The program strives to keep the languages of English and ASL separate, although each language may be used to support the learning of the other through a technique called "sandwiching," in which an utterance presented through cueing may be followed by the same utterance signed for clarification, and then followed by cueing the utterance again.

English is not taught as a "second language" as in the English as a Second Language (ESL), or English Language Learning (ELL), approaches to instruction for hearing, non-English-speaking learners in the public schools. These learners typically come to school with an intact first language (L1) due to access to the home language through normal hearing. For learners who are deaf, such access to the home language of the parents cannot be assumed. A deaf learner coming from an English-speaking home typically is referred for special education services because the lack of access to the home language due to the hearing loss has resulted in language and communication delays. For the approximately 95% of deaf learners whose parents are hearing and whose home language is not ASL, but English or another spoken language (Mitchell & Karchmer, 2004), the program typically regards the spoken language of the home as the target L1. Thus, the L1 for a learner in the program may be Spanish, English, or ASL, depending on the parents' native language. The L2 may be English for a learner whose home language is ASL, ASL for a learner whose home language is English, or perhaps both ASL and English for a learner from a non-English-speaking hearing family.

The increased access and exposure to English, being the majority language of most of the learners in the program, is continued in the school setting for a preschool learner through the use of English via spoken/cued English as the language-of-instruction. English is provided consistently as a conversational and academic language, and students are given as much opportunity as is deemed appropriate to interact with that language, be it spoken, cued, or written. English is used as the language of instruction for the subjects of reading, writing, and spelling, as well as for the English-text, English-vocabulary, and language aspects of other subjects. Typically, cued English is paired with spoken English. However, the learners in the program with profound hearing losses who do not benefit from auditory input have sometimes received English via cued English only (i.e., with no paired vocalized spoken English, but with appropriate CAE mouth movements) from staff who are themselves deaf and fluent in cued English. This method of language delivery is based on the program's conclusions that: (1) internalization and mastery in a language occurs most effectively and efficiently through natural communication and discourse via immersion in a target language, and (2) children must acquire an internalized mastery of a traditionally spoken language *first* in order to acquire phonemic awareness and the learned skill to decode the printed form of the language for reading, and encode it for writing.

It is deemed critical to the program to have staff who are themselves deaf to serve as both language and role models for its learners. Currently there are three teachers and a program assistant who are deaf, all with superior skills in ASL. As ASL models, they are not expected to become fluent cuers; however, one teacher who is deaf also has superior skills in CAE and several others have learned to cue. ASL has no voice component, and therefore, the staff in the program communicating in ASL do so in "voice-off mode." Typically, the staff who are hearing and fluent in English serve as the English models via cued and spoken English. Teachers who are hearing and serve as the English language models have intermediate to advanced skills in ASL.

Orientation to Literacy Instruction

Reading Level ≠ Language Level

The program strives to keep separate the concepts of reading level and language level. A *reading level* is a person's ability to read and understand the *printed* form of a language. A *language level* is the proficiency a child has in conversing in a language via *nonprinted* forms (e.g., speaking, cueing, signing). Reading scores of children exposed to signing versus cueing typically start to look very dissimilar to hearing learners' scores at the third- or fourth-grade reading level, even if they may appear similar in earlier grades. On-grade-level reading scores for young deaf children in the early elementary years must be interpreted carefully, as on-grade-level English language abilities cannot be assumed from on-grade-level reading scores. For example, a learner can have a "second-grade reading level" without having a 7- or 8-year-old's English *language level*.

English and Phonemic Awareness Instruction

Emphasis on phonemic awareness and phonics is integrated into language arts reading and writing instruction with the assistance of several curricula designed to provide skill development in these areas, including, but not limited to, the Lindamood Phoneme Sequencing Program for Reading, Spelling and Speech (Lindamood & Lindamood, 1998), Scott Foresman Reading series, (Afflerbach et al., 2004) and the Sopris West Language! (Green, 2000) curriculum. The use of cued English allows for the acquisition of skills in these areas due to its inherent ability to convey the phonological linguistic features of a consonant-vowel language.

Assessment of English Achievement

Measurement of student achievement is conducted using formal measures on a yearly basis in the ISD 917 program, as well as during the federally required three-year special education re-evaluation process. The program is currently utilizing the following formal measures normed on hearing students, in addition to other formal and informal measures, to assess receptive and expressive English language development and reading achievement: the Test of Auditory Comprehension of Language, Third Edition (TACL-III) (Carrow-Woolfolk, 1999); the Clinical Evaluation of Language Fundamentals, Fourth Edition (CELF-4) (Semel, Wiig, & Secord, 2004), the Peabody Picture Vocabulary Test, Fourth Edition, (PPVT-IV) (Dunn & Dunn, 2006), the Cottage Acquisition Scales for Listening, Language and Speech (CASLLS) (Wilkes, 2001); and the Gates-MacGinitie Test of

Reading, Fourth Edition (MacGinitie & MacGinitie, 2003). All tests measuring English competency are administered in English via cued/spoken English.

Evidence From Learners Who Are Deaf

Evidence for the efficacy of the program comes from aggregate achievement data collected over a period of years, and from cases of specific learners.

Program Language and Reading Achievement Data

In the aggregation of results of all the learners served in the program 2001 to 2006 reflected in Figure 10–1, the 2005 to 2006 population of learners in the program reflected the following demographic information:

- *Hearing Loss*—21% profound; 29% severe-profound with cochlear implant; 24% moderate-severe; 8% mild-moderate;

Outcomes from Intermediate District 917
Deaf and Hard of Hearing Program

The data collected below has been gathered on deaf and hard of hearing learners whose exposure to English included participation in the 917 D/HH English Preschool Program starting anywhere from age 2 to 4 years old since the 2001-2002 school year.

Assessment	Number of Children (N)	% of children who made one year of progress (or more) in one year of time	% of children with Standard Score equal to, or greater than, 85 (within, or above, average range)
Peabody Picture Vocabulary Test – Receptive (PPVT – Receptive)	20* (*Includes a learner served home-based who came in to the preschool with average language development who was not tested.)	95%	67%
Clinical Evaluation of Language Fundamentals – 4 - Receptive (CELF-4-Receptive)	12	100% (9 out of 9 learners who have received the CELF on consecutive years)	67%* (*One of the learners took the Preschool Language Scale, and received a 50 PR, indicating a language level in the average range. Including this learner makes the number of learners achieving in the average range or above **73%**.)

NOTE: Expressive English language is evaluated using various assessment tools, including the CASLLS (Cottage Acquisition Scales for Listening, Language and Speech), EVT (Expressive Vocabulary Test), and TEEM (Test Examining Expressive Morphology) due to their ability to provide diagnostic information to determine and target language, speech and auditory development goals on the IFSP/IEP. The 917 D/HH preschool program has begun to also use the Clinical Evaluation of Language Fundamentals-Preschool (CELF-PRE) to monitor expressive English language development.

Figure 10–1. Aggregate data from ISD 917 program.

- *Deaf/Hearing Parents*—21% with parents who are deaf; 79% with parents who are hearing;
- *Home Language/Communication Mode*—17% ASL; 12% PSE; 21% cued English; 42% spoken English only; 8% other spoken language only;
- *Socioeconomic Status*—33% on free/reduced lunch.

Annual tracking of student language and reading growth on standardized tests over the past 10 years has revealed that students in the program make at least one year of gain in their reading and language skills per each year of instruction, including learners whose parents do not cue at home. Some students make significantly larger gains of up to three years in one year. While many learners in the program achieve the 1:1 standard, for those who do not, the program aims for significant growth in that direction.

Figures 10–2A and 10–2B indicate results from the Gates-MacGinitie Test of Reading for a representative sample of program learners. Figures 10–3A and 10–3B indicate results from the PPVT-IV (a test of receptive English vocabulary) for a representative sample of program learners. Figures 10–4A and 10–4B indicate results from the CELF-4 (a test of English language development) for a representative sample of program learners.

The program starts tracking the English language development of its learners at the preschool level. Performance on a standardized measure of receptive English vocabulary indicates virtually 100% of learners achieving at least one year of gain per one year of instruction, and a significant percentage of learners scoring in

the average range compared to same-grade hearing peers. Many learners transfer to general education settings in different school districts after participation in the preschool and/or early elementary years in the program, at which time their performance no longer can be tracked.

The numbers reflect the performance for a mix of learners, including those with and without additional learning challenges, those who transfer into the program at various ages, and those with varied previous language and communication experiences at school and/or at home.

ISD 917 Versus National Deaf Reading Achievement Performance

Because reading achievement is the more commonly reported measure of deaf learners' achievement to reflect their skills in English, the program compiles the reading achievement scores of its learners to determine the degree of impact its practices is having on its learners as a whole. Figure 10–5 indicates the average grade-equivalent (GE) net gain per year in reading of students served in the ISD 917 program from 2001–2002 to 2005–2006. Compared to previous findings that, on average, it takes a deaf child five years to increase one year on a standardized reading test (LaSasso, 1999), thus an average of 0.2 grade equivalent net gain per one year of instruction, the program's data indicating an average net gain of 1.0 grade equivalent per one year of instruction reflects practices resulting in a robust impact on the reading achievement of its learners.

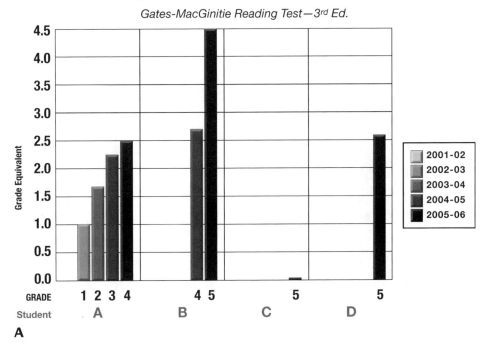

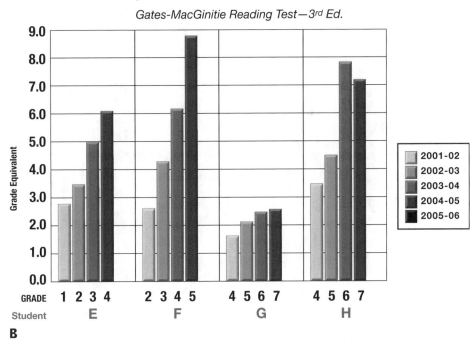

Figure 10–2. A. Sample Gates-MacGinitie Test of Reading standardized testing results, students A through D. **B.** Sample Gates-MacGinitie Test of Reading standardized testing results, students E through H.

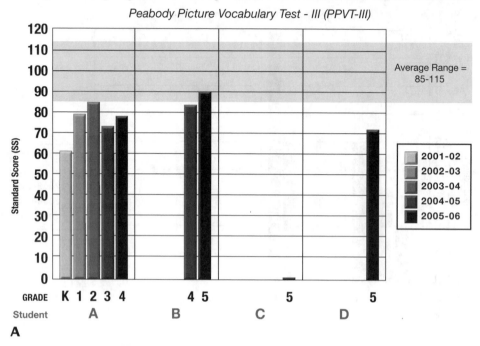

English Language-Vocabulary Scores of District 917 D/HH Students

Peabody Picture Vocabulary Test - III (PPVT-III)

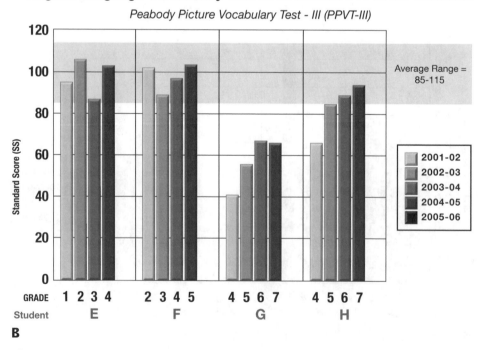

English Language-Vocabulary Scores of District 917 D/HH Students

Peabody Picture Vocabulary Test - III (PPVT-III)

Figure 10–3. A. Sample PPVT-IV standardized testing results, students A through D. **B.** Sample PPVT-IV standardized testing results, students E through H.

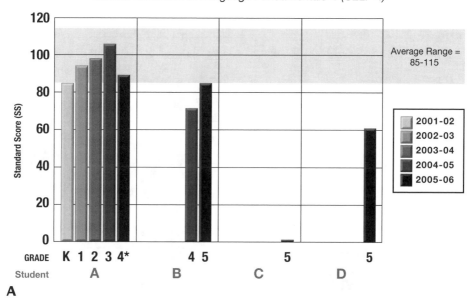

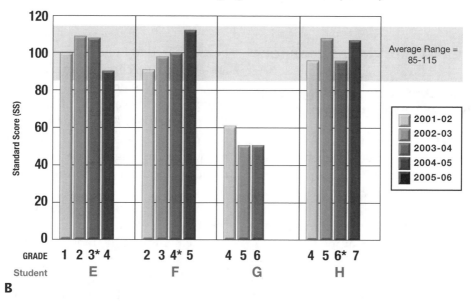

Figure 10–4. A. Sample CELF-4 and TACL-3 standardized testing results, students A through D. **B.** Sample CELF-4 and TACL-3 standardized testing results, students E through H.

*Indicates switch from TACL-3 to CELF-4.

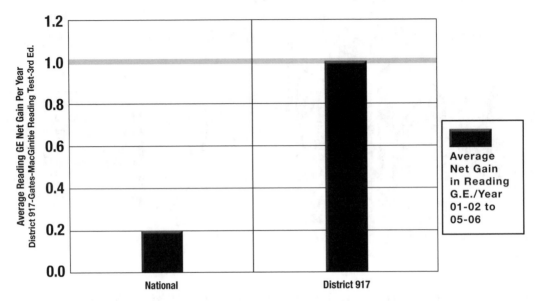

Figure 10–5. District 917 program versus national reading achievement results.

Cases of Individual Learners

Tessa: On-Grade Reading Level Masking Low Language Level

The situation where on-grade-level reading scores can mask actual English language levels is illustrated by the case of "Tessa," who attended the program through middle school, and is now in high school in the general education setting with minimal special education support.

Tessa, who has a congenital severe-profound hearing loss, had on-grade-level reading scores in both second and fifth grades, but, when tested on English language measures using cued English at the age of 8, was found to have the English language level of a 4-year-old. Tessa had

been exposed to English via cued English and ASL in the school setting in preschool and the early elementary years. Pidgin signed English was, and still is, used in the home setting. Tessa's parents and professional team decided to increase her immersion in English via cued English from two hours a day to the majority of her school day starting in third grade. She maintained this exposure throughout fourth grade. When she was retested at the beginning of fifth grade, English vocabulary scores revealed a five-year gain attained in three school years, as illustrated in Figures 10–6A and 10–6B. Figure 10–7 provides a graphic representation of the relationship between Tessa's measured reading level and measured language level at the two testing periods. Significant

Reading Achievement
Standardized Reading Inventory-2 Test

When Tessa was 11 years and 5 months old and in her second month of 5th grade, she achieved the scores below. At right are her percentile rank scores in both 5th grade and 2nd grade. Tessa's reading achievement scores appeared on-grade-level both in 2nd & 5th grades. The 2nd-grade average reading scores masked an extremely low language level.

Category	5th Grade Age Equivalent SCORE	5th Grade Grade Equivalent SCORE	5th Grade PR SCORE	2nd Grade PR SCORE
Passage Comprehension	10 yrs-3 mos	4th gr-5 mos	25	25
Word Recognition	11 yrs-3 mos	5th gr-5 mos	50	37
Vocabulary in Context	11 yrs-6 mos	5th gr-8 mos	50	50

Average range for percentile ranks (PR) is 25–75.

A

English Language Vocabulary Achievement
Peabody Picture Vocabulary Test-III
Testing conducted in English via cued/spoken English

Whereas Tessa's reading level appears to be in the average range for both 2nd & 5th grades, her English vocabulary scores for 2nd grade were significantly below average. Immersed in cued English in school for two years in 3rd and 4th grades, she made a five-year gain in English vocabulary by 5th grade.

Date	Age	Grade	Age-Equivalent SCORES	Percentile Rank SCORES
Fall, 1999	8 yrs-5 mos	2nd	4 yrs-8 mos	0.5
Fall, 2002	11 yrs-5 mos	5th	9 yrs-1 mo	16

Average range for percentile ranks (PR) is 25 - 75.

B

Figure 10–6. A. Tessa's reading achievement test scores. **B.** Tessa's English language vocabulary scores.

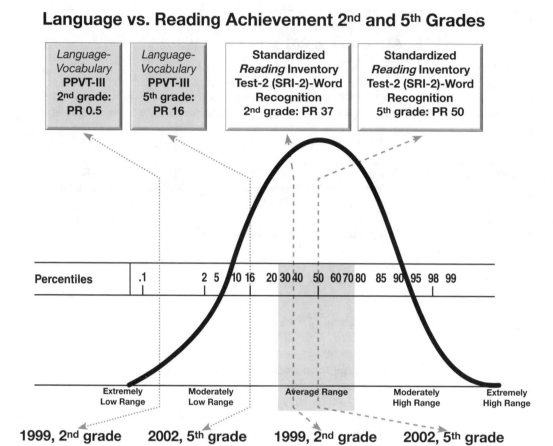

Figure 10–7. Relationship between Tessa's reading and language levels.

growth in written English skills occurred as well, as illustrated in Figures 10–8A and 10–8B, representing writing samples taken when Tessa was in the second and fifth grades, respectively.

Peter: The Importance of Parental Involvement

The case of "Peter," a young 4-year-old in the program with one more preschool year remaining prior to entering kindergarten, illustrates the collaborative teamwork of parents and staff, and the input from parents in making language-of-instruction decisions. Peter entered the program at age 2 with very minimal spoken English skills, no previous exposure to CAE, and only minimal prior exposure to signing. Peter has a severe bilateral sensorineural hearing loss, and began consistently using appropriate hearing aids at age 2. When Peter was in his second year in the program, his parents' input was sought to assist the team in determining IEP goals and a language-of-instruction plan.

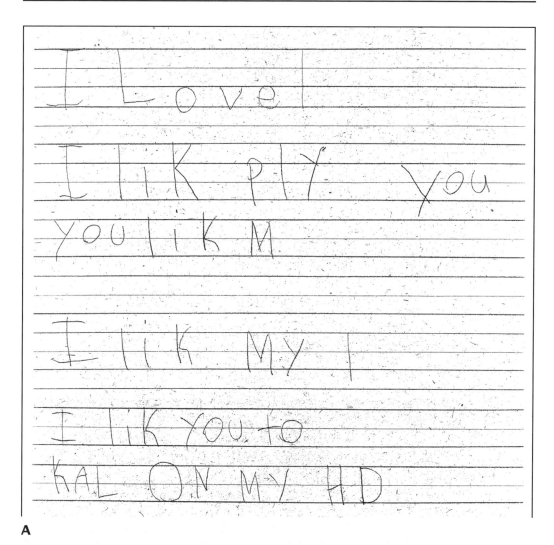

A

Figure 10–8. A. Tessa's 2nd grade writing sample. *continues*

The IEP team, including the parents, determined that Peter's language-of-instruction plan for that year would be approximately 50% English via spoken/cued English, and 50% ASL in the school setting. The plan the next year for the school year when Peter would turn 4 years old was determined to be approximately 60% English, and 40% ASL during his school day. At home, the parents communicate with Peter primarily in spoken English with some cueing and signing support. Peter's progress in English vocabulary development during his two and a half years in the program, illustrated in Figures 10–9A and 10–9B, indicate significant growth in his acquisition of English language skills from a below average level to an above average level compared with same-age hearing peers in just one year.

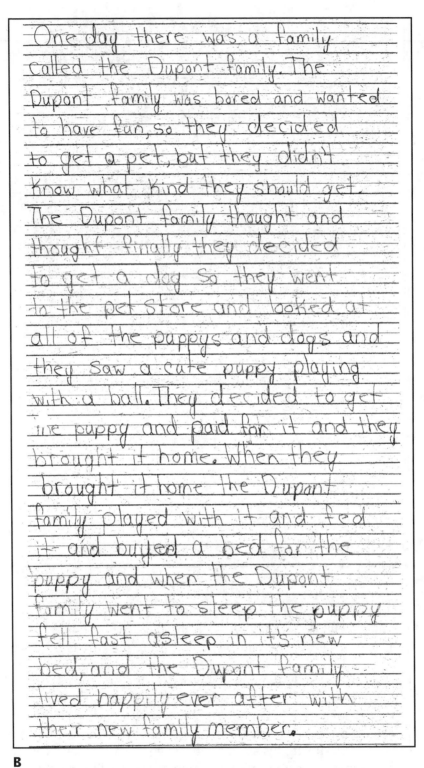

One day there was a family called the Dupont family. The Dupont family was bored and wanted to have fun, so they decided to get a pet, but they didn't know what kind they should get. The Dupont family thought and thought finally they decided to get a dog so they went to the pet store and looked at all of the puppys and dogs and they saw a cute puppy playing with a ball. They decided to get the puppy and paid for it and they brought it home. When they brought it home the Dupont family played with it and fed it and buyed a bed for the puppy and when the Dupont family went to sleep the puppy fell fast asleep in it's new bed, and the Dupont family lived happily ever after with their new family member.

B

Figure 10–8. *continued* **B.** Tessa's 5th grade writing sample.

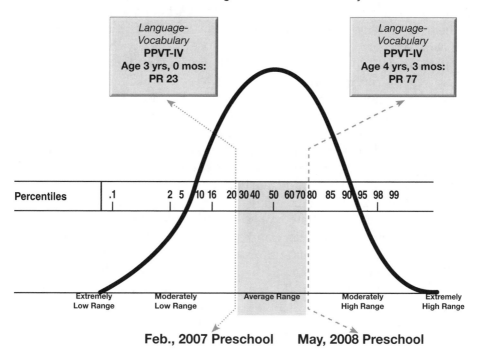

**Receptive English Vocabulary Language
Performance of a District 917 Preschooler**
Peabody Picture Vocabulary Test-IV
Testing conducted in English via cued/spoken English

*Whereas Peter's receptive English vocabulary level was in the below average range
when tested at age 3, his scores spiked to above the average range one year later.
Immersed in cued/spoken English in the District 917 D/HH Preschool program,
he made a 2.5-year gain in English vocabulary from age 3 to 4.*

Date	Age	Age-Equivalent SCORES	Standard SCORES	Percentile Rank SCORES
Feb, 2007	3 yrs-0 mos	2 yrs-6 mos	89	23
May, 2008	4 yrs-3 mos	5 yrs-1 mo	111	77

Average range for percentile ranks (PR) is 25 - 75.

A

**Receptive English Vocabulary Language Achievement
District 917 Preschooler – Age 3 to Age 4**
Below to above average achievement in one year

Language-
Vocabulary
PPVT-IV
Age 3 yrs, 0 mos:
PR 23

Language-
Vocabulary
PPVT-IV
Age 4 yrs, 3 mos:
PR 77

Percentiles   .1   2 5   10 16   20 30 40   50   60 70 80   85   90 95 98 99

Extremely
Low Range   Moderately
Low Range   Average Range   Moderately
High Range   Extremely
High Range

Feb., 2007 Preschool   May, 2008 Preschool

Average range for percentile ranks (PR) is 25 - 75.

B

Figure 10–9. A. Peter's preschool receptive language test results. **B.** Peter's language gain compared to normal hearing peers normative sample.

Scott: The Impact of CAE Immersion on Academic Achievement

The case of "Scott" illustrates the positive impact of exposure to, and immersion in spoken/cued American English on linguistic and academic achievement. Scott enrolled in the program in the beginning of fourth grade, having previously attended another large metro program for deaf students, which utilized Pidgin Sign English (PSE) with spoken English in the school setting. Both parents had learned and used sign language with Scott from an early age. Scott had a severe-profound bilateral sensorineural hearing loss and cerebral palsy from birth. He received a cochlear implant at age 3 years, 9 months. He received an AD/HD diagnosis at age 5, for which he takes medication. He began hearing aid use for his nonimplanted ear at age 7.

Scott was evaluated upon entering the program in his fourth-grade year. He scored in the average range on a standardized measure of intelligence. However, reading and language scores on standardized tests indicated scores significantly below same-grade hearing peers, with a 2.7 grade-equivalent, 19th percentile rank scores on the Gates-MacGinitie Reading Test-3, and very to extremely low scores on standardized English vocabulary and language measures: 12th percentile rank on the PPVT-III, 23rd percentile rank on the Expressive Vocabulary Test (EVT), and 1st percentile rank score on the CELF-4 (Stoesz, 2006).

Word-recognition testing at that time, with Scott's use of his cochlear implant and hearing aid through auditory input only in a quiet setting, was 56%, and in noise 32%, indicating the critical need for access to visual input for full access to spoken language (Stoesz, 2006).

Scott initially received most direct instruction from deaf program staff fluent in signing and cued English, with only his "specialist" classes in art, music, physical education, and science in the general education setting with a sign language interpreter. All language arts classes in the 917 program classroom setting were conducted in spoken/cued English, with "sandwiching" using signing to support comprehension as necessary. Speech-language therapy sessions were conducted in spoken/cued English for additional vocabulary and English language development, and for instruction in the system of Cued Speech.

Gradually, with the increased level of immersion in English via spoken/English both at school and home, as Scott's parents became fluent in cued English also, the use of "sandwiching" in sign language diminished and Scott's receptive and expressive skills in English increased. By fifth grade, Scott was functioning with a cued language transliterator (CLT) for his classes in the general education setting, and by his fourth year in the program he spent his entire school day in the general education setting with a CLT, with the exception of one class period to provide continued content-related vocabulary and language support. Figures 10–10A through 10–10C reflect the rise in Scott's gains in language, vocabulary, and reading achievement.

The spontaneous writing samples collected from Scott annually illustrate this development most dramatically. Figures 10–11A and 10–11B illustrate writing samples from Scott at the beginning of his first year in the program and in the spring of his fourth year in the program, respectively.

Receptive English *Language* Scores for "Scott"

Clinical Evaluation of Language Fundamentals-4 (CELF-4)

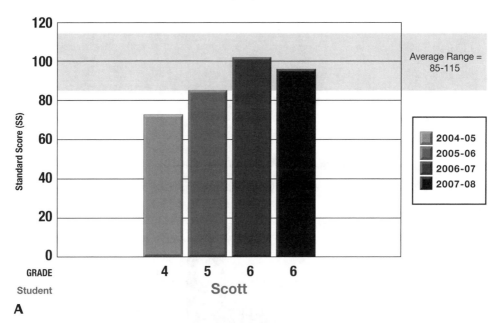

A

English Language-*Vocabulary* Scores for "Scott"

Peabody Picture Vocabulary Test - III, IV

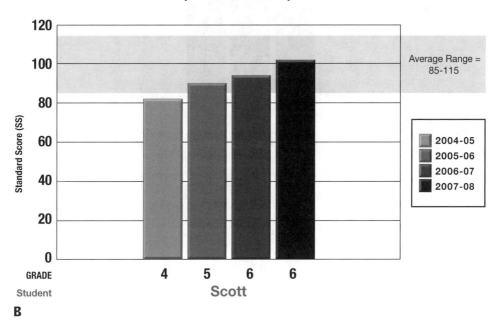

B

Figure 10–10. A. Scott's language gains. **B.** Scott's vocabulary gains. *continues*

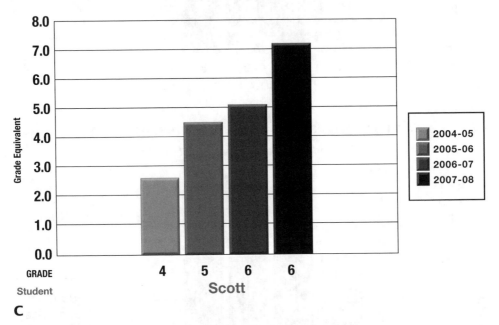

Reading Scores for "Scott"

Gates-MacGinitie Reading Test—3rd Ed.

C

Figure 10–10. *continued* **C.** Scott's reading achievement.

Writing Sample
Beginning of Year One (4th grade)—"Scott"
September 24, 2004

The wolf fell off big pail down, down, down he goes. He tumbling. "OW" He said! "He is dead" Tao said. He strating to die. "YES" Shang, Tao, and Paotze

A

Writing Sample
Spring of Year Four (6th grade)—"Scott"

A boy named Rudi climbed the mountains in Switzerland. He was climbing on the glaciers, when he saw a black dot on the mountain, it appeared to be a hut and he decided to stop there to sleep several times. Next day, while he was climbing he heard a voice, it appeared to him, and it was faint voice that was coming from the crack in the glacier. The man was stuck in the crack for three hours, asked Rudi to go to look for help but, Rudi refused to go. Then the man asked him if he had a rope but, Rudi didn't have one! Rudi took of his clothes to make a rope and tied to his staff, then dropped it down to the man. Rudi pulled the staff until the figure came out of the crack. The man helped Rudi to get dressed. Rudi relized he saved Caption John Winter.

B

Figure 10-11. A. Writing sample from Scott's first year in the program. **B.** Writing sample from Scott's fourth year in the program.

Discussion

The data presented in this chapter point to the need for professionals in the field of deaf education to rethink certain long-standing beliefs and paradigms regarding language access, language learning, literacy development, and bilingualism as they relate to learners who are deaf.

Beliefs Regarding Immersion in English as a Prerequisite to Literacy

The field of deaf education must first acknowledge and address the prevalent situation of ambiguous and absent access to natural English language acquisition inherent in the majority of current educational linguistic environments for deaf learners before it can enter into discussions of "best practices in reading" and address the issue of the acquisition of phonemic awareness skills in deaf children. It is premature to talk about reading development and strategies absent the creation of linguistic environments that allow deaf learners to acquire an internalized mastery of the English language before coming to the task of reading and writing.

If developing an internalized mastery and complete linguistic mapping of English is indeed a goal for deaf learners, then it appears that the majority of current educational environments for learners who are deaf continue to provide instructional linguistic environments that prevent the realization of such a goal. The PSE and MCE systems commonly in use in deaf education today provide incomplete, deficient, and ambiguous visual access to English in discourse due to the absence of English phonemic and other lin-guistic information. The popular bilingual approach of immersion in ASL-first, then exposure to English via ASL-translation and access-to-English-via-print-only meth-odologies (LaSasso & Lollis, 2003) do not allow for the prerequisites to the natural language learning of English to occur, including: (1) constant and consistent immersion in the target language of English through natural communication with fluent English language models, and (2) exposure to complete visual representations of English provided through natural discourse. Moreover, inherent in that currently prevalent bilingual model is delayed exposure to English, which, when it does occur, is through print only. Such a model is at odds with the goal of students having an internalized mastery of the English language *prior* to coming to the task of reading at an early elementary age.

Beliefs Regarding Visual Access to English

It is important to note that the ISD 917 program views the use of signs and cues as vehicles for exposure to specific languages. As this relates to the use of CAE, the program recognizes the need to emphasize and define "sufficient early exposure." The program maintains that phonological awareness of a traditionally spoken language can be established best when a deaf child is immersed in a language-rich environment that uses cueing to make the linguistic information of that language visually accessible. The program's use of cued English contrasts with other programs that may incorporate the use of cueing for English phonics, phonemic drills or spelling, as opposed to the use of cueing for broader access to English in conversational and other instructional contexts for a significant portion of the school day. Programs incorporating cueing on such a sporadic and isolated basis may indeed erroneously conclude that the use of cueing does not work to achieve English proficiency, even if such drills are used on a daily basis, due to failing to recognize the degree of sufficient early exposure and immersion necessary to acquire proficiency in another language.

Paradigm Shift: From Competition to Coexistence

The use of cueing with learners who are deaf cannot be discussed without acknowledging the emotional and personal reactions its use evokes among many members of the Deaf and professional communities. The system of Cued Speech initially looks odd and unnatural to the eye accustomed to sign communication, and can appear incongruent with the more prevalent, traditional educational linguistic environments for deaf children. Because the system of Cued Speech historically has seen limited use in isolated locations in the United States, its efficacy has long been confused with its popularity.

There are many highly literate, highly educated and successful deaf adults who acquired their English literacy skills without exposure to CAE, particularly those raised in homes with deaf parents who modeled ASL as L1. The existence of such individuals is often used as an argument against considering the use of cueing. The critical question the field must address is: How can we best provide immediate and complete visual access to the home language of the *majority* of deaf children who are born to hearing parents with no previous ASL experience? Language learning for children who are deaf should not be a

struggle. It appears to not be a struggle for deaf children of deaf parents, and it *need not* be a struggle for deaf children of hearing parents. A visual means is available for deaf learners to acquire English skills at an early age, following an age-appropriate developmental sequence, and through natural discourse, and it is incumbent on the field of deaf education to take notice without further delay. It should and need not be an issue of ASL and English competing for dominance in the education and lives of deaf individuals. Rather, the natural acquisition of *both* languages should be available to all deaf individuals.

Paradigm Shift: Bilingualism and Deafness

As is evidenced by the ISD 917 program, learners who are deaf are capable of developing the two very visually distinct languages and systems of ASL and CAE, just as hearing children are capable of developing two auditorily distinct spoken languages. Rather than believing deaf children are being deprived of ASL by immersion in CAE, the program believes these learners are being afforded opportunities to meet their language, academic, and vocational potential while simultaneously experiencing a linguistic learning environment to acquire proficiency in ASL and English.

Conclusion

Practitioners in deaf education have choices to make. The status of underachievement among the majority of learners who are deaf in the United States and worldwide continues to exist. As a result, the negative impact on academic and vocational opportunities and performance for many learners prevails. Against this backdrop, the field can choose to look at the growing body of research on the powerful tool of cued English and its success in providing English language proficiency, phonemic awareness, and literacy for learners who are deaf, or it can continue current practices to perpetuate the legacy of underachievement of the population of deaf learners.

There is a critical and immediate need to examine the linguistic environments in which deaf learners are expected to acquire English language proficiency and literacy. In addition, there is a need to include strategies that make natural language acquisition of English possible at an early age in a developmentally appropriate sequence similar to hearing children. It is critical that educators in the field of deaf education not lose sight of the prerequisites for natural language learning and seek to address the development of vocabulary, phonemic awareness, and other language skills in the context of immersion in English via means which provide unambiguous linguistic access to the language. It is hoped that the information provided in this chapter can serve as a catalyst for reflection and thoughtful discussions between and among service providers and administrators in the field of deaf education and the parents of deaf children to whom they are ultimately accountable. Such discussions should result in improved outcomes for all deaf learners.

References

Afflerbach, P., Beers, J., Blachowicz, C., Boyd, C., Cheyney, W., Diffily, D., . . . Wixson, K. K. (2000). *Scott Foresman Reading* series. Glenview, IL: Pearson Education.

Carrow-Woolfolk, E. (1999). *Test for Auditory Comprehension of Language* (3rd ed.). Austin, TX: Pro-Ed.

Doenges, K. (2003). *How cued English impacts learning to read and write English for deaf and hard of hearing students.* Unpublished manuscript, Intermediate School District 917. Rosemount, MN.

Doenges, K., & Kyllo, K. (2001). *Cued English: A bridge to literacy for deaf and hard of hearing children.* Presentation, Cue Camp Minnesota, 2001. Collegeville, MN: St. John's University.

Dunn, D., & Dunn, L. (2007). *Peabody Picture Vocabulary Test* (4th ed.). Circle Pines, MN: American Guidance Service Publishing.

Fleetwood, E., & Metzger, M. (1998a). *Cued language structure: An analysis of cued American English based on linguistic principles.* Silver Spring, MD: Calliope Press.

Fleetwood, E., & Metzger, M. (1998b). *What's the difference between Cued Speech, cued English, cued language, and cuem.* Silver Spring, MD: Calliope Press.

Green, J. (2000). *Language: A language intervention curriculum* (2nd ed.). Longmont, CA: Sopris West.

Intermediate District 917 Program for DHOH Learners. (1997) *Program for deaf and hard-of-hearing learners language-of-instruction program practices.* Unpublished manuscript. Rosemount, MN.

Kyllo, K. (2003). Phonemic awareness through cued American English. *Odyssey, 5,* 36–44.

Kyllo, K., & Doenges, K. (2001). *A different approach to the education of deaf and hard of hearing children: Bilingualism through ASL and cued English.* Unpublished manuscript. Rosemount, MN: Intermediate District 917.

LaSasso, C. (1999). Test-taking abilities: A missing component of the curriculum for deaf students. *American Annals of the Deaf, 144,* 35–43.

LaSasso, C., & Lollis, J. (2003). Survey of residential and day schools for the deaf in the United States that identify themselves as bilingual-bicultural programs.

Journal of Deaf Studies and Deaf Education, 8, 71–91.

Lindamood, P., & Lindamood, P. (1998). *The Lindamood phoneme sequencing program for reading, spelling, and speech: Classroom version* (3rd ed.). Austin, TX: Pro-Ed.

MacGinitie, W., & MacGinitie, R. (2003). *Gates-MacGinitie Reading Tests* (4th ed.). Itasca, IL: Riverside Publishing.

Mitchell, R., & Karchmer, M. (2004). Chasing the mythical ten percent: Parental hearing status of deaf and hard of hearing students in the United States. *Sign Language Studies, 4,* 138–163.

Semel, E., Wiig, E., & Secord, W. (2004). *Clinical Evaluation of Language Fundamentals* (4th ed). San Antonio, TX: Psychological Corporation, Harcourt Brace.

Stoesz, H. (2006). *Bilingualism: Transitioning deaf students to a second language.* Presentation, 2006 ASHA Convention, Miami, FL.

WETA-TV. (2007). A chance to read: Signs of literacy. *PBS Reading Rockets: Launching Young Readers, Episode 9.* WETA-TV, Washington, DC.

Wilkes, E. (2001). *Cottage Acquisition Scales for Listening, Language and Speech* (2nd ed.). San Antonio, TX: Sunshine Cottage School for Deaf Children.

Section IV

CUED LANGUAGE FOR THE DEVELOPMENT OF READING

Chapter 11

CUED SPEECH FOR THE DEAF STUDENTS' MASTERY OF THE ALPHABETIC PRINCIPLE

Jacqueline Leybaert, Stephanie Colin, and Carol J. LaSasso

Reading—an extraordinary ability, peculiarly human and yet distinctly unnatural . . . acquired in childhood, forms an intrinsic part of our existence as human beings, and is taken for granted by most of us.
(Shaywitz, 2003, p. 3)

Broad and Narrow Views of Reading

Reading can be defined narrowly or broadly. Narrow definitions consider reading as application of the alphabetic principle or a set of discrete skills to decode printed words. Broader definitions consider reading as: (1) a theoretical con-struct, largely unobservable directly, or theoretically as comprehension or (2) more tangibly as performance on reading comprehension tests. Entire volumes (cf. Kamil, Mosenthal, Pearson, & Barr, 2000); are devoted to describing and discussing various theoretical views of reading, which can be variously categorized as top-down, bottom-up, or interactive (Kelly, 1995). Numerous standardized reading tests, with varying links to theoretical views of reading, exist to measure reading comprehension. These are discussed at greater length in Chapter 12.

The standardized test used most with deaf[1] students in the United States since the early 1970s when the MCE sign systems

---

[1]In this chapter, the term *deaf* refers to individuals who are deaf or hard of hearing

and Cued Speech were created is the Stanford Achievement Test (SAT). The reading comprehension subtest of the SAT, normed on both deaf and hearing students, requires students to read short narrative and/or expository passages and answer multiple-choice questions about those passages. Scaled scores on the SAT can be compared across the various levels of the test and are typically reported as grade level equivalents. More recently, due largely to the No Child Left Behind (NCLB) Act of 2001 accountability legislation, states have been developing their own standardized reading tests that are similar in format to the SAT reading comprehension test but often not normed on deaf students (Lollis & LaSasso, 2009).

Deaf students tend to plateau on standardized reading comprehension tests around the third- to fourth-grade reading level, which is comparable to that of 8 to 9-year-old hearing students. Traxler (2000), for example, found that half of 17-year-old deaf and hard of hearing students were reading at a fourth grade reading level. Fewer than 1% of hearing peers taking the same test scored at that level (Marschark, 2006).

In this chapter we focus on a *narrow* view of reading, as decoding, from a cognitive psychology perspective. Specifically, we focus on the learning and application of the alphabetic principle, which involves both phonological awareness and awareness of the relationship between phonemes and graphemes in alphabetic languages. Most of the empirical research related to reading achievement of deaf students has focused on reading as decoding. Chapter 12 focuses on reading more broadly as *comprehension* or *measured comprehension* and discusses reading and deaf students in an educational context.

The Paradox in Learning to Read

Learning to read is paradoxical. First, for most children, reading is considered a *visual* activity; however, children who are blind do not have particular difficulties in learning to read Braille characters through the tactile modality, whereas children who have intact visual abilities but who have been deaf from birth typically experience great difficulty in learning to read. The second paradox is that while reading seems to be an effortless and automatic activity for adult skilled readers, learning to read can be a challenging task, one which often takes many years. Unfortunately, some children never achieve fluency and reading comprehension comparable to that of skilled readers. This is often the case for hearing children who are dyslexic and for many (nondyslexic) deaf children. This situation is worrisome given the fact that literacy is essential to achieving success in societies like ours, where vast amounts of information are conveyed by written words. In order to promote the full integration of deaf children into the academic, industrial, and/or commercial jobs they seek, it is important to understand the source of their reading difficulties and how to overcome them. To achieve this goal, parents, practitioners, and other stakeholders need to understand the preconditions for learning to read, the task of learning to read an alphabetic script, and the multimodal nature of many of the specific processes related to reading.

We begin by discussing the alphabetic principle and related theoretical perspectives of: Frith (1985), Jorm and Share (1983), and Perfetti (1992, 1997). Next, we counter the claim that there is little research related to the effectiveness of Cued Speech for the development of abilities related to fluent reading by describing findings of studies with deaf children from cued language backgrounds related to phonemic awareness, phonics, phonological recoding, and spelling. Finally, we link these research findings back to the views of Frith, Jorm and Share, and Perfetti related to the alphabetic principle, and discuss the theoretical support and empirical evidence of Cued Speech for the development of reading in deaf students.

Reading as Grapheme-Phoneme Decoding

The Alphabetic Principle

Writing systems connect to the spoken language in a systematic way. The written form, including graphemes (letters), words, and punctuation, does not encode meanings directly. Elementary writing units can correspond to three types of units of spoken language: (1) phonemes, which are abstract "speech sound"[2] units that contrast minimal pairs in a language, (e.g., /b/ which contrasts *bat* from *pat*), (2) syllables, and (3) morphemes. Morphemes are the smallest linguistic units associating form with *meaning*.

Three types of mapping between spoken and written languages give rise to the different writing systems that are found in the world's languages, some-

times in inter-mixed form: *alphabetic, syllabary,* and *morphosyllabic* (Gelb, 1952). English, Italian, Spanish, Swedish, and French orthographies are examples of *alphabetic* writing systems in which the written units (letters or letter groups) are mapped with phonemes as abstract language units.[3] The letter *c* in the written English word *car* corresponds to the phoneme /k/ in the spoken English word /kar/ or the phoneme /s/ in *cent*; the letter *f* and the letter group *ph* both correspond to the phoneme /f/ such as in *female* or *elephant*.

The beginning reader must learn how a given writing system relates to spoken units in his or her language. Compared to syllabary (e.g., Mycenaean Greek and Cherokee) writing systems and morphosyllabic (e.g., Kanji, Chinese) writing systems, alphabetic writing systems offer both advantages and difficulties. An alphabetic system gains economy by mapping written units (i.e., the letters or letter groups) onto a small set of elements (i.e., the phonemes) rather than to a much larger set of morphemes comprising the language. The association between letters and phonemes is called the *alphabetic principle,* and it allows the alphabet to be *generative.* That is, with a small set of symbols, (i.e., the letters), an unlimited number of morphemes can be generated. For example, no more than four different letters are required to generate the 15 different words *to, so, tot, tots, pop, pops, pot, pots, stop, spot, spots, tops, post, posts,* and *stops.* This difference in economy makes learning

---

[2]As reflected in Chapters 2 through 4 in this volume, the example of Cued Speech illustrates that phonemes exist in the absence of either speech or sound.

[3]In the context of the present chapter, we limit our discussion to the *alphabetic* orthographies because there are no comparative studies investigating the difficulties encountered by deaf children learning to read syllabic or morphosyllabic writing systems.

to read much easier in an alphabetic writing than in a morphosyllabic writing system such as Kanji or Chinese. Although learning to phonically decode an alphabetic writing system typically requires, on average, 2 to 3 years for a hearing child from a western culture, depending on how consistent, or transparent, the relationship is between graphemes and phonemes, learning to read takes much more time and effort in Chinese. It takes, on average, six years for Chinese children to learn 3,500 characters, and several years more to achieve the 5,000 to 7,000 characters vocabulary that is typical of literate Chinese adults (Rayner, Foorman, Perfetti, Pesetsky, & Seidenberg, 2001).

There are two major limitations of alphabetic writing systems. First, the language units represented by the letters are *phonemes*, which are abstract units of traditionally spoken language. Indeed, phonemes like /b/ or /d/ do not correspond to an invariant acoustic signal (Liberman, Cooper, Shankweiler, & Studdert-Kennedy, 1967). For example, the /b/ in ball is different acoustically from the b in *cab*, because of the *coarticulation* phenomenon, meaning that the acoustic realization of a consonant is highly dependent on the vowels that precede and follow it. Subsequent to the pioneering work done by Liberman, Shankweiler, Fischer, and Carter (1974), numerous studies have demonstrated that phonemes are much more difficult to manipulate than syllables for young children (see Castles & Coltheart, 2004, for a review). The development of phonological awareness, which is especially important for learning to read in alphabetic writing systems (National Reading Panel, 2000), is examined in greater detail below.

A second difficulty inherent to alphabetic writing systems is that there are more phonemes (i.e., 40 or so in English) than graphemes (i.e., 26 in the English alphabet). This is particularly true for vowels, but also, to a lesser extent, for consonants. In American English for example, there are more than a dozen vowel sounds for only five standard vowel graphemes (*a, e, i, o,* and *u*), meaning that each vowel letter is associated with more than one vowel sound. For example, the vowel grapheme *a* is used to represent different phonemes in words like *car, cat, cake,* and *above*. Conversely, the same vowel can be represented by different graphemes. For example, the phoneme /i/ could be represented by *-e-* or *-ea-* as in *repeat*, by *-ee-* as in *feel*, by *-ie-* as in *field*, or by *-ei-* as in *ceiling*. Similarly, the phonological rime /ɛr/ could be represented by *-air* as in *hair*, or *-ear* as in *bear*, or *-err* as in *error*. These examples are illustrative of the fact that in English, there is an inconsistent phoneme-grapheme relationship. Some of these inconsistencies can be reduced by considering the graphemic context. For example, the pronunciation of the grapheme *a* is consistent in the rime *-ake*. To sum up, the strengths of writing systems based on the alphabetic principle relate to their economy of effort and generative nature. The limitations of alphabetic writing systems relate to their degree of abstractness and lack of phoneme-grapheme consistency.

Learning to Read an Alphabetic Orthography: Hearing Children

In order to utilize an alphabetic writing system, children must learn which graphemes or grapheme groups (e.g., bigraphs, trigraphs) correspond to abstract phonemes or phoneme groups. To the extent that young readers cannot match abstract phonemes with specific graphemes or grapheme groups, they will not be able to take advantage of the economic-generative alphabetic principle and will be forced to process written words by: (1) memorizing arbitrary associations of written words with traditionally spoken words, as in the Chinese writing system, which can be quite costly in terms of memory load, or (2) by using contextual analysis, which requires knowledge of the syntactic structure of a language as well as background knowledge related to the content in the text.

Several stage and nonstage theories about the development of the reading process in hearing children are helpful in understanding the difficulties encountered by deaf children in learning to read as well as the benefit of Cued Speech for ameliorating those difficulties. These include: (1) Frith's (1985) stage theory; (2) Jorm and Share's (1983) theory related to the role of phonological recoding for self-teaching; and (3) Perfetti's (1992, 1997) theory about the development of specificity and redundancy.

Before discussing these theories, it is important to note that written graphemes or words do not encode meanings *directly*. In alphabetic writing (e.g., English orthography) as in morphosyllabic writing systems (e.g., Kanji, or Chinese orthographies), written words correspond to other linguistic units (e.g., traditionally spoken words in traditionally spoken languages). For deaf children, written words can relate to *signs* from sign languages such as American Sign Language (ASL), *fingerspelled words*, or *cued words* in cued languages (e.g., Cued American English or Cued French). Spoken words, ASL signs, fingerspelled words, or cued words are related to the meaning, but in only an arbitrary manner, except in onomatopoeia (e.g., *buzz, meow, clank*).

Frith's (1985) Stage Theory of Reading Development

Frith's three-stage model of the developmental reading process describes the evolution of the relationship between the *written* word and the *spoken* word as the developing hearing reader progresses from the logographic stage, through the alphabetic stage, to the orthographic stage. In this context, we will discuss the evolution of the relationship between the *written word* and *signed, fingerspelled*, or *cued words* for children who are deaf.

Logographic Stage. The first stage in Frith's model is *logographic*. In this stage, hearing prereaders do not yet understand that printed words represent spoken words at the phonemic and morphemic levels. Prereaders associate the printed word with the spoken word in an arbitrary way. Their visual system tries to recognize the printed words in the same manner as it recognizes faces and objects: by identifying salient visual characteristics like word length, ascending or descending letters, visual form, or color. In this stage, children recognize their first name, the names of their classmates, and brand names such as Coca-Cola or McDonalds. The size of the "logographic lexicon" seems to vary by language (Wimmer & Hummer, 1990). That is, in very transparent languages (e.g., Italian, German), with fairly consistent phoneme-grapheme relationships, the logographic lexicon could be nonexistent, while in more opaque languages, characterized by inconsistent phoneme-grapheme relationships (e.g., English), the logographic lexicon could be more developed. The logographic lexicon represents, after all, prereading, or "pseudoreading," which does not require any formal reading (i.e., decoding) instruction. Logographic reading has more to do with guessing or visual matching (LaSasso, 1985) than with real reading (i.e., decoding), as exemplified by the following observations: Prereaders will not recognize the word Coca-Cola if not presented in the familiar font; they will not generalize to new, visually similar words, like Coco, Laco, or Lola, even if the first two are made by permutations of the syllables of the initial target. Furthermore, they will "read" (i.e., give the same pronunciation) semantically related words like *Mom* and *Mummy*.

Alphabetic Stage. The second stage in Frith's model is the *alphabetic* stage. In order to overcome the disadvantages of the logographic stage, children must imperatively develop the alphabetic route of word reading, which associates each letter chain to its pronunciation by systematic conversions from graphemes to phonemes. This procedure typically appears during the first months of formal schooling of hearing children, who then typically cease to process words as whole entities. Rather, hearing children learn to pay attention to and process small visual constituents: syllables, letters, grapheme groups, such as *ph* that correspond to a single phoneme such as /f/. This is realized by visual processing. In addition, hearing children learn to associate each grapheme or grapheme group (e.g., bigraph or trigraph) with the phonemes of the language, and to assemble these phonemes in order to produce words. They will first make errors when reading words containing complex graphemes, like *-ough* in rough; by recovering the correct word pronunciation, they will learn how to pronounce the complex graphemes. They will also make

errors when reading irregular words, like *pint* in English which, according to phonics rules, should have a short vowel sound (as in *pin*) but rather has a long vowel sound (as in *mind*).

The advantage of the alphabetic strategy over the logographic strategy is most obvious when words are visually similar. Conrad (1979) reported that among the first "key words" typically included in initial instructional reading materials, 70% have either three or four letters, looking similar. In addition, 20% of these begin with either *b*, *d*, or *p*, known to present problems of visual discrimination for young children (Dehaene, 2007; Orton, 1937). Although these key words would present difficulties if read logographically, they would not if read with the alphabetic strategy.

Proper application of the alphabetic principle requires awareness of the internal morphophonological structure of words that the alphabet represents. What the child assembles during reading is not the letter *names*, but the phonemes which are abstract units corresponding to letters or letter groups. Children must realize that the speech stream may be parsed into phonemes, for example that the word /ski/ may be decomposed into /s/, /k/, and /i/. The emergence of "phonological awareness" corresponds to a *mental revolution* in which children discover the "molecules of language" (Dehaene, 2007, p. 267) that can be combined to form new words. For example, words such as *pots, tops,* and *stop* consist of the same language molecules (i.e., phonemes) assembled in different orders, and words like *cut* and *but* only differ by one molecule (i.e., one phoneme). Unfortunately, this important discovery is not an automatic consequence of speaking a language.

José Morais and his colleagues have revealed that this mental revolution is favored by the analytic (i.e., phonics) mode of reading instruction, as opposed to the whole-word method of instruction, where children are led to memorize printed forms of spoken words (see Alegria & Morais, 1979; Leybaert & Content, 1995; Morais, Bertelson, Cary, & Alegria, 1986; Morais, Cary, Alegria, & Bertelson, 1979). Children exposed to an analytic method of reading instruction learn to analyze words into phonemes. In contrast, prereading children exposed solely to a whole-word method, and most adults incapable of reading are not able to analyze spoken words into phonemes. Chinese readers who have only learned the traditional Chinese writing do not succeed in tasks involving phoneme manipulation, whereas the readers who have learned to read the alphabetic pinyin writing do succeed in these tasks (Read, Zhang, Nie, & Ding, 1986).

In sum, the alphabetic stage involves a change from the logographic stage in terms of the visual and phonological processing requirements. Visually, the reader must now learn to parse the word into graphemes or grapheme clusters, including digraphs (e.g., *ph* in phone) or trigraphs (e.g., *sch* in schilling); phonologically, the reader has to link these graphemes to the areas of the brain involved in speech processing, which now must represent *phonemes*.

The Orthographic Stage: The Competent Reader. The orthographic stage is characterized by the reader having a vast repertoire of visual units of various sizes (e.g., syllables, bigrams, rimes, morphemes). Upon reaching this stage, the child's brain has registered thousands of statistics about frequency of usage of each word, letter, bigram, syllable, or morpheme. The time taken to read a word is no longer determined solely by the number of its letters

or the complexity of its graphemes. Rather, the time needed to read a word increasingly depends on the nature of the word and more precisely on the frequency of the word in the language: rare words are read more slowly, and spelled with less accuracy. Irregular words like *pint* are no longer regularized, and are read fluently or automatically with the correct pronunciation. These effects reflect the emergence of a second route to reading: the lexical (or orthographic) route, which progressively supplants the grapheme-to-phoneme decoding route.

The salient characteristics of the orthographic stage for word reading (as well as for word spelling) are the presence of frequency effect and the reduction of both length effect and regularity effect (i.e., the difference between performance for regular and irregular words, or short and long words, which are all read using the orthographic procedure). The orthographic stage is characterized by an increasing parallelism of the grapheme-to-phonemes route with the orthographic route: the visual system provides an increasingly compact code for words, which represents, at once, the totality of the letters.

Other Nonstage Theories of Reading Development

The universality of the "logographic stage" has been challenged (Wimmer & Hummer, 1990). In orthographies with more transparent correspondences between phonemes and graphemes (e.g., French or Spanish), hearing children seem to use these correspondences from the very beginning. Furthermore, the idea that children learn to read by progressing through a series of stages defined by different decoding strategies also has been challenged. Other theories emphasize that children use *multiple* strategies simultaneously, and that qualitative shifts in strategy occur depending on the complexity of the information, the frequency of occurrence of words, and so forth. For frequent and regular words, children may progress very rapidly from an early logographic processing strategy, in which printed words are directly associated with pronunciation, to an alphabetic processing strategy, in which they are increasingly sensitive to the internal structure of words and the correspondences between subword components and pronunciation.

Jorm and Share (1983) developed the idea that *phonological recoding* (i.e., internal grapheme to phoneme translation) and the opportunities to associate print with sound that this recoding provides is essential in the building of orthographic representations. According to their hypothesis: "phonological recoding acts as a *self-teaching* device, or built-in teacher, enabling a child to independently develop the word-specific orthographic representations essential to skilled reading and spelling" (Share, 1999, p. 96). The self-teaching hypothesis is consistent with findings from numerous studies that have shown that efficient phonological processing is a necessary (but not sufficient) condition for orthographic learning: virtually no child with deficient phonological processing skills develops reading ability (Juel, Griffith, & Gough, 1986). The self-teaching hypothesis has important implications for deaf children's learning to read.

Perfetti's (1992) theory provides interesting insights about the development of orthographic representations. In Perfetti's view, learning to read: (1) involves the acquisition of increasing numbers of word representations that can be accessed by their spellings (i.e., quantity change);

and (2) is accompanied by a change in the *specificity* and *redundancy* (i.e., quality change) of individual words' representations. Increasing *specificity* means that as a child progresses in learning to read, his or her representations of words increasingly has specific letters in their correct positions. These representations become *phonologically redundant* because the addition of specific grapheme-phoneme correspondences is redundant with the word-level pronunciation of the word. When both letter-level and word-level processes concur to produce a word's pronunciation, reading (i.e., decoding) is facilitated. Increasing specificity and redundancy allow high-quality word representations that can be reliably activated by the orthographic input. Perfetti's hypotheses have important implications for deaf children's development of written word representations.

Learning to Read an Alphabetic Orthography: Deaf Children

Frith's developmental theory, as well as those of Jorm and Share (1983) and Perfetti (1992) are useful for understanding the difficulties encountered by deaf children in using alphabetic and orthographic modes of processing and how exposure to cued language can ameliorate these difficulties.

Logographic Stage: Available to All Deaf Children

Whether their first language (L1) is spoken, signed, or cued, deaf children pass through a *logographic* stage of printed word processing in the same way as hearing children: by associating, in an arbitrary way, the written word with a representation in their L1. No advantage (or sensory impairment disadvantage) would be expected of one language background over the other at the logographic stage of processing. All things being equal, the visual system of deaf children is able to process characteristics such as word length, word visual form, and color. Similar errors to those observed in hearing children would be expected in deaf children.

Alphabetic Stage: The Importance of Language Background

Is it necessary, advantageous, or even possible for children born deaf to go from the logographic to the *alphabetic* stage? The different linguistic backgrounds clearly do not offer the same possibilities regarding the *mental revolution* of phonological and phonemic awareness. In this section, we first discuss the case of deaf children whose L1 is a signed language which includes fingerspelling, and then discuss the case of deaf children whose L1 is cued.

Signed Languages and the Alphabetic Principle. Consider the example of a deaf child whose lexicon is limited to only sign representations from signed languages such as ASL, without any other linguistic representation, based on spoken articulation, or fingerspelling.[4] This hypothetical child would not be able to make correspondences between the graphemes in alphabetic English[5] and corresponding units of their primary signed language. Indeed, the phonological units of signs,

including: hand configuration, hand placement, hand movement, and hand location (Stokoe, 1971) do not have any systematic correspondence with graphemes. The link between a written word and a sign could only be arbitrary, as in the logographic stage. Important consequences for children who cannot make associations between the phonemes and graphemes of a language include the following: (1) they cannot be "autonomous readers" (in Jorm & Share's 1983 terminology) meaning that they cannot independently access the meaning of "new" written words that they have not encountered in print before; (2) they will not develop "redundancy" in Perfetti's terms; (3) they will be at risk of not developing orthographic representations of high quality. Such children must either *guess* the meaning of novel print words, via contextual analysis, for example; use a dictionary; or ask the help of a more skilled reader. The way that reading is taught in some classes in which a signed language is the instructional language well illustrates this possibility: the teacher first translates the written text into the signed language, which is understood by the children; and then, the children try to *read* the written text by associating the written words with the corresponding signs. It should be noted that although the signing children in this scenario may be experiencing pleasure in learning to read when they are provided a signed translation, they are *not* presenting as autonomous readers.

Fingerspelling and the Alphabetic Principle. Most (if not all) children who are native signers have representations of

---

[4]It should be noted that ASL linguists consider fingerspelling to be part of ASL.
[5]We do not discuss here the attempts to invent writing systems for sign languages.

articulated words and fingerspelled words in their lexicon in addition to signed representations.[6] Fingerspelling is a means of manually representing graphemes of a spoken language (Wilcox, 1992). The words represented are necessarily derived from a spoken/written language. Fingerspelling is used when (1) no sign is readily known to the people conversing; (2) the sign is too generic, or nonspecific (e.g., bird for crow); or (3) the sign available has multiple meanings. For example, the same ASL sign might be used for *expert, expertise, skill, skills, skilled,* or *skillful.* Fingerspelling may be used formally as a medium of instruction for deaf people learning to read. Indeed, each manual configuration corresponds to a letter of the printed word. From a fingerspelling experience, deaf children may get a hint about the "molecular nature" of written language, because fingerspelling *is* a representation of the alphabet. In fingerspelling, as in written language, the words *apt, pat,* and *tap* consist of the same written molecules assembled in different sequences, and the words *cut* and *but* only differ by one molecule. The close link between *fingerspelling* and *alphabetic writing,* if not discovered spontaneously, can easily be taught to young deaf children.

Fingerspelling may thus constitute a visual tool from which the awareness that words in print are comprised of small, discrete constituents (or molecules). Of course, fingerspelling may also possibly interact with representations of spoken language articulation (e.g., lipreading and mouthing) in the development of awareness about "sound" segments in deaf signers. In that sense, exposure to an MCE sign system or a signed language (including

fingerspelling) is by no means incompatible with the idea that deaf children may go through the alphabetic stage, if one is ready to accept that a certain amount of the phonology of English and other traditionally spoken languages could be derived from visual information such as lipshapes or fingerspelling.

Padden and colleagues (Padden & Hanson, 1999; Padden & Ramsey, 2000) argue that specific aspects of signed language, such as fingerspelling and initialized signs, *can* be used in learning to read printed words. In fingerspelling, signers execute, in rapid sequence, handshapes that correspond to each letter in the word. Initialized signs involve replacing the handshape of an ASL sign with the handshape corresponding to a letter (typically the first letter) of the English translation of the sign. An example of an initialized sign in ASL is *"development,"* which is made with a fingerspelled *d* handshape instead of the traditional ASL sign made with four fingers, moving in an upward movement along the other hand. Initialized signs and fingerspelling are used together in the classroom when teachers are emphasizing a word's spelling or attempting to represent a specific English word. For example, one teacher wanting to sign *volcano* might substitute an initialized MCE sign for the traditional ASL sign *mountain.* That is, instead of using an ASL compound sign incorporating the sign for ROCK and a classifier for the slope of a mountainside, the teacher might use a *V* handshape for the sides of a mountain, and then immediately fingerspell the word V-O-L-C-A-N-O. Padden and Ramsey found that young children with a hearing impairment, who were better able to write down

---

[6]Users of MCE sign systems would be expected to have even more representations of articulated or fingerspelled words in their lexicon.

words that were fingerspelled to them and who were able to translate initialized signs, also did better on reading tests. These skills were more likely to be found among children with hearing impairment who had grown up with ASL, such as those whose parents were deaf ASL users; however, they were also used by deaf children with hearing parents who performed well on tests of ASL ability. Padden and Ramsey interpreted their results as indicating that signing readers who are deaf may take advantage of the explicit links between ASL and written English, such as fingerspelled or initialized signs.

We do not refute the value inherent in various aspects of language exposure or instruction based on signed languages, such as ASL. Deaf children of ASL signing parents, compared to nonsigning deaf children who have difficulty communicating with their parents, are relatively advantaged in acquiring general world knowledge or "fund of information" knowledge[7] prior to reading instruction which will be very helpful in formal reading instruction. Furthermore, as previously discussed, a signed educational background does not necessarily preclude the mastering of the alphabetic principle by deaf children. Obviously, the use of signing activities to supplement phonics instruction may make reading more enjoyable and meaningful for deaf children. Such activities may be most beneficial to children from backgrounds where Cued Speech is used very little, or not at all.

Cued Language and the Alphabetic Principle. Children exposed to a cued language (e.g., Cued American English or Langage Parlé Complété) via Cued Speech are in a radically different situation from children exposed to an MCE sign system or a signed language such as ASL. During the period from 0 to 5 years, children exposed to Cued Speech have stored cued representations in which the phonological contrasts are clearly marked, both at the syllabic level and at the phonemic level. For example, the cued representation of the word *but* is different from the cued representation of the word *cut* and from the cued representation of the word *bat* (see Chapter 2 in this volume). The fact that the cued representations of words are clearly distinct does not mean that speech needs to be involved. As Metzger and Fleetwood argue in Chapter 3, distinct word representations in cued languages can be acquired on a purely *visual* basis. That is, when cueing, deaf children are taught to pay attention to isolated graphemes, complex graphemes, or syllables. They can associate each of these elements to the phonemes (or phoneme clusters, or syllables) and assemble these language units to form words. For example, children who know that the word *bit* consists of handshape 4 at the throat placement, followed by handshape 5 at the side placement (with the attendant mouthshapes) have the possibility of learning the correspondence between the letter group *bi* and its handshape/placement configuration or, conversely, the correspondence between the phoneme /t/ and its handshape/placement configuration. The advantages are threefold: (1) once children have learned the correspondences between graphemes and the manual cues from Cued Speech, they can be "autonomous readers" (Jorm & Share, 1983) in the sense that they can get the meaning of

---

[7]The importance of fund of information knowledge, or background knowledge, will be discussed in greater detail in Chapter 12 where reading is discussed in a broader context.

words they never encountered in print before (for evidence, see Alegria, Aurouer, & Hage, 1997 described below); (2) children exposed to Cued Speech will be able to use grapheme-to-phoneme correspondences for reading printed words and the phoneme-to-grapheme correspondences for word spelling (for evidence, see Leybaert, 2000; Leybaert & Charlier, 1996; Leybaert & Lechat, 2001); and (3) the use of correspondences between graphemes and corresponding visual "phonemes" (i.e., manual cues and mouthshapes) makes possible the development of phonological awareness (see Charlier & Leybaert, 2000).

Orthographic Stage

In the discussion of Frith's orthographic stage in the development of reading, we now turn to the organization of the brain in *deaf* skilled readers (i.e., readers for whom word recognition is an effortless, efficient, and rapid skill). There are multiple pathways for deriving meaning from print in the case of deafness. The brain of a deaf child can register thousands of statistics about frequency of usage of each letter, bigraph or trigraph, syllable, morpheme, or word in a particular alphabetic writing system. These hints to English graphotactics can be uncovered from the print data alone, without any access to the spoken language. Some of these English graphotactics are rooted in English phonology, morphology, and syntax (e.g., plural marking, rules for subject-verb agreement), but they are also *visual* cues. Whether or not their mastery is correlated with phonemic awareness in deaf readers is still an open question. The fact that deaf children exposed to Cued Speech can develop efficient storage of orthographic representations of words has been repeatedly demonstrated by studies of the spell-

ing abilities of deaf children (for evidence, see Leybaert, 2000; Leybaert & Lechat, 2001; described below).

Research Supporting Cued Speech and Cued Language for the Development of Deaf Readers' Phonological Abilities Related to Reading

The National Reading Panel (2000) identified phonemic awareness and phonics as two of the five critical abilities linked to reading achievement. These two abilities, as well as phonological recoding (often referred to as "internal speech"), typically are problematic for deaf readers from oral and signing backgrounds (see Leybaert, 1993; Paul, 1984). In this section, research related to phonemic awareness, phonological recoding, and phonics of deaf children from cueing backgrounds is discussed. We include a discussion of research related to spelling of deaf students because spelling, like phonics, includes phoneme-grapheme relationships.

Research Supporting Cued Speech for the Development of Phonemic Awareness in Deaf Students

As previously noted, a central problem in learning to read English or French is that although discovering and applying the alphabetic principle is a key to success, this is not an easy achievement for beginning readers. One key difficulty in acquiring the alphabetic principle relates to the fact that phonemes are abstract categories, the representations of which have not been fully developed through the use of speech by the time the reading instruction begins.

The terms *phonological awareness* and *phonemic awareness* refer to children's knowledge of the internal sound structure of spoken words. The concept of *rhyme awareness* refers to the ability to be aware of and manipulate sublexical units (i.e., the onset and the rhyme) in the speech stream. For example, the spoken English word *bear* consists of two parts: the onset /b/ and the rhyme, or rime /ɛr/. There is a large amount of literature examining how children's level of phonological awareness and rhyme awareness relates to their success learning to read. Children who perform well on such tasks do markedly better in early reading than those who do not. Conversely, children who score poorly on phonological awareness tests prior to entering school are much more at risk for not learning to read than children who score well (Bradley & Bryant, 1978; 1983; Bryant, MacLean, & Bradley, 1990; Bryant, MacLean, Bradley, & Crossland, 1990; Lundberg, Olofsson, & Wall, 1980; Maclean, Bryant, & Bradley, 1987). Bryant et al. (1990) found a *causal* link between early rhyming abilities and later reading. Bowey and Francis (1991) speculate that children's experiences with rhyme allow them to form categories of words that share common sounds; and that later, they are able to make connections between these categories and words that might share common spelling patterns. For example, knowing that *rough*, *tough*, and *enough* rhyme might help children understand that these words share a common spelling sequence as well as a common rhyme (LaSasso & Metzger, 1998). Goswami (1993) provides evidence that English-speaking children do link rhyming categories with spelling categories as soon as they begin to learn to read and spell.

Given the importance of rhyming abilities as an indicator of adequate phonological representations and development of phonological sensitivity, one might be preoccupied by findings showing that deaf children *not* exposed to Cued Speech experience difficulty in making rhyming judgments about written words or pictures (Campbell & Wright, 1988; Dodd & Hermelin, 1977; Hanson & Fowler, 1987; Hanson & McGarr, 1987). For example, Campbell and Wright (1988) showed that orally educated children performed quite well when deciding whether two pictures rhyme when the names were spelled similarly (like *dream* and *team*); however, they were at chance level (50% of correct responses) when the names of the pictures were spelled differently (like *hair-bear*). Convergent findings for deaf college students who were good readers and users of sign language were reported by Hanson and Fowler (1987), Hanson and McGarr (1987) as well as by Sterne (1996) and Sterne and Goswami (2000). Leybaert (1993) conjectures that phonological representations in deaf students from oral or signing backgrounds may be insufficiently robust to support rhyme judgment; thus, these students must rely on orthographic or speechread information (p. 302).

Cornett designed Cued Speech in order to "insure that the deaf child comes to think in the phonemic equivalent of spoken English; that is, in words comprehended in their phonemic content" (Cornett, 1967; p. 9). Several studies (Charlier & Leybaert, 2000; D'Hondt & Leybaert, 2003; LaSasso, Crain, & Leybaert, 2003) have examined rhyming abilities of deaf subjects from cueing backgrounds, both in French and in English, with the following reasoning: if early experience with Cued Speech has a strong impact on the development of accurate phonological representations (as supposed by Cornett, 1967), one might expect that this experience gives the child the opportunity to notice the phonological similarities between words. Deaf children exposed to cueing would thus be able to develop rhyming skills before learning to read, as do normally-hearing children. Their rhyming judgments would not be affected by the word's spelling. In contrast, children educated orally or with signs would develop rhyming ability *after* reading instruction. These children would be good at judging that two words spelled similarly do rhyme (like *dream* and *team*), but they would perform poorly when the words do rhyme but are spelled differently (like *hair-bear*).

Charlier and Leybaert (2000) speculated that rhyming and lipread similarity have always been confounded in the *previous* research. Words that do rhyme also have similar images on the lips; words that do not rhyme have different lipread images. But words that do have similar lipread images do not necessarily rhyme. Charlier and Leybaert (2000) used pictures as stimuli to elicit rhyming judgments about pairs of pictures from deaf children from oral, signing, and cueing backgrounds. The word pairs were presented in one of four conditions: the rhyming pairs were either: (1) orthographically similar (*chaise/fraise*) or (2) dissimilar (*tasse/glace*); and nonrhyming pairs had either (3) similar speechread representations (*lit/nez*) or (4) dissimilar speechread representations (*lit/roi*). It was supposed that (1) if early exposure to cueing leads to the development of accurate phonological representations on the basis of the lips *and* manual cues, early Cued Speech users would not be mislead by lipread similarity, and would not be influenced by spelling similarity; (2) children from signing and oral backgrounds would be

mislead by speechread similarity (i.e., they would have a tendency to judge that words with the same lipread images do rhyme), and by spelling similarity (i.e., they would have a tendency to judge that words with different spellings, like *lit* and *riz* do not rhyme).

Results of the Leybaert and Charlier (2000) study support these expectations. Specifically, early Cued Speech users (mean age: 10;1 years) achieved a high level of accuracy in making rhyme judgment about pairs of pictures, and their performance was not influenced by spelling similarity between the names of the pictures. They were only slightly influenced by lipread/articulatory similarity: pairs like *lit/nez* were sometimes inadvertently judged as rhyming. These children seem thus to rely on phonological representations, giving perhaps more attention to the articulatory/lipread cues than hearing children of the same age. Children from signing and oral backgrounds, as well as children exposed at Cued Speech only at school achieved good performance when the names of the pictures rhymed and were spelled similarly (e.g., *bouche/mouche*) and when the pictures' names did not rhyme and were spelled differently (e.g., *poule/bain*), but they were more prone to errors when the pictures' names rhymed and were not spelled similarly (e.g., *lit-riz*) and the pictures' names did not rhyme and had similar lipread images. These children seemed thus to rely on spelling and lipread information to judge whether two words rhyme.

Rhyming judgment was also studied in 10- to 14-year-old emerging readers of English who had been exposed at an early age to Cued Speech (Crain, 2003). As reflected in Chapter 14, results of this study suggest that deaf emerging readers of English orthography who are from

Cued Speech backgrounds have developed rhyming abilities comparable to those of their hearing peers. These results are important, given the fact that Spencer and Marschark (2006, p. 16) urge caution when interpreting results of phonological awareness studies of French readers to English readers due to differences in the phonology-to-orthography consistency of the two languages. That is, French has a much more consistent phonology-to-orthography than English. For example, in French, there is a single pronunciation of the graphemes *eau* /o/ (as in *bateau, gateau*); however, in English, the grapheme *ou* has different pronunciations in *cough, out,* and *route*. It should be noted, however, that the degree of consistency of the phonology-to-orthography should not influence the development of rhyming sensitivity if children rely on phonological representations and *not* on orthographic representations.

The fact that both young readers of French and English who were exposed to Cued Speech have been found to develop genuine rhyming abilities is consistent with the hypothesis that the critical factor in this development is not, as Marschark and Spencer (2006) speculate, related to the *transparency or degree of consistency of the orthography*, but is rather related to the possibility of *having complete and consistent access to the phonemic contrasts of the primary language*. Charlier and Leybaert (2000) found that the rhyming scores, both average and individual, of children educated with Cued Speech at home were within the range of the scores of normally hearing children of the same chronological age. The high level of performance on rhyming judgment tasks exhibited by early Cued Speech users had not previously been reported in the literature about profoundly deaf children. This leaves open the possibility that rhyming ability can emerge spontaneously in the course of cued language development in deaf children, provided that Cued Speech is used early at home.

Research Supporting a Causal Relationship Between Phonological Awareness and Learning to Read in Deaf Children

The nature of the causal relationship between phonological awareness and learning to read has raised a polemic discussion in the literature related to hearing children, often referred to as a "chicken and egg" problem. The issue is whether it is *necessary* for children to first analyze the speech stream into phonemes in order to be able to learn the written code or, alternatively, whether they must first understand the existence of letters to realize that speech is made of discrete units, the phonemes (see for example Rayner et al., 2001).

A *causal* relationship between phonological awareness and learning to read is supported by numerous studies showing that hearing children who are more skilled in phonological awareness tasks requiring manipulation of phonemes learn to read faster than those who are less skilled in phonological awareness (see Adams, 1990; Wagner & Torgesen, 1987, for reviews). Furthermore, exercises which train children to manipulate, or play with, phonemes improve not only phonemic awareness but also reading scores (Ehri et al., 2001). Therefore, a number of theorists have argued that the discovery of phonemes precedes the discovery of graphemes (Goswami & Bryant, 1990; Gough & Hillinger, 1980; Hulmes, Caravolas, Malkova, & Brigstocke, 2005; Mattingly, 1972).

The causal relationship between learning to read and discovery of phonemes is also supported by findings from studies of illiterate adults from Portugal or Brazil (Morais, Cary, Alegria, & Bertelson, 1979) and literate readers of the Chinese writing (Read et al., 1986). Participants in these studies were not able to perform tasks requiring manipulation of phonemes, although previously illiterate Portuguese adults and Chinese readers who learned the pinyin writing system were able to do so. This suggests that instruction in an alphabetic orthography is a necessary condition for the emergence of phonological awareness (for more discussion, see Castles & Coltheart, 2004).

At present, the best model of phonological learning is likely to be a model of *reciprocal* interactions between knowledge of phonological structure and ability to read. That is, the learning of graphemes favors attention to phonemes, and analysis of phonemes favors the learning of graphemes and reading achievement. This reciprocal interaction sets the stage for the emergence of the graphemic code and the phonemic representation of speech (Perfetti, Beck, Bell, & Hughes, 1987).

In the case of deaf children, this "chicken and egg" issue is highly critical. Indeed, some authors have raised the question of whether phonological awareness *precedes* or *follows* excellence in reading in profoundly deaf individuals. That is, do profoundly deaf individuals become excellent readers because they know something about the sound system of English? Or do they learn something about the sound system of English after having become excellent readers of English orthography? (Goldin-Meadow & Mayberry, 2001). Deaf readers may gain access to phonological units such as syllables and phonemes represented visually in Cued Speech as a result of how reading is taught to them. On the other hand, awareness of syllables and phonemes developed through experience with Cued Speech could precede, and indeed favor, the acquisition of word recognition in deaf children. The best way to address this question is via *longitudinal research*, examining whether early phonological skills measured in kindergarten do predict later word recognition and word spelling development.

Recently, Colin, Magnan, Ecalle, and Leybaert (2007) examined the relationship between early phonological awareness of deaf children from a Cued Speech background and hearing peers and subsequent phonics abilities in a two-year longitudinal study of children in kindergarten and first grade. These researchers were interested in determining whether it is critical for deaf children to have the phonological representations in their mental lexicon *before* learning to read in order for the rate of reading acquisition to be efficient.

Colin et al. (2007) assessed 21 hearing subjects and 21 deaf subjects twice: first in kindergarten, from April to June, and the second time in first grade, in June, after 10 months of reading instruction. In kindergarten, children completed a pictured rhyme decision task and a rhyme generation task. Twelve months later, in first grade, the same children were given three new experimental tests: a new rhyme decision task, a phonological common unit identification task, and a word recognition task. Data were analyzed by two methods: a classical comparison between the mean of the hearing children and the mean of the deaf children (Colin, Magnan, Ecalle, & Leybaert, 2007), and an analysis of deviance in which the individual performance of each deaf child was placed within (or outside) a confidence interval computed on the basis of the data of the hearing children (Colin, Leybaert, Ecalle, & Magnan, 2008).

Findings from the Colin et al. (2007) study suggest that while the mean score of the deaf children in kindergarten was significantly below that of the hearing children, both in rhyme detection and rhyme generation, only two of the 21 deaf children were outside the confidence interval based on the data of the hearing children. In first grade, the deaf children had on average lower performances than those of the hearing children on both the rhyme decision test and the phonological common unit identification task. However, in the phonological common unit identification task taken in the first grade, which required an explicit ability to manipulate and identify the phonological units of spoken language, the majority of children, who were educated orally or who had received Cued Speech only at school, were outside the confidence interval, whereas the performances of all children who were exposed to Cued Speech at home (but one) were within the confidence interval. Taken together, the results suggest that *early exposure* to Cued Speech at home facilitates *an implicit organization* of the lexicon according to phonological similarities. However, it is not before the first grade, when children are under pressure of learning to read, that this knowledge about phonological similarities between words can be manipulated *more explicitly* and can be used in learning phoneme-to-grapheme correspondences.

Deaf children in the Colin et al. (2007) study also reached, on average, lower scores than hearing children on the word recognition task in first grade, which is consistent with the literature (Harris & Beech; 1998; Kyle & Harris, 2006). The examination of individual scores reveals that all children educated orally or with Cued Speech only at school present a deviant score compared to the confidence interval of hearing children of the same age; their mean reading level was 8 months inferior to that of the hearing children (6;7 versus 7;5 years). Children who were exposed to Cued Speech at home, however, reached a lexical age similar to that of hearing children (7;3 years). When making an error in the choice of a written word, the children with Cued Speech at home chose a pseudo-homophone (e.g., *"bato"* instead of *bateau*; an English equivalent would be *"brane"* instead of *brain*), while those educated orally or with Cued Speech only at school tended to choose words *visually similar* to the target (e.g., *"baleau"* instead of *bateau*; *"braim"* instead of *brain*). In this first year of learning to read, deaf children from home cueing backgrounds, thus, seem to recognize words by grapheme-to-phoneme correspondences, and most of them have word recognition abilities comparable to hearing peers.

Colin et al. (2007) also examined the relations between rhyming performance (measured in kindergarten and first grade) and word recognition level in first grade. In hearing children, the results at the rhyme detection and rhyme generation tasks administered in kindergarten explained 31% of the variance of the word recognition score in first grade. The contribution of chronologic age, nonverbal IQ, and scores at the phonological tasks in first grade was not significant. In deaf children, a different pattern of relations emerged. Specifically, the word recognition score in first grade was predicted both by the scores on the phonological tasks in kindergarten (28% of the variance explained), and in addition, by the score at the common unit detection task in first grade (17% of supplementary variance explained). This finding suggests that the potential contribution of phonological scores to reading variability is already measurable and captured in kindergarten in hearing children; however, sensitivity to rhyme and other phonological units develops more slowly in deaf children than in hearing children. That is, for deaf children, the variability in phonological ability measured in kindergarten captures *only part* of the variability of later reading. When pressure is exerted for learning to read, children begin to refine, or sharpen, phonological representations by taking into account phonemic segments. When children are forced to make finer discriminations and to represent speech in terms of ordered, or sequential segments (Studdert Kennedy, 1986), interindividual differences between deaf children regarding phonological knowledge are accentuated, and these differences capture an additional source of variance of reading ability. This explanation is consistent with the notion that the changes induced by early exposure to Cued Speech do not massively affect children's behavior before the first grade (i.e., before pressure is typically exerted to use phonological skills to decipher an alphabetic orthography).

According to the above hypothesis, age of exposure to Cued Speech would not predict the level of development of phonological skills in kindergarten, because these skills are still at an *implicit* level; however, this variable should predict phonological knowledge and word recognition level subsequently, in first grade. This is exactly what was found in multiple regressions in which chronologic age, nonverbal IQ, hearing loss, and speech intelligibility were entered first, and then the predictive power of age of exposure to cueing was tested as a second predictor. Age of exposure to cueing did not contribute significantly to the phonological scores

measured in kindergarten, but *did* contribute to the explanation of variance of the two phonological tasks and the word recognition task administered in first grade (Colin, Magnan, Ecalle, & Leybaert, 2007). This very coherent pattern suggests that the effect of cued language, including early and later exposure to cued language, on phonological skills and reading development should be tracked very precisely at different periods in the developmental process. When deaf children are still manipulating global representations of phonology, mainly based on gross articulatory movements, the effect might not be apparent. However, when children are forced, in the context of formal reading instruction, to become conscious of the structure of phonological representations and their relation to the structure of written words, the effect of Cued Speech exposure becomes more obvious.

Research Related to Cued Speech for the Development of Phonics Abilities of Deaf Students

Phonics involves mapping one's knowledge about the phonemes of a language to the graphemes of that language to "sound out," or decode, that word. To the extent that an orthography is phonically-regular (i.e., there is an exact, one-to-one correspondence between the graphemes and the phonemes), readers can "phonologically assemble," or "sound out" words previously not encountered in print. Although English is not as phonically regular as some languages (e.g., Spanish or French), much of English *is* phonically regular. Typically, structured reading programs in the United States focus on helping young readers develop phonics generalizations through third grade and subsequently focus instruction on reading comprehension. The fact that deaf children tend to plateau in reading at the third to fourth grade suggests that the problems readers who are deaf experience with reading go beyond phonics or basic word recognition and are more closely linked to linguistic or experiential variables (LaSasso, 1996).

Studies of phonics abilities of deaf subjects *from oral or signing backgrounds* have utilized a variety of methodologies, including: (1) *letter cancellation* tasks (Dodd, 1987; Locke, 1978), (2) *Stroop* tasks (Leybaert & Alegria, 1993), (3) *lexical decision* tasks (Hanson, 1986; 1989; Hanson & Fowler, 1987; Waters & Doehring, 1990), (4) *spelling* tasks (Burden & Campbell, 1994; Hanson, Shankweiler, & Fisher, 1983; Leybaert, 2000; Leybaert & Alegria, 1995; Leybaert & Lechat, 2001), (5) *semantic acceptability* tasks (Hanson, Goodell, & Perfetti, 1991), and (6) *read-aloud* tasks (see Leybaert, 1993; Marschark, 1993 for an extensive review of these studies). Findings from phonics studies, taken collectively, suggest that deaf individuals from oral and signing backgrounds can acquire knowledge of phoneme-grapheme relationships; however, there is more variability in phonics usage among deaf children than among hearing children. Furthermore, deaf children are less likely to take full advantage of the phoneme grapheme relationship. This may be related to the underspecified nature of deaf individuals' phonological representations (Leybaert, 1993).

One stringent test of the notion that deaf children use grapheme-to-phoneme correspondences to get semantic access via a phonological representation consists of measuring deaf children's ability to identify novel written words encountered for the first time. Let us suppose that the child possesses a phonological representation of a word and that this word has

never been seen before. If the child is able to "phonologically assemble" the individual phonemic elements and blend those elements into something that has been perceived previously and associated with meaning, this could be considered as strong evidence regarding the psychological reality of phonological processing of orthographic information.

Alegria, Aurouer, and Hage (1997) conducted an experiment designed to test this hypothesis with 8 to 12-year-old deaf children from oral and cueing backgrounds. The participants were first presented with drawings representing unfamiliar items (for example a *banjo*). The drawings were paired with four different sequences of letters: *banjo* (real word), *taireu*, *pachaud* (distractor with similar lipread image), *lincat*. In the pretest, children were asked to underline the correct sequence of letters; it was expected that participants' choices would be at random (because they did not know these words). Then the children were given a lesson including the name of the objects. After the lesson, children once again needed to choose the correct sequence of letters. If children had learned about the phonological representation of the item during the lesson, they would be able to choose the correct spelling (*banjo*) more often in the posttest than in the pretest. Two experimental conditions were introduced: the lesson via lipreading alone or via Cued Speech. Results show a reliable increase of the percentage of correct written word identification responses from the pretest to the posttest. Children had thus profited from the lessons to elaborate phonological representations of the words. These representations constrained the possible orthographic representations and allowed the exclusion of distractors with similar lipread images. The role of cueing in the elaboration of the internal representations of words was evidenced by the fact that the improvement induced by the lessons was greater when cueing was used in addition to lipreading than when it was not. This finding is interpreted to mean that phonological representations were more accurate when cueing was involved in the lesson than when only lipreading was available.

Research Related to Cued Speech for the Development of Phonological Recoding Abilities of Deaf Students

In addition to phonological awareness and phonics, *phonological recoding* has been found to be related to reading achievement in hearing children. In the present chapter, phonological recoding, also known as *"internal speech,"* refers to how the reader communicates to himself or herself while reading or memorizing. Most of the studies of phonological, or "speech"-based, codes in working memory of deaf subjects have utilized serial retention tasks in which subjects have been presented stimuli, including: *letters* (Hanson, Liberman, & Shankweiler, 1984; Locke & Locke, 1971), *words* (Conrad, 1979; Hanson, 1982; Krakow & Hanson, 1985), or *sentences* (Garrison, Long, & Dowaliby, 1997). Findings of studies with deaf subjects from oral or signing backgrounds on working memory tasks, taken collectively, indicate that: (1) working memory capacity is as strong a predictor of reading achievement for deaf students as it is for hearing students (Daneman, Nemeth, Stainton, & Huelsmann, 1995), and a stronger predictor of reading achievement than degree of hearing loss; (2) deaf individuals, from both oral or signing backgrounds, tend to have smaller working memory capacities than hearing individuals on temporal sequential working memory tasks, with their working memory resembling that of younger hearing children (Bavelier, Newport, Hall, Supalla, & Boutla, 2008; Boutla, Supalla, Newport, & Bavelier, 2004), (3) deaf students use a variety of coding strategies (Lichtenstein, 1998; MacSweeney, Campbell, & Donlan, 1996; Waters & Doehring, 1990), (4) with one exception (Waters & Doehring, 1990), phonological abilities enhance working memory capacity of deaf individuals (Conrad, 1979; Hanson, 1982; Hanson et al., 1984; Lichtenstein, 1998; Wandel, 1989), and (5) the use of a speech-based code, unlike use of a sign code, is related to reading achievement in most of the studies that have examined this relationship (Conrad, 1979; Hanson et al., 1984; Lichtenstein, 1998; Wandel, 1989). It is tempting to speculate that phonological recoding abilities explain the superior performance of relatively competent readers who are deaf.

Research conducted with children who are deaf from Cued Speech backgrounds demonstrates that these early Cued Speech users achieve memory span similar to that of hearing children, and superior to that of other deaf individuals not exposed early to Cued Speech (Ketchum, 2001; Leybaert & Charlier, 1996; Wandel, 1989). Wandel (1989) utilized Conrad's (1979) methods and materials to investigate whether the deaf students' propensity to code phonologically in short term memory varied in terms of hearing loss, communication method (i.e., oral, total communication, Cued Speech), gender, age, or cognitive ability. Subjects for Wandel's study consisted of 90 deaf subjects, ranging in age from 7 to 16 years, and a control group of 30 hearing subjects. Deaf subjects came from three communication backgrounds

(Cued Speech, oral, and total communication) in public school programs serving deaf students. Total communication was described as the use of amplification, speechreading, and "simultaneous communication." Simultaneous communication was defined as the use of speech with a form of MCE signing and fingerspelling for proper nouns (Wandel, p. 25). All subjects came from homes in which parents had normal hearing, and English was the language primarily used. Subjects in each communication group and the control group were balanced for blocking factors of age, hearing loss, general cognitive ability, years in the manual mode, gender, schooling in programs with all three communication modes, and parental education background. All deaf subjects were prelingually deaf (i.e., had become deaf prior to the age of two years) and had bilateral severe-to-profound hearing losses with a pure-tone average for the better ear being greater than 65 dB. The 30 subjects in the comparison group were randomly selected from a group of 57 subjects who met the criteria of possessing normal hearing and balancing deaf subjects in terms of blocking factors. Measures used by Wandel included: (1) the Raven Standard Progressive Matrices (Raven, Court, & Raven, 1983), which is a nonverbal, paper and pencil, group intelligence test, normed on deaf students, and used by Conrad in his 1979 study, (2) reading comprehension subtests of the 7th edition (1982) of the Stanford Achievement Test, and (3) Conrad's (1979) internal speech materials. Conrad calculated internal speech (IS) ratios based on subjects' abilities to accurately write down homophones (H) or nonhomophones (NH) presented briefly on cards to the subjects. Homophones were words such as *do, few, who, blue,* and *through* which are phonetically similar but

orthographically different. Nonhomophones consisted of words such as *bear, bean, door, furs, have, home, farm,* and *lane* which all contain four letters and a single syllable and are visually similar but have different phonetic features. Wandel, like Conrad, calculated internal ratio (IS) ratios by comparing subjects' scores reflecting correctly reported homophones with those of correctly reported nonhomophones. IS ratios could range from 0 to 100. An IS ratio of 100 meant that a subject made memory errors only on the H sets. Conversely, an IS ratio of 0 meant that a subject made memory errors only on the NH-sets. An IS ratio of 50 meant an equal number of H-set and non-H sets memory errors. Wandel found that hearing subjects and deaf subjects from oral and Cued Speech backgrounds had higher IS ratios than deaf children with sign backgrounds, meaning that the former made more memory errors on the H set than on the NH set. This is a particularly interesting finding because the cuers had not been exposed to cued English during the preschool (i.e., critical language learning) years. Wandel's finding suggests that deaf cuers utilize internal speech more extensively to memorize than deaf students exposed to MCE sign systems.

Leybaert and Charlier (1996) compared deaf children raised orally, those raised with cueing at home and at school, and those raised with cueing only at school on their use of phonological representations (i.e., the way a word is pronounced) for remembering a series of words. Picture stimuli were used to avoid the possibility of giving the children pronunciation clues based on spelling or lipreading. The three groups were asked to recall series of pictures representing words in two sets of conditions: (1) rhyming versus nonrhyming and (2) one-syllable versus multiple syllables. The hearing children and the children who were exposed to cueing both at home and at school were able to recall more words than the oral group, and showed a difference in their ability to remember words based on word length and on phonological similarity (it is harder to remember a list of words if they rhyme, and it is harder to remember a list of long words than short words) suggesting that the children exposed to Cued Speech both at home and at school process the phonological structure of spoken words in much the same way as hearing children.

Ketchum (2001) compared the working memory capacity and the type of phonological coding of deaf individuals from cueing background, to that of a group of hearing controls. The study explored the recall of participants when presented with cued and printed word stimuli in conditions of oral and cued articulatory suppression. Ketchum found that deaf cuers use internal speech recoding similar to hearing individuals in working memory tasks, and do not show reduced working memory capacity relative to hearing individuals.

Taken together, these three studies consistently indicate that exposure to Cued Speech induces the use of "internal speech" in short-term memory experiments.

Spelling Development in Hearing Children

Spelling and phonics can be viewed to be different sides of the same coin, in that each involves utilizing knowledge of both phonemes and graphemes; however, whereas phonics utilizes phoneme-grapheme knowledge to sound out (or cue out) unfamiliar words, spelling utilizes phoneme-grapheme conventions to graphically represent spoken words. According to theorists of reading and spelling acquisition (Ehri, 1991; Frith, 1985; Perfetti, 1992, 1997; Perfetti & Sandak, 2000; Rayner et al., 2001), children's initial expression of the alphabetic principle appears *more often* in spelling than in reading. Reading involves *recognition*, whereas spelling involves *production*. For reading, the child may use phoneme-to-grapheme knowledge, but also partial guessing, in order to access a linguistic representation and a meaning from a written word. For spelling, the child is forced to access his or her lexical representations. If the child does not have full representation of the way words are spelled, he or she must produce the letters or letter groups from the phonological representation. Spelling is thus very important to consider, in the view of many theorists:

> One underestimates the child's potential grasp of the alphabetic principle—or at least the idea that speech sounds are associated with letters—if one considers only decoding. Spelling is the primary early indicator of this potential and can form the basis of later expression of the alphabetic principle in decoding. (Rayner et al., 2001, p. 41)

It is also clear that early spellings are guided by more than the child's attempts to map sounds onto letters. At an early age, children become sensitive to both the orthographic structures and the morphological structures that are present in spellings (Nunes, Bryant, & Bindman, 1997); Treiman, 1993; Treiman & Cassar, 1996). In the early grades, children's use of morphology is very incomplete; many of their errors reflect a preference for spelling a sound over spelling a morpheme. However, as soon as literacy instruction is underway, children begin to show an awareness that both phonological and morphological structures, as well as orthographic constraints, are present in conventional spellings.

In many languages, the learner confronts an important fact about spelling; specifically, that the mapping from pronunciation to spelling is less consistent than the mapping from spelling to pronunciation. For example, in English, the rime unit /ir/ is spelled variously as *eer*, *ear*, *ier*, or *ere*, whereas *eer* is always pronounced (read) as /ir/. In French too, vowels like /ɛ̃/ at the end of words can be spelled in different ways (*in, ain, ym, ein*), as do consonants like /s/ at the beginning of words (*s, c, sc*). These different phoneme-to-grapheme correspondences have different frequencies in French orthography (Véronis, 1986). For example, the phoneme /ɛ̃/ at the end of words is most frequently transcribed by the grapheme *in* (the most dominant transcription) and less frequently by *ain, ym* (the less dominant transcription). With progress in literacy, the child must learn not only that a particular unit (vowel, rime, or consonant) could be spelled with the dominant graphemes, but also the same unit could be spelled with other graphemes, and the particular words in which a particular grapheme is used. The first part of this learning thus concerns the mastery of *dominant* phoneme-to-grapheme correspondences (i.e., phonics rules), and the second part concerns learning of *word-specific* orthography (i.e., exceptions).

Spelling Development in Deaf Children: Our Perspective

For a long time, for several reasons, we have been convinced that the spelling abilities of deaf children are important to understand. One reason is that spelling is the primary early indicator of the potential for acquiring the alphabetic principle and can form the basis for later expression of the use of the alphabetic principle for deaf as well as for hearing children. A second reason, more specific to deaf children, is that deaf children's acquisition of spoken language phonology is largely influenced by visual experiences such as speechreading, and by articulatory experience such as speaking. In speechreading, there is a similarity in appearance of speech elements sharing the same place of articulation, like /p/, /b/, and /m/ (Erber, 1979; Walden, Prosek, Montgomery, Scherr, & Jones, 1977), and some phonemes are nearly invisible (like /r/) or highly confusable (like /k/, /g/, or /t/, /s/). As a consequence, phonological representations developed by deaf children solely from only speechread input tend to be incomplete, inaccurate, and underspecified (Leybaert, 1993).

The process of extracting regularities between orthographic units and phonological units is possible only when relatively systematic relationships between the phonological forms and the written forms of the words exist. The capacity to use the alphabetic principle productively thus requires accurate, fully-specified, phonological representations which allow any phoneme to be distinguished from all others. Underspecified phonological representations are an obstacle to learning to spell (and to read) in an alphabetic orthography. If deaf children only have underspecified phonological representations, they will be hindered in their ability to use the alphabetic principle generatively, not because they are unable to appreciate the mapping between written and spoken language, but because these mappings are less transparent for them than they are for hearing peers. Suppose that the English word *tree* is orally (sound + lipreading) presented to a deaf child (or the French word *armoire*). A child who cannot perceive the phoneme /r/ in the English word *tree* or in the French word *armoire* will have difficulty associating it with the specific grapheme (such as *r*) and will tend to *omit* this grapheme. Suppose now that the word French word *pyjama* (/piʒama/) is presented to a child, who cannot perceive the difference between the phonemes /ʒ/, /s/, or /tʃ/. When asked to spell *pyjama*, the child will likely transcribe the phoneme /ʒ/ with the graphemes *ch* or *s*, producing *pychama* or *pysama*. A child who cannot perceive the difference between voiced and voiceless phonemes (because this distinction is invisible in speechreading) will likely produce *oufert* for the word *ouvert* (an English-language example of this error type would be a spelling of *ofen* for the word *oven*). These types of errors have been found in spelling studies with orally educated deaf children (Leybaert & Alegria, 1995; see also Alamargot, Lambert, Thebault, & Dansac, 2006).

It is important to distinguish deaf children's phonological processing difficulties from those experienced by dyslexic children. Deaf children suffer from a deficit of *accessing* phonological information, not a phonological *processing* deficit such as might exist in some forms of dyslexia (see Rayner et al., 2001, p. 44). Therefore, it can be assumed that the addition of complementary visual information, which fully specifies, disambiguates, or resolves the ambiguity of the speechread signal, could improve accuracy of deaf children's phonological representations, and consequently, their ability to exploit the relationship between phonology and orthography. Our argument here

is twofold. First, experience with Cued Speech allows deaf children to identify the abstract phonemes (French examples include /r/ in *armoire*, /v/ in *ouvert*, /ʒ/ in *pyjama*; English examples include /h/ in *happy*, /k/ in *excellent*, /t/ in *washed*), and this will help them to associate these "visual phonemes" with specific graphemes. Second, the use of phoneme-to-grapheme correspondences constitutes the main learning mechanism available to the deaf child. That is, each time the child attempts to spell a word by using phoneme-to-grapheme correspondences, the child gets feedback from this attempt. This feedback may be simply the correct visual production, or it may be the reaction of the teacher or a parent. The feedback from these attempts gradually builds up the orthographic representation of specific words. In that sense, as posited by Jorm and Share (1983), the role of phonology is a *self-teaching* mechanism, which influences the development of word-specific orthographic representations. Conversely, the fact that the deaf child not exposed to Cued Speech repeatedly produces incorrect spellings for a given word (for example *amoire* instead of *armoire*) will reinforce the underspecificity of his or her orthographic representations. This underspecified orthographic representation will become automatically activated when the child wants to spell this particular word.

Empirical Data Related to Spelling Abilities of Deaf Students

Spelling Development of Deaf Children Educated Orally or with Signs. Deaf children educated orally or with signs must write a language whose primary mode (i.e., spoken) they cannot neither completely access nor easily produce.

Given the strong relationship between phonological abilities and reading acquisition, it is not surprising to find a strong delay, generally, in deaf children's reading and spelling development. At the beginning of the 20th century, Gates and Chase (1926) found that deaf youngsters aged 13 to 18 years were delayed by 2 to 5 years in spelling and by 6 to 8 years in reading. They concluded that:

> The deaf are incapable of thinking first of the sounds and then recalling a combination of letters which represent them . . . it seems probable that they depend mainly on . . . a more careful visual study of the word forms . . . [They] attempt to recall not the lip-movement-letter combination associations but the visual appearance of the word . . . (Gates & Chase, 1926, p. 300)

In contrast to the assumption of Gates and Chase that deaf children do not attempt to recall the lip movement–letter combination associations, Dodd (1987) assumed that prelingually, profoundly deaf individuals could, through lipreading, gain sufficient information about the phonological structure of language to acquire reading and phonics-based spelling skills. Dodd also believed that a phonological code is likely to be amodal (i.e., existing irrespective of whether the phonemes perceived are heard or lipread) (Dodd, 1987). However, as noted earlier, information from lipreading is not specific enough to allow the development of precise phonological representations, and the orthographic representations acquired by deaf children are also underspecified (Burden & Campbell, 1994; Hanson, Shankweiler & Fischer, 1983; Hoemann, Andrews, Florian, Hoemann, & Jensema, 1976; Sutcliffe, Dowker, & Campbell, 1999).

Spelling Development of Deaf Children Educated with Cued Speech: the Alphabetic Principle. The use of phoneme-to-grapheme correspondences in word spelling has been examined in several studies (Leybaert, 2000; Leybaert & Lechat, 2001). Leybaert (2000) sought to determine whether deaf cuers utilize phonology-to-orthography mappings for word spellings to the same extent as hearing peers. They tested three groups of children: children educated early with Cued Speech at home (CS-home), children educated with Cued Speech later at school (CS-school), and hearing children. The participants were asked to spell high and low-frequency words. It was reasoned that if the CS-home group possesses accurate phonological representations, they could extract regularities between letters (or letter groups) and specific combinations of manual cues and lip movements. They should be able to produce a similar rate of phonologically acceptable responses as hearing children, for high-frequency as well as for low-frequency words. It was further reasoned that the performance of the CS-home children would contrast with that of CS-school children, who have underspecified representations of phonology (Leybaert, 2000).

The three groups in the Leybaert (2000) study were matched for general spelling level. Interestingly, the children from the CS-home group achieved a similar reading score as the hearing, at the same chronologic age (8;3). In contrast, children in the CS-school group, although being older (11 years) were reading-delayed. As expected, most of the spelling errors of the hearing and the CS-home groups were phonological substitutions (e.g., sigarette for *cigarette*), whereas the errors of the CS-school group were a mixture of phonological substitutions and nonphonological errors (e.g., tigarette for *cigarette*). Leybaert (2000) concluded that for CS-home children, spelling a word for which the child does not have an orthographic representation, involves first considering the word's phonological form and then producing a combination of letters that represent it. Leybaert further concluded that the data clearly indicate that the development of phonology-to-orthography mappings does not in any way necessarily depend on the perception of auditory information (Leybaert, 2000, pp. 311–312).

Findings related to intensive exposure to Cued Speech from the Leybaert (2000) study were confounded with the total amount of language exposure. Specifically, early exposure to a fully accessible language may be the critical factor, rather than exposure to Cued Speech per se. In a second experiment, Leybaert and Lechat (2001) compared the spelling of the CS-home children to that of children exposed early in life to a visual language, albeit of a different nature (i.e., French sign language, langue des signes française). Leybaert and Lechat (2001) compared CS-home and Sign Language (SL) home children, CS-school and SL-school children to hearing controls. The five groups of children were matched for reading score; the hearing and the CS-home children were younger (107 months and 98 months, respectively) than the CS-school (130 months), the SL-home (135 months), and the SL-school (141 months). As predicted, most of the errors made by the CS-home children and the hearing children were phonologically accurate errors. When required to spell a word for which they did not have a fully detailed orthographic representation, hearing and CS-home children started from accurate phonological representations and applied dominant correspondences be-

tween phonemes and graphemes. The CS-school, SL-home, and SL-school children performed differently in spelling than did the CS-home and hearing children. The former made fewer phonologically accurate misspellings, indicating a lower ability to use accurate phoneme-to-grapheme mappings. Their performance may have resulted from inaccuracy at the level of phonological representations, deficiency in segmentation of these representations, or a difficulty in attributing graphemes to phonemes. CS-school children and children educated with sign language were found to have underspecified representations of phonology (Charlier & Leybaert, 2000). Inaccuracy of their phonological representations hindered these children in applying phoneme-to-grapheme correspondences.

Spelling Development of Deaf Children Educated with Cued Speech: the Orthographic Principle. According to Perfetti's (1992) framework described earlier in this chapter, learning to read involves the acquisition of increasing numbers of word representations that change in *specificity* and *redundancy*. Increasing specificity means that as a child learns to read, his or her representations of words increasingly have specific letters in their correct positions. Increasing redundancy means that these representations become phonologically redundant: the addition of specific grapheme-to-phoneme correspondences for a word is redundant with the word-level pronunciation of the word. According to this framework, the precision of the orthographic representation could be variable, even for phonemes that have entirely predictable spellings. In the case of consonant clusters for example, liquids (e.g., /l/ or /r/) that follow initial stops or fricatives (e.g., *truck*, *slip*) are more likely to be omitted when spelled

(Bruck & Treiman, 1990; Leybaert & Content, 1995; Perfetti, 1992; Sprenger-Charolles & Siegel, 1997). Cluster reduction has also been observed in deaf children's written productions (Dodd, 1980; Leybaert & Alegria, 1995). The fact that the second consonant is nearly invisible via speechreading increases the difficulty represented by consonant clusters. Cued Speech, by making consonant clusters highly visible, could lead deaf children to include the two consonants in the phonological representation, thereby facilitating the development of a full orthographic representation. Therefore, Leybaert (2000) asked CS-home, CS-school, and hearing children to spell /r/ and /l/ either in consonant clusters (like in *fleur* or *grenouille*) or at the beginning of a syllable (like in *lapin* or *revolver*). The results revealed that hearing children spelled the /r/ and /l/ equally well in the two phonological structures; for CS-home children, spelling /r/ or /l/ was slightly easier at the beginning of words than as the second consonant in a cluster; for CS-school children, the spelling of /r/ and /l/ was much more difficult in consonant clusters than at the word's beginning. It was concluded that children who perceive spoken words via Cued Speech get a representation of *all* the phonemes, including those embedded in consonant clusters. Furthermore, when learning to read and spell, children exposed to Cued Speech develop representations of words that have increasing specificity (i.e., specific letters in their correct positions).

To sum up, the experimental data reported here consistently show very strong similarities between prelingually, profoundly deaf children exposed early to Cued Speech and hearing children. Specifically, (1) deaf cuers achieved the same reading level and spelling level as their hearing peers of the same chronologic age, (2) the use of phoneme-to-grapheme correspondences was found to be similar in deaf cuers and their hearing peers, and (3) the acquisition of orthographic representations was nearly as precise in deaf cuers as in hearing. The deaf cuers surpassed the other groups of deaf children in all of these aspects.

Evidence from Cognitive Neuroscience Studies of Deaf Readers

Over the last few decades, the functional neuroanatomy of reading has been increasingly researched, thanks to the improvement of techniques allowing the capture of the brain's activity. In the past, the visual hemifield presentation paradigm has been successfully used to investigate the differences between the left and the right hemispheres in processing the semantics and the phonology of written words (Abernethy & Coney, 1996; Grossi, Coch, Coffey-Corina, Holcomb, & Neville, 2001; Rayman & Zaidel, 1991). This paradigm is based on behavioral responses to words, pictures, or objects presented to the desired hemisphere. Indeed, the nerve fibers carrying information about stimuli presented to the right visual hemifield (RVF) project to the visual cortex of the left cerebral hemisphere, whereas the fibers carrying information about stimuli presented to the left visual hemifield (LVF) project to the visual cortex of the right cerebral hemisphere (RVF). Hearing subjects generally show an advantage in semantic and phonological processing for words presented in the RVF (thus processed preferentially by the left hemisphere).

D'Hondt and Leybaert (2003) compared the lateralization pattern of deaf youngsters who are skilled readers and who have been exposed to Cued Speech for the processing of written stimuli with that of hearing subjects matched for gender, reading level, and linguistic competence. In this study, participants had to compare a stimulus presented at the center of the screen (hereafter: central) to a stimulus presented next for 250 milliseconds in the left or right visual hemifield (hereafter: lateral), together with a digit presented centrally in order to fixate subjects' attention. Three tasks were used: two linguistic and one nonlinguistic. The nonlinguistic task involved a visual judgment, that is, determining whether "EeeE" (central stimulus) and "Eeee" (lateral stimulus) were the same or not. Performance on this task did not differ between left and right hemispheres, either in the deaf or the hearing participants. The first linguistic task involved semantic judgments, such as determining whether *cat* (central stimulus) and *rabbit* (lateral stimulus) belong to the same semantic category. A right visual field (left hemisphere) advantage was observed for this semantic decision task in deaf as well as in hearing subjects. The second linguistic task involved judging whether two orthographically dissimilar words rhymed, such as: do *feu* (central stimulus) and *noeud* (lateral stimulus) rhyme (in English: do *blue* and *few* rhyme?). In line with previous findings (Grossi, Coch, Coffey-Corina, Holcomb, & Neville, 2001; Rayman & Zaidel, 1991), hearing subjects showed a right visual field (left hemisphere) advantage. A surprising finding was that *no* hemifield advantage was observed in cuers who were good at rhyming in a controlled paper-and-pencil task. The authors suggested that the neural substrate activated

during rhyme judgment could be different in deaf cuers from that activated by hearing subjects.

Methods such as functional magnetic resonance imaging (fMRI) and positron emission tomography (PET) are being used increasingly to provide converging information about the functional neuroanatomy of reading. These imaging methods provide good spatial information about what "lights up" in the brain when words are read, but they provide poor information about the time course of these events. Questions about the temporal course of processing information are better addressed by event-related potential (ERP) methods. These brain-imaging methods might yield evidence for the role of phonological processes involved in deaf students' word identification that have proved to be so important for hearing subjects.

Research related to the functional neuroanatomy network underlying reading in hearing subjects has identified three brain regions that play a role in word reading: the inferior frontal cortex, the left temporoparietal cortex, and the left basal temporal cortex (next the occipitotemporal boundary) (Fiez, Balota, Raichle, & Petersen, 1999; Pugh, Shaywitz, Shaywitz, & Shankweiler, 1997; see also Rayner et al., 2001). These three areas appear to provide a major part of the functional neuroanatomy underlying the orthographic, phonological, and semantic components that are needed in word reading. The visual areas in the occipital cortex that are used for object recognition support the orthographic component in the brain. The search for an area that is dedicated to printed words (a *word-form* area) has lead to the identification of areas near the occipitotemporal border, the left middle fusiform gyrus.

The conversion of an orthographic form into a phonological form is a central part of reading, as we have argued in the section of this chapter on phonological recoding. Two brain regions where lesions lead to deficits in phonological decoding are the left inferior frontal lobe and the temporoparietal cortex. Lesions in one or both of these areas are associated with difficulty in reading pseudowords (Fiez & Petersen, 1998). Recent evidence shows that the ability of normal readers to read aloud pseudowords, which constitutes a signature for the sublexical processing, is disrupted by stimulation of the temporoparietal region, while the ability to read words is not (Simos et al., 2000). The frontal regions have also shown greater activation for pseudowords than for real words in some studies; thus both left frontal and temporoparietal regions are active in reading in tasks that require or encourage phonological processing (Demonet, Fiez, Paulesu, Petersen, & Zatorre, 1996).

In order to compare deaf and hearing subjects's neural activity in functional regions of interest engaged in reading, Aparicio, Gounot, Demont, and Metz-Lutz (2007) used a rhyme decision task. The material consisted of rhyming pairs which were either consistent (*bouche-mouche*) or inconsistent (e.g., *poêle-toile*) in orthography and nonrhyming pairs which were spelled similarly (e.g., *hamac-tabac*) or not (e.g., *poêle- hamac*). The fMRI session consisted of alternating blocks of experimental and baseline conditions. This means that the neural activity of the rhyming and nonrhyming, consistent and inconsistent trials was measured at once. The group of deaf participants was comprised of 12 congenitally, profoundly deaf participants who had a bilingual French oral and sign language background. Four of them were exposed to Cued Speech at school for a short period only, but none of them used it for everyday verbal com-

munication. On average, their reading age was 15 months lower than that of the hearing control participants.

The accuracy of deaf subjects in the rhyming task was lower than that of the hearing subjects (72.6% versus 88.5%, respectively), confirming previous findings about deaf people who are *not* Cued Speech-users to manage a rhyming task (Campbell & Wright, 1988; Charlier & Leybaert, 2000; Hanson & Fowler, 1987). Accuracy rate was thus introduced as a covariate in the analysis of the difference of activation in the regions of interest. The significant differences in activation in these regions thus likely reflect different cognitive strategies.

In comparison to hearing subjects, the deaf readers showed significantly greater activation in the left and right IFG (inferior frontal gyrus) and the left inferior parietal lobe in the rhyming judgment task. It is interesting to note that in addition to more activation in the *left* IFG, the deaf readers recruited the *right* IFG. These results are in line with those of D'Hondt & Leybaert (2003), suggesting that the rhyming-related cortical network in less lateralized in deaf individuals than in hearing individuals. The recruitment of the right IFG in addition to the left IFG by deaf readers whose single word reading performances were similar to those of the hearing subjects might be interpreted as being a compensatory mechanism for phonological recoding relying on speech articulation and inner speech (BA 44), and even lexical identification (BA 45).

The second area that was more activated in the deaf group in the Aparicio et al. (2007) study, the left inferior parietal lobe, has been associated with the spelling-to-sound conversion required in phonological tasks (Paulesu, Frith, & Frackowiack, 1993). Together with the left BA 44, greater activation in this area would suggest that deaf readers relied more strongly on the indirect route. Deaf subjects had significantly more activation in the pMFC (premotor frontal cortex), a region playing a role in cognitive control. Indeed, activation in this area is elicited by decision uncertainty, response conflict, and errors. In the visual rhyming task, the reader could actually experience the orthographically or phonologically incongruent word pairs as a source of decision uncertainty, or even as response conflict (Aparicio et al., 2007).

To sum up, various methods, including hemifield presentation and brain-imaging studies, converge on a picture of the rhyming decision task as inducing partly similar and partly different cognitive strategies in deaf and in hearing subjects. Deaf participants can transform the graphic input into the phonological representation, distributed across functional brain regions; however, the functional regions seem partly different, at least in those participants who have not been exposed to Cued Speech intensively and precociously. Much remains to be learned about the specific regions that support both the processing of Cued Speech information (see Chapter 24) and about the specific neuroanatomo-functional network developed by those deaf who are early Cued Speech-users. This research is currently in progress.

Cued Speech and Cochlear Implants

During the past several decades, an increasing number of children born with profound deafness have been fitted with a cochlear implant. The aim of cochlear implantation is to restore auditory percep-

tion. According to numerous studies, the earlier the fitting, the greater the probability that children achieve language development and academic achievement similar to those of normally hearing children (Svirsky, Robbins, Kirk, Pisoni, & Miyamoto, 2000).

Besides age of implantation, the method of communication (oral versus sign supported speech) has been found to be an important variable in the development of speech perception and phonological memory (Burkolder & Pisoni, 2006; O'Donoghue, Nikolopoulos, & Archbold, 2000). This suggests the existence of an important brain *plasticity* following the fitting with a cochlear implant. Those children stimulated with spoken language are better able to process acoustic speech information than those who are poorly stimulated.

It is important to consider the multimodal characteristic of speech perception through the cochlear implant (Leybaert & Colin, 2007). The stimulation delivered by the cochlear implant is not as precise as the acoustic stimulation delivered by the natural ear. Phonemic contrasts such as place of articulation remain poorly discriminated through the cochlear implant, and speech perception is deteriorated under noise conditions. These phonetic features must be clarified through visual means in order to provide deaf children with accurate phonological information. Therefore, a number of parents and practitioners in France, Belgium, Spain, and the United States (see Chapter 8) have opted for the use of Cued Speech with the deaf children, conjointly with the use of a cochlear implant. Given the fact that the combination of lips + hands in Cued Speech delivers an unambiguous message, the processing of cued information should help cochlear implant recipients exploit the auditory clues related to the visual cues, for example, clues related to the place of articulation. As the movement of the cueing hand precedes the opening of the mouth, which precedes the arrival of the sound (see Chapter 19), cueing should also allow deaf children to better focus his or her attention and reduce the uncertainty of the auditory perception resulting from the implant stimulation (see Chapter 6 for more detailed arguments).

Children who are fitted with a cochlear implant and are exposed to Cued Speech process auditory speech information better, and have an advantage over implanted children who do not use Cued Speech regarding the use of grapheme-to-phoneme conversions in word reading and word spelling. Leybaert, Bravard, Sudre, and Cochard (2009) found that reading and spelling achievement of children with cochlear implants and Cued Speech were closer to that of hearing peers, and that children with cochlear implants but without Cued Speech were more delayed compared to their hearing peers. The three groups of children were extracted from the same classrooms, excluding the possibility to explain the results by a difference of instruction or socioeconomic backgrounds.

Summary and Conclusions

In this chapter, we have focused on a *narrow view* of reading as decoding, or more precisely, utilization of the alphabetic principle, and we discussed several topics related to how deaf children exposed to Cued Speech learn to read. We supported our argument about the effectiveness of Cued Speech with findings from research related to phonological awareness, development of word recognition and of spelling, and brain activity during reading. From all these perspectives, several conclusions emerge related to: (1) the importance of mastering the alphabetic principle, (2) the importance of deaf children having an L1 prior to formal reading instruction, and (3) the relevance of cued language for deaf children with a cochlear implant.

The Importance of Deaf Children Mastering the Alphabetic Principle

Mastering the alphabetic principle is as essential for deaf children as it is for hearing children in becoming proficient in decoding and spelling. Mastery of the alphabetic principle is entirely possible via Cued Speech and cued language. The advantage of a cued language over a spoken or signed language for deaf children is that cueing fully specifies, or distinguishes, phonemes of a traditionally spoken language which better prepares children to learn the alphabetic principle in an easy and efficient way. The combination of cued language and phonics instruction places deaf children less at risk for becoming poor readers or poor spellers because the phonology of the language in phonics instruction is visually clarified.

The Importance of Deaf Children Having an L1 Prior to Formal Reading Instruction

Having an L1 prior to formal reading instruction is as important for deaf children as it is for hearing children for formal reading instruction and reading achievement. This L1 could be a signed, spoken, or cued language. Neural structures and brain organization are specified for language, but not for spoken language exclusively. It is through language experience, including its communicational and pragmatic aspects, that the network of getting meaning from (or bringing meaning to) linguistic stimuli (e.g., spoken, signed, or cued words and morphosyntax) develops and automatizes. Children who acquire a good command of a language prior to formal reading instruction will be better readers. This implies early, clear, complete, and intensive exposure to that language. It can be hypothesized that such exposure to a cued language can provide the language foundation upon which all reading comprehension is ultimately built.

The relative advantage of cued language over traditionally spoken language for natural L1 acquisition prior to formal reading instruction is that cueing *fully* specifies the phonemes of English and other traditionally spoken languages, thereby conveying English and other traditionally spoken languages as clearly to deaf individuals as speech conveys them to hearing individuals. Deaf cuers who have been exposed early and consistently to cued languages have been found to acquire those languages in the same ways and rates as hearing peers.

The relative advantage of cued English as L1 over ASL as L1 for the development of English literacy is that cued English corresponds to the language encoded in print. As discussed in Chapter 12, cued English offers deaf children the same advantage in learning to read that English-speaking children have, compared to children who are learning to read via English as a Second Language (ESL) methods. That is, learning to read a language is much simpler for children who are familiar with the conversational form of that language

before formal reading instruction than it is for children who are learning to read while *simultaneously* learning the language. Materials and instructional procedures used to develop deaf cuers' reading abilities, including those related to developing the alphabetic principle, *do not need to differ from those used with hearing peers*. The only difference in educating deaf and hearing children in the same reading class needs to be the *communication method* used by the teacher (i.e., Cued Speech). The process of developing reading abilities of deaf children whose L1 is ASL or another signed language is more similar to that used with ESL (English as Second Language) learners.

The Relevance of Cued Language for Deaf Children with a Cochlear Implant

While one might think that Cued Speech and cued language are less important now that cochlear implants are the new reality, we have argued in this chapter that despite the fact that cochlear implants represent a revolution for the spoken language development of deaf children, they do not currently (nor are they projected to do so in the near future) provide sufficient acoustic information about the fine-grained phonology. Therefore, for optimum speech perception, it is necessary to clarify the underspecified acoustic phonological contrasts provided by cochlear implants with visual tools, such as Cued Speech. Findings from research reported in this chapter and in Chapter 6 demonstrate that deaf children with cochlear implants who use Cued Speech and cued language have better speech perception scores than those who do not use Cued Speech.

Conclusion

Accurate phonological representations and phonics instruction are critically important because they help the beginning reader understand the alphabetic principle and apply it to reading and spelling. It should be clear that educators of young deaf children who make the alphabetic principle explicit to their students are helping these students to become skilled and independent readers. In Chapter 12, Cued Speech and Visual Phonics (Trezak, Wang, Woods, Gampp, & Paul, 2007; Waddy-Smith & Wilson, 2003) are compared for their effectiveness in developing deaf students' reading abilities.

References

Abernethy, M., & Coney, J. (1996). Semantic category priming in the left cerebral hemisphere. *Neuropsychologia, 34,* 339–350.

Adams, M. (1990). *Beginning to read: Thinking and learning about print.* Cambridge, MA: MIT Press.

Alamargot, D., Lambert, E., Thebault, C., & Dansac, C. (2006). Text composition by deaf and hearing middle school students: Effects of working memory. *Reading and Writing, 20,* 333–360.

Alegria, J., Aurouer, V., & Hage, C. (1997, December 4–5). *How do deaf children identify written words encountered for the first time: Phonological representations and phonological processing.* Working paper presented at the International Symposium "Integrating Research and Practice in Literacy," London, UK.

Alegria, J., & Morais, J. (1979). Le développement de l'habileté d'analyse phonétique consciente de la parole et l'apprentissage de la lecture. *Archives de Psychologie, 47,* 251–270.

Aparicio, M., Gounot, D., Demont, E., & Metz-Lutz, M. (2007). Phonological processing in relation to reading: An fMRI study in deaf readers. *Neuroimage, 35,* 1303–1316.

Bavelier, D., Newport, E., Hall, M., Supalla, T., & Boutla, M. (2008). Ordered short-term memory differs in signers and speakers: Implications for models of short-term memory. *Cognition, 107,* 433–459.

Boutla, M., Supalla, T., Newport, E., & Bavelier, D. (2004). Short-term memory span: Insights from sign language. *Nature Neuroscience, 7,* 997–1002.

Bowey, J., & Francis, J. (1991). Phonological analysis as a function of age and exposure to reading instruction. *Applied Psycholinguistics, 12,* 91–121.

Bradley, L., & Bryant, P. (1978). Differences in auditory organization as a possible cause for reading backwardness. *Nature, 271,* 746–747.

Bradley, L., & Bryant, P. (1983). Categorizing sounds and learning to read—a causal connection. *Nature, 301,* 419–421.

Bruck, M., & Treiman, R. (1990). Phonological awareness and spelling in normal children and dyslexics: The case of the initial consonant clusters. *Journal of Experimental Child Psychology, 50,* 156–178.

Bryant, P., MacLean, M., & Bradley, L. (1990). Rhyme, language, and children's reading. *Applied Psycholinguistics, 11,* 237–252.

Bryant, P., MacLean, M., & Bradley, L., & Crossland, J. (1990). Rhyme and alliteration, phoneme detection, and learning to read. *Developmental Psychology, 26,* 429–438.

Burden, V., & Campbell, R. (1994). The development of word coding skills in the born deaf: An experimental study of deaf school leavers. *British Journal of Psychology, 72,* 371–376.

Burkholder, R., & Pisoni, D. (2006). Working memory capacity, verbal rehearsal speed, and scanning in deaf children with cochlear implants. In: P. Spencer & M. Marschark (Eds), *Advances in the spoken language development of deaf and hard-of-hearing children* (pp. 328–357). New York, NY: Oxford University Press.

Campbell, R., & Wright, H. (1988). Deafness, spelling and rhyme: How spelling support written word and picture rhyming skills in deaf subjects. *Quarterly Journal of Experimental Psychology, 40A,* 771–788.

Castles, A., & Coltheart, M. (2004). Is there a causal link from phonological awareness to success in learning to read? *Cognition, 91,* 107–139.

Charlier, B., & Leybaert, J. (2000). The rhyming skills of deaf children educated with phonetically augmented speechreading. *Quarterly Journal of Experimental Psychology, 53A,* 349–375.

Colin, S., Leybaert, J., Ecalle, J., & Magnan, A. (2008). The influence of implicit and explicit phonological knowledge on deaf and hearing children's beginning of literacy. *Revista Portuguesa de Psicologia, 40,* 51–72.

Colin, S., Magnan, A., Ecalle, J., & Leybaert, J. (2007). A longitudinal study of the development of reading in deaf children: Effect of Cued Speech. *Journal of Child Psychology and Psychiatry, 48,* 139–146

Conrad, R. (1979). *The deaf school child.* London, UK: Harper & Row.

Cornett, R. O. (1967). Cued Speech. *American Annals of the Deaf, 112,* 3–13.

Crain, K. (2003). *The development of phonological awareness in moderately-to-profoundly deaf developing readers: The effect of exposure to cued American English.* Unpublished doctoral dissertation. Gallaudet University, Washington, DC.

Daneman, M., Nemeth, S., Stainton, M., & Huelsmann, K. (1995). Working memory as a predictor of reading achievement in orally educated hearing-impaired children. *Volta Review, 97,* 225–241.

Dehaene, S. (2007). *Les neurones de la lecture.* Paris, France: Odile Jacob.

Demonet, J., Fiez, J., Paulesu, E., Petersen, S., & Zatorre, R. (1996). PET studies of phonological processing: A critical reply to Poeppel. *Brain and Language, 55,* 352–379.

D'Hondt, M., & Leybaert, J. (2003). Lateralization effects during semantic and rhyme judgment tasks in deaf and hearing subjects. *Brain and Language, 87,* 227–240.

Dodd, B. (1980). The spelling abilities of profoundly, pre-linguistically deaf children. In U. Frith (Ed.), *Cognitive processes in spelling* (pp. 423–443). New York, NY: Academic Press.

Dodd, B. (1987). Lip-reading, phonological coding, and deafness. In B. Dodd & R. Campbell (Eds.), *Hearing by eye: The psychology of lipreading* (pp. 177–189). London, UK: Lawrence Erlbaum Associates.

Dodd, B., & Hermelin, B. (1977). Phonological coding by the prelinguistically deaf. *Perception and Psychophysics, 21,* 413–417.

Ehri, L. (1991). Learning to read and to spell words. In L. Rieben & C. Perfetti (Eds.), *Learning to read: Basic research and its implications* (pp. 57–73). Hillsdale, NJ: Erlbaum.

Ehri, L., Nunes, S., Willows, D., Schuster, B., Yaghoub-Zadeh, Z., & Shanahan, T. (2001). Phonemic awareness instruction helps children learn to read: Evidence from the National Reading Panel's meta-analysis. *Reading Research Quarterly, 36,* 250–287.

Erber, N. (1979). Speech perception in profoundly hearing-impaired children. *Journal of Speech and Hearing Research, 44,* 225–270.

Fiez, J., Balota, D., Raichle, M., & Petersen, S. (1999). Effects of lexicality, frequency, and spelling-to-sound consistency on the functional anatomy of reading. *Neuron, 24,* 205–218.

Fiez, J., & Petersen, S. (1998). Neuroimaging studies of word reading. *Proceedings of National Academy of Sciences, USA, 95,* 914–921.

Frith, U. (1985). Beneath the surface of developmental dyslexia. In K. Patterson, J. Marshall, & M. Coltheart (Eds.), *Surface dyslexia: Neuropsychological and cognitive studies of phonological recoding* (pp. 301–330). London, UK: Erlbaum.

Garrison, W., Long, G., & Dowaliby, F. (1997). Working memory capacity and comprehension processes in deaf readers. *Journal of Deaf Studies and Deaf Education, 2,* 78–94.

Gates, A., & Chase, E. (1926). Methods and theories of learning to spell tested by studies of deaf children. *Journal of Educational Psychology, 17,* 289–300.

Gelb, I. (1952). *A study of writing.* Chicago, IL: University of Chicago Press.

Goldin-Meadow, S., & Mayberry, R. (2001). How do profoundly deaf children learn to read? *Learning disabilities research and practice (Special issue: Emergent and early literacy: Current status and research directions), 16,* 221–228.

Goswami, U. (1993). Toward an interactive analogy model of reading development: Decoding vowel graphemes in beginning reading. *Journal of Experimental Child Psychology, 56,* 443–475.

Goswami, U., & Bryant, P. (1990). *Phonological skills and learning to read.* London, UK: Erlbaum.

Gough, P., & Hillinger, M. (1980). Learning to read: An unnatural act. *Bulletin of the Orton Society, 30,* 179–196.

Grossi, G., Coch, D., Coffey-Corina, S., Holcomb, P., & Neville, H. (2001). Phonological processing in visual rhyming: A developmental ERP study. *Journal of Cognitive Neuroscience, 13,* 610–625.

Hanson, V. (1982). Short-term recall by deaf signers of American Sign Language: Implications of encoding strategy for order recall. *Journal of Experimental Psychology: Learning, Memory and Cognition, 8,* 572–583.

Hanson, V. (1986). Access to spoken language and the acquisition of orthographic structure: Evidence from deaf readers. *Quarterly Journal of Experimental Psychology, 38A,* 193–212.

Hanson, V. (1989). Phonology and reading: Evidence from profoundly deaf readers. In D. Shankweiler & I. Liberman (Eds.), *Phonology and reading disabilities* (pp. 69–89). Ann Arbor, MI: University of Michigan Press.

Hanson, V., & Fowler, C. (1987). Phonological coding in word reading: Evidence from deaf and hearing readers. *Memory and Cognition, 15,* 199–207.

Hanson, V., Goodell, E., & Perfetti, C. (1991). Tongue-twister effects in the silent reading of hearing and deaf college students. *Journal of Memory and Language, 30,* 319–330.

Hanson, V., Liberman, I., & Shankweiler, D. (1984). Linguistic coding by deaf children in relation to beginning reading success. *Journal of Experimental Child Psychology, 37,* 378–393.

Hanson, V., & McGarr, N. (1989). Rhyme generation by deaf adults. *Journal of Speech and Hearing Research, 32,* 2–11.

Hanson, V., Shankweiler, D., & Fischer, F. (1983). Determinants of spelling ability in deaf and hearing adults: Access to linguistic structure. *Cognition, 14,* 323–344.

Harris, M., & Beech, J. R. (1998). Implicit phonological awareness and early reading development in prelingually deaf children. *Journal of Deaf Studies and Deaf Education, 3,* 205–216.

Hoemann, H., Andrews, C., Florian, V., Hoeman, S., & Jensema, C. (1976). The spelling proficiency of deaf children. *American Annals of the Deaf, 121,* 489–493.

Hulmes, C., Caravolas, M., Malkova, G., & Brigstocke, S. (2005). Phoneme isolation ability is not simply a consequence of letter-sound knowledge. *Cognition, 97,* B1–B11.

Jorm, A., & Share, D. (1983). Phonological recoding and reading acquisition. *Applied Psycholinguistics, 4,* 103–147.

Juel, C., Griffith, P., & Gough, P. (1986). Acquisition of literacy: A longitudinal study of children in first and second grade. *Journal of Educational Psychology, 78,* 243–255.

Kamil, M., Mosenthal, P., Pearson, P., & Barr, R. (2000). *Handbook of reading research: Vol III.* Mahwah, NJ: Lawrence Erlbaum Associates.

Kelly, L. (1995). Processing of bottom-up and top-down information by skilled and average deaf readers and implications for whole language instruction. *Exceptional Children, 61,* 318–334.

Ketchum, K. (2001). *Implications of working memory strategies in deaf native cuers: Hearings cuers, and hearing non-cuers.* Doctoral dissertation, Washington DC: Gallaudet University.

Krakow, R., & Hanson, V. (1985). Deaf signers and serial recall in the visual modality: Memory for signs, finger spelling, and print. *Memory and Cognition, 13,* 265–272.

Kyle, F., & Harris, M. (2006). Concurrent correlates and predictors of reading and spelling achievement in deaf and hearing school children. *Journal of Deaf Studies and Deaf Education, 11*, 273–288.

LaSasso, C. (1985). Visual matching test-taking strategies used by hearing impaired readers. *Journal of Speech and Hearing Research, 28*, 2–7.

LaSasso, C. (1996). Foniks for deff tshildrun? *Perspectives in Education and Deafness, 14*, 6–9.

LaSasso, C., Crain, K., & Leybaert, J. (2003). Rhyme generation in deaf students: The effect of exposure to Cued Speech. *Journal of Deaf Studies and Deaf Education, 8*, 250–270.

LaSasso, C., & Metzger, M. (1998) An alternate route to bilingualism: The home language as L1 and Cued Speech for conveying traditionally spoken languages. *Journal of Deaf Studies and Deaf Education, 3*, 264–289.

Leybaert, J. (1993). Reading in the deaf: The roles of phonological codes. In M. Marschark & D. Clark (Eds.), *Psychological perspectives on deafness.* Hillsdale, NJ: Lawrence Erlbaum Associates.

Leybaert, J. (2000). Phonology acquired through the eyes and spelling in deaf children. *Journal of Experimental Child Psychology, 75*, 291–318.

Leybaert, J., & Alegria, J. (1993). Is word processing involuntary in deaf children? *British Journal of Developmental Psychology, 11*, 1–29.

Leybaert, J., & Alegria, J. (1995). Spelling development in hearing and deaf children: Evidence for the use of morpho-phonological regularities in French. *Reading and Writing, 7*, 89–109.

Leybaert, J., Bravard, S., Sudre, O., & Cochard, N. (2009). La adquisicion de la lectura y la orthographia en ninos sordos con implante coclear: Efectos de la Palabra Complementada. In: M. Carillo & A. B. Dominguez (Eds.), *Lineas actuales en el estudio de la lengua escrita y sus dificultades: Dislexia y sordera. Libro de lecturas en honor de Jésus Alegria.* Malaga, Spain: Aljibe.

Leybaert, J., & Charlier, B. (1996). Visual speech in the head: The effect of Cued Speech on rhyming, remembering and spelling. *Journal of Deaf Studies and Deaf Education, 1*, 234–248.

Leybaert, J., & Colin, C. (2007). Le rôle des informations visuelles dans le développement du langage de l'enfant sourd muni d'un implant cochléaire. *Enfance, 57*, 245–253.

Leybaert, J., & Content, A. (1995). Reading and spelling acquisition in two different teaching methods: A test of the independence hypothesis. *Reading and Writing, 7*, 65–88.

Leybaert, J., & Lechat, J. (2001b). Variability in deaf children's spelling: The effect of language experience. *Journal of Educational Psychology, 93*, 554–562.

Liberman, A., Cooper, F., Shankweiler, D., & Studdert-Kennedy, M. (1967). The perception of the speech code. *Psychological Review, 24*, 431–461.

Liberman, I., Shankweiler, D., Fischer, F., & Carter, B. (1974). Explicit syllable and phoneme segmentation in the young child. *Journal of Experimental Child Psychology, 18*, 201–212.

Lichtenstein, E. (1998). The relationships between reading processes and English skills for deaf students. *Journal of Deaf Studies and Deaf Education, 3*, 80–134.

Locke, J. (1978). Phonemic effects in the silent reading of hearing and deaf children. *Cognition, 6*, 175–187.

Locke, J., & Locke, V. (1971). Deaf children's phonetic, visual and dactylic coding in a grapheme recall task. *Journal of Experimental Psychology, 89*, 142–146.

Lollis, J., & LaSasso, C. (2009). The appropriateness of the NC state-mandated reading competency test for deaf students as a criterion for high school graduation. *Journal of Deaf Studies and Deaf Education, 14*(1), 76–98.

Lundberg, I., Olofsson, A., & Wall, S. (1980). Reading and spelling skills in the first school years predicted from phonemic awareness skills in kindergarten. *Scandinavian Journal of Psychology, 21*, 159–173.

Maclean, M., Bryant, P., & Bradley, L. (1987). Rhymes, nursery rhymes, and reading in early childhood. *Merrill-Palmer Quarterly, 33*, 255–281.

MacSweeney, M., Campbell, R., Calvert, G., McGuire, P., David, A., Suckling, J., . . . Brammer, M. J. (2001). Dispersed activation in the left temporal cortex for speech-reading in congenitally deaf people. *Proceedings of Royal Society of London, 268,* 451–457.

MacSweeney, M., Campbell, R., & Donlan, C. (1996). Varieties of short-term memory coding in deaf teenagers. *Journal of Deaf Studies and Deaf Education, 1,* 249–262.

Marschark, M. (1993). *Psychological development of deaf children.* New York, NY: Oxford University Press.

Marschark, M., (2006). *Educating deaf students: Is literacy the issue?* Paper presented at the 2006 PEPNet conference Roots and Wings. Proceedings available from the University of Tennessee, Postsecondary Education Consortium Web site, http://sunsite.utk.edu/cod/pec/products.html

Mattingly, I. (1972). Reading, the linguistic process and linguistic awxareness. In J. Kavanagh & I. Mattingly (Eds.), *Phonological awareness in reading: the evolution of current perspectives* (pp. 31–71). New York, NY: Springer-Verlag.

Morais, J., Bertelson, P., Cary, L., & Alegria, J. (1986). Literacy training and speech analysis. *Cognition, 24,* 45–64.

Morais, J., Cary, L., Alegria, J., & Bertelson, P. (1979). Does awareness of speech as a sequence of phones arise spontaneously? *Cognition, 7,* 323–331.

National Reading Panel. (2000). *Teaching children to read: An evidence-based assessment of the Scientific literature on reading and its implications for reading instruction.* United States Department of Health and Human Services.

No Child Left Behind Act of 2001. 20 U.S.C. 6301 et seq (2002).

Nunes, T., Bryant P., & Bindman, M. (1997). Morphological spelling strategies: Developmental stages and processes. *Developmental Psychology, 33,* 637–649.

O'Donoghue, G., Nikolopoulos; T., Archbold, S. (2000). Determinants of speech perception in children after cochlear implantation. *The Lancet, 356,* 466–468.

Orton, S. (1937). *Reading, writing, and speech problems in children.* New York, NY: Norton.

Padden, C., & Hanson, V. (1999). Search for the missing link: The development of skilled reading in deaf children. In H. Lane & K. Emmorey (Eds.), *The signs of language revisited: An anthology to honor Ursula Bellugi and Edward Klima* (pp. 435–449). Hillsdale, NJ: Lawrence Erlbaum.

Padden, C., & Ramsey, C. (2000). American sign language and reading ability in deaf children. In C. Chamberlain, J. Morford, & R. Mayberry (Eds.), *Language acquisition by eye* (pp. 165–189). Mahwah, NJ: Lawrence Erlbaum Associates.

Paul, P. (1984). *Literacy and deafness: The development of reading, writing, and literate thought.* New York, NY: Psychology Press.

Paulesu, E., Frith, C., & Frackowiack, R. (1993). The neural correlates of the verbal component of working memory. *Nature, 362,* 342–345.

Perfetti, C. (1992). The representation problem in reading acquisition. In P. Gough, L. Ehri, & R. Treiman (Eds.), *Reading acquisition* (pp. 145–174). Hillsdale, NJ: Erlbaum.

Perfetti, C. (1997). The psycholinguistics of spelling and reading. In C. Perfetti, L. Rieben, & M. Fayol (Eds.), *Learning to spell: Research, theory, and practice across languages* (pp. 21–38). Mahwah, NJ: Erlbaum.

Perfetti, C., Beck, I., Bell, L., & Hughes, C. (1987). Phonemic knowledge and learning to read are reciprocal: A longitudinal study of first-grade children. *Merrill-Palmer Quarterly, 33,* 283–319.

Perfetti, C., & Sandak, R. (2000). Reading optimally builds on spoken language: Implications for deaf readers. *Journal of Deaf Studies and Deaf Education, 5,* 32–50.

Pugh, K., Shaywitz, B., Shaywitz, S., & Shankweiler, D. (1997). Predicting reading performance from neuroimaging profiles: The cerebral basis of phonological effects in printed word identification. *Journal of Experimental Psychology: Human Perception and Performance, 23,* 299–318.

Raven, J., Court, J., & Raven, J. (1983). *Manual for Raven's Progressive Matrices and Vocabulary Scales (Section 3)—Standard Progressive Matrices (1983 edition).* London, UK: Lewis.

Rayman, J., & Zaidel, E. (1991). Rhyming and the right hemisphere. *Brain and Language, 40,* 89–105.

Rayner, K., Foorman, B., Perfetti, C., Pesetsky, D., & Seidenberg, M. (2001). How psychological science informs the teaching of reading. *Psychological Science in the Public Interest, 2,* 31–74.

Read, C., Zhang, Y., Nie, H., & Ding, B. (1986). The ability to manipulate speech sounds depends on knowing the alphabetic principle. *Cognition, 24,* 31–45.

Share, D. (1999). Phonological recoding and orthographic learning: A direct test of the self-teaching hypothesis. *Journal of Experimental Child Psychology, 72,* 95–129.

Shaywitz, S. (2003). *Overcoming dyslexia: A new and complete science-based program for reading problems at any level.* New York, NY: Knopf.

Simos, P., Breier, J., Wheless, J., Maggio, W., Fletcher, J., Castillo, E., & Papanicolaou, A. (2000). Brain mechanisms for reading: The role of the superior temporal gyrus in word and pseudoword naming. *Neuroreport, 11,* 2443–2447.

Smith, F. (1997) *Reading without nonsense* (3rd ed.). New York, NY: Teachers College Press.

Spencer, P., & Marschark, M. (2003), Cochlear implants: Issues and Implications. In M. Marschark & P. Spencer (Eds.), *Oxford handbook of deaf studies, language and education* (pp. 434–448). New York, NY: Oxford University Press.

Sprenger-Charolles, L., & Siegel, L. (1997). A longitudinal study of the effects of syllabic structure on the development of reading and spelling skills in French. *Applied Psycholinguistics, 18,* 485–505.

Sterne, A. (1996). *Phonological awareness, memory, and reading in deaf children.* Cambridge, UK: University of Cambridge.

Sterne, A., & Goswami, U. (2000). Phonological awareness of syllables, rhymes, and phonemes in deaf children. *Journal of Child Psychology and Psychiatry, 41,* 609–625.

Stokoe, W. (1971). *The study of sign language.* Silver Spring, MD: National Association of the Deaf.

Studdert-Kennedy, M. (1986). Sources of variability in early speech development. In J. Perkell & D. Klatt (Eds.), *Invariance and variability in speech processes* (pp. 58–84). Hillsdale, NJ: Erlbaum.

Sutcliffe, A., Dowker, A., & Campbell, R. (1999). Deaf children's spelling: Does it show sensitivity to phonology? *Journal of Deaf Studies and Deaf Education, 4,* 111–123.

Svirsky, M., Robbins, A., Kirk, K., Pisoni, D., & Miyamoto, R. T. (2000). Language development in profoundly deaf children with cochlear implants. *Psychological Science, 11,* 153–158.

Traxler, C. (2000). The Stanford Achievement Test, 9th edition: National norming and performance standards for deaf and hard-of-hearing students. *Journal of Deaf Studies and Deaf Education, 5,* 337–348.

Treiman, R. (1993). *Beginning to spell: A study of first-grade children.* New York, NY: Oxford University Press.

Treiman, R., & Cassar, M. (1997). Spelling acquisition in English. In C. Perfetti, L. Rieben, & M. Fayol (Eds.), *Learning to spell: Research, theory, and practices across languages* (pp. 61–80). Mahwah, NJ: Erlbaum.

Trezek, B., Paul, P., & Wang, Y. (2009). *Reading and deafness: Theory, research, and practice.* Clifton Park, NY: Delmar Cengage Learning.

Trezak, B., Wang, Y., Woods, D., Gampp, T., & Paul, P. (2007) Using Visual Phonics to supplement beginning reading instruction for students who are deaf or hard of hearing. *Journal of Deaf Studies and Deaf Education, 12,* 373–384.

Véronis, J. (1986). Etude quantitative sur le système graphique et phono-graphique du francois. *Cahiers de Psychologie Cognitive, 6,* 501–531.

Waddy-Smith, B., & Wilson, V. (2003). See that sound! Visual Phonics helps deaf and hard of hearing students develop reading skills. *Odyssey, 5,* 14–17.

Wagner, R., & Torgesen, J. (1987). The nature of phonological processing and its causal role in the acquisition of reading skills. *Psychological Bulletin, 101,* 192–212.

Walden, B., Prosek, R., Montgomery, A., Scherr, C., & Jones, C. (1977). Effect of training on the visual recognition of consonants. *Journal of Speech and Hearing Research, 20*, 130–145.

Wandel, J. (1989). *Use of internal speech in reading by hearing and hearing impaired students in oral, total communication, and Cued Speech programs.* Unpublished doctoral dissertation, Teacher's College, Columbia University, New York, NY.

Waters, G., & Doehring, D. (1990). Reading acquisition in congenitally deaf children who communicate orally: Insights from an analysis of component reading, language, and memory skills. In T. Carr & B. Levy (Eds.), *Reading and its development: Component skills approaches* (pp. 323–373). San Diego, CA: Academic Press.

Wilcox, S. (1992). *The phonetics of finger spelling.* Amsterdam, the Netherlands: John Benjamins.

Wimmer, H., & Hummer, P. (1990). How German speaking first graders read and spell: Doubts on the importance of the logographic stage. *Applied Psycholinguistics, 11*, 349–368.

Chapter 12

CUED LANGUAGE FOR THE DEVELOPMENT OF DEAF STUDENTS' READING COMPREHENSION AND MEASURED READING COMPREHENSION[1]

Carol J. LaSasso and Kelly Lamar Crain

Reading is a term that lacks a single, universal definition. A parent who boasts that her young child is able to read before kindergarten is defining reading in a narrow sense, as the alphabetic principle. A parent of a 9 to 10-year-old child who expresses concern that the child is not a good reader *may* be referring to mastery of the alphabetic principle, but more likely, the parent is referring to the child's comprehension. Parents or teachers who refer to a particular child's "reading level" are referring to the child's measured reading comprehension, that is, performance on a formal or informal reading test, which may or may not correspond to what the child actually comprehended (LaSasso, 1987).

Most of the experimental research related to reading abilities of deaf students has focused on reading in a narrow sense, as decoding, or the alphabetic principle. Practitioners responsible for developing reading abilities of deaf (or hearing)

[1]Portions of this chapter are reprinted in part from, "An alternate route to preparing deaf children for bilingual-bicultural programs: The home language as L1 and Cued Speech for conveying English and other traditionally spoken languages" by Carol LaSasso and Melanie Metzger, originally published in *Journal of Deaf Studies and Deaf Education*, 3, 264–289. Copyright 1998, Oxford University Press. Used with permission.

students, however, realize that the alphabetic principle is only part of what students need to learn to be successful readers. Readers of this book may be surprised to learn that reading problems of deaf readers in the United States beyond the primary (K–3) grades are related less to phonological awareness and the alphabetic principle and are more related to: (1) the language encoded in print, (2) background knowledge presumed of readers, and/or (3) test-taking skills. In other words, what impedes deaf readers the most beyond the primary grades on reading tests is what would impede them the most if the text and reading test were conveyed to them conversationally via spoken, fingerspelled, or signed English (see Marschark et al., 2009 for a discussion of the critical role of language comprehension on measures of learning).

Early in the conceptualization of this book, due to the multiple uses of the term "reading," by parents, teachers, policy makers, and reading scholars and the keen interest among stakeholders in improving deaf students' reading levels, we decided to devote *two* chapters to reading: one focusing on reading in the narrow sense as mastery of the alphabetic principle and a second focusing on reading in the broader sense as comprehension or measured reading comprehension. Chapter 11 addresses reading in a narrow sense and focuses on the role played by Cued Speech and cued language in *beginning reading instruction* in the kindergarten to 12th grade (K to 12) educational continuum; that is, on the development of fundamental phonological and graphemic skills, including: phonemic awareness, phonological recoding, phonics, and spelling, each of which employs the alphabetic principle. Chapter 12 focuses on the role of Cued Speech on reading more broadly defined as *reading comprehension* or *measured*

reading comprehension (including performance on standardized tests). Karchmer and Mitchell (2003) note that "the issue of standardized reading assessment performance remains the primary focus of deaf education" (p. 21). The focus of this chapter is on variables besides the alphabetic principle that impact on deaf students' comprehension and performance on reading tests, including: linguistic abilities, background knowledge, and test-taking abilities. Included in this chapter is support for our view that deaf children do not need to be considered disabled in terms of acquiring English and other traditionally spoken languages naturally, learning to read with the same instructional materials and procedures used with hearing peers, and taking the same standardized tests as hearing peers without special accommodations. Cued speech and cued language are compared to MCE sign systems for natural language acquisition, and Cued Speech and Visual Phonics are compared for the development of deaf students' reading abilities. As background for our discussion of the merits of Cued Speech for the development of deaf students' reading abilities, we begin by discussing the range of perspectives related to the construct of reading comprehension, and we discuss issues related to formal and informal measures of reading comprehension used with deaf students.

Reading Comprehension

Reading comprehension involves an intricate intertwining of: (1) *reader* characteristics, including perceptual, cognitive, metacognitive, and linguistic abilities, as well as memory, background knowledge, motivation, and questions about what is being read, (2) *text* characteristics, including structure and cohesion, (3) *test* charac-teristics, related to test format and type of comprehension being assessed, and (4) a "tricky mix" (Nelson & Camarata, 1996) of learning conditions, including self-esteem and related factors. Because reading is a covert process, one that cannot be observed directly, numerous theories have been developed to try and describe or explain it (see Kamil, Mosenthal, Pearson, & Barr, 2000 for a review of reading theories). It is vital for teachers of reading to be able to articulate a clear construct of reading and the factors that influence it. Without a clear construct of the reading process, teachers of deaf (or hearing) students are at risk of focusing too much time on one aspect of the reading process (e.g., decod-ing) and not enough on others (e.g., lan-guage comprehension or performance on reading tests). It is, therefore, a goal of this chapter to provide a clear and useful theory of reading upon which to base instruction and assessment.

Reading theories vary in terms of their *relative* emphases on different aspects of the process (Purcell-Gates, 1997). Some theories emphasize the role of letter and word recognition, such as Gough's (1972) theory related to informational process-ing, and LaBerge and Samuels' (1974) the-ory related to automaticity. Others, such as Goodman's (1974) psycholinguistic "guessing game" theory, emphasize the role of *comprehension* over letter and word identification. More recent theories em-phasize the role of phonemic awareness to word recognition and automaticity, such as that espoused by Adams (1990), or the role of social and cultural context and the relationship between reader and text, such as Rosenblatt's (1994) transactional theory or Rumelhart's (1977) interactive theory. Ehri (1995) proposes a series of phases through which the developing reader progresses in the development of word automaticity, from pre-alphabetic, through partial and full alphabetic, and finally to the consolidated alphabetic phase, wherein readers recognize printed words by letter patterns that occur across different words.

Reading Comprehension Based on Readers' Questions

A simple yet surprisingly comprehensive view of reading, found by many parents and teachers of deaf (and hearing) chil-dren to be helpful in diagnosing and addressing children's reading difficulties, conceptualizes reading comprehension as a process that goes forward or is impeded in terms of readers' questions about what they read (LaSasso, 1990; Smith, 2004). In this view, reading comprehension is defined as the "reduction of uncertainty." Specifically, reading comprehension is enhanced or impeded by the reader's uncertainty, or questions, about what is being read (Smith, 2004). Readers either read for their *own* purpose (i.e., to answer their own questions) or they read for the *teacher's* or other *test-maker's* purpose. Questions of readers who are reading for their own purpose can be categorized as being about: (1) the written code, (2) the lan-guage encoded in print, or (3) the content of print material. Readers *in instructional situations* who are reading in preparation for a test constructed by a teacher or another test-constructor face two addi-tional types of questions related to the *task*, specifically: the test constructor's *purpose* for reading and the *format* of the reading test (LaSasso, 1996). These addi-tional questions will be discussed later in this chapter in the section addressing measured reading comprehension.

Questions About the Code

Readers' questions about the code pertain to the printed form of the language, including the printed words and punctuation. If a reader encounters a word that is not a sight word (i.e., not instantly recognized), the reader may be able to identify it by applying word attack skills such as phonics, contextual analysis or structural analysis.

Phonics Analysis. Phonics involves using one's knowledge of the relationship between the phonemes and graphemes of a language (i.e., the alphabetic principle, see Chapter 11) to "sound out" (or in the case of deaf cuers, "cue out"), or decode, an unfamiliar print form of a word that is in the reader's vocabulary. *Preezgribe* and *ahrunj* are examples of phonically regular nonwords whose meaning can be determined by analyzing them phonically.[2]

Phonics has been identified by the National Reading Panel (NRP) as being one of five critical abilities related to reading comprehension (NRP, 2000). In terms of the alphabetic principle, written French and Spanish are considered to be fairly *transparent* languages due to a fairly consistent phoneme-grapheme (i.e., phonics) relationship; however, written English is characterized as being much less transparent due to the many phonic irregularities. For example, children who learn the English pronunciation of *ow* in the written word *cow* (/kaʊ/) will not pronounce *ow* in *low* (/loʊ/) in its written form correctly.

Much of the early reading instruction with hearing children in the United States focuses on teaching phonics rules (i.e., generalizations) and exceptions to those rules. Phonics generalizations allow hearing readers of English to employ an auditory feedback system to *sound out* unfamiliar print forms of words they have in their "auditory" vocabulary. For example, readers of the English word *cat* who know the phonics rule that the grapheme *c* followed by the grapheme *a* usually has a /k/ pronunciation instead of a /s/ pronunciation, might say to themselves: *kuh-ah-tuh* several times and increasingly quickly until they pronounce *cat* (/kæt/) and have a mental picture of a small furry animal with a long tail. In another example, readers of a phonically regular spelling of an English phrase, such as *waunsuppun-nuhtyem*, can vocally or subvocally experiment with different possible syllables and pronunciations of the letters and letter groups in those syllables and blend the letter "sounds" together until they vocalize or subvocalize a phrase that they have heard before and associated with meaning (i.e., *once upon a time*).

Traditionally, phonics has been conceptualized as an ability that *requires* an auditory feedback system, however, deaf children who use American Sign Language (ASL) who have limited, if any, auditory feedback capability, report using phonics; however, they report that they use a *tactile-kinesthetic feedback system* rather than an auditory feedback system (LaSasso, 1996). Using the example of cat (/kæt/) again, in the same way that hearing readers try different combinations of sounds, or auditory sensations, until they produce an auditory sensation that evokes the mental picture of a cat, deaf signers and deaf cuers report that they try different combinations of tactile-kinesthetic sensations in their vocal tract until they arrive

---

[2]Prescribe and orange.

at a familiar combination of sensations that evokes the mental picture of a cat. It should be noted that it does not appear to be necessary for deaf signers or cuers to pronounce the word *correctly* to be able to phonically decode it. What appears to be critical is *consistency* in pronunciation. Deaf cuers, who are asked to decipher, or decode, a phonically regular word, such as *cat* or *waunsuppunnuhtyem*, are observed to not *sound out*, but rather *cue out*, a word until they arrive at words in their visual or tactile-kinesthetic *cue vocabulary* (La-Sasso, 1996). Typically, cuers will produce a lipreadable form of the word; however, because cued language requires no use of sound, a deaf person's ability to produce the related speech constitutes a separate skill (see Chapter 3).

Readers who master the phoneme-grapheme relationship of a language have an advantage when they come to unfamiliar print forms of words they already know. An advantage of having a *cue-read vocabulary* versus an *MCE sign vocabulary* is that cue-read vocabulary will have a *phonological* component which, like that of hearing readers, when combined with the graphemic or orthographic component during reading, will enable the formation of a phonological assembly system which can be used to independently decipher, or decode, words not previously encountered in print (see Chapter 11). To the extent that a reader can phonologically assemble words, the reader does not need to memorize a large number of sight words. It can take dozens of exposures to a word before it becomes a sight word. An additional advantage of the phonological component of phonics is that it assists in the storage of the surface structure of written text in working memory while that text is being processed. Refer to Chapter 11 for a discussion of studies supporting the effi-cacy of cueing for the development of working memory abilities.

Contextual Analysis. Contextual analysis involves using pictures or other words encoded in the sentence or paragraph to help the reader determine the meaning of an unknown word. For readers who have mastered the alphabetic code, contextual analysis is the word recognition strategy used most often by readers to determine the meaning of an unknown printed word. The meaning of *flim* and *bliks* can be determined through contextual clues in the following sentences (LaSasso, 1994).

1. A *flim* is a closed figure with three straight sides.
2. Oranges, pineapples, and lemons are some of the *bliks* grown in Florida.

Contextual analysis can be a particularly effective strategy when the unknown written word is not phonically regular, such as in the following English words: *come, have, were, does, laugh, eight,* all of which are on the list of the 220 most common English words (Dolch, 1948). Effective use of contextual analysis, however, requires that readers understand how words are assembled *syntactically* in English to convey meaning. Knowledge of English syntax has been found to be challenging for deaf students from noncueing backgrounds. Numerous studies have shown that deaf children from oral and signing backgrounds do not perform as well as hearing peers on tests of knowledge of the following English syntactic structures: negatives, relative clauses, passive voice, question forms, pronominalization, and complementation (see King & Quigley, 1985; and Paul, 1998 for a review). However, as reflected in Chapter 11, deaf children, like hearing children, *can* acquire morphosyntactic rules *naturally* when they have early clear complete visual access to that language. Deaf cuers whose parents cued to them early, during the critical language learning years, have been found to have morphosyntactic abilities comparable to those of their hearing peers (Hage & Leybaert, 2006). This may explain the superior performance of deaf cuers, compared to noncuers, on reading comprehension tests (Wandel, 1989).

Structural Analysis. Structural analysis involves using sublexical morphemes, such as inflections, other *affixes*, and *syllables* as clues for identifying the meaning of unfamiliar printed words. To the extent that readers can use their knowledge of sublexical units of English, they will have fewer questions about the *meaning* of English words containing those structures.

Creators of MCE sign systems, recognizing the importance of sublexical morphemic information not readily available from ASL base signs, invented separate signed units such as *pre-, -ment, -ing, -s, -ed*. There are at least three limitations of these invented markers for such sublexical units. First, separate and discrete sign markers were not created for every English affix, making it necessary to use a single sign marker and rely on speechread information to disambiguate such affixes as *–ish* and *–esque*, (as in *mannish* and *statuesque*) or *–ette* and *-ina* (as in *launderette* and *czarina*). Second, adding "signs" to the beginning and/or end of ASL signs becomes cumbersome and affects the fluency of signing as compared to the spoken English message. Third, many fundamental *bound morphemes* are embedded within their root words; for example, the English word *ran* contains two morphemes that are conveyed simultaneously and cannot be extricated from one another. Example 12–1 shows an illustration of the inability of MCE sign systems to convey embedded morphemes.

Example 12–1

English   (4 words):
HE LOCKED THE DOOR

MCE   (5 signs):
HE LOCK PAST-TENSE MARKER THE DOOR

Deaf cuers have an advantage over users of MCE sign systems in that their exposure to (and acquisition of) all sublexical morphemic units of English mirrors the way that the phonemes are pronounced, whether as conjoined free + bound morphemes, or as bound morphemes embedded within lexical units.

Questions About the Language

From the literature related to hearing readers, we know that language skills contribute substantial and unique variance to reading development, in addition to phonological processing skills (Nation, 2005). Studies measuring language and phonological processing skills in hearing students have found that language development plays a protracted and central role in reading development. In first and second grades, language difficulties are strongly associated with reading problems, over and above phonics skills. Students who exhibit reading problems beyond the primary grades have been found to have impaired listening comprehension (Nation & Angell, 2006).

Deaf children from noncueing backgrounds generally present delays in phonology, vocabulary development, morphosyntactic development, and pragmatic development (see Paul, 1998, 2008; and

Quigley & Paul, 1984, for reviews). Deaf children's underachievement in a first language is generally cited as the primary reason for their difficulty in learning to read (Conrad, 1979, 2006; Paul, 2008).

Readers' questions about the language encoded in print include questions about: the vocabulary, figurative language, or syntax, including Wh-question forms that are encoded in test passages and/or related test items. A young deaf reader might have vocabulary-related questions while reading *"A warm-blooded, feathered vertebrate is pursued by the domesticated, feline quadruped"* (Smith, 2004, p. 33) while having few vocabulary-related questions with *"The cat is chasing the bird,"* which has virtually the same meaning.

Figurative expressions, such as *"He drives me up a wall," "Don't beat around the bush,"* or *"Don't cry over spilt milk"* can be problematic for literal readers, young readers whose first language is not English, and for readers who are deaf (Fruchter, Wilbur, & Fraser, 1984; Rittenhouse & Kenyon, 1990). It is not unusual for even highly educated deaf or foreign-born adults to not be able to supply the word replaced by a nonsense word in the following sentences: (1) *"It has been one of those tidtads"* and (2) *"In this case, two is company, but three is a gul."* Familiarity with English figurative expressions is required to understand that *tidtads* refers to days or weeks and *gul* refers to crowd. Prereading vocabulary and figurative language acquisition in hearing and cueing children typically occurs naturally, without formal instruction, in play-based interactions with parents and others in the child's environment.

English syntax refers to how words are arranged in English to convey meaning. A deaf reader who is unfamiliar with *passive voice* in the following sentence: *"The lion was killed by the hunter"* might have a question about whether the lion or hunter was killed. A deaf student who has difficulty with *question forms* might respond with *"Eggs, oil, flour, and water"* to the question: *"Who brought the cake?"* The following syntactically complex sentence would tax the working memory of listeners or readers who process the words one at a time without grouping the words into syntactically acceptable propositions: *"Mark Watkins' big, white, farmhouse, on the tree-lined cul-de-sac, on Hedge Avenue, behind the church, was recently demolished by a hurricane."* There are at least nine propositions in this sentence, including: (1) a hurricane demolished the house recently; (2) Mark Watkins has a house, (3) the house is big, (4) the house is white, (5) the house is a farm house, (6) the house is on a cul-de-sac, (7) the cul-de-sac is tree-lined, (8) the house is on Hedge Avenue, and (9) the house is behind the church. These units of meaning are related but are expressed in a sentence of more than 20 words with a passive verb, which puts the subject (hurricane) at the end of the sentence. The point of this sentence (i.e., that the farmhouse was demolished) might be missed by a reader who tries to hold each piece of information in working memory until the end of the sentence.

Syntax typically is not *taught* to young children; rather, children typically *acquire*, or *deduce*, syntactic rules naturally, in linguistic interactions with parents and other adults when they have clear, complete visual access to their home language, such as that provided by Cued Speech. The advantage of deaf readers or test-takers from Cued Speech backgrounds versus non-Cued Speech backgrounds is that they tend to have fewer questions about the language encoded in print and are better able to focus their attention on their questions related to the code, content, or reading task.

Questions About the Content

Readers may have questions about the *content* of the text that are separate from their questions about the code or language. Consider, for example, students who read the following inferential test item:

> Mrs. Grodinsky, the Kindergarten teacher, sent Aron to the principal's office. Why?"
>
> _____ (1) to get a pencil
> _____ (2) to be reprimanded.

It is not uncommon for a foreign college student to select the first response option to the inferential question. Foreign students' lack of background knowledge about the role and normal functions of a school principal may prevent them from selecting a correct answer whereas English readers, more familiar with the role of a school principal, tend to have no trouble selecting the second response option as the "correct" answer. Similarly, deaf students' lack of general world knowledge or background knowledge often prevents them from connecting that knowledge to information in the text being read and making appropriate inferences while reading (Andrews & Mason, 1991; Walker, Munro, & Rickards, 1998). The classic example illustrating the power of relevant background knowledge is that of Bransford and Johnson (1972), shown in Example 12–2. Read the passage and reflect on why it is difficult to understand. Next, look at the illustration in Appendix 12-A. Finally, reread the passage.

Example 12–2

If the balloons popped, the sound wouldn't be able to carry since everything would be too far away from the correct floor. A closed window would also prevent the sound from carrying. Since the whole operation depends on a steady flow of electricity, a break in the middle of the wire also would cause problems. Of course, the fellow could shout, but the human voice is not loud enough to carry that far. An additional problem is that a string could break on the instrument. Then there could be no accompaniment to the message. It is clear that the best situation would involve less distance. Then there would be fewer problems. With face to face contact, the least number of things could go wrong.

As this example illustrates, regardless of how familiar the vocabulary and figurative expressions, how basic and understandable the syntax, and how familiar the printed code is to the reader, nothing substitutes for having requisite *background knowledge* for being able to comprehend a linguistic message, regardless of how it is communicated (e.g., spoken, cued, fingerspelled, signed, or written). In the experience of the authors of this chapter, deaf cuers, who have had early, clear English language interaction with parents and others in natural play-based situations, tend to come to school with background knowledge more comparable to that of hearing peers than deaf peers from noncueing backgrounds.

Measured Reading Comprehension

In the previous section, we described reading comprehension as a complicated perceptual, linguistic, cognitive process, influenced by readers' background knowledge and other factors. We discussed a particular view that conceptualizes reading comprehension as a process that is directly influenced by readers' questions in three categories related to the language, content, and code. Readers who get answers to their own questions while reading can be said to have comprehended what they read. In this section, we discuss reading comprehension in the context of *instructional situations* where students need to read to answer the *teacher's* questions (which may or may not be the same as the student's questions) and *produce* something that can be measured and evaluated by the teacher to determine whether the student has comprehended. We begin with a discussion of two additional types of questions readers may have in instructional situations that they do not have when reading for their own purposes. Next, we describe two common types of reading tasks used by teachers to assess deaf students' reading comprehension: informal "read aloud" protocols and more formal standardized reading tests. We discuss the advantages of deaf cuers compared to noncuers on each type of test.

Two Additional Categories of Readers' Questions in Instructional Contexts

Readers in instructional situations potentially have questions in the same three categories (i.e., language, content, and code) as when they are reading for their own purpose. In instructional situations, however, readers may have questions in two additional categories related to the nature of the *reading task*: (1) the *test-maker's purpose for reading* (e.g., to answer questions posed by the teacher or another test-maker) and (2) the *format* of the reading test. Impor-

tantly, to the extent that readers' questions do not match those of the test-maker, the reader (deaf or hearing) may not be able to demonstrate comprehension. For this reason, it is important for teachers to inform their students about the questions they will be expected to answer at the completion of a reading task.

Equally important as knowing the test-maker's purpose for reading is knowing what to expect in terms of the *test format*. Readers who prepare for one type of test format may not be able to demonstrate comprehension on a test with a different format. For example, reading in a way to be able to produce written responses to *essay* questions on a reading test is different from reading in a way to be able to recognize the correct answer from among the alternatives on multiple-choice test questions. Teachers should always be clear with their students about the format of a reading test that will be used to measure reading comprehension.

Formal and Informal Measures of Reading Comprehension and Fluency

Assessment of reading comprehension can either be informal via informal reading inventories (LaSasso & Swaiko, 1983), cloze tests, or read aloud procedures (Easterbrooks & Huston, 2008), or they can be more formal via standardized reading comprehension tests (Lollis & LaSasso, 2009). We will limit our discussion of informal measures here to read aloud assessments of fluency because of a widely held assumption that this type of assessment is not suitable for deaf students who do not have intelligible speech (see Easterbrooks & Huston, 2008).

Informal Read Aloud Assessments

One common informal method used to assess hearing readers' comprehension and to diagnose readers' questions while reading involves having readers read aloud printed words, sentences, or passages and assessing the reader's fluency, which includes: *speed, accuracy,* and *proper expression* (NRP, 2000). Reading *speed* typically is reported as the number of words read aloud per minute, while *accuracy* refers to the number of words read correctly. Reading speed has been positively correlated to hearing readers' measured reading comprehension (Jenkins, Fuchs, van den Broek, Epsin, & Deno, 2003; Swanson & Howell, 2001). Reading *accuracy* typically is calculated either in the context of connected text or isolated words. The first method for calculating reading accuracy involves: having a student read a passage aloud; making a verbatim transcription of the read-aloud; analyzing the transcription in terms of reading syntactic, semantic, and/or orthographic miscues; and reporting the number or proportion of miscues in each category. The second method involves having students read aloud a specified number of printed words in isolation or in word lists and calculating the time needed to recognize those words. This latter method, involving measures of both accuracy (correct pronunciation) and rate (number of words in a number of minutes), is referred to as a measure of *automaticity* (Kelly, 2003). To the extent that a reader recognizes words instantly and does not need to analyze them phonically, the burden on working memory is lessened and the reader can focus more attention on other aspects of reading, such as the content or reading task.

Prosodic expression, referring to pitch, stress, and juncture of the spoken word, requires that a reader group words together in phrases, rather than reading word-for-word. Readers who read aloud with appropriate emphasis, phrasing, and other prosodic elements reflect that they are actively engaged in interpreting or constructing meaning from the passage (Rasinski, 2004). Readers who read word-for-word are at risk for over-burdening working memory until they arrive at the end of a sentence. For example, in the previous example of the farmhouse destroyed by the hurricane, the reader needs to hold more than 20 words in working memory before arriving at the final word in the sentence (hurricane), which could burden the reader's working memory if the reader cannot *chunk* the individual words into larger units, such as phrases, and hold a smaller number of phrases in short term memory than individual words.

Teachers and other practitioners working with noncueing deaf students know that the assessment of their reading fluency can be challenging if not impossible. To the extent that the speech of deaf noncuers is unintelligible, practitioners are handicapped in judging fluency on traditional read aloud tasks. Frustration with traditional read aloud methods that depend on speech intelligibility for assessing reading fluency led Easterbrooks and Huston (2008) to devise a compensatory *signed fluency* test for deaf students. This assessment attempts to circumvent the presumed dependence upon traditionally oral language abilities and speech intelligibility, but necessarily sacrifices calculations of rate and accuracy, which are standard among traditional *reading fluency* measures.

Deaf cuers, regardless of speech intelligibility, *are* able to demonstrate to cueing teachers all three aspects of reading fluency traditionally assessed in hearing readers: rate, accuracy, and proper expression (including prosodic expression). They do so by cueing aloud a portion of a text (either with or without speech), and the cueing teacher can determine *solely from the visual information* from the cues, mouth movements, and facial expression whether the student is reading words correctly at an appropriate rate and with appropriate prosody. Importantly, the accurate assessment of reading fluency of deaf cuers is possible in the absence of speech or *regardless of speech intelligibility*. In the sole study of reading fluency of deaf students from a variety of language and communication backgrounds (see Chapter 13), deaf cuers were found to have superior reading fluency scores compared to those of peers from oral and signing backgrounds. A clear advantage of cued English over signed English, spoken English, or ASL is that it *is* possible via cued English to assess deaf students' expressive reading fluency, including rate, accuracy, and prosody in real time and in the language encoded in the text.

Standardized Reading Comprehension Tests

Despite the lack of a one-to-one correspondence between what a reader (deaf or hearing) comprehends and what the reader produces on a reading test, standardized reading comprehension tests have been commonplace in education in the United States for nearly a century (National Research Council [NRC], 1999; Valencia & Wixson, 2000). For much of that time, these tests have been administered to deaf students, despite the fact that the tests were not designed for special educa-

tion students (Cawthon, 2004, 2006, 2007; Martin & Mounty, 2005). Findings from a recent national survey of assessment practices, conducted by Luckner and Bowen (2006), indicate that statewide annual reading assessments are the most often reported type of reading assessment used with deaf students, followed by the Stanford Achievement Test and Woodcock Johnson III Test of Achievement. Standardized test scores are used for different purposes, including gauging program effectiveness, determining student placement, and planning instruction (Scheuneman & Oakland, 1998).

Typically, standardized reading comprehension tests are comprised of short narrative or expository passages with related test items consisting of either Wh-question stems (beginning with *who, what, where, when, why,* or *how*) or incomplete statement stems (e.g., *A _____ is an example of a fruit*). Students select from among 3–5 response options consisting of 3 to 4 foils (distractors) and the correct answer. Standardized tests are typically timed and administered in a prescribed manner. Students' raw scores are converted to grade level equivalents, or "reading levels." A fourth-grade "reading level" is interpreted to mean the student performed like the average 9-year-old fourth grade student who took the test. Typically, standardized tests have been subjected to various psychometric procedures to determine validity and reliability for the general population.

A fundamental problem related to standardized reading tests is that there is not a one-to-one relationship between what a reader *comprehends* during the process of reading and what the reader *produces* (i.e., the reading product) on the reading test/task to demonstrate comprehension. For example, a reader might fully comprehend what is read but fail to demonstrate that comprehension on a reading test due to factors such as: fatigue, memory required to answer the questions, or insufficient time to complete the test. Another reader might not comprehend much of the text but be able to make good guesses on the reading test or use visual matching, which is described later in this chapter (Brauer, Braden, Pollard, & Hardy-Braz, 1998; LaSasso, 1999).

It is beyond the scope of this chapter to discuss all psychometric considerations in constructing, evaluating, and/or selecting a standardized reading test; however, one principle related to testing deaf students, which is often overlooked, relates to the test's *appropriateness* or *fairness*, for all groups required to take the test. Test fairness, in psychometric terms, refers to a lack of bias for groups of students that differ from the general population of students in terms of gender, race-ethnicity, family income, or other characteristics (see, for example, Berk, 1982; Kunnan, 2008; National Research Council, 1999; Scheuneman & Oakland, 1998). During the past three decades, test fairness has received considerable attention in the courts, legislatures, schools, and employment settings (Pratt & Moreland, 1998). A criterion for a test being "fair" or "unbiased" is that the meaning of the test scores does not differ across individuals, groups, or settings (NRC, 1999); that is, if one population, based on gender, race-ethnicity, or family income, for example, is favored over another on a test item, the item is considered to be not fair and the test is considered to be biased. Much of the research related to test fairness for different populations, including noncueing deaf students (Lollis, 2002; Martin, 2005), has focused on the appropriateness of *language, content,* or *test format.*

Language Bias. Language bias in reading test passages or test items has received considerable attention in the research literature related to test fairness. The bulk of that research relates to second language learners, or English language learners, who are less than proficient with the English language (Abedi, 2004; Abedi & Dietel, 2004; Abedi, Leon, & Mirocha, 2001; Bailey, 2000; Butler & Stevens, 2001; Cunningham & Moore, 1993; Kopriva, 2000; Messick, 1989; Sandoval & Duran, 1998). Findings from these studies collectively suggest that English language learners score considerably lower on standardized reading tests than their native speaking peers; content reading assessment scores typically correlate with students' language proficiency scores; second language learners are more apt to interpret questions differently than native speakers who are familiar with the host culture; and the language of reading achievement tests is often beyond the proficiency level of many of the English language learners. Cunningham and Moore (1993) found that when the language of a reading test was modified for English language learners, their performance increased; that is, when everyday language and vocabulary were used in written comprehension questions, rather than academic language and vocabulary, the students' performance increased. Cunningham and Moore (1993) speculate that English language learners may become frustrated when, despite having mastered the content knowledge being assessed, they are stymied by the language requirements of the test.

In many regards, deaf readers from noncueing backgrounds are similar to hearing students who are English language learners. Numerous studies have compared vocabulary, figurative language, and syntax of noncueing deaf and hearing peers on tests of written language (see Lollis & LaSasso, 2009; Paul, 1998 for an overview). Findings from these studies consistently reveal that deaf students from oral and signing backgrounds lag behind their hearing age-mates in each of these linguistic dimensions. In addition, the length and linguistic complexity of reading test items have been shown to differentially influence hearing and (noncueing) deaf students' performance on reading tasks. Trybus and Buchanan (1973) found a positive correlation between the difficulty of the question for deaf students and the number of words in the question stem (i.e., probe or question) as well as the length of the passage. Rudner (1978) analyzed the data used by Trybus and Buchanan (1973) and concluded that the following linguistic structures created more difficulty for deaf test takers than their hearing peers when matched for reading level: (1) conditionals (e.g., *if* clauses), (2) comparatives (e.g., *greater than, the most*), (3) negatives (e.g., *not, without, answer not given*), (4) inferentials (e.g., *should, could, because, since*), (5) low information pronouns (e.g., *it, something*), and (6) lengthy passages. DiFrancesca and Carey (1972) found that differential performance between deaf and hearing readers on multiple-choice reading tests was related to some distracters not being as effective for (noncueing) deaf readers. For example, if one of the distracters were phonically similar to the correct answer, a hearing reader might select it, whereas a deaf reader might not.

Language bias on standardized tests was formally examined by Lollis (2002) on a high stakes state-mandated reading comprehension test designed for the general population of students in North Carolina but also administered to deaf students in that state. Results of the North Carolina test are a criterion for receiving a high school diploma. Lollis used the same procedures originally used to determine the appropriateness of the test for the general population of students in North Carolina: having curriculum specialists for the general population of students examine test passages and related test items (i.e., multiple choice questions) for test bias (i.e., differential impact) for different groups of readers, which did *not* include students who were deaf or hard of hearing. Lollis replicated that procedure with experienced teachers of deaf students and found test bias against deaf students related to both the language of the *passages* and the *test items* (Lollis, 2002). In a follow up study, Martin (2005) found the same language bias against deaf students in a high stakes, state-required reading comprehension test in New York. To the extent that deaf children taking a reading test comprehend the language and content of the passages and test items, they are more likely to perform like hearing peers on those tests. Stated differently, readers with fewer questions about the language, content, and code (e.g., readers from Cued Speech backgrounds) can focus more attention to their questions about the reading test.

Content Bias. The content of standardized reading test passages also has been found to differentially influence test performance of different groups of students and therefore, the test's fairness, or appropriateness. Content bias exists when: (1) the content of the test does not match the content of the curriculum (National Research Council, 1999) and/or (2) the content of reading passages assumes general world knowledge on the part of the reader (LaSasso, 1979). To the extent that the content of the test does not match the curriculum, a student's performance may be negatively affected (Benning, 2000; Lollis & LaSasso, 2009).

A form of content bias on standardized reading tests, referred to as *fund of information bias*, exists when the content of an achievement test reflects the test-taker's exposure to and familiarity with background knowledge, or general world knowledge, such as that derived from the radio, overhearing others' conversations, or informal play based situations, as opposed to what is learned in school (Brauer, Braden, Pollard, & Hardy-Braz, 1998, p. 305). Due to reduced sensory input, fund of world knowledge of deaf children typically is less extensive than that of hearing peers (Oakhill & Cain, 2000). Lollis (2002) and Martin (2005) found fund of information bias against deaf students in each of the state-mandated tests they assessed. Differential fund of information knowledge may explain why noncueing deaf children tend to plateau around the 3rd to 4th grade reading levels. Reading tasks in the primary (K to 3) grades focus on text-explicit (literal) questions to assess decoding skills of readers. Beginning in 4th grade, however, greater emphasis is placed on assessing readers' text implicit (inferential) knowledge which requires the reader to combine their background knowledge with knowledge on the printed page to answer the inferential question.

The often cited advantage of deaf children of (presumably ASL signing) deaf parents on early reading achievement tests (see Marschark, 1993) can be attributed to these children being able to interact naturally via a visual language with parents, which provides them general background knowledge presumed of readers by developers of early reading materials for young readers. Similarly, the advantage on reading achievement tests that deaf children of cueing parents have on reading tests (Wandel, 1989) can be attributed, in part, to their being able to interact via a complete visual language (e.g., cued English, cued French, or cued Spanish) with parents, thereby providing them with the background knowledge expected of hearing peers by developers of reading materials. Like deaf children of (presumably ASL signing) deaf parents, deaf children of hearing or deaf parents who cue English (or other traditionally spoken languages) with their children are likely to have fewer questions about the content of what they are reading than deaf children who cannot interact linguistically with their parents (see Chapter 8). The two advantages that deaf cuers have over ASL signers for reading instruction are that deaf cuers are likely to have fewer questions about: (1) the English language encoded in print and (2) the relationship between the phonemes and graphemes of a language (i.e., alphabetic code) and therefore can focus their attention on their questions related to the reading task.

Test Format Bias. A third type of bias that can impact deaf students' performance on standardized reading tests relates to test format. Research comparing (noncueing) deaf and hearing test takers on *format* variables (Bornstein, 1971; Davey & LaSasso, 1984; Davey, LaSasso, & Macready, 1983; DiFrancesca & Carey, 1972; LaSasso, 1979; McKee & Bondi-Wolcott, 1982; Osguthorpe, Long, & Ellsworth, 1977; Rudner, 1978; Trybus & Karchmer, 1977) collectively suggest that a number of test variables differentially affect deaf and hearing peers' reading comprehension test performance. These variables include: (1) the ability to reinspect, or look back at, the text while answering questions, (2) the *production* versus *recognition* response mode of the task, and (3) the placement of the correct answer in the list of response options on multiple-choice tests (see LaSasso & Lollis, 2009; & Paul, 1998 for a review).

Compensatory Test-Taking Strategies. Deaf students from oral and signing backgrounds also have been found to use specific, *compensatory* test-taking strategies more often than hearing peers on reading tests when (presumably) they are not comprehending what they are reading (LaSasso, 1985; 1986; Webster, Wood, & Griffiths, 1981; Wolk & Schildroth, 1984). Strategies, including guessing and the use of visual matching, often result in the student getting a correct answer to the question without comprehending.

LaSasso (1985, 1986) found that deaf students used visual matching extensively on a short answer, reading test when reinspection of the passage was permitted (LaSasso, 1985, 1986). The strategy, presumably employed when a test taker is not able to answer a test question, involves responding by writing a verbatim word or series of words in close proximity (i.e., within two lines above or below) to a word in the text that matches a word or words in the question. In a study of 50 deaf participants matched for reading level with 50 hearing participants, LaSasso (1985) found that 76% of deaf participants used the strategy at least 25% of the time, 33% used it at least 50% of the time, and 17% of the participants used it at least 67% of the time. The average number of responses suggesting visual matching on the 24-item test used in that study was 4.2 for deaf participants and 0.1 for hearing participants matched for reading level with the deaf participants (LaSasso, 1985). Similar visual matching strategies have been observed with deaf readers in Greece (Savvides & LaSasso, 1988) and with deaf and hearing

readers matched for both age and reading level (LaSasso, 1986). Example 12–3 shows an example of visual matching.

Example 12–3

Partial Text

The electric *eel* is a fish which is native to South America. It defends itself from *attacks from enemies* by a natural electronic battery. A discharge from this battery is powerful. It can stun even the largest animals. In South America, roads often pass . . .

Question: How is the eel used by the Indians?
Response: attacks from enemies.

In the context of the discussion of reading in this chapter, to the extent that deaf students have fewer questions about the code, content, and language encoded in print, they are less likely to use compensatory test-taking strategies such as visual matching (LaSasso, 1986). As discussed earlier in this chapter, deaf students exposed early to Cued Speech tend to have fewer questions about the language, content, and code than their noncueing peers who lack clear complete conversational access to the language encoded in print and can therefore focus more of their attention to the reading test.

Large-Scale Initiatives Designed to Improve Reading Levels

A consistent finding of comparative studies of deaf and hearing peers on standardized reading comprehension test performance for the past 90 years is that scores of students from oral or signing backgrounds are much lower than those of hearing age-mates (Allen, 1986; DiFrancesca & Carey, 1972; Furth, 1966; Fusfeld, 1955; Goetzinger & Rousey, 1959; Holt, 1993; Karchmer & Mitchell, 2003; Pintner & Patterson, 1916; Pugh, 1946; Traxler, 2000; Trybus & Karchmer, 1977; Wrightstone, Aronow & Moskowitz, 1963). Furthermore, the average reading level on the Stanford Achievement Test (SAT) for 17- to 18-year-old 12th graders has remained virtually static (i.e., 3rd to 4th-grade reading level) since the early 1970s before the creation of MCE sign systems and *Reading Milestones* (Quigley & King, 1981-1984; Quigley, McAnally, Rose, & King, 1992). In the most recent administration of the SAT, approximately 50% of 17 to 18-year-old 12th grade deaf students in the United States scored below a fourth grade level on the Reading Comprehension subtest (Karchmer & Mitchell, 2003). Fewer than 1% of *hearing* peers scored below a fourth grade level (Marschark, 2006).

Unimproved standardized reading levels of deaf students have been the major impetus for a number of bold, well-intentioned initiatives during the past 40 years designed to address the low reading levels of deaf students. The initiatives vary in terms of whether they address: (1) fundamental language (ASL or English) issues in Deaf Education, (2) instructional materials and procedures for developing deaf students' reading abilities, or (3) reading tests or testing accommodations for deaf students.

Paradigm Shifts Related to the Language of Instruction for Deaf Students

There have been a number of major paradigm shifts related to the language of instruction in deaf education during the last 40 years. In this section we discuss two such shifts: the 1970s shift away from spoken English toward MCE sign systems and the late 1980s to 1990s shift away from spoken and signed English and toward ASL-written English bilingual programs in residential schools.

1970s Shift Toward MCE Sign Systems

In the 1970s, dissatisfaction with the continued low reading levels of deaf students at the time, which were approximately 3rd grade, led to a shift away from oral-aural methods toward signed English, via MCE sign systems such as Seeing Essential English, or SEE I (Anthony, 1971); Signing Exact English, or SEE II (Gustason, Pfetzing, & Zawolkow, 1972) and Signed English (Bornstein & Saulnier, 1981). The creators of the MCE sign systems reasoned that deaf students' lack of mastery of English was the major obstacle in their learning to read. The creators further reasoned that if English could be better conveyed visually than by spoken language methods, deaf children could develop English more naturally in preparation for formal reading instruction. The developers of MCE sign systems attempted to overcome the visual limitations of spoken language (oral-aural) methods by combining ASL signs, English word order, and invented signs for English morphemes. The advantage of MCE sign systems over ASL for nonsigning deaf parents is that the syntax of MCE sign systems corresponds more closely to that of English. Despite widespread usage for almost four decades, the MCE sign systems have failed to have a large-scale impact on deaf students' reading levels on standardized tests. As discussed in Chapter 1, the limitations of MCE sign systems relate to: (1) the inherit difficulty of signing and speaking at the same time which results in the dropping of some signs and (2) the lack of fundamental phonemic information about English in MCE sign systems needed to generalize rules of English naturally (Drasgow & Paul, 1995; LaSasso & Metzger, 1998). Later in this chapter, Cued Speech and MCE sign systems are compared in terms of their structural capability of conveying English clearly and completely as well as task differences related to the memory required to learn each system and the cognitive energy required to use each system.

Late 1980s Shift Toward ASL

A second paradigm shift related to nature of the instructional language for deaf students occurred in the late 1980s after the federally appointed Commission on the Education of the Deaf (COED) supported bilingual education and ASL in the classroom to address the chronic low reading achievement levels of deaf students at the time (COED, 1988). Leaders of the ASL-written English bilingual initiative of the 1990s reasoned that, based on the limited effectiveness of MCE sign systems for improving deaf students' reading achievement, English was neither a visual conversational language nor a language that can be acquired naturally by deaf children (Johnson, Liddell, & Erting, 1989). ASL-written English bilingual programs occur primarily in residential and day schools for deaf students and are characterized by: suppressed spoken and signed English, ASL as the language of instruction, and written English developed via reading and fingerspelling (LaSasso & Lollis, 2003). To date, despite widespread implementation of ASL-written English bilingual methods in residential schools for deaf students for

nearly 20 years, there are no published data related to the effectiveness of these methods for improving deaf students' reading achievement (Moores, 2008).

Special Instructional Materials and Procedures for Deaf Students

Another type of initiative during the past 40 years designed to address deaf students' low reading achievement levels was *Reading Milestones*, a commercially available developmental reading program with strict controls on vocabulary and syntax. The creators of *Reading Milestones* (Quigley & King, 1981-1984) concluded that the fundamental problem related to deaf students' low reading achievement was the lack of linguistic suitability of basal reading programs designed for the general population of students. Quigley and associates found that deaf students have relatively greater difficulty than hearing peers with specific English syntactic constructions, including: passive voice, conjunctions, pronouns, relative clauses, and question forms (see King & Quigley, 1985). They further determined that these same linguistic constructions occurred early and extensively in commercially available basal reading systems designed for the general population of students (Russell, Quigley, & Power, 1976). Quigley and associates reasoned that if vocabulary and syntactic structures were controlled more strictly than in basal readers developed for the general population, deaf children could be taught to read. Accordingly, they created *Reading Milestones,* which has been in widespread use since its creation. By 1997, *Reading Milestones* was used by 30% of programs educating deaf students in the United States, more than three times as much as the next most frequently cited basal reader in a national survey of materials and procedures used to develop deaf students' reading abilities (LaSasso & Mobley, 1997).

Advocacy for Test Accommodations

A third type of initiative that has occurred during the past 40 years to address deaf students' low reading achievement levels has targeted reading tests themselves. For example, the National Task Force on Equity in Testing Deaf and Hard of Hearing Individuals was created in 1987 to promote equity in testing deaf and hard of hearing individuals of all ages (retrieved June 20, 2009, from http://gri.gallaudet .edu/TestEquity). This task force collaborates with state and federal licensure bodies to influence policies about using tests for professional access. In addition, the task force networks with college and university admissions offices to promote better understanding of reasons behind possible discrepancies between standardized admissions test scores and other aspects of applicants' academic or professional profiles to make equitable admissions decisions. The task force also works with testing companies to determine appropriate accommodations for deaf candidates, devise guidelines for alternative assessment procedures, and ensure equity in the development of new tests.

Despite the limitations and criticisms of standardized reading tests, especially for deaf students, it is likely that these tests will continue to be used in the foreseeable future. Increasingly, states are constructing and administering standardized reading competency tests to all stu-

dents in the state, including students who are deaf (Cawthon, 2004, 2006; Luckner & Bowen, 2006; Martin & Mounty, 2005). This is due, in large part, to accountability measures mandated by the No Child Left Behind Act of 2001 (2002) and the Individuals with Disabilities Education Act Amendments of 1997 (2001). In our view, rather than advocating for special tests or testing accommodations for deaf students, parents and other stakeholders should advocate for fully visual (i.e. cued) access to the same curriculum provided to hearing peers (in the same language as all curricular materials and texts), which would provide deaf students with the same opportunities to acquire the fundamental linguistic, reading, and test-taking abilities needed to successfully compete with hearing peers on standardized reading and content area achievement tests.

A Shift in Perspective: Viewing Deaf Children as Capable

All of the initiatives described in the previous section can be characterized as bold, well-meaning attempts to address the reality at the time they were created, that is, the persistent low reading and academic achievement levels of deaf students at the time the initiatives were implemented. The initiatives differ in terms of whether they addressed: (1) fundamental language (ASL or English) issues, (2) the nature of materials and instructional methods to teach reading to deaf students, or (3) reading tests. What the initiatives have in common is that they all approach deaf students reading achievement from a *defi-*

ciency model perspective. That is, an undergirding assumption or premise of each initiative is that children who are deaf *cannot* learn English naturally, develop comparable reading abilities in the same ways and rates as hearing peers, and/or take the same standardized achievement tests in the same conditions as hearing peers.

We view deaf children differently: not as innately deficient, but as innately *capable* of acquiring English and other traditionally spoken home languages naturally; developing reading abilities in the same ways and at the same rates as hearing peers; and performing as well as hearing peers on the same unmodified or unadapted reading achievement tests—as long as they have functionally equivalent sensory access to English or other traditionally spoken home languages. Due to the multimodal nature of speech perception (see Chapter 5), deaf children who lack clear, complete *auditory* access to spoken language, are still biologically predisposed to acquiring English and other traditionally spoken home languages naturally when they have early, clear, complete *visual* access to that language and opportunities to interact with fluent language models. In this section we support this view by: (1) discussing the biological disposition to language acquisition, (2) countering the view that signed languages are the only natural languages of deaf children, (3) describing the advantages of Cued Speech over MCE sign systems for natural language acquisition and the development of reading abilities, and (4) discussing advantages of Cued Speech over Visual Phonics for the development of reading in both the narrow sense as decoding and in the broader sense as reading comprehension or performance on reading tests.

The Biological Predisposition to Acquire Language

Children are biologically predisposed to acquire a spoken language (Gee & Goodhart, 1988; Goldin-Meadow & Mylander, 1990; Klima & Bellugi, 1979; Lenneberg, 1967; Marler, 1990; Petitto & Marentette, 1991). This is true, regardless of children's hearing status (deaf or hearing), nature of the language (signed or spoken), national origin, or complexity of the phonology and syntax of a language. In fact, it is the *unusual* child with sensory access to the "continuous phoneme stream" of a language and sufficient opportunities to interact with that language, who does not discover the rules of that language in a very short period of time (LaSasso & Metzger, 1998). Furthermore, children in all parts of the world, regardless of the complexity of their home language, acquire the rules of that language in remarkably similar patterns related to the phonological contrasts of the language and rules governing its morphology, syntax, semantics, and pragmatics (see de Boysson-Bardies, 1999; Pinker, 1994; Tomasello, 2006) well before formal reading instruction begins at 5 to 6 years of age. Specifically, children in different parts of the world tend to utter their first word around the time they take their first steps, lose the ability to produce phonemes not in their native language by the time they are two years of age, and acquire the major components of their native language by the time they are 3 to 4 years old (Berko-Gleason, 1993; Rayner, Foorman, Perfetti, Pesetsky, & Seidenberg, 2001). For example, by the age of 6 years, children regularly exposed to the English language typically master all of the regular morphological inflections of English; use compound and complex sentences, and have receptive vocabularies estimated to be as large as 25,000 words (Just & Carpenter, 1987).

Sensory *access* to the continuous phoneme stream is only one element in acquiring native competence in a language naturally. Also important are *early* exposure to the language and regular opportunities to interact with fluent language models. Findings related to both feral and neglected children suggest that there is a critical period (0 to 6 years), or sensitive age, for first-language learning (Curtiss, 1977; Lane, 1976; Rymer, 1992).

Children acquire language naturally when they have access to and interaction with fluent language users during the preschool years. Typically, those language models are the child's parents. Parents, regardless of whether their child is hearing or deaf, ultimately are responsible for providing the optimum language learning environment for their child, which can be characterized as: (1) fully accessible; interactive; spontaneous and natural (as opposed to contrived or formal); (2) conducive to numerous opportunities for developing linguistic competence through games, daily living activities, excursions with family members and friends, storytelling and reading of stories, and other age-appropriate activities; and (3) one in which the parents feel empowered to develop their child's language (LaSasso & Metzger, 1998). Schlesinger (1988) found that hearing mothers of (noncueing) deaf children reported feelings of powerlessness over their ability to parent or communicate with their child. Schlesinger reported that such feelings of powerlessness have been found to be a powerful predictor of (noncueing) deaf children's later academic achievement.

Most parents of hearing children are not faced with decisions related to *which*

language should be modeled for their hearing child. Parents whose home language is a traditionally spoken language are able to model their language to their hearing child. Similarly, deaf parents whose home language is a signed language, such as ASL, British Sign Language (BSL), or la Langue des Signes Québécoise (LSQ), are able to model that language for their deaf child. However, nonsigning *deaf or hearing* parents, whose home language is a traditionally spoken language, need to decide whether to attempt to model the home language, a signed language, or a combination of the two for their deaf child (LaSasso & Metzger, 1998). An additional issue for nonsigning deaf or hearing parents of children who are deaf is how to convey English and other traditionally spoken languages conversationally (e.g., via oral methods, MCE sign systems, fingerspelling, or Cued Speech) to their deaf child.

Visual Language Options for Deaf Children

In the view of some (cf. Lane, Hoffmeister, & Bahan, 1996), ASL and other signed languages are the only complete visual language options for deaf children. This view is often cited by day and residential schools as support for ASL-written English bilingual (formerly bilingual-bicultural, or BiBi) approaches that discourage signed or spoken English and approach reading instruction via reading and writing (LaSasso & Lollis, 2003). A view supported in this book is that *cued languages* are also complete visual languages for children who are deaf (see Chapters 3 and 4). Deaf children who have been exposed to cued English or another cued language prior to the onset of their schooling and formal reading instruction acquire that language naturally, including phonologically distinguishable internal, or mental, word representations needed for accurate identification of written words (see Chapter 11). Different phonological representations for American English words such as *dumber* and *upper*, which are undistinguishable on the lips, *are* visually distinct when cued. In addition, exposure to cued language in the context of social interaction allows deaf children to naturally acquire vocabulary, morphosyntax, and social and communicative uses of language.

A second view supported in this book is that deaf children who are in the best position for formal reading instruction are those with a well-developed first language, including those with a well-developed *signed* language (e.g., ASL) or a well-developed *cued* language (e.g., cued English, cued French, or cued Spanish). Two primary differences, however, between cued English and ASL are that cued English is capable of providing clear, complete visual access to: (1) vocabulary and the grammar of English and other traditionally spoken languages encoded in print and (2) the phonology of the spoken language, which allows cueing children, in contrast to children from noncueing backgrounds, to more easily grasp the alphabetic principle (LaSasso & Metzger, 1998).

A Comparison of Cued Speech and MCE Sign Systems for Linguistic Access

In order for deaf children to realize their biological predisposition to acquire English and other traditionally spoken languages naturally, they need clear, complete access to the target language at the phoneme level. As discussed in previous chapters, spoken language is neither fully accessible to deaf children via speechreading (see Chapter 5) nor current hearing enhancement technology, including cochlear implants (see Chapter 6). MCE sign systems, created to convey English more visually than oral-aural methods, combine ASL signed vocabulary with English syntax and invented signs to convey sublexical English morphemes. Despite widespread use of MCE sign systems since the early 1970s, reading levels of 17-year-old deaf students remain static at the 3rd to 4th grade levels (Karchmer & Mitchell, 2003; Traxler, 2000). Although Cued Speech might be considered by some to be a manual code on English (MCE) system, it differs significantly from MCE *sign* systems in terms of: (1) how clearly and completely it conveys English, including the phonological aspects of English; (2) the memory involved in learning it, and (3) the cognitive requirements involved.

Differences in Structural Capability to Convey English

Although MCE sign systems were designed to convey English syntax by combining ASL signs, English word order, and MCE-specific signs for sublexical morphemes, a number of studies suggest that MCE sign systems have limitations in helping deaf children internalize rules of English (Davidson, Newport, & Supalla, 1996; Stack, 1996; Supalla, 1991). A number of 'degraded input' hypotheses and 'structural limitation' hypotheses have been put forth to explain the limited success of MCE sign systems for improving deaf students' reading levels (Drasgow & Paul, 1995; LaSasso & Metzger, 1998). According to degraded input hypotheses (Baker, 1978; Erting, 1985; Geers, Moog, & Schick, 1984; Johnson & Erting, 1989; Kluwin, 1981; Luetke-Stahlman, 1988; Marmor & Petitto,

1979; Strong & Charlson, 1987; Swisher & Thompson, 1985; Woodward & Allen, 1988), some or much of spoken English is deleted or incorrectly coded into sign by both parents and teachers using MCE sign systems due to the difficulty of signing and speaking at the same time.

According to structural limitation hypotheses (Bellugi, Fischer, & Newkirk, 1979; Leybaert & Charlier, 1996; Fleetwood & Metzger, 1991, 1998; Maxwell, 1983, 1987; Schick & Moeller, 1992; Supalla, 1990, 1991), the signed portion of MCE systems may not provide enough structured input for learners to use their innate biological language-learning capabilities to learn English. The task of learning English via MCE sign systems has been described as being similar to that of a hearing child trying to learn English in a (hypothetical) system that presents French or Japanese vocabulary in English word order with English prefixes and suffixes added to the French or Japanese words (personal communication, Robert E. Johnson, Linguistics Department, Gallaudet University, May, 1997).

Fleetwood and Metzger (1991, 1998) and Leybaert and Charlier (1996) note that a major structural limitation of MCE systems for developing English language competence, including reading, relates to the inherent inability of MCE sign systems to convey English at the *phonological* level (Fleetwood & Metzger, 1991, 1998; Leybaert & Charlier, 1996). Fleetwood and Metzger (1991, 1998) note that ASL phonology (handshapes and movements) incorporated in MCE systems bear no relationship to the English phonology (consonants and vowels). For example, the index finger-and-thumb-tapping-together sign (borrowed from ASL), which can be translated as the English word "bird," conveys no phonological (consonant-vowel) informa-

tion about the form of the English word. Thus, none of the phonemes comprising "bird" are present in the ASL sign referencing the same animal (just as none of the ASL phonology is present in the English word). As a result, a deaf child (like a hearing child) could only equate the ASL sign and the English word by: (1) performing an exercise in translation, which requires competence in both of the relevant languages, or (2) being explicitly taught and memorizing this particular pairing (LaSasso & Metzger, 1998).

Besides conveying no information about the phonology of English, MCE sign systems do not completely convey *morphological* information about English (Johnson, Liddell, & Erting, 1989; Fleetwood & Metzger, 1990; Supalla, 1991). In MCE sign systems, the *number* of ASL and MCE-specific morphemes conveyed neither systematically nor predictably corresponds to the *number* of morphemes in the English translation (Fleetwood & Metzger, 1991, 1997, 1998). For example, as indicated in Example 12–1, sometimes the number of MCE sign units needed to convey its English equivalent words exceeds, or is less than, the number of English morphemes. The point here is that deaf children, whose linguistic exposure is limited to visual information from MCE sign systems, are provided no systematic and predictable exposure to the morphological structures and rules of English embedded in its lexicon. These structures and rules are foundational to English grammar, building the phrase structure and clauses that constitute English. To use the example cited earlier, children who try to learn English in a system that uses French or Japanese vocabulary with English inflections and English word order simply are not conveyed enough key aspects of English to be able to develop English language competence.

Cueing English has neither of the limitations of signing MCE systems described above. Unlike MCE sign systems, cueing English and other traditionally spoken languages visually conveys functionally equivalent phonological and prosodic information to deaf individuals that is conveyed by speech to hearing people (see Chapter 2). This enables functionally equivalent morphological, syntactic, semantic, and pragmatic information to be received visually by deaf individuals as is received auditorially by hearing individuals (LaSasso & Metzger, 1998).

Task Differences Related to Learning to Cue or Sign English

In addition to differences between Cued Speech and MCE sign systems for clearly and completely conveying English, clear *task* differences exist related to: (1) the memory involved in learning to convey English via cues or signs and (2) the cognitive effort required to cue or sign English.

Memory Requirements. The task for new-to-signing parents learning MCE sign systems involves learning an extensive sign vocabulary to match the English vocabulary needed by preschool children. Estimates of the receptive vocabulary of 6-year-old hearing children range as high as 25,000 words (Just & Carpenter, 1987), which is an average of 14 new words a day, from birth through age five (25,000 words/6 years with 365 days in a year). This can be a daunting task for new-to-signing parents who do not have resources to learn that many new signs that quickly (LaSasso & Metzger, 1998).

For the competent English user whose goal is to provide the deaf child exposure to English, the memory required to learn the combinations of cues (i.e., handshapes

and placements) that equate to the vowels and consonants of English is far less than that required for learning ASL signs that equate with every English word. Assuming that the person wishing to serve as an English model has already internalized its phonology (and is a competent English user), the task of learning to cue American English is merely one of equating that phonologic knowledge with the eight handshapes and four placements that visibly distinguish among the 40 or so American English phonemes comprising all English words (see Figure 1–1).

Estimates of the time needed to learn the fundamentals of cueing (i.e., matching the handshapes and placements with the phonemes of a language) range from 10 hours to several weeks (Charlier, 1992; Cornett, 1990; Cornett & Daisey, 1992; Kipila & Williams-Scott, 1990), with fluency depending on the motivation of the cuer and the amount of practice. Torres, Moreno-Torres, and Santana (2006) found that the mother in their study could cue close to her normal rate of speech in less than three months. One of the authors of this chapter (LaSasso) has supervised numerous student teachers in cued English classes with 8- to 14-year-old deaf children. In each situation, at the beginning of the student teaching practicum, the student teacher was judged by the cooperating teacher as not yet being a fluent cuer (i.e., able to cue at the same rate as or slightly slower than normal speech); however, by the end of six weeks, each of the students was judged by their cooperating teacher as being fluent. Although Cornett and Daisey (1992) indicate that it is not uncommon for adults immersed in a cueing environment to become fluent within six weeks, this area needs research. Similarly, research is needed to determine how long it takes an adult immersed in an MCE sign environment to become a fluent user of that system (LaSasso & Metzger, 1998).

Cognitive Processing Demands. Although the linguistic needs of a deaf child are, by far, the most important consideration for parents in selecting between or among various options for conveying a traditionally spoken language, *practical* considerations are often a factor for parents in their selecting a mode of communication. One practical consideration for some parents of a deaf child may be the cognitive processing requirements involved in the various options. New parents, who may be experiencing stress related to having an infant in the home, may find themselves particularly vulnerable to cognitive burden, or cognitive overload, if required to learn an extensive new MCE sign vocabulary while simultaneously trying to cope with a new infant. Cummins (1987) defines *cognitive burden* as the volume of information that must be processed in order to carry out the activity (p. 63). Jankowski (1990) discusses the cognitive processing burden of MCE sign systems related to translation requirements. Specifically, MCE users are required to think constantly about *how* to express ideas, as opposed to spontaneously conveying those ideas in a free-flowing manner (p. 57).

The cognitive processing requirements of a task include the *number* and *type* of decisions facing the conveyor of the language (Smith, 2004). Tasks requiring *fewer* decisions can be viewed as less cognitively demanding than those requiring *more* decisions. For example, consider the relative difficulty of guessing a letter of the alphabet versus guessing a word that someone has in mind. Clearly, the task of correctly guessing the letter of the alphabet is easier because of the chance factor;

the chance of guessing the *letter* correctly, is 1 in 26, whereas the chance of getting the *word* correctly is one in 50,000 to 100,000, based on estimates of hearing adults' vocabulary (Just & Carpenter, 1987).

Fluent signers of MCE systems face different decisions than fluent cuers of English. Processes involved in signing a signed language (e.g., ASL) or speaking or cueing English or another traditionally spoken language can and typically do become fairly automatic; however, with MCE sign systems, because the sign vocabulary is adapted from one language to represent the vocabulary of another language, *translation* decisions are involved. For example, at the lexical level, the fluent MCE-user needs make translation decisions about which of several signs adapted from ASL is contextually appropriate for English words (e.g., "right"). By way of illustration, in SEE II (Gustason, Pfetzing, & Zawolkow, 1972), different signs would be used for signing the following sentences: (1) Turn *right* into the parking lot, (2) You are *right*, of course, or (3) It is my *right* to be here. Additional decisions that MCE signers need to make relate to those English words for which the signer knows no sign or cannot recall a sign, in which case, the signer needs to mentally search his or her sign lexicon and select that which comes closest in meaning to the English word. Other translation decisions that fluent MCE signers need to make relate to metacognitive decisions about the degree of translation specificity desired by the receiver, including whether to use a generalized sign, such as *candy* for fudge or caramels, *bug* for insect, or *meat* for steak or pork chop. The cuer of English would not face these decisions. Unlike the fluent signer of MCE systems, the fluent *cuer* of English and the fluent *signer* of ASL are not concerned with translating between two languages; and thus, they have fewer lexical decisions to make than MCE signers who have translation decisions. Cuers of English and other traditionally spoken languages are concerned solely with conveying the visible consonant-vowel phoneme-equivalents and the accompanying prosodic information. The cuer would cue "right" the same way, regardless of its meaning[3] and leave it to the deaf individual to determine its meaning, in the same way that hearing individuals determine the meaning of such words.

In theory, the fluent cuer of English, who is faced with fewer lexical decisions than the fluent signer of MCE systems, has more residual energy to concentrate on the pragmatic, semantic, and syntactic aspects of communication. It can be speculated that the relative energy drain related to *signing* English, via MCE sign systems, may result in reduced linguistic interactions between the MCE-signing parent and deaf child, thereby resulting in fewer opportunities for the deaf child to generalize the morphosyntactic rules of English. It can be further speculated that the energy drain resulting from the translation requirements of signing MCE systems may be an additional explanation for the observation of Bornstein (1990) and others that some hearing parents and teachers drop some signs while signing English.

The fact that cueing does not involve translation decisions may be one explanation for the observation that cued English, once learned, becomes as automatic as speaking English or signing ASL (Cornett & Daisey, 1992). In fact, for new-to-cueing hearing parents, learning to cue English has been compared to learning to *type* English; that is, once the keyboard has

been learned, the typist need only to type to gain fluency (Cornett & Daisey, 1992). Similarly, once the cuer learns the eight handshapes and four placements, the cuer needs only to cue to gain fluency. The only decisions a cuer needs to make, besides those described above, are metalinguistic decisions related to whether a phoneme has been cued correctly or whether the receiver can see the cued message. Similar metacognitive decisions need to be made by MCE signers of English; however, MCE signers, unlike cuers, must constantly be aware of the contextual appropriateness of the sign selected to represent the English word as well as the need of the receiver for specificity of the vocabulary. This can be a daunting task for an adult and even more daunting for a young deaf child without the cognitive abilities of adult MCE signers (LaSasso & Metzger, 1998).

In conclusion, Cued Speech, compared to MCE sign systems has three advantages for the natural acquisition of English and clearly and completely conveying English to deaf children. These advantages relate to the structural capability to convey English completely, the memory required to learn each system, and the cognitive effort required to use each system. In the next section, advantages of Cued Speech, compared to Visual Phonics, are described for developing deaf students' reading abilities.

Advantages of Cued Speech Over Visual Phonics

Visual Phonics is an instructional tool designed to make the phonemes of English visually and tactile-kinesthetically acces-

---

[3]A cuer would cue "right" in keeping with the cuer's dialect. Although dialects differ among cuers, the cueing of one's own dialect does not require a conscious decision.

sible to deaf children, via hand coding and written symbols (Narr, 2008; Trezak, Wang, Woods, Gampp, & Paul, 2007; Waddy-Smith & Wilson, 2003). It can be used in instructional programs where the language of instruction is spoken, signed, or a combination of the two. Developed in 1989, Visual Phonics is comprised of 45 manual representations (i.e., hand signals) plus 45 written symbols corresponding to the 45 phonemes of English, and a 46th hand signal (two hands crossed over the mouth) to indicate a silent *e*. The moving hand signals are used in conjunction with speech and speechreading and are designed to look and feel like the individual phonemes they represent (Waddy-Smith & Wilson, 2003). The mouth movements of Visual Phonics are mirrored in a hand gesture. The hand gesture is then represented in a written symbol. Each hand signal and corresponding written symbol in Visual Phonics corresponds to a single phoneme of English. For example, the manual representation for /f/ consists of four fingers of the hand placed on the thumb of that hand with the palm facing one's mouth then quickly flicking the fingers upward off the thumb, representing movement of lips and teeth (Waddy-Smith & Wilson, 2003). The printed symbol for each manual representation in Visual Phonics is a visual representation of the handshape and represents the same sound regardless of the spelling. For example, the /f/ manual representation and written symbol are used to signal the pronunciation of the first /f/ phoneme in the English words *phone* and *fun*. The manual representations and written symbols are designed to help students make sense of the various spellings and reinforce the sound/symbol connection. For example, the grapheme *ow* represents two different phonemes

in the words *low* and *cow* and can be distinguished by either the manual or printed representations of the phonemes that are represented by the grapheme. Furthermore, the phoneme /i/ (which has a "long e" sound) can be produced by various graphemes as illustrated in the following words: *bean, relief, feet*, and *here*.

Despite years of anecdotal support, there is relatively little published evidence regarding the impact of Visual Phonics on reading achievement. Trezak et al. (2007) examined the effectiveness of using Visual Phonics as a supplement to another phonics-based reading curriculum for students who are deaf or hard of hearing. Twenty students with various degrees of hearing loss in kindergarten and first grade as well as four teachers participated in the study. Findings from this study indicated that after one year of instruction in a phonics-based reading curriculum supplemented by Visual Phonics, deaf and hard of hearing students demonstrated statistically significant improvements in beginning reading skills as measured by standardized assessments. In a second study, Narr (2008) examined the relationship between performance on a phonological awareness task, performance on a decoding task, reading ability, and length of time in literacy instruction with Visual Phonics for 10 deaf and hard of hearing children in kindergarten to grade 3 who receiving academic instruction with sign-supported English and American Sign Language. Narr found that subjects were able to use phonological information to make rhyme judgments and to decode; however, no relationship was found between reading ability and length of time in literacy instruction with Visual Phonics. Importantly, both of these studies examined the effectiveness of Visual Phonics for reading in a narrow sense: as mastery of the alphabetic principle.

In contrast to Visual Phonics, Cued Speech is a manual communication tool for clear, complete visual expression and reception of English and other traditionally spoken languages at the fundamental phoneme level, in the absence of speech and/or hearing. Cued Speech employs a combination of eight handshapes, four hand placements, and natural mouth movements to fully distinguish, or specify, the 40 or so phonemes of English (see Chapter 2 for a detailed description of Cued Speech). Cued Speech has been adapted to 63 alphabetic and tonal languages and dialects (http://www.cuedspeech.org/sub/cued/language.asp). Chapter 11 discusses extensive research related to the effectiveness of Cued Speech and cued language for the development deaf students' mastery of the alphabetic principle.

Proponents and instructors of both Cued Speech and Visual Phonics note that the fundamentals of each system can be initially learned in a weekend; however, they caution that proficiency (and, for Cued Speech, ultimately fluency) will require considerable practice. Estimates of the time needed to be a fluent user of Cued Speech (i.e., cue at or near the same rate as speaking) range from 6 weeks to 3 months when cuers have the opportunity to interact with other cuers (see Chapter 7). No information could be found regarding the time needed to be a proficient user of Visual Phonics or what would be involved in being judged to be "proficient." An advantage of Cued Speech over Visual Phonics for opportunities to practice the system is that Cued Speech is a natural means of expressing thoughts and feelings in authentic contexts; thus, there is no limit to the situations and contexts in which a parent can practice and build fluency with the system while simultaneously engaging the deaf child in meaningful, authentic, language-rich experiences. Daily routines (e.g., waking, feeding, play, bathing) can become cueing practice (i.e., gaining fluency with the 8 handshapes and 4 placements) for the parent while providing *language* exposure for the deaf child.

The effectiveness of Cued Speech over Visual Phonics for developing deaf students' reading abilities is best understood in the context of reading defined more broadly as comprehension or measured reading comprehension. While Cued Speech and Visual Phonics are structurally capable of impacting readers' questions about the alphabetic principle, Visual Phonics was not designed to develop the other abilities related to reading comprehension. Specifically, Visual Phonics does not address readers' questions about the language encoded in print, including the vocabulary, morphosyntactic, and pragmatic aspects of reading, which are essential for reading comprehension nor can Visual Phonics be used as a communication tool for conveying English conversationally. To try and communicate English via Visual Phonics would be "slow, laborious, and cumbersome if at all possible" (Woolsey, Satterfield, & Roberson, 2006). Cued Speech, on the other hand is intended to provide, from the earliest age, visual access to a traditionally spoken language, allowing the deaf child to naturally acquire not only the phonemic/phonological foundation of that language for later application in the explicit teaching of the alphabetic principle, but also the vocabulary, morphosyntactic, and pragmatic rules of that language, which are critical for reading comprehension. Cued Speech, unlike Visual Phonics, allows the deaf child to *see* the larger (syntactic and words) and smaller (morphemes, phonemes) units of language as they occur in natural language contexts. Explicit phonics instruction, typically occurring during the primary (K–3) grades, can be carried out with cueing children in the manner traditionally experienced by hearing children; that is, by pairing phonemes, already known to the child, with graphemes that appear in printed words and phrases that are already known to the child via conversational language.

Deaf children from cueing backgrounds typically have an advantage in phonics instruction (either with or without Visual Phonics) over deaf children from noncueing backgrounds. That is, by the time formal, explicit phonics instruction begins (typically kindergarten or 1st grade), five to six years of language exposure and experience have transpired. The typical deaf child from spoken language or MCE sign backgrounds has received incomplete access to the language encoded in print and is, therefore, already at a disadvantage compared to hearing or cueing peers when attempting to learn not only the phonemes and graphemes of the language (even with supplemental instruction via Visual Phonics), but also the global language structures and rules of the language, and the language-specific labels for the concepts referred to in printed materials. Deaf cuers with early exposure to cued language, however, have had the opportunity to naturally acquire all aspects of that language, and can take advantage of the language-specific labeling of concrete objects and abstract notions. Deaf cuers also have the educational advantage of being able to use general world knowledge and knowledge of English syntax and apply contextual analysis when decoding unfamiliar print forms, theoretically learning phonics in a more efficient manner, and

saving cognitive resources for addressing questions related to the reading task.

Conclusion

Reading is discussed broadly in this chapter as comprehension or *measured reading comprehension*. The focus of this chapter is on: (1) variables besides the alphabetic principle that impact students' reading comprehension and performance on reading tests beyond the primary grades and (2) the applications of Cued Speech and cued language for developing those abilities. While Cued Speech has been shown to be effective for teaching deaf children the alphabetic principle (see Chapter 11), its benefit is even greater for developing the other critical abilities needed for fluent reading, including: cognitive and linguistic abilities and fund of information knowledge that children typically develop during the preschool years when they have clear, complete access to the home language, and opportunities to interact with fluent language models.

Reading comprehension is conceptualized in this chapter as a process that progresses or is impeded by readers' questions about the language, content, alphabetic code, and/or the nature of the reading task. All other things being equal, deaf children exposed early and consistently to cued English will have fewer questions related to the vocabulary, morphosyntax, and pragmatic aspects of the language encoded in print than their noncueing deaf peers and will be better able to interact with English language models to develop background knowledge presumed of readers engaged with beginning reading materials. Like hearing peers, deaf cuers with early exposure to cued English can focus their attention, in relative measure, on their questions related to all aspects of the reading comprehension task, including the code, language, content, and the reading test or task. In this way, Cued Speech is a comprehensive, flexible tool for phonics decoding, as well as a viable means of language acquisition for reading comprehension and performance on reading tests.

This chapter described a number of large scale initiatives during the past 40 years that have been designed to improve deaf students' reading levels. These initiatives vary in terms of whether they focus on the language of instruction (ASL or English), instructional reading materials and procedures, or standardized test accommodations for deaf students. What all of these initiatives have in common is that they view deaf children with a *deficiency model* perspective, reflecting a historical view by many teachers, school administrators, and other stakeholders that deaf students are innately *incapable* of acquiring English naturally and requiring special schools, special reading programs, and/or special reading tests or test accommodations.

In this chapter, deaf children are viewed not as disabled, but rather as *capable* of learning to read and progress through the reading and content area curricula with the same instructional materials, instructional procedures, and reading tests as their hearing peers when they arrive at school with cued English abilities comparable to those of spoken language abilities of hearing peers and are afforded full visual access to the curriculum via cued English. Similarly, deaf children who come to school with a cued language that is different from English (e.g., cued Spanish), can be can expected to learn to read with the same English as Second Language (ESL) instructional materials and

procedures as hearing peers when they are afforded clear, complete visual (cued) access to the ESL curriculum.

Advantages of Cued Speech over MCE sign systems for communicating English and Visual Phonics for phonics instruction were described in this chapter. Cued Speech, unlike MCE sign systems, is structurally capable of conveying English clearly and completely to deaf individuals because cueing conveys English at the fundamental *phoneme* level whereas the most fundamental aspect of English conveyed by MCE sign systems is morphemic. Two additional advantages of Cued Speech over the widely used MCE sign systems for the natural acquisition of English relate to the memory required to learn the system to be fluent language models and the cognitive energy required to use it. The advantage of Cued Speech over Visual Phonics is clear when reading is defined in the broader sense as *comprehension* or *measured reading comprehension*. Cued Speech addresses the *same* deaf readers' questions as Visual Phonics about the alphabetic principle, but in addition, Cued Speech addresses the other critical abilities needed for reading comprehension, not the least of which are language abilities, including vocabulary, morphosyntax, and pragmatic aspects of English upon which fluent reading depends.

References

Abedi, J. (2004). The No Child Left Behind Act and English language learners: Assessment and accountability issues. *Educational Researcher, 33*, 4–14.

Abedi, J., & Dietel, R. (2004). Challenges in the No Child Left Behind Act for English language learners. *Phi Delta Kappan, 85*, 782–785.

Abedi, J., Leon, D., & Mirocha, J. (2001). *Impact of students' language background on standardized achievement test results: Analyses of extant data.* Los Angeles, CA: University of California, Los Angeles, National Center for Research on Evaluation, Standards, and Student Testing.

Adams, M. (1990). *Beginning to read: Thinking and learning about print.* Cambridge, MA: MIT Press.

Allen, T. (1986). A study of the achievement patterns of hearing-impaired students: 1974–1983. In A. Schildroth & M. Karchmer (Eds.), *Deaf children in America* (pp. 161–206). San Diego, CA: College-Hill Press.

Andrews, J., & Mason, J. (1991). Strategy usage among deaf and hearing readers. *Exceptional Children, 57*, 536–545.

Anthony, D. (1971). *SEE I* (Vols. 1–2). Anaheim, CA. Educational Services Division, Anaheim Union School District.

Bailey, A. (2000). Language analysis of standardized achievement tests: Considerations in the assessment of English language learners. In J. Abedi, A. Bailey, F. Butler, M. Castellon-Wellington, S. Leon, & J. Mirocha (Eds.), *The validity of administering large-scale content assessments to English language learners: An investigation from three perspectives (2000) (CSE Rep. No. 663)* (pp. 85–105). Los Angeles, CA: University of California, National Center for Research on Evaluation, Standards, and Student Testing.

Baker, C. (1978). How does "sim-com" fit into a bilingual approach to education? In F. Caccamise & D. Hicks (Eds.), *American Sign Language in a bilingual/bicultural context: Proceedings of the Second National Symposium on Sign Language Research and Teaching, USA* (pp. 13–26). Silver Spring, MD: National Association of the Deaf.

Bellugi, U., Fischer, S., & Newkirk, C. (1979). The rate of speaking and signing. In E. Klima & U. Bellugi (Eds.), *The signs of language* (pp. 181–194). Cambridge, MA: Harvard University Press.

Benning, V. (2000, November 1). Blacks, Hispanics still lag on tests. *The Washington Post*, B1, B5.

Berk, R. (1982). *Handbook of methods for detecting test bias.* Baltimore, MD: The Johns Hopkins University Press.

Berko-Gleason, J. (1993). *The development of language* (3rd ed.). New York, NY: Macmillan.

Bornstein, H. (1971). Some effects of verbal load on achievement tests. *American Annals of the Deaf, 16*, 44–48.

Bornstein, H. (1990). Signed English. In H. Bornstein (Ed.), *Manual communication: Implications for education* (pp. 128–138). Washington, DC: Gallaudet University Press.

Bornstein, H., & Saulnier, K. (1981). Signed English: A brief follow-up to the first evaluation. *American Annals of the Deaf, 126*, 69–92.

Bornstein, H., Saulnier, K., & Hamilton, L. (1973–1984). *The Signed English series.* Washington, DC: Gallaudet College Press.

Bransford, J., & Johnson, M. (1972). Contextual prerequisites for understanding. Some investigations of comprehension and recall. *Journal of Verbal Learning Behavior, 11*, 717–726.

Brauer, B., Braden, J., Pollard, R., & Hardy-Braz, S. (1998). Deaf and hard-of-hearing people. In J. Sandoval, C. Frisby, K. Geisinger, J. Ramos-Grenier & J. Dowd-Scheuneman (Eds.), *Test interpretation and diversity: Achieving equity in assessment* (pp. 297–315). Washington, DC: American Psychological Association.

Butler, F., & Stevens, R. (2001). Standardized assessment of the content knowledge of English language learners in K–12: Current trends and old dilemmas. *Language Testing, 18*, 409–427.

Cawthon, S. (2004). Schools for the deaf and the No Child Left Behind Act. *American Annals of the Deaf, 149*, 314–323.

Cawthon, S. (2006) National survey of accommodations and alternate assessments for students who are deaf or hard of hearing in the United States. *Journal of Deaf Studies and Deaf Education, 11*, 337–359.

Cawthon, S. (2007). Hidden benefits and unintended consequences of No Child Left Behind policies for students who are deaf or hard of hearing. *American Educational Research Journal, 44*, 460–497

Charlier, B. (1992). *Complete signed and cued French: An original signed language-Cued Speech combination* (unpublished manuscript).

Commission of Education of the Deaf. (1998). *Toward equality: Education of the deaf.* Washington, DC: U.S. Government Printing Office.

Conrad, R. (1979). *The deaf school child.* London, UK: Harper & Row.

Cornett, R. O. (1990). The complete deaf person. *Communication issues among the deaf. A Deaf American monograph.* Silver Spring, MD: National Association of the Deaf.

Cornett, R. O., & Daisey, M. (1992). *The Cued Speech resource book for parents of deaf children.* Raleigh, NC: National Cued Speech Corporation.

Cummins, J. (1987). Bilingualism, language proficiency, and metalinguistic development. In P. Homel, M. Palij, & D. Aaronson (Eds.), *Childhood bilingualism: Aspects of linguistic, cognitive, and social development* (pp. 57–73). Hillsdale, NJ: Lawrence Erlbaum.

Cunningham, J., & Moore, D. (1993). The contribution of understanding academic vocabulary to answering comprehension questions. *Journal of Reading Behavior, 25,* 171–180.

Curtiss, S. (1977). *Genie: A psycholinguistic study of a modern-day "wild child."* New York, NY: Academic Press.

Davey, B., & LaSasso, C. (1984). The interaction of reader and task factors in the assessment of reading comprehension. *Journal of Experimental Education, 52,* 199–206.

Davey, B., LaSasso, C., & Macready, G. (1983). Comparison of reading comprehension task performance for deaf and hearing readers. *Journal of Speech and Hearing Research, 26,* 622–628.

Davidson, M., Newport, E., & Supalla, S. (1996). *The acquisition of natural and unnatural linguistic devices: Aspect and number marking in MCE children.* Paper presented at the Fifth International Conference on Theoretical Issues in Sign Language Research, Montreal, Canada.

de Boysson-Bardies, B. (1999). *How language comes to children: From birth to two years.* Cambridge, MA: MIT Press.

DiFrancesca, S., & Carey, S. (1972). *Academic achievement test results of a national testing program for hearing impaired students, United States, Spring, 1971.* Washington, DC: Gallaudet College, Office of Demographic Studies.

Dolch, E. (1948). *Teaching primary reading.* Champaign, IL: Garrard Press.

Drasgow, E., & Paul, P. (1995). A critical analysis of the use of MCE systems with deaf students: A review of the literature. *Association of Canadians Educators of the Hearing Impaired, 21,* 80–93.

Easterbrooks, S., & Huston, S. (2008). The signed reading fluency of students who are deaf/hard of hearing. *Journal of Deaf Studies and Deaf Education 13,* 37–54.

Ehri, L. (1995). Phases of development in learning to read words by sight. *Journal of Research in Reading, 18,* 116–125.

Erting, C. (1985). Sociocultural dimensions of deaf education: Belief systems and communicative interaction. *Sign Language Studies, 47,* 11–126.

Fleetwood, E., & Metzger, M. (1990). *Cued Speech transliteration: Theory and application.* Silver Spring, MD: Calliope Press.

Fleetwood, E., & Metzger, M. (1991). *ASL and cued English: A contrastive analysis,* Paper presented at the Deaf Awareness Conference, Dothan, Alabama.

Fleetwood, E., & Metzger, M. (1997). *Does Cued Speech entail speech? A comparison of cued and spoken information in terms of distinctive features.* Unpublished manuscript, Gallaudet University.

Fleetwood, E., & Metzger, M. (1998). *Cued language structure: An analysis of cued American English based on linguistic principles.* Silver Spring, MD: Calliope Press.

Fruchter, A., Wilbur, R., & Fraser (1984). Comprehension of idioms by hearing impaired students. *Volta Review, 86,* 7–19.

Furth, H. (1966). A comparison of reading test norms of deaf and hearing children. *American Annals of the Deaf, 111,* 461–462.

Fusfeld, I. (1955). The academic program of schools for the deaf. *Volta Review, 57,* 63–70.

Gee, J., & Goodhart, W. (1988). American Sign Language and the human biological capacity for language. In M. Strong (Ed.), *Language learning and deafness* (pp. 49–74). New York, NY: Cambridge University Press.

Geers, A., Moog, J., & Schick, B. (1984). Acquisition of spoken and signed English by profoundly deaf children. *Journal of Speech and Hearing Disorders, 49,* 378–388.

Goetzinger, C., & Rousey, C. (1959). Educational achievement of deaf children. *American Annals of the Deaf, 104,* 221–231.

Goldin-Meadow, S., & Mylander, C. (1990). Beyond the input given: The child's role in the acquisition of language. *Language, 66,* 323–355.

Goodman, K. (1974). A psycholinguistic guessing game. In H. Singer (Ed.), *Theoretical models and processes of reading* (2nd ed., pp. 497–508). Newark, DE: International Reading Association.

Gough, P. (1972). One second of reading. In J. Kavanagh & I. Mattingly (Eds.), *Language by ear and eye* (pp. 331–358). Cambridge, MA: The MIT Press.

Gustason, G., Pfetzing, D., Zawolkow, E. (1972). *Signing exact English.* Rossmore, CA: Modern Signs Press.

Hage, C., & Leybaert, J. (2006). The development of oral language through Cued Speech. In: P. Spencer & M. Marschark (Eds.), *The development of spoken language in deaf children* (pp. 193–211). New York, NY: Oxford University Press.

Holt, J. (1993). Stanford Achievement Test (8th Edition): Reading comprehension subgroup results. *American Annals of the Deaf, 138,* 172–175.

Individuals with Disabilities Education Act Amendments of 1997. 20 U.S.C. 1400 et seq. (2001).

Jankowski, K. (1990). Am I communicating? In M. Garretson (Ed.), *Communication issues among deaf people: A Deaf American monograph* (pp. 55–57). Silver Spring, MD: National Association of the Deaf.

Jenkins, J., Fuchs, L., van den Broek, P., Espin, C., & Deno, S. (2003). Accuracy and fluency in list and context reading of skilled and RD groups: Absolute and relative performance levels. *Learning Disabilities Research and Practice, 18,* 237–245.

Johnson, R., & Erting, C. (1989). Ethnicity and socialization in a classroom for deaf children. In C. Lucas (Ed.), *The sociolinguistics of the Deaf community* (pp. 41–83). New York, NY: Academic Press.

Johnson, R., Liddell, S., & Erting, C. (1989). *Unlocking the curriculum: Principles for achieving access in deaf education (Working Paper #89-3).* Washington DC: Gallaudet University.

Just, M., & Carpenter, P. (1987). *The psychology of reading and language comprehension.* Boston, MA: Allyn and Bacon.

Kamil, M., Mosenthal, P., Pearson, P., Barr, R. (2000). *Handbook of reading research* (Vol. III). Mahwah, NJ: Lawrence Earlbaum Associates.

Karchmer, M., & Mitchell, R. (2003). Demographic and achievement characteristics of deaf and hard of hearing students. In M. Marschark & P. Spencer (Eds.), *Oxford handbook of deaf studies, language, and deaf education* (pp. 21–27). New York, NY: Oxford University Press.

Kelly, L. (2003). The importance of processing automaticity and temporary storage capacity to the differences in comprehension between skilled and less skilled college-age deaf readers. *Journal of Deaf Studies and Deaf Education, 8,* 230–249.

King, C., & Quigley, S. (1985). *Reading and deafness.* Austin, TX: Pro-Ed.

Kipila, B. & Williams-Scott, B. (1990). Cued Speech. In H. Bornstein (Ed.), *Manual communication: Implications for education* (pp. 139–150). Washington DC: Gallaudet University Press.

Klima, E., & Bellugi, U. (1979). *The signs of language.* Cambridge, MA: Harvard University Press.

Kluwin, T. (1981). A rationale for modifying classroom signing systems. *Sign Language Studies, 31,* 179–187.

Kopriva, R. (2000). *Ensuring accuracy in testing for English language learners.* Washington, DC: Council of Chief State School Officers.

Kunnan, A. (2008). Test fairness, test bias and DIF. *Language Assessment Quarterly, 4,* 109–112.

LaBerge, D., & Samuels, S. (1974). Toward a theory of automatic information processing in reading. *Cognitive Psychology, 6*, 293–323.

Lane, H. (1976). *The wild boy of Aveyron.* Cambridge, MA: Harvard University Press.

Lane, H., Hoffmeister, R., & Bahan, B. (1996). *A journey into the deaf-world.* San Diego, CA: Dawn Sign Press.

LaSasso, C. (1979). The effect of WH question format versus incomplete statement format on deaf students' comprehension of text-explicit information. *American Annals of the Deaf, 124*, 833–837.

LaSasso, C. (1985). Visual matching test-taking strategies used by hearing impaired readers. *Journal of Speech and Hearing Research, 28*, 2–7.

LaSasso, C. (1986). A comparison of test-taking strategies of comparably-aged hearing and hearing-impaired readers with comparable reading levels. *Volta Review, 88*, 231–241.

LaSasso, C. (1987). What parents need to know about reading levels of hearing impaired students. *American Annals of the Deaf, 132*, 218–220.

LaSasso, C. (1990). Developing the ability of hearing-impaired students to comprehend and generate question forms. *American Annals of the Deaf, 135*, 409–411.

LaSasso, C. (1994). Reading comprehension of deaf readers; The impact of too many or too few questions. *American Annals of the Deaf, 138*, 435–441.

LaSasso, C. (1996). Foniks for deff tshildrun? *Perspectives in Education and Deafness, 14*, 6–9.

LaSasso, C. (1999). Test-taking abilities: A missing component of the curriculum for deaf students. *American Annals of the Deaf, 144*, 35–43.

LaSasso, C., & Lollis, J (2003). National survey of residential and day schools serving deaf students that identify themselves as bilingual-bicultural programs. *Journal of Deaf Studies and Deaf Education, 8*, 79–91.

LaSasso, C., & Metzger, M. (1998). An alternate route to bilingualism: The home language as L1 and Cued Speech for conveying traditionally spoken languages. *Journal of Deaf Studies and Deaf Education, 3*, 264–289.

LaSasso, C., & Mobley, R. (1997). National survey of reading instruction for deaf and hard of hearing students in the U.S. *Volta Review, 99*, 31–60.

LaSasso, C., & Swaiko, N. (1983). Considerations in selecting and using commercially prepared informal reading inventories with deaf students. *American Annals of the Deaf, 128*, 449–452.

Lenneberg, E. (1967). *Biological foundations of language.* New York, NY: Wiley.

Leybaert, J., & Charlier, B. (1996). Visual speech in the head: The effect of Cued Speech on rhyming, remembering, and spelling. *Journal of Deaf Studies and Deaf Education, 1*, 234–248.

Lollis, J. (2002). *The appropriateness of the North Carolina state mandated reading competency test as a criterion for high school graduation for deaf students.* Unpublished doctoral dissertation, Gallaudet University, Washington DC.

Lollis, J., & LaSasso, C. (2009). The appropriateness of the NC State-Mandated Reading Competency Test for deaf students as a criterion for high school graduation. *Journal of Deaf Studies and Deaf Education, 14*, 76–98.

Luckner, J., & Bowen, S. (2006). Assessment practices of professionals serving students who are deaf or hard of hearing: An initial investigation. *American Annals of the Deaf, 151*, 410–417.

Luetke-Stahlman, B. (1988). The benefit of oral English-only as compared with signed input to hearing-impaired students. *Volta Review, 90*, 349–361.

Marler, P. (1990). Innate learning preferences: Signals for communication. *Developmental Psychobiology, 23*, 557–569.

Marmor, G., & Petitto, L. (1979). Simultaneous communication in the classroom: How well is English grammar represented? *Sign Language Studies, 23*, 99–136.

Marschark, M. (1993). *Psychological development of deaf children.* New York, NY: Oxford University Press.

Marschark, M., (2006). *Educating deaf students: Is literacy the issue?* [Electronic version]. Paper presented at the 2006 PEPNet conference

Roots & Wings. Proceedings available from the University of Tennessee, Postsecondary Education Consortium Web site.

Marschark, M., Sapere, P., Convertino, C., Mayer, C., Waters, L., & Sarchet, T. (2009). Are deaf students' reading challenges really about reading. *American Annals of the Deaf, 154*, 357–370.

Martin, D., & Mounty, J. (2005) Overview of the challenge. Assessing deaf adults: Critical issues in testing and evaluation. In J. Mounty & D. Martin (Eds.), *Assessing deaf adults: Critical issues in testing and evaluation* (pp. 3–10). Washington, DC: Gallaudet University Press.

Martin, P. (2005). *An examination of the appropriateness of the New York State English language arts: Grade 8 test for deaf students.* Unpublished doctoral dissertation, Washington, DC: Gallaudet University.

Maxwell, M. (1983). Language acquisition in a deaf child of deaf parents: Speech, sign variations and print variations. In K. Nelson (Ed.), *Children's language* (Vol. 4, pp. 283–313). Hillsdale, NJ: Lawrence Erlbaum.

Maxwell, M. (1987). The acquisition of English bound morphemes in sign form. *Sign Language Studies, 57*, 323–352.

McKee, B., & Bondi-Wolcott, J. (1982). Three studies of the relation of item format and estimates of achievement for hearing-impaired postsecondary students. In F. Solano, J. Egelston-Dodd, & E. Costello (Eds.), *Focus on infusion* (pp. 146–154). Silver Spring, MD: Convention of American Instructors of the Deaf.

Messick S. (1989). Validity. In R. Linn (Ed.), *Educational measurement 3rd edition* (pp. 13–103). New York, NY: Macmillan.

Moores, D. (2008). Research on BiBi Instruction. *American Annals of the Deaf, 153*, 3–4.

Narr, R. (2008). Phonological awareness and decoding in deaf/hard-of-hearing students who use Visual Phonics. *Journal of Deaf Studies and Deaf Education, 13*, 405–416.

Nation, K. (2005). Children's reading comprehension difficulties. In: M. Snowling, C. Hulme, & M. Seidenberg (Eds.), *The science of reading: A handbook* (pp. 248–265). Oxford, UK: Blackwell.

Nation, K., & Angell, P. (2006). Learning to read and learning to comprehend. *London Review of Education, 4*, 77–87.

National Reading Panel. (2000). *Teaching children to read: An evidence-based assessment of the scientific literature on reading and its implications for reading instruction.* United States Department of Health and Human Services.

National Research Council (NRC). (1999). *High stakes: Testing for tracking, promotion, and graduation.* Washington, DC: National Academy Press.

Nelson, K., & Camarata, S. (1996). Improving English literacy and speech-acquisition learning conditions for children with severe to profound hearing impairments. *Volta Review, 98*, 17–21.

No Child Left Behind Act of 2001. 20 U.S.C. 6301 et seq (2002).

Oakhill, J., & Cain, K. (2000). Children's difficulties in text comprehension: Assessing causal issues. *Journal of Deaf Studies and Deaf Education, 5*, 51–59.

Osguthorpe, R., Long, G., & Ellsworth, R. (1977). *The effect of reviewing class notes for deaf and hearing students.* Rochester, NY: National Technical Institute for the Deaf.

Paul, P. (1998). *Literacy and deafness: The development of reading, writing, and literate thought.* Boston, MA: Allyn and Bacon.

Paul, P. (2008). *Language and deafness* (4th ed.). Sudbury, MA: Jones & Bartlett.

Petitto, L., & Marentette, P. (1991). Babbling in the manual mode: Evidence for the ontogeny of language. *Science, 251*, 1493–1496.

Pinker, S. (1994). *The language instinct: How the mind creates language.* New York, NY: William Morrow.

Pintner, R., & Patterson, D. (1916). A comparison of deaf and hearing children in visual memory for digits. *Journal of Experimental Psychology, 2*, 76–78.

Pratt, S., & Moreland, I. (1998). Individuals with other characteristics. In J. Sandoval, C. Frisby, K. Geisinger, J. Scheuneman, & J. Grenier, (Eds.), *Test interpretation and diver-*

sity. Washington, DC: American Psychological Association.

Pugh, G. (1946). Summaries from appraisal of the silent reading abilities of acoustically handicapped children. *American Annals of the Deaf, 35*, 331–345.

Purcell-Gates, V. (1997). *Other people's words. The cycle of low literacy*. Cambridge, MA: Harvard University Press.

Quigley, S., & King, C. (1981–1984). *Reading milestones*. Beaverton, OR: Dormac.

Quigley, S., McAnally, P., Rose, S., & King, C. (1992). *Reading milestones*. Austin, TX: Pro-Ed.

Quigley, S., & Paul, P. (1984). *Language and deafness*. San Diego, CA: College-Hill Press.

Rasinski, T. (2004). *Assessing reading fluency*. Honolulu, HI: Pacific Resources for Education and Learning.

Rayner, K., Foorman, B., Perfetti, C., Pesetsky, D., & Seidenberg, M. (2001). How psychological science informs the teaching of reading. *Psychological Science in the Public Interest, 2*, 31–74.

Rittenhouse, R., & Kenyon, P. (1990) Teaching idiomatic expressions: A comparison of two instructional methods. *American Annals of the Deaf, 135*, 322–326.

Rosenblatt, L. (1994). The transactional theory of reading and writing. In R. Ruddell, M. Ruddell, & H. Singer (Eds.), *Theoretical models and processes of reading. Fourth edition.* (pp. 1057–1092). Newark, DE: International Reading Association.

Rudner, L. (1978). Using standard tests with the hearing impaired: The problem of item bias. *Volta Review, 80*, 31–40.

Rumelhart, D. (1977). Toward an interactive model of reading. In S. Dornio (Ed.), *Attention and performance VI* (pp. 573–603). Hillsdale, NJ: Lawrence Erlbaum and Associates.

Russell, W., Quigley, S., & Power, D. (1976). *Linguistics and deaf children: Transformationals syntax and its application*. Washington, DC: The Alexander Graham Bell Association for the Deaf, Inc.

Rymer, R. (1992). Annals of science: A silent childhood-I. *The New Yorker*, pp. 41–81.

Sandoval, J., & Duran, R. (1998). Language. In J. Sandoval, C. Frisby, K. Geisinger, J. Scheuneman, & J. Grenier (Eds.), *Test interpretation and diversity: Achieving equity in assessment* (pp. 181–212). Washington, DC: American Psychological Association.

Savvides, G., & LaSasso, C. (1988). Visual matching: A strategy employed by deaf readers in Greece and Cyprus when dealing with a reading comprehension task. *Hope* (Greek newspaper), pp. 13–14.

Scheuneman, J., & Oakland, T. (1998). High stakes testing in education. In J. Sandoval, C. Frisby, K. Geisinger, J. Scheuneman, & J. Grenier (Eds.), *Test interpretation and diversity: Achieving equity in assessment* (pp. 77–103). Washington, DC: American Psychological Association.

Schick, B., & Moeller, M. (1992). What is learnable in manually-coded English sign systems? *Applied Psycholinguistics, 13*, 313–340.

Schlesinger, H. (1988). Questions and answers in the development of deaf children. In M. Strong (Ed.), *Language learning and deafness* (pp. 261–292). New York, NY: Cambridge University Press.

Smith, F. (2004). *Understanding reading* (6th ed.). Mahwah, NJ: Lawrence Erlbaum Associates.

Stack, K. (1996). *The development of a pronominal system in the absence of a natural target language*. Paper presented at the Fifth International Conference on Theoretical Issues in Sign Language, Montreal, Canada.

Stanford Achievement Test. (1996). *Norms Booklet* (9th ed.). Houston, TX: Psychological Corporation: Harcourt Brace Jovanovich.

Strong, M., & Charlson, E. (1987). Simultaneous communication: Are teachers attempting an impossible task? *American Annals of the Deaf, 132*, 376–382.

Supalla, S. (1990). *Segmentation of manually-coded English: Problems in the mapping of English in the visual/gestural mode*. Unpublished doctoral dissertation, University of Illinois.

Supalla, S. (1991). Manually-coded English: The modality question in signed language development. In P. Siple & S. Fischer (Eds.), *Theoretical issues in sign language research* (pp. 85–109). Chicago, IL: University of Chicago Press.

Swanson, H., & Howell, M. (2001). Working memory, short term memory, and speech rate as predictors of children's reading. *Journal of Educational Psychology, 93,* 720–734.

Swisher, V., & Thompson, M. (1985). Mothers learning simultaneous communication: The dimensions of the task. *American Annals of the Deaf, 130,* 212–217.

Tomasello, M. (2006). Acquiring linguistic constructions. In D. Kuhn & R. Siegler (Eds.), *Handbook of child psychology* (pp. 255–298). New York, NY: Wiley.

Torres, S., Moreno-Torres, I., & Santana, R. (2006). Quantitative and qualitative evaluation of linguistic input support to a prelingually deaf child with Cued Speech: A case study. *Journal of Deaf Studies and Deaf Education, 11,* 438–448.

Traxler, C. (2000). The Stanford Achievement Test, 9th edition: National norming and performance standards for deaf and hard-of-hearing students. *Journal of Deaf Studies and Deaf Education, 5,* 337–348.

Trezak, B., Wang, Y., Woods, D., Gampp, T., & Paul, P. (2007) Using Visual Phonics to supplement beginning reading instruction for students who are deaf or hard of hearing. *Journal of Deaf Studies and Deaf Education, 12,* 373–384.

Trybus, R., & Buchanan, G. (1973). Patterns of achievement test performance. *Studies in achievement testing hearing-impaired students. United States, 1971* (Series D, No. 11). Washington, DC: Gallaudet College, Office of Demographic Studies.

Trybus, R., & Karchmer, M. (1977). School achievement scores of hearing impaired children: National data on achievement status and growth patterns. *American Annals of the Deaf Directory of Programs and Services, 122,* 62–69.

Valencia, S., & Wixson, K. (2000). Policy-oriented research on literacy standards and assessment. In M. Kamil, P. Mosenthal, P. D. Pearson, & R. Barr (Eds.), *Handbook of reading research* (Vol. 3, pp. 909–935). Mahwah, NJ: Lawrence Erlbaum Associates.

Waddy-Smith, B., & Wilson, V. (2003). See that sound! Visual Phonics helps deaf and hard of hearing students develop reading skills. *Odyssey, 5,* 14–17.

Walker, L., Munro, J., & Rickards, F. (1998). Literal and inferential reading comprehension of students who are deaf. *Volta Review, 100,* 87–103.

Wampler, D. (1971). *Linguistics of Visual English: An introduction.* Santa Rosa, CA: Santa Rosa City Schools.

Wandel, J. (1989). *Use of internal speech in reading by hearing and hearing-impaired students in oral, total communication and Cued Speech programs.* Unpublished doctoral dissertation, Teachers College, Columbia University, New York, NY.

Webster, A., Wood, D., & Griffiths, A. (1981). Reading retardation or linguistic deficit? I: Interpreting reading test performance of hearing impaired adolescents. *Journal of Research in Reading, 4,* 136–147.

Wolk, S., & Schildroth, A. (1984). Consistency of an associational strategy used by hearing-impaired students. *Journal of Research in Reading, 7,* 135–142.

Woodward, J., & Allen, T. (1988). Classroom use of artificial sign systems by teachers. *Sign Language Studies. 61,* 405–518.

Woolsey, M., Satterfield, S., & Roberson, L. (2006). Visual Phonics: An English code buster? *American Annals of the Deaf, 151,* 452–457.

Wrightstone, J., Aronow, M., & Moskowitz, S. (1963). Developing reading test norms for deaf children. *American Annals of the Deaf, 108*, 311–316.

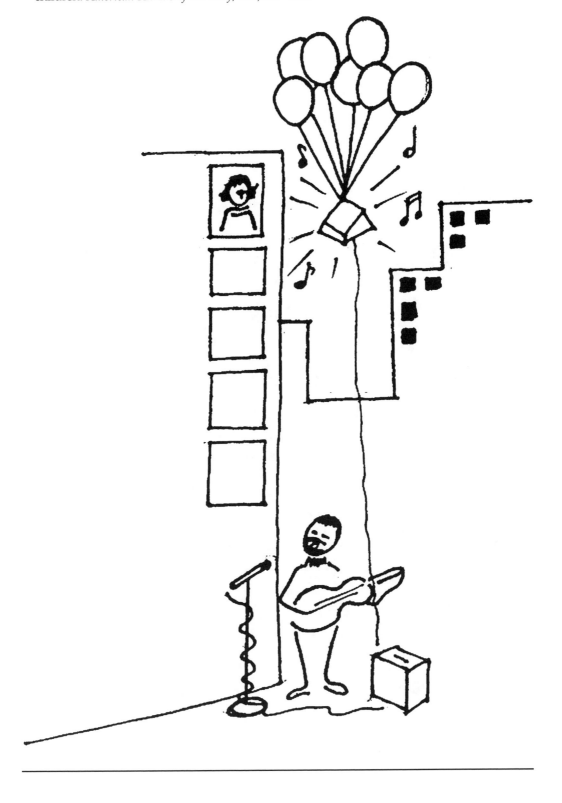

Chapter 13

PHONOLOGICAL AWARENESS, SHORT-TERM MEMORY, AND FLUENCY IN HEARING AND DEAF INDIVIDUALS FROM DIFFERENT COMMUNICATION BACKGROUNDS[1]

Daniel S. Koo, Kelly L. Crain, Carol J. LaSasso, and Guinevere F. Eden

Previous work in deaf populations on phonological coding and working memory, two skills thought to play an important role in the acquisition of written language skills, have focused primarily on signers or did not clearly identify the subjects' native language and communication mode. In the present study, we examined the effect of sensory experience, early language experience, and communication mode on the phonological awareness skills and serial recall of linguistic items in deaf and hearing individuals of different communicative and linguistic backgrounds: hearing nonsigning controls, hearing users of ASL, deaf users of ASL, deaf oral users of English, and deaf users of Cued Speech. As many current measures of phonological awareness skills are inappropriate for deaf populations due to the verbal demands in the stimuli or response, we devised a nonverbal phonological measure that addresses this limitation. The Phoneme Detection Test revealed that deaf cuers and oral-users, but not deaf signers, performed as well as their hearing peers when detecting phonemes not transparent in the orthography. The second focus of the study

[1]Reprinted with permission from The New York Academy of Sciences.

examined short-term memory skills and found that in response to the traditional digit span as well as an experimental visual version, digit span performance was similar across the three deaf groups yet deaf subjects' retrieval was lower than that of hearing subjects. Our results support the claim (Bavelier et al., 2006) that lexical items processed in the visual-spatial modality are not as well retained as information processed in the auditory channel. Together these findings show that the relationship between working memory, phonological coding, and reading may not be as tightly interwoven in deaf students as would have been predicted from work conducted in hearing students.

Introduction

In languages with alphabetic writing systems, individuals typically acquire reading by matching knowledge of the phonological content of their spoken language to the corresponding orthographic representation. This process of applying the alphabetic principle, combined with phonemic awareness and rules of phonics, allows for decoding of words which eventually leads to reading fluency and comprehension of text (Juel, 1988). Phonological coding or phonological awareness (PA), which is the ability to recognize that words in spoken languages are composed of a set of meaningless discrete segments called phonemes (Scarborough & Brady, 2002), has been shown in hearing children to be a powerful predictor of subsequent reading achievement (Adams, 1990; Bradley & Bryant, 1985; Ehri & Sweet, 1991; Goswami & Bryant, 1992; Olson, Forsberg, Wise, & Rack, 1994; Schatschneider, Carlson, Francis, Foorman, & Fletcher, 2002; Snow, Burns, & Griffin, 1998; Torgeson, Wagner, &

Rashotte, 1994; Wagner & Torgeson, 1987). In addition, investigations of the relation between early oral language proficiency and later reading outcome have repeatedly shown that comprehension of oral language is a strong predictor of reading ability (Bishop & Adams, 1990; Catts, Hogan, Fey, 2003; Scarborough, 1989).

In contrast, congenitally deaf children generally do not have sufficient auditory access to spoken languages and for them learning to read is an entirely different endeavor. Many studies have consistently shown that profoundly and prelingually deaf individuals lag significantly behind their hearing peers in standardized measures of reading achievement (Conrad, 1979; Furth, 1966; Karchmer, Milone, & Wolk, 1979; Mitchell & Karchmer, 2004; Traxler, 2000). Their reading abilities vary widely but national surveys indicate an average of third or fourth grade reading level (Allen, 1986; Furth, 1966; Quigley & Paul, 1986; Traxler, 2000; Trybus & Karchmer, 1977). One explanation for this performance deficit is that deafness prevents access to spoken phonology (Perfetti & Sandak, 2000; Shankweiler, Liberman, Mark, Fowler, & Fischer, 1979) and by extension, the use of phonetic coding in working memory, phonological awareness, and phonetic recoding in lexical access, which are considered to be interdependent hallmarks of successful reading development in hearing children (Tractenberg, 2002; Wagner & Torgeson, 1987). This claim, however, is not without dispute as certain deaf individuals demonstrate evidence of phonological coding (Conrad, 1979; Hanson, 1989; Hanson & Fowler, 1987; Hanson & Lichtenstein, 1990; LaSasso, Crain, & Leybaert, 2003; Leybaert, 1993). Still, others have argued that the reason for limited reading achievement among many deaf students is the lack of higher order language skills, not phonological decoding (Chamberlain & Mayberry, 2000), and that levels of comprehension required at the higher grade levels presents an obstacle to reading development. To complicate matters further, there is considerable variability in the use of communication systems among deaf students and their use is usually determined by whether they are born into families of deaf or hearing parents. Unfortunately, many early studies on reading outcomes have not considered the role of the various communication systems available to the deaf population, each of which may independently influence the degree to which deaf students access written English.

Communication Choices

Generally, deaf and hard-of-hearing individuals living in the United States have four visually-based language/communication choices available to them: (1) sign communication (e.g., American Sign Language), (2) oral/aural communication (the exclusive use of audition, speech/lipreading, and speech production), (3) Cued Speech, which is a communication system designed to visually convey the phonology of spoken languages, and (4) manually-coded English (MCE) sign systems, which combine signs borrowed from ASL in English word order with invented signs for sublexical morphemes such as affixes. This chapter is limited to discussing ASL, oral-aural methods, and Cued Speech. For a detailed discussion of MCE sign systems, see Chapter 12.

American Sign Language (ASL) is a widely used manual form of communication in the North American deaf community and is recognized by linguists as a fully autonomous natural language, because it contains the same complex linguistic elements as spoken languages: phonology, morphology, syntax, semantics, and prosody (Klima & Bellugi, 1979; Lane & Grosjean, 1980; Lucas, 1990; Wilbur, 1987). In ASL, signs are produced by a combination of parameters (e.g., handshape, place of articulation, movement, and orientation) (Bellugi, Klima, & Siple, 1975; Stokoe, Casterline, & Croneberg, 1965). ASL is one of a class of signed languages indigenous to deaf communities around the globe. Other signed languages include British Sign Language and French Sign Language. Signed languages are structurally distinct from one another.

Oral/aural communication, which includes speech reading (lipreading), is an approach that places great emphasis and training on the use of speech, residual hearing, and speechreading with the goal of developing intelligible speech, optimal use of residual hearing (generally with the assistance of a hearing aid or cochlear implant), and communicative independence. A national survey reported that 47.8% of more than 37,000 American deaf and hard-of-hearing children use "speech only" as a primary mode of communication (Gallaudet Research Institute, 2005). However, the amount of linguistic information conveyed using the oral method is extremely limited. Research has shown that lipreading single words is only 30% accurate, even in contextual sentences or phrases (Clarke & Ling, 1976; Nicholls & Ling, 1982). Skilled speechreaders often use their grammatical and semantic knowledge to infer messages when the information seen on the lips is ambiguous; this is often referred to as top-down processing (Goodman, 1985).

A much smaller subgroup of deaf individuals uses a communication system commonly known as Cued Speech. This manual system utilizes a set of handshapes to indicate and distinguish (receptively and expressively) the consonants that appear similar on the lips of the "speaker" and a set of hand locations to distinguish vowels that are visibly similar on the mouth of the speaker (Cornett, 1967). For instance, the consonant phonemes /b/, /p/, and /m/ are visually indistinguishable when articulated without the benefit of sound, but are fully specified, or differentiated in Cued Speech via different hand shapes for each phoneme. Similarly, the vowel phonemes /ɪ/ and /ɛ/ are easily misperceived in the absence of sound, but are fully distinguished in Cued Speech via different hand placements. Cued Speech is designed to provide the deaf or hard-of-hearing person with clear and unambiguous visual access to the phonemic information of spoken language by combining the different hand shapes and locations with natural mouth movements inherent in speech. As a result, deaf children who are exposed to Cued Speech from an early age have demonstrated comparable phonological knowledge to their hearing counterparts (Crain, 2003) (see Chapter 14). A national survey reports that 0.3% of more than 37,000 deaf and hard-of-hearing students use Cued Speech (Gallaudet Research Institute, 2005).

Phonology, Reading, and Deafness

Because of the predictive power of phonological skills in determining reading outcome in hearing students, the role of phonology in deaf students vis-à-vis reading has been a subject of great interest. Historically, the definition of a phoneme has often been characterized as sound-based units in part because much of the literature on phonology has focused on spoken languages (e.g., Wagner & Tor-

geson, 1987). In reality, phonemes are abstract cognitive units whose physical (or phonetic) forms typically are manifested via speech or cued gestures (Fleetwood & Metzger, 1998; Hanson, 1989; Scarborough & Brady, 2002).

Studies investigating the role of phonology and reading in deaf individuals have focused largely on the recognition or generation of rhymes (as rhyming is seen as an indicator of PA). For example, in a UK-based study of orally raised deaf students, Conrad (1979) found better readers recalled fewer items from rhyming lists of printed letters than from corresponding nonrhyming lists, suggesting that the more proficient deaf readers had access to phonetic coding that interfered with their recall. Campbell and Wright (1988), in a British study of orally raised deaf adolescents and hearing controls, found that deaf children performed poorly on a rhyme judgment task as a consequence of being susceptible to orthographic similarity. Moreover, in an effort to match the two groups on reading-age (using the Neale reading test), the investigators found that the average chronologic age of deaf subjects was almost twice that of their hearing counterparts (14.6 and 7.6, respectively).

In deaf users of sign language, Hanson and Fowler (1987) conducted a series of experiments employing a speeded lexical decision task in which college-aged deaf and hearing participants made decisions as to whether pairs of written items contained words or pseudowords. They found that phonological similarity between word pairs reduced the reading rate of both the hearing and the signing deaf participants, suggesting a similar phonetic coding strategy in the deaf and hearing participants. In another study, Hanson and McGarr (1989) found that signing deaf college students were able to demonstrate a certain level of PA in a rhyme generation task, but not as extensively as those expected of hearing peers, producing only 50% correct responses to written words. Because the participants were considered good readers, the authors speculated that PA abilities in these deaf adults may have developed as a consequence of reading experience and that in general, PA skills might not be expected to be present in young developing readers. It should be noted that these studies by Hanson and colleagues did not identify whether deaf subjects were native users of ASL, making it difficult to infer possible relationships between deafness, signing experience, and PA skills.

In one of the few comparative studies investigating the phonological skills of children from oral, signing, and cueing backgrounds, Charlier and Leybaert (2000) conducted two experiments examining the rhyming abilities of deaf children in Belgium. In the first experiment, children were asked to make rhyme judgments in their native French based on picture stimuli. They found no differences between the hearing group and the group with extensive Cued Speech exposure (use of Cued Speech both at home and at school) and both of these groups outperformed all other deaf groups (including those who only used Cued Speech at school). In the second experiment, a different group of French deaf cuers and hearing children (mean age = 10.1) were asked to generate rhyming words for pictured and written target items. The results again indicated that the group of children who used Cued Speech at home and school performed similarly to (although slightly lower than) the hearing control group. More recently, LaSasso and colleagues (LaSasso et al., 2003) used a similar rhyme generation task as Hanson and McGarr (1989) to

compare PA performance of college students matched on reading levels (using the Stanford Achievement Test-9, 1996). They compared three groups of skilled readers, hearing, deaf cuers and deaf noncuers, and found that the deaf cuers had PA skills comparable to their hearing peers and superior to that of the deaf noncuers.

Taken together, these studies generally indicate lower performance on measures of PA in deaf compared to hearing students with evidence of strong PA skills among the more accomplished deaf readers, regardless of communication background. However, there is emerging evidence that the performance gap in measures of reading and PA between hearing and deaf students is considerably less in deaf students who have extensive exposure to Cued Speech.

Short-Term Memory and Deafness

In addition to PA, phonetic coding of linguistic items (digits, words, etc.) into short-term memory (STM) is also an important predictor of reading development in hearing children (Wagner & Torgeson, 1987). Hearing individuals have been shown to use a phonetic code during short-term recall of linguistic stimuli (Conrad, 1964, 1973, 1977; Healy, 1982); however, the encoding strategy employed by deaf individuals during STM tasks is less clear. An early STM study by Conrad (1970) claimed that deaf subjects, particularly those who are prelingually deaf, do not use this speech-based phonetic coding. However, other studies have noted some evidence of phonetic coding memory in deaf populations during short-term recall of linguistic items (Conrad, 1979; Hanson, 1982, 1990) which are thought to be advantageous in their reading achievement (Hanson, Liberman, & Shankweiler, 1984; Lichtenstein, 1985, 1998). Specifically, Conrad (1979) tested deaf oral subjects on short-term recall of rhyming printed letters and found decreased performance with rhyming letters compared to unrhymed letters. Hanson (1982) found a similar effect in skilled deaf readers who were native users of ASL when their short-term recall of printed word-items decreased with phonetically similar lists, but not orthographically similar lists. Later, Hanson (1990) examined deaf and hearing adults' temporal (and spatial) recall of letters following an articulatory interference task using letter sets that were designed to confuse subjects on the basis of phonetic, manual, and visual similarity. Both deaf and hearing groups were affected by phonetic similarity in the letters and showed no evidence of manual or visual coding during temporal recall.

Whereas the above studies examined the encoding strategies employed by deaf individuals, a number of studies have focused extensively on the number of linguistic items that subjects recall. Although Tractenberg (2002) found comparable digit recall performance between deaf signers and hearing nonsigning subjects, most other studies consistently indicate that deaf individuals recall fewer items than their hearing counterparts (i.e., Bavelier, Newport, Hall, Supalla, & Boutla, 2006; Bellugi et al., 1975; Boutla, Supalla, Newport, & Bavelier, 2004; Conrad, 1970; Coryell, 2001; Hanson, 1982, 1990; Wallace & Corballis, 1973). Using a computer for stimuli presentation, Coryell (2001) compared the digit span of deaf signers and deaf cuers to age-matched hearing controls and found that deaf signers recalled significantly fewer digit items than did hearing subjects, consistent with previous findings (Bellugi et al., 1975; Conrad, 1970; Wallace & Cor-

ballis, 1973). Additional studies have shown that this lower capacity for recall in deaf signers compared to hearing subjects occurs even when rate of articulation and phonological similarity in item presentation is controlled for (Bavelier et al., 2006; Boutla et al., 2004). However, this discrepancy seems to be limited to serial recall, as deaf subjects exhibit recall performance comparable to that of hearing controls during free recall of linguistic items (Boutla et al., 2004; Hanson, 1982).

Deaf cuers, on the other hand, showed comparable performance to hearing controls and significantly greater digit recall than deaf signers (Coryell, 2001). However, it should be noted that this study employed only the forward recall list of the test and that mental reordering skills, such as those required to perform the backward list, were not the focus of the study.

One criticism of these memory capacity studies described above is that differences in linguistic modality and the formational properties between ASL and spoken languages, rather than lack of audition, might account for the differences observed in STM capacities between hearing and deaf participants. More recent studies have addressed this issue with the inclusion of hearing native signers who share the same early ASL experience as deaf signers (Bavelier et al., 2006; Boutla et al., 2004; Wilson & Emmorey, 1998). These studies have found that hearing native signers of ASL recalled fewer items when stimuli were presented in ASL compared to English, suggesting that sign language, and not sensory experience, can negatively affect STM capacity. Considerable debate continues over whether the sequential nature of spoken languages is most advantageous for temporal-order STM tasks compared to the visuospatial nature of signed languages. Wilson and

Emmorey (2006a, 2006b) have argued that memory capacity is not affected by language modality but is restricted by processing load and that items taking longer to produce, as in the case of signs, will result in a smaller capacity. In a study carefully controlling for intrinsic factors such as word length, articulation rate, and phonological similarity, hearing nonsigners and deaf signers demonstrated comparable STM span using letter stimuli presented in English and ASL respectively (Wilson & Emmorey, 2006a). In contrast, another study (Bavelier et al., 2006) has asserted that the shorter span for ASL-presented items in deaf and hearing native users of ASL exists independently of such manipulations and is attributed to the differences between the auditory and visual modality during serial memory encoding. Their conclusions arose from their findings that deaf and hearing signers persist in showing decreased digit spans despite efforts to control for rate of stimulus presentation and phonological similarity across languages (Bavelier et al., 2006). Taken together, the STM capacity of deaf individuals has largely been shown to be reduced, but the reason for this difference, whether it is attributed to language modality or cross-linguistic differences, is still poorly understood.

Present Study Questions

In short, the conclusions on the nature of PA and verbal STM in deaf populations remain unsettled. Importantly, these studies have been limited in their inclusion or description of the diverse communication backgrounds available to deaf people, thereby hindering a clear determination of whether any differences observed among hearing and deaf subjects in these two

skills can be ascribed to the absence of audition or to their communication modality. Whereas LaSasso and colleagues compared rhyme generation in deaf adult cuers with deaf noncuers (LaSasso et al., 2003), the present study focuses on detection of phonemic units in lexical items and takes a step further by distinguishing deaf noncuers into two groups of oral and signing backgrounds. Likewise, even though the empirical literature is rife with STM studies of deaf oral-users and ASL signers (Bavelier et al., 2006; Boutla et al., 2004; Conrad, 1979; Hanson, 1982, 1990), the present study includes deaf cuers and extends the findings of Coryell (2001) to include backward digit span recall (in addition to forward digit span) during verbal presentation of the stimuli in deaf groups of various communication backgrounds. American deaf adults from distinct language/communication backgrounds, ASL, oral English, and Cued English, were recruited and compared with one another as well as with two groups of hearing subjects, hearing nonsigners, and hearing native signers. In order to specifically address the role of sensory and early language experience on phonemic knowledge and short-term memory, these groups were matched on their reading performance (measured by a test of word recognition) as well as performance IQ. The study of adults, as opposed to children, has the advantage of examining a population whose reading and reading-related skills have reached a mature stage and whose cognitive and linguistic abilities are reflective of their lifelong experience with their auditory and communicative systems.

We made several predictions with regards to phonemic knowledge and short-term memory in skilled readers of distinct sensory and language backgrounds. First, because Cued Speech provides deaf users with unambiguous visual access to English phonology, we predicted that deaf cuers would do well in measures of phonological awareness. By comparison, orally raised deaf adults who without manual cues depend primarily on speechreading to access English and have incomplete visual access to English phonology were predicted to be less proficient in phonological awareness than cuers. Deaf native users of ASL were predicted to have the least access to English phonology and hence the lowest PA skills of the three deaf groups. Second, we predicted that the examination of STM capacity in the three aforementioned deaf groups compared to hearing subjects would provide valuable insight into potential differences in STM capacity between hearing and deaf proficient readers. Importantly, the present study allows us to examine the interplay of language modality and memory encoding skills. If deaf users of Cued Speech and oral-users, whose visual communication system retains the sequential structure of spoken language, demonstrated comparable performance to that of hearing subjects, then Wilson and Emmorey's (2006a) claim of equal spans across language modalities (while taking language-specific differences into account) would be supported. In other words, as long as the individuals share the same native language (English), STM may be preserved even in the absence of audition. Such a finding could suggest that the lower digit span scores seen in deaf signers might be attributed to articulatory differences between the two languages and not sensory differences per se. If, on the other hand, deaf cuers exhibited lower digit span capacity than their hearing counterparts, this would support the claim made by Bavelier et al. (2006) that linguistic information presented in the visuogestural modality is not compatible with the temporal properties of STM in the auditory modality. To address these competing hypotheses, the present study employed two different versions of the digit span, verbal and visual, with the assumption that the visual version of the digit span negates any language-specific differences in stimulus item presentation, such as articulatory rate, duration, and mode of presentation. Although it has already been established that digit span capacity in deaf signers is significantly lower than that of hearing speakers for a number of possible reasons (Bellugi et al., 1975; Conrad, 1970; Hanson, 1982; Wallace & Corballis, 1973), concerns about differences in articulatory rate and word length effect across languages (Wilson & Emmorey, 2006a, 2006b) are not an issue here because deaf cuers and oral users share English with hearing speakers as their native language.

Methods

Participants

A total of 51 subjects from five different categories of language and sensory backgrounds were recruited from the metropolitan Washington, DC area: deaf native users of American Sign Language (DA) ($n = 14$), deaf users of Cued Speech (DC) ($n = 9$), deaf oral users of English (DO) ($n = 8$), hearing native users of American Sign Language (HA) ($n = 10$), and hearing native speakers of English (H) ($n = 10$). Hearing controls were recruited from Georgetown University and deaf and hearing native signers were recruited via flyers posted at Gallaudet University (all participants were college educated with a minimum of 12 years of education). All deaf subjects were born deaf or became deaf before the age of two years, with greater than 85 db hearing loss in the better ear. Subjects reported continuous use of their native languages and communication mode from before the age of five years until adolescence or beyond. All subjects were healthy with no reported history of reading, mental, or neurological disorders. All subjects were participants in a larger study involving functional brain imaging and the tests given to subjects were part of a larger battery of neuropsychological tests spanning two sessions of three hours each. For this analysis, subjects were chosen on the basis of their compatibility with regards to performance IQ and reading accuracy; to attain this goal four subjects with performance IQ standard scores of 127 or more were excluded from the analysis. IRB approval was obtained from Georgetown and Gallaudet Universities.

Neuropsychological and Behavioral Tests

All tests were administered in the subjects preferred language/communication mode by a hearing research assistant fluent in spoken English, ASL, and cued English, unless described otherwise.

Intelligence Quotient

Performance IQ (PIQ) was measured using the Wechsler Abbreviated Scale of Intelligence (WASI) test (Wechsler, 1999). This instrument contains four subtests, each measuring different aspects of intelligence and using items of increasing difficulty. The Performance IQ score was derived for each participant from the Block Design and the Matrix Reasoning subtest scores. A Verbal IQ score was also obtained in four of the five groups using the WASI, but will not be reported for the purpose of the current study as it was not obtained for the deaf ASL group.

Word Identification Fluency

The Test of Silent Word Reading Fluency (TSWRF) (Pro-Ed, Inc.) assesses word identification fluency "as a valid estimate of general reading ability [which] can be used with confidence to identify poor readers" (Mather, Hammill, Allen, & Roberts, 2004). Subjects were presented with rows of words with no spaces between them and asked to draw lines between the boundaries of as many words as possible within 3 minutes. The TSWRF yielded raw scores for accuracy, which were then converted to standard scores through tables provided in the manual.

Reading Comprehension

The Passage Comprehension subtest of the Woodcock-Johnson III test measures silent reading comprehension without time constraints (Woodcock, McGrew, & Mather, 2001). The present reading achievement level of the subject dictates the starting point of the test and the level of difficulty of the test increases by increasing the level of vocabulary, the passage length, and the syntactic and semantic complexity of the items. The recommended starting point for an average adult requires the person to silently read a sentence or short paragraph and verbally supply the missing word that appropriately completes the sentence. This subtest yields raw scores and standard scores.

Phoneme Detection Test (PDT)

Although rhyming tasks are often used as an indicator of phonological awareness, more direct measures of phonological awareness have been difficult to obtain in deaf populations in large part due to insensitive test administration protocols. Many current measures (e.g., Rosner Test of Auditory Analysis Skills, the Lindamood Auditory Conceptualization Test, or the Comprehensive Test of Phonological Processing) require stimulus items or the subject's responses to be spoken or verbalized, which can be problematic for deaf subjects who do not speech-read or use speech to communicate. Here we introduce a computer-based phonological awareness measure, the Phoneme Detection Test (PDT), which addresses these administrative confounds. This test was developed to measure phonemic awareness via detection of the presence of a single phoneme in individual, visually presented words (computer generation of these stimuli was achieved with Presentation version 0.81, http://www.neurobs.com). The test includes 150 high-frequency words with multiple or opaque orthography-to-phonology correspondences (e.g., "c" maps to /s/ and /k/ phonemes such as *cent* and *call*), divided into five target-phoneme sets of 30 items each: /s/, /g/, /dʒ/, and /k/ (/k/ repeated for "ch" and "c" sets). Half the items contained target phonemes appearing in initial, medial, or word-final positions and the other half served as orthographic foils in which an alternative grapheme-to-phoneme correspondence was used. Subjects were instructed to respond as quickly and accurately as possible with keyboard buttons indicating "Yes" or "No" if an item contained the target phoneme. Nonverbal stimuli and response modality remove undesirable confounds from subjects' different communication modes and allow between-group comparisons of accuracy and reaction time. Explicit instructions and examples were given at the beginning of the test to ensure subjects understood that the task was not to detect orthographic units, but phonemic units. In addition, each set was preceded by a four-item practice session. The order of set presentation was counterbalanced across subjects.

Spatial Memory Span

The Spatial Span (SS) subtest from the Wechsler Memory Scale-III measures the ability to hold a visual-spatial sequence of events in working memory (Wechsler, 1997). A three-dimensional board of nine cubes positioned on a base is used to administer visual-spatial sequences, ranging in difficulty from two to nine movements with two trials at each level. Subjects are instructed to manually respond by touching the blocks in correct sequences, either forwards or backwards for Spatial Span Forward and Spatial Span Backward. Total raw score (from Forward and Backward trials) is converted to an age-referenced scaled score. This test was included to provide a spatial analogue to the verbal memory span.

Verbal Digit Span

The Wechsler Adult Intelligence Scale-III (WAIS-III) Digit Span subtest requires repetition of numbers in sequences of increasing length, from 2 to 9 numbers with two trials at each difficulty level (Wechsler, 1999). The subject is given two strings of each length, the length increasing with each pair. If the subject repeats both sequences correctly, he or she receives a score of 2, if only one is correct a score of 1, and if neither is correct no points are earned. Hence, it is these scores that are reflected in the raw score (not the longest correctly repeated sequence). The score from forward and backward lists were combined and converted to an age-reference scaled score. As is typical for this test, an experimenter administered the DST in English for hearing and deaf oral subjects. Prior to taking the test, deaf oral subjects were given opportunities to be familiarized with the experimenter's mouth movements. Deaf signers and deaf cuers viewed a prerecorded Quicktime video in which the experimenter presented the digits in their respective languages, ASL and English (via Cued Speech). Subjects were given opportunity to respond in their preferred mode or language.

Visual Version of the Digit Span

Because of difficulties in interpreting between-group differences for the traditional version of the Digit Span described above and the existence of sensory and language differences during task presentation (Boutla et al., 2004; Wilson & Emmorey, 1998, 2006a, 2006b), we also administered a visual version of the Digit Span to our subjects. Written task instructions and practice sessions were presented on a computer screen at the beginning of the test to ensure subjects understood the task. Digits were presented centrally on the screen in large black font and at the same pace as the traditional verbal version of the Digit Span (Presentation version 0.81, http://www.neurobs.com). Immediately following the presentation of number strings, a red square flashed briefly on the screen to signal the end of the trial and begin recall. To visually simulate the falling intonation used when the last digit in a string is uttered in the verbal Digit

Span, the last digit in a string was presented using a different colored font (red), to prompt the subject that the sequence is about to end. Subjects responded using the number keypad and were given opportunities to delete their response if they made keyboard errors.

Data Analysis

We compared the five groups (deaf users of ASL, oral English, and cued English as well as hearing nonsigners and hearing native signers) on each behavioral measure using one-way ANOVAs with significance defined as alpha <0.05. Where main effect of group was observed, pairwise multiple comparisons were made among each of the five groups. To estimate intermeasure reliability, the traditional Verbal Digit Span and the experimental visual version of the Verbal Digit Span were entered into a correlation analysis (with forward and backward raw scores combined). In addition, to establish the relationship between measures of reading with measures of STM and PA, measures from the PDT and the Digit Span (both the traditional verbal version as well as for the experimental visual version) were entered into nonparametric correlation analyses with passage comprehension and word identification fluency scores.

Results

Neuropsychological and Behavioral Tests

Table 13–1 shows the groups' demographics as well as their behavioral scores. As described above, subjects were selected in

Table 13–1. Demographics, Neuropsychological, and Behavioral Measures Expressed as Mean Score (Standard Deviation)

	Hearing	Hearing ASL	Deaf ASL	Deaf CS	Deaf Oral	Significance
Number	8	9	13	9	8	
Demographics						
Age (years)	22.6 (3.1)	30.4 (5.8)	23.1 (3.6)	29.4 (3.6)	25.0 (3.5)	0.000
Gender	4F	9F	7F	4F	2F	
Neuropsychological and Behavioral Scores						
Performance IQ	117.75 (6.7)	114.89 (10.5)	109.92 (10.0)	112.88 (8.8)	112.50 (8.7)	n.s.
Reading (accuracy)						
TSWRF (word identification)	115.62 (13.6)	108.56 (14.0)	105.15 (16.9)	122.55 (8.4)	113.87 (12.1)	n.s.
WJ-III Comprehension	119.5 (11.2)	112.67 (13.1)	100.15 (11.9)	106.0 (4.6)	102.5 (7.9)	0.001
Short-Term Memory						
Spatial Span (SS)	109.37 (9.8)	106.67 (8.3)	108.85 (11.4)	97.77 (14.2)	101.87 (6.5)	n.s.
Digit Span Verbal (SS)	121.88 (16.2)	108.89 (14.5)	96.92 (13.9)	105.00 (10.3)	97.37 (10.0)	0.002
Digit Span Verbal (Raw)	23.75 (4.7)	19.78 (3.8)	16.46 (4.0)	18.22 (2.7)	16.75 (2.9)	0.001
Visual Version of Digit Span (Raw)	22.33 (2.4)	21.44 (3.9)	15.81 (3.7)	15.87 (3.0)	11.86 (2.3)	0.000
Phonemic Awareness						
PDT Accuracy (%)	93.7 (7.3)	93.4 (5.2)	65.2 (14.5)	86.4 (12.3)	87.6 (6.9)	0.000
PDT RT (in ms)	1156 (335)	1854 (665)	2848 (1027)	1819 (777)	2577 (1332)	0.002

such a way that they were matched for Performance IQ ($F(4, 42) = .985$, $p < 0.426$) and reading fluency as measured by TSWRF ($F(4, 42) = 2.461$, $p = 0.060$). However, despite their generally equivalent performance on word recognition fluency, we found a main effect of group in the Passage Comprehension subtest ($F(4, 42) = 5.313$, $p < 0.001$). Post hoc comparisons revealed that performance of the hearing nonsigning group was significantly higher on reading comprehension than the deaf signing (Tukey's HSD = 19.34, $p < 0.002$) and oral (Tukey's HSD = 17.00, $p < 0.018$) groups, but not the hearing signers or deaf cuers ($p > 0.05$). Hearing signers were not significantly different from any of the three deaf groups ($p > 0.05$), nor were there significant differences when comparing any of the three deaf groups with each other. Therefore, the hearing nonsigning group was the only group at odds compared to the others with a significant advantage for reading comprehension.

Phoneme Detection Test (PDT)

Computer difficulties resulted in data loss from six subjects for this test (H = 2, DC = 1, DO = 1, and DA = 2). Main effect of group was observed in the remaining PDT data on measures of performance accuracy ($F(4,36) = 12.26$, $p < 0.001$) and reaction time ($F(4,36) = 4.33$, $p = 0.006$). Posthoc comparisons revealed that the deaf signing group was significantly less accurate (Tamhane's T2, $p < 0.05$) on phoneme detection compared to the other four groups. However, deaf signers reported no significant difference in reaction times when compared to the other groups ($p > 0.05$) except for the hearing nonsigners, who were faster than the deaf signers (Tamhane's T2, $p < 0.01$). Accuracy and reaction

times for the deaf cueing group was comparable to that of the hearing control group, hearing signers, and deaf oral users (Tamhane's T2, $p > 0.05$). The deaf oral group also demonstrated statistically indistinguishable accuracy and reaction times when compared to the hearing nonsigning group and hearing signing group (Tamhane's T2, $p > 0.05$).

Spatial Memory Span

WMS-Spatial Span revealed no significant group differences among the five groups ($F(4, 42) = 2.054$, $p > 0.05$).

Verbal Digit Span

The traditional verbal version of Digit Span test from the WAIS-III revealed significant group differences in raw scores ($F(4, 42) = 5.67$, $p < 0.001$). Post hoc comparisons between the three deaf and two hearing groups showed that the hearing nonsigners performed significantly better (Tukey's HSD, $p < 0.05$) than all other groups except hearing signers (Tukey's HSD = 3.97, $p > 0.05$). The hearing ASL signers did not differ significantly from any of the deaf groups and no significant differences were found among the three deaf groups (Tukey's HSD, $p > 0.05$).

Visual Version of the Digit Span

Computer difficulties resulted in some data loss for the Visual Digit Span (H = 2; DA = 2; DC = 1; DO = 1). For the remaining data, significant between-group differences were observed in raw scores ($F(4, 36) = 12.63$, $p < 0.001$). Post hoc comparisons indicated that all three deaf groups performed significantly lower than the two hearing groups in all pair-wise contrasts (Tukey's HSD, p <0.01). However, all deaf groups showed no significant differences with each other (Tukey's HSD, p >0.05). Hearing nonsigners were not significantly different from hearing signers (Tukey's HSD = .889, p >0.05).

Correlation Analyses

To assess the relationship between the standard verbal versions of the digit span and our experimental visual version of this test, we entered the data into a non-parametric correlation analyses and found that the two measures were significantly correlated to each other (t = .602, p <0.001).

To estimate the relationship between phonemic awareness skills (as measured by the PDT) and reading ability, nonparametric correlation analysis (Kendall's tau) was performed between PDT accuracy scores and performance on the TSWRF as well as passage comprehension scores. Surprisingly, the first revealed no significant correlation between PDT accuracy and TSWRF. The second, showed a positive correlation (t = .305, p <0.01; two-tailed) between PA skills and reading comprehension. Reaction time from the PDT was negatively correlated to the above same measures (TSWRF: t = −.291, p <0.01; two-tailed and Passage Comprehension: t = −.248; p <0.05, two-tailed).

To estimate the relationship between STM memory and reading measures, both the traditional Verbal Digit Span and the experimental visually presented version of the Verbal Digit Span were entered into nonparametric correlation analyses and found to be significantly correlated with the Passage Comprehension (DS-Verbal:

t = .323; DS-visual version of the verbal: t = .409, p <0.01; two-tailed). However, neither version of the Digit Span was correlated to word identification fluency as measured by TSWRF (DS-Verbal: t = .114; DS-Visual: t = .082, p >0.05).

Discussion

With a few exceptions (i.e., Charlier & Leybeart, 2000; LaSasso et al., 2003), previous empirical studies examining the impact of deafness on skills that support reading have focused on deaf signers, making it difficult to dissociate the effect of deafness from early language experience. Inclusion of deaf individuals who acquired English natively via visual means (oral communication or Cued Speech) along with deaf users of ASL will help us disentangle the effect of deafness and language experience on phonological awareness and verbal short-term memory, two of the three core predictors of reading achievement (Wagner & Torgeson, 1987). The first aim of the present study was to explore the PA skills of deaf cuers (who have full, unambiguous access to the phonological structure of traditionally spoken languages) relative to other deaf and hearing groups. Then, by examining verbal working memory of deaf nonsigners as well as the more traditionally studied group of deaf signers, the second aim was to gain further insight into the role visual language plays in the capacity to retain lexical items in short-term memory.

Phonemic Awareness

Because commercially available measures of phonological awareness are not suitable for deaf populations (see Tractenberg, 2002), the PDT was developed to probe phonological coding skills in deaf participants using visual stimuli and nonverbal responses. As expected, deaf native signers of ASL did not perform well on phonemic detection of English words, reflecting their lack of experience with spoken English phonology. Specifically, the deaf signing group was significantly less accurate on the PDT than all other groups. Mean reaction time for the deaf signers was longer on the PDT, but this difference was significant only in comparison to the hearing nonsigning group. Only two deaf signers showed greater than 85% accuracy on the PDT and deaf signers in general performed at or slightly above chance during the detection of phonemic units, despite being good readers.

On the other hand, deaf cuers and deaf oral users had accuracy scores that were statistically indistinguishable from those of either hearing groups. With an average accuracy above 85% on the PDT, both of the English-native deaf groups (cuers and oral-users) clearly demonstrated robust awareness of the phonological structure of English lexical items even when certain phonemes were not explicitly revealed in the orthography. To our surprise, deaf cuers and oral-users were not different from each other during this phonological coding task (based on accuracy and reaction times). More direct access to the phonemic stream of English in deaf cuers would have predicted an advantage for this group over the oral group (cuers had shorter but not statistically different reaction times), but such a benefit was not observed on this test.

Correlation analyses revealed that although accuracy on the PDT was not correlated to performance on word identification fluency (measured by the TSWRF), it was correlated with passage comprehension; and reaction time on the PDT was correlated with both the TSWRF as well as reading comprehension, suggesting that a relationship does exist between reading and PA skills in the context of the speed by which subjects perform the PDT task. The absence of a correlation between accuracy in word recognition fluency and PA is somewhat surprising, as studies of hearing populations frequently report that measures of phonemic coding skills correlate with word reading accuracy. The reason for a lack of a correlation between the PA test and the TSWRF is most likely due to the fact that the TSWRF task relies more on sight word recognition than addressed phonology. Addressed phonology is probed more directly during tests of reading aloud, especially the reading of pseudowords.

In sum, we found that PA skills are not well developed in deaf users of sign language in our study, even though they have acquired proficient reading skills. This suggests that under some circumstances proficient reading can be attained in the absence of PA skills. Future studies will need to determine whether there are other skills, linguistic or otherwise, that are more strongly developed in deaf signers with good reading ability and how these facilitate their reading. We also found that deaf cuers performed more like hearing subjects and significantly better than deaf signers on the PA test. Their ability to detect phonemic units suggests they have been facilitated by lifelong use of manual cues to visually access English phonology. However, since our oral subjects performed equally well as the cuers, it seems that access to the phonological representation of English can also be obtained without the use of cues.

Short-Term Memory

There has been an ongoing debate as to whether retention spans in short-term verbal memory are lower in people who are deaf. Some have argued that studies in which differences have been observed in deaf population may be confounded by the delivery of the tests, that is, administration in sign language compared to English may introduce other variables that lead to shorter retention spans. Here we addressed this question using a two-pronged approach. First, the inclusion of deaf participants who use English to perform the task (instead of ASL) allows for a more comparable assessment between hearing and deaf groups. Second, we devised a visual version of the traditional Verbal Digit Span, as a way to equalize the stimuli presentation and response mode between hearing and deaf groups. Together this allowed us to examine whether verbal STM is affected by sensory experience, language experience, or modality of tests presentation.

Our overall finding was that although all five groups were comparable on the Spatial Span tests, there were profound group differences on performance of the Verbal Digit Span. All three deaf groups showed shorter digit retention when compared to the nonsigning hearing group during the traditional version of the Digit Span, and further, all three deaf groups showed shorter digit retention when compared to both hearing groups in an experimental visual version of the Digit Span where subjects responded to visual stimuli using a keyboard.

Our first observation of lower performance on the Digit Span is consistent with recent findings (Bavelier et al., 2006; Boutla et al., 2004), that deaf signers exhibit shorter digit span for numbers presented

in ASL compared to hearing nonsigners. When examining the longest correct digit length attained, our hearing subjects achieved spans of 7.2 (nonsigners) and 6.3 (signers) and our deaf subjects had spans of 4.9 (signers), 5.4 (cuers) and 5.0 (oral). These findings are largely consistent with the digit spans described by Bavelier and colleagues (2006) for signers. In addition to this observation, Boutla and colleagues also reported decreased serial item recall in hearing signers when they viewed the stimuli in ASL compared to when they heard the stimuli in English. Together, these results suggest a detrimental effect of ASL on measures of verbal retention, but perhaps somewhat surprisingly, our deaf cueing and oral groups also exhibited significantly lower digit spans than the hearing nonsigners. As both the cueing and oral groups received the stimuli in their native English language and linguistic modality (cued or orally), the discrepancy in short-term recall of digits described in the literature cannot be solely attributed to signed languages. Our second test of verbal short-term verbal memory was given in the visual modality to all participants and resulted in all three deaf groups performing similarly to one another and significantly lower than the two hearing groups. Together these results suggest that even when language experience or modality of tests presentation are taken into consideration, there are differences among hearing and deaf subjects in ability to retain digits.

These findings suggest that the use of the visual-spatial modality (rather than the auditory modality used by hearing subjects) to receive and hold linguistic items in working memory presents a greater processing load, and results in lower item recall. This conclusion is consistent with the view put forward by

Bavelier and colleagues, suggesting that visual modality is a limiting factor in working memory (Bavelier et al., 2006; Boutla et al., 2004). In this context it is also worth considering that deaf subjects did not only differ from the hearing subjects in their retention span and that all deaf groups performed similarly to one another, but also that the deaf signers did not show any improvements in performance on the experimental visual version of the digit span compared to the traditional verbal version. Specifically, our efforts to remove any linguistic or modality bias in stimuli presentation and recall responses, had little positive effect on the performance of our deaf participants. This is consistent with findings where visually presented nonnameable items have reduced hearing subjects' capacity for serial item recall (Alvarez & Cavanagh, 2004; Cowan, 2001).

Finally, it is of interest to examine working memory spans in the context of our other measures. Deaf cuers performed similarly to the hearing subjects on word identification fluency and phonemic awareness, but they had significantly lower digit span performance, suggesting that: (1) good reading skill can be attained in the absence of strong working memory skills, and (2) skills traditionally thought of as predicting reading outcome in hearing subjects (Wagner & Torgeson, 1987) may not be suitable in gauging reading achievement in deaf students.

In sum, we found that deaf subjects regardless of communication or language background had lower digit span retention than hearing subjects, while spatial span was comparable amongst all groups. Further, we found no differences in performance among all three deaf groups even though their language background might have predicted differential ability on memory span. The findings suggest that longer digit recall in hearing compared to deaf subjects can be explained by the availability of the articulatory loop that is utilized for the sequential nature of the auditory channel in working memory.

Conclusion

The goal of the present study was to gain some insight into the cognitive and linguistic abilities of deaf people who are skilled readers yet have been raised with a variety of language/communication systems, namely ASL, Cued Speech, or the oral-aural method. We found deaf native signers of ASL did not do well on detection of hidden English phonology in visually presented words, while deaf cuers and deaf oral-users had phonological performance comparable to that of hearing subjects. Second, we examined the digit span of deaf and hearing subjects and found that all three deaf groups performed similarly to one another and weaker than hearing subjects. As deaf cuers and oral-users receive the digit stimuli in the same language as hearing groups via a different visual medium, we conclude that the use of sign language does not have a detrimental effect on serial recall of linguistic items. Instead, it appears that linguistic information processing in the visual channel creates additional processing burden on short-term memory capacity and subsequent recall. This was confirmed by a second measure of digit span that did not involve the use of manual languages in its administration. Taken together, the findings support the idea put forward by Bavelier et al. (2006) that the articulatory loop in working memory is most advantageous when speech articulation is used to encode linguistic items and that the visual nature of linguistic stimuli triggers a decrease in STM span. Finally, our results demonstrate that among deaf subjects skilled reading can be attained despite lower working memory abilities and in the case of signers, despite lower STM and phonemic awareness skills. This strongly suggests that deaf subjects' reading skills are facilitated by abilities other than those traditionally considered to be important in hearing students.

Acknowledgments. This work was supported by the National Institutes of Health (NICHD Grant HD40095, NIDCD Grant F32 DC007774) and the General Clinical Research Center Program of the NCR-Resources (M01-RR13297). This material is based upon work supported by the National Science Foundation under Grant No.SBE 0541953 for the Science of Learning Centers Program. We wish to thank Lynn Flowers, Eileen Napoliello, Jill Weisberg, Ashley Wall, and Alina Engelman for their help. We also thank our subjects for their participation.

References

Adams, M. (1990). *Beginning to read: Thinking and learning about print*. Cambridge, MA: MIT Press.

Allen, T. (1986) Patterns of academic achievement among hearing impaired students: 1974 and 1983. In A. Schildroth & M. Karchmer (Eds.), *Deaf children in America* (pp. 161–206). San Diego, CA: College-Hill.

Alvarez, G., & Cavanagh, P. (2004). The capacity of visual short-term memory is set both by visual information load and by number of objects. *Psychological Science, 15*, 106–111.

Bavalier, D., Newport, E., Hall, M., Supalla, T., & Boutla, M. (2006). Persistent difference in short-term memory span between sign and speech. *Psychological Science, 17*, 1090–1092.

Bellugi, U., Klima, E., & Siple, P. (1975). Remembering in signs. *Cognition, 3*, 93–125.

Bishop, D., & Adams, C. (1990). A prospective study of the relationship between specific language impairment, phonological disorders and reading retardation. *Journal of Child Psychology and Psychiatry and Allied Disciplines, 31*, 1027–1050.

Boutla, M., Supalla, T., Newport, E., & Bavelier, D. (2004). Short-term memory span: Insights from sign language. *Nature Neuroscience, 7*, 997–1002.

Bradley, L., & Bryant, P. (1985). *Rhyme and reason in reading and spelling (IARLD Monographs, No. 1)*. Ann Arbor, MI: University of Michigan Press.

Campbell, R., & Wright, H. (1988). Deafness, spelling, and rhyme: How spelling supports written word and picture rhyming skills in deaf subjects. *Quarterly Journal of Experimental Psychology, 40A*, 771–788.

Catts, H. W., Hogan, T. P., & Fey, M. E. (2003). Subgrouping poor readers on the basis of individual differences in reading-related abilities. *Journal of Learning Disabilites, 36*(2), 151–164.

Chamberlain, C., & Mayberry, R. I. (2000). Theorizing about the relationship between American Sign Language and reading. In C. Chamberlain, J. P. Morford, & R. I. Mayberry (Eds.), *Language acquisition by eye* (pp. 221–260). Mahwah, NJ: Lawrence Erlbaum.

Charlier, B., & Leybaert, J. (2000). The rhyming skills of deaf children educated with phonetically augmented lipreading. *Quarterly Journal of Experimental Psychology, 53A*, 349–375.

Clarke, B., & Ling, D. The effects of using Cued Speech: A follow-up study. *Volta Review, 78*, 23–34.

Conrad, R. (1964) Acoustic confusions in immediate memory. *British Journal of Psychology, 55*, 75–84.

Conrad, R. (1970). Short-term memory processes in the deaf. *British Journal of Psychology, 61*, 179–195.

Conrad, R. (1973). Some correlates of speech coding in the short-term memory of the deaf. *Journal of Speech and Hearing Research, 16*, 375–384.

Conrad, R. (1977). The reading ability of deaf school-leavers. *British Journal of Educational Psychology, 47*, 138–148.

Conrad, R. (1979). *The deaf school child*. London, UK: Harper and Row.

Cornett, R. O. (1967). Cued Speech. *American Annals of the Deaf, 112*, 3–13.

Coryell, H. (2001). *Verbal sequential processing skills and reading ability in deaf individuals using Cued Speech and signed communication.* Unpublished dissertation. Gallaudet University, Washington, DC.

Cowan, N. (2001). The magical number 4 in short-term memory: A reconsideration of mental storage capacity. *Behavioral Brain Science, 24*, 87–185.

Crain, K. L. (2003). *The development of phonological awareness in moderately-to-profound deaf developing readers: The effect of exposure to cued American English.* Unpublished doctoral dissertation, Gallaudet University, Washington DC.

Ehri, L., & Sweet, J. (1991). Fingerpoint-reading of memorized text: What enables beginners to process the print? *Reading Research Quarterly, 24*, 442–462.

Fleetwood, E., & Metzger, M. (1998). *Cued language structure: An analysis of cued American English based on linguistic principles.* Silver Spring, MD: Calliope Press.

Furth, H. (1966). A comparison of reading test norms of deaf and hearing children. *American Annals of the Deaf, 111*, 461–462.

Gallaudet Research Institute. (2005). *Regional and National Summary Report of Data from the 2004–2005 Annual Survey of Deaf and Hard of Hearing Children and Youth.* Washington, DC: Gallaudet University.

Goodman, K. (1985) Unity in reading. In H. Singer & R. Ruddell (Eds.), *Theoretical models and processes of reading* (3rd ed., pp. 813–840). Newark, DE: International Reading Association.

Goswami, U., & Bryant, P. (1992). Rhyme, analogy, and children's reading. In P. Gough, L. Ehri, & R. Treiman (Eds.), *Read-ing acquisition* (pp. 49–64). Hillsdale, NJ: Lawrence Erlbaum Associates.

Hanson, V. (1982). Short-term recall by deaf signers of American Sign Language: Implication of encoding strategy for ordered recall. *Journal of Experimental Psychology, 8*, 572–583.

Hanson, V. (1989). Phonology and reading: Evidence from profoundly deaf readers. In D. Shankweiler & E. Liberman (Eds.), *Phonology and reading disability: Solving the reading puzzle* (pp. 67–89). Ann Arbor, MI: University of Michigan Press

Hanson, V. (1990). Recall of order information by deaf signers: Phonetic coding in temporal order recall. *Memory & Cognition, 18*, 604–610.

Hanson, V., & Fowler, C. (1987). Phonological coding in word reading: Evidence from hearing and deaf readers. *Memory & Cognition, 15*, 199–207.

Hanson, V., Liberman, I., & Shankweiler, D. (1984). Linguistic coding by deaf children in relation to beginning reading success. *Journal of Experimental Child Psychology, 37*, 378–393.

Hanson, V., & Lichtenstein, E. (1990) Short-term memory by deaf signers: The primary language coding hypothesis reconsidered. *Cognitive Psychology, 22*, 211–224.

Hanson, V., & McGarr, N. (1989). Rhyme generation in deaf adults. *Journal of Speech and Hearing Research, 32*, 2–11.

Healy, A. (1982). Short-term memory for order information. In G. Bower (Ed.), *The psychology of learning and motivation* (Vol. 16, pp. 191–238). New York, NY: Academic Press.

Juel, C. (1988). Learning to read and write: A longitudinal study of 54 children from first through fourth grades. *Journal of Educational Psychology, 80*, 437–447.

Karchmer, M., Milone, M., & Wolk, S. (1979). Educational significance of hearing loss at three levels of severity. *American Annals of the Deaf, 124*, 97–109.

Klima, E., & Bellugi, U. *The signs of language.* Cambridge, MA: Harvard University Press.

LaSasso, C., Crain, K., & Leybaert, J. (2003). Rhyme generation in deaf students: The effect of exposure to Cued Speech. *Journal of Deaf Studies and Deaf Education, 8,* 250–270.

Lane, H., & Grosjean, F. (Eds.). (1980). *Recent perspectives on American Sign Language.* Hillsdale, NJ: Erlbaum.

Leybeart, J. (1993). Reading in the deaf: The roles of phonological codes. In M. Marcshark & M. Clark (Eds.), *Psychological perspectives on deafness* (pp. 269–309). Hillsdale, NJ: Lawrence Erlbaum Associates.

Lichtenstein, E. (1985). Deaf working memory processes and English language. In D. Martin (Ed.), *Cognition, education and deafness* (pp. 111–114). Washington, DC: Gallaudet College Press.

Lichtenstein, E. (1998). The relationship between reading processes and English skills of deaf college students. *Journal of Deaf Studies and Deaf Education, 3,* 80–134.

Lucas, C. (Ed.) (1990). *Sign language research.* Washington, DC: Gallaudet University Press.

Mather, N., Hammill, D., Allen, E., & Roberts, R. (2004) *Test of Silent Word Reading Fluency.* Austin, TX: Pro-Ed.

Nicholls, G., & Ling, D. (1982). Cued Speech and the reception of spoken language. *Journal of Speech and Hearing Research, 25,* 262–269.

Olson, R., Forsberg, H., Wise, B., & Rack, J. (1994). Measurement of word recognition, orthographic, and phonological skills. In R. Lyon (Ed.), *Frames of reference from the assessment of learning disabilities* (pp. 243–277). Baltimore, MD: Brookes.

Perfetti, C., & Sandak, R. (2000) Reading optimally builds on spoken language. *Journal of Deaf Studies and Deaf Education, 5,* 32–50.

Quigley, S., & Paul, P. (1986) A perspective on academic achievement. In D. Luterman (Ed.), *Deafness in perspective* (pp. 55–86). San Diego, CA: College-Hill.

Scarborough, H. (1989). Prediction of reading dysfunction from familial and individual differences. *Journal of Educational Psychology, 81,* 101–108.

Scarborough, H., & Brady, S. (2002). *Toward a common terminology for talking about speech and reading: A glossary of the "phon" words and some related terms.* (Unpublished manuscript).

Schatschneider, C., Carlson, C. D., Francis, D. J., Foorman, B. R., & Fletcher, J. M. Relationship of rapid automatized naming and phonological awareness in early reading development: implications for the double-deficit hypothesis. *Journal of Learning Disabilities, 35*(3), 245–256.

Shankweiler, D., Liberman, I., Mark, L., Fowler, C., & Fischer, F. (1979). The speech code and learning to read. *Journal of experimental psychology: Human learning and memory, 5,* 531–545.

Snow, C., Burns, S., & Griffin, P. (Eds.). (1998). *Preventing reading difficulties in young children.* Washington, DC: National Academy Press.

Stokoe, W., Casterline, D., & Croneberg, C. (1965). *A Dictionary of American Sign Language.* Washington, DC: Gallaudet College Press.

The Psychological Corporation (1996). *The Stanford Achievement Test* (9th ed.). Houston, TX: Harcourt Educational Measurement.

Torgeson, J., Wagner, R., & Rashotte, C. (1994). Longitudinal studies of phonological processing and reading. *Journal of Learning Disabilities, 27,* 276–286.

Tractenberg, R. (2002). Exploring hypotheses about phonological awareness, memory, and reading achievement. *Journal of Learning Disabilities, 35,* 407–424.

Traxler, C. (2000). The Stanford Achievement Test, 9th edition: National norming and performance standards for deaf and hard-of-hearing students. *Journal of Deaf Studies and Deaf Education, 5,* 337–348.

Trybus, R., & Karchmer, M. (1977). School achievement scores of hearing impaired children: National data on achievement status and growth patterns. *American Annals of the Deaf Directory of Programs and Services, 122,* 62–69.

Wagner, R., & Torgeson, J. (1987). The nature of phonological processing and its causal role in the acquisition of reading skills. *Psychological Bulletin, 101,* 192–212.

Wallace, G., & Corballis, M. (1973). Short-term memory and coding strategy of the deaf. *Journal of Experimental Psychology, 99,* 334–348.

Wechsler, D. (1997). *Wechsler Memory Scale—Third Edition (WMS-III) Spatial Span.* San Antonio, TX: Psychological Corporation, Harcourt Brace and Company.

Wechsler, D. (1999). *Wechsler Abbreviated Scale of Intelligence.* San Antonio, TX: Psychological Corporation, Harcourt Brace and Company.

Wilbur, R. (1987). *American Sign Language: Linguistic and applied dimensions* (2nd ed.). Boston, MA: Little, Brown.

Wilson, M., & Emmorey, K. (1998). A "word length effect" for sign language: Further evidence for the role of language in structuring working memory. *Memory and Cognition, 26,* 584–590.

Wilson, M., & Emmorey, K. (2006a). Comparing sign language and speech reveals a universal limit on short-term memory capacity. *Psychological Science, 17,* 682–683.

Wilson, M., & Emmorey, K. (2006b). No difference in short-term memory span between sign and speech. *Psychological Science, 17,* 1093–1094.

Woodcock, R., McGrew, K., & Mather, N. (2001). *Woodcock-Johnson III Tests of Achievement.* Itasca, IL: Riverside.

Chapter 14

GENERATIVE RHYMING ABILITY OF 10- TO 14-YEAR-OLD READERS WHO ARE DEAF FROM ORAL AND CUED SPEECH BACKGROUNDS

Kelly Lamar Crain and Carol J. LaSasso

Phonological Awareness

Phonological awareness (PA) refers to an individual's ability to consider the discrete segments comprising words in a language. Such segments may be individual phonemes or larger units, such as consonant-vowel (C-V) or vowel-consonant (V-C) syllables, rimes, or consonant cluster onsets. The interest in PA by linguists, psychologists, and other researchers stems from the relationship of PA to: (1) children's natural acquisition of English and other traditionally spoken languages (Paul & Jennings, 1992; Velleman, 1988), (2) working memory, and (3) phonics, all three of which are critical to reading comprehension (Wagner, Torgeson, & Rashotte, 1994). It has been speculated that deaf children's relatively

lower scores on reading comprehension tests (Karchmer & Mitchell, 2003; Traxler, 2000) relate to their difficulties with PA (Colin, Magnan, Ecalle, & Leybaert, 2007; Dyer, MacSweeney, Szczerbinski, Green, & Campbell, 2003).

Phonological awareness plays an important role in natural language acquisition. Children in all parts of the world tend to acquire traditionally spoken home languages naturally, without formal instruction, regardless of the nature (e.g., alphabetic, tonal) or complexity of the language. Two conditions that have been found to be essential for natural language acquisition include: (1) early, clear, complete access to the "continuous phoneme stream" of the language and (2) opportunities to interact, in age-appropriate ways, with fluent models of the language (see

Chapter 12). This universally observed phenomenon supports the view of Chomsky (1975) and others that children are biologically predisposed to acquire language; however, children will not do so in the absence of key environmental factors, including sensory stimulation and opportunities to interact with fluent users of the language. For example, children with auditory deficits typically do not acquire traditionally spoken languages naturally at the same rate as their hearing peers (Sterne & Goswami, 2000). It is not the deafness, per se, that is directly implicated. Children with profound degrees of deafness *can* naturally acquire spoken language visually (e.g., via Cued Speech), and children with normal hearing can experience disruptions in their acquisition of spoken language.

Children who are deaf or hard-of-hearing, lack certain sensory input, to varying degrees; and therefore, provide an excellent opportunity to study the effects of sensory differences on the natural acquisition of English and other traditionally spoken languages and the development of reading. Findings from studies of PA, vocabulary, and morphosyntactic abilities of students who are deaf from oral and signing backgrounds indicate that, in comparison to hearing peers, children who are deaf tend to arrive at kindergarten with lower PA, vocabulary, morphosyntactic abilities and other linguistic abilities (see Paul, 2001, 2003 for a review of research); and they graduate from high school with reading comprehension scores comparable to 8- to 9-year-old hearing children (Mitchell & Karchmer, 2006; Traxler, 2000). In contrast, studies conducted with students who are deaf from Cued Speech backgrounds indicate that they have PA, vocabulary, and morphosyntactic abilities that are comparable to hearing peers (Koo, 2003; LaSasso, Crain, & Leybaert, 2003; Leybaert, Alegria, & Foncke, 1983; Leybaert & Lechat, 2001).

Rhyming as an Indicator of Phonological Awareness

The abilities to recognize that two words rhyme and produce words that rhyme with a spoken word are among the first expressions of children's ability to appreciate the phonological structure of spoken language (Maclean, Bryant, & Bradley, 1987). Children who are 2 to 3 years old with normal hearing produce and judge rhymes spontaneously (Read, 1978; Slobin, 1978), the precise age linked to individual differences related to the quality of their oral productions (Webster & Plante, 1995). Results of metaphonological awareness studies, including rhyming, show that metaphonological ability is a strong predictor of early reading success of hearing students (Bradley & Bryant, 1978), and more recently, deaf students from Cued Speech backgrounds (Colin et al., 2007).

Studies investigating the role of PA in individuals who are deaf have focused largely on the *recognition* or *generation* of rhymes. Our review of the literature revealed 11 studies that have examined rhyming abilities of deaf students (Campbell & Wright, 1988; Charlier & Leybaert, 2000; Colin et al., 2007; Dodd & Hermelin, 1977; Dyer et al., 2003; Hanson & Fowler, 1987; Hanson & McGarr, 1989; Harris & Beech, 1998; LaSasso et al., 2003; Sterne & Goswami, 2000; Waters & Doehring, 1990). These studies vary in terms of the nature of the *stimulus* (written words or pictures), nature of *response mode* (recognition or generation), *age* (adult or child), *communication background* (signing or nonsigning), and *home language* of deaf participants; as well as findings related to whether PA exists in individuals who are deaf.

Prior to the study described here (Crain, 2003), rhyme generation studies of individuals who are deaf have either involved adults, or have involved children from non-English speaking countries. The three generative rhyming studies conducted in the United States (Hanson & Fowler, 1987; Hanson & McGarr, 1989; LaSasso et al., 2003) involved *adult deaf* participants. Findings from all three studies indicated that rhyming ability existed in deaf adults. Two additional studies (Charlier & Leybaert, 2000; Colin et al., 2007) employed generative rhyming tasks and found sensitivity to rhyme in deaf children; however, the children spoke French. Spencer and Marschark (2006, p. 16) urge caution when interpreting results of PA studies of French readers to English readers due to differences in the transparency of the two languages. That is, French is considered to be more transparent than English because French has a much more consistent orthography-to-phonology than English. For example, in French, there is a single pronunciation of the graphemes *ou* /u/ (as in *bouche, mouche*); however, in English, the grapheme *ou* has different pronunciations in *cough, out*, and *route*. To date, no one has examined the generative rhyming abilities of younger, *emerging* deaf readers of English.

Purpose of the Study

The purpose of the study described in this chapter was to determine: (1) whether 10- to 14-year-old developing deaf readers of English from Cued Speech backgrounds differ from deaf age-mates from oral back-

grounds in their PA performance on a generative rhyming task, and (2) whether PA performance is related to: degree of deafness, measured reading comprehension, and/or speech intelligibility for either group.

Methods

Thirty 10- to 14-year-old participants from a single large county public school system in the Washington, DC area participated in the study. These included 20 participants, referred to as *deaf* in this chapter, who were enrolled in their county's special education program for students who are deaf and hard of hearing, and 10 hearing participants. According to the Individuals with Disabilities in Education Act (IDEA), a deaf student is one with hearing impairment severe enough to affect the student's academic performance if intervention is not provided (IDEA, 2004). Of the 20 deaf participants, 10 (cueing group) were educated with Cued Speech, and 10 (oral group) were educated with oral-aural methods. Participants' hearing losses ranged from moderate to profound, based on participants' most recent audiogram (Table 14–1).

Cueing participants were all prelingually deaf, that is, they were diagnosed prior to the age of two years. All received educational services either in a self-contained classroom where they received instruction directly from a certified teacher of deaf students who communicated directly via Cued Speech or in a mainstream classroom with a Cued Speech transliterator (CST).

Oral participants received educational services either in a self-contained oral classroom or in mainstream settings. Due to the difficulty of finding an equal num-

Table 14–1. Audiologic Characteristics of Participants Based on Most Recent Audiogram

	Age	Degree of Deafness	Hearing Aids? Since What Age?	Cochlear Implant? Since What Age?
Cueing 1	12.11	Severe	Yes	No
Cueing 2	12.8	Profound	Yes	Yes—12
Cueing 3	12.5	Severe	Yes	No
Cueing 4	14.8	Severe	Yes	Yes—13
Cueing 5	13.6	Profound	No	Yes—9
Cueing 6	12.5	Severe	Yes	No
Cueing 7	10.1	Moderate	Yes	No
Cueing 8	10.3	Severe	Yes	No
Cueing 9	10.9	Severe	Yes	No
Cueing 10	14.4	Profound	No	No
Oral 1	10.11	Severe	Yes	No
Oral 2	11.4	Moderate	Yes	No
Oral 3	12.8	Severe	Yes	No
Oral 4	12.7	Moderate	Yes	No
Oral 5	12.4	Severe	Yes	No
Oral 6	12.1	Severe	Yes	No
Oral 7	12.9	Severe	Yes	No
Oral 8	13.3	Moderate	Yes	No
Oral 9	13.9	Severe	Yes	Yes—13
Oral 10	13.5	Moderate	Yes	No

ber (i.e., 10) of age-matched prelingually deaf participants from oral backgrounds whose parents were interested in participating, it was necessary to include participants in the oral group whose hearing loss was *adventitious and/or progressive.* Children with adventitious deafness are born hearing and either become deaf subsequently, or gradually lose hearing ability. This difference in regard to onset of deafness and/or diagnosis made certain analyses difficult, including correlation between degree of deafness and measured PA and the impact of early auditory experience across groups; however, certain between-group comparisons could be made, and other within-group analyses could be conducted.

Measures used in this study consisted of: (1) the Stanford-9 Reading Comprehension subtest (SAT-9) (The Psychological Corporation, 1996), (2) the NTID Speech Intelligibility Rating Scale (Subtelny, Orlando, & Whitehead, 1981), and (3) a generative rhyming task adapted from Hanson (1987) and LaSasso et al. (2003). The SAT-9 was used as the measure of reading comprehension. Similar to the current SAT-10, the SAT-9 is a paper-and-pencil reading comprehension test where students read short passages and answer Wh- questions (e.g., who, what, why) in incomplete statements in an untimed-lookback condition. The SAT-9 was administered in group settings within participants' schools. Raw scores, consisting of the total correct responses, were calculated and converted to scaled scores (i.e., transformed scores, which can be used to compare participants' measured reading achievement, across levels of the test).

The NTID Speech Intelligibility Rating Scale (Subtelny, Orlando, & Whitehead, 1981) was used to rate participants' speech intelligibility. The NTID scale is a Likert-like 5-point scale, which rates speech intelligibility from 1 (speech cannot be understood) to 5 (speech is intelligible). It has been found to be a reliable measure of listeners' judgment of speech skills, with a .74 correlation to a monosyllabic word write-down procedure and a .87 correlation to a sentence context write-down procedure (Subtelny, 1977). Speech intelligibility ratings were done by one of three school-based certified speech/language pathologists (CCC-SLP), each of whom had been trained to use the NTID scale and had at least three years' experience providing assessment and intervention to deaf and hard of hearing children. The three raters first independently rated all of the deaf participants, and then they met to reach consensus on all study participants.

The generative rhyming task, a measure of PA, was adapted from that used by Hanson and McGarr (1989) and LaSasso

et al. (2003). It consists of a 4-page packet with 54 typed target words, listed in two columns on each page, with instructions to write in the space below and next to the target word as many rhyming words as possible for each target. The rhyming task was administered in group settings within participants' schools. Researchers first judged responses as being words or nonwords, including for analysis only those responses spelled correctly as words or spelled in such as way as to be pronounceable as English words (e.g., *roap* for *rope*). Second, responses judged to be words were rated as to whether or not they rhymed with the targets. Third, correct rhyming responses were classified as being either orthographically similar (OS) or orthographically dissimilar (OD) to the targets. Fourth, error responses were classified into categories (two of which have subcategories) used by Hanson and McGarr (1989), and by LaSasso et al. (2003).

Responses judged to be words by the researchers were then judged as to whether or not they rhymed with the target. Nonrhyming responses were counted as errors. Some responses had more than one possible pronunciation. For example, the word "read" can be pronounced with a long e̱ /i/ (rhyming with "weed") or short e̱ /ɛ/, (rhyming with "bed"), depending on whether the intended word is in the present or past tense. In such situations for the purpose of rhyming judgment, participants were given the benefit of the doubt. Correct rhyme responses for targets were then classified as either: (1) orthographically similar (OS) to the target (e.g., BLUE-glue; or SCHOOL-cool) or (2) orthographically dissimilar (OD) (e.g., SHOE-few; or BEAR-fare).

Incorrect rhyme responses were classified as *errors*. Errors were then further classified depending on: whether the vowel was orthographically similar (VO) or dissimilar (V) to the target; whether the rime (e.g., -ood) was orthographically similar (O); whether the response bore some other orthographic similarity (SO); whether the response may have been due to speech-read similarity to the target (SR). Error responses that could not be so classified were deemed unclassifiable (U).

Results

Before the primary questions in this study were addressed, a series of discrete one-way ANOVAs were run with groups (two levels: cueing and oral) to determine whether the two groups of deaf participants differed on any of the following variables of interest: SAT-9 reading comprehension, speech intelligibility, and degree of deafness. There was no difference in SAT-9 reading comprehension; however, the groups differed significantly in: speech intelligibility and degree of deafness. A Pearson chi-square test determined that the cueing group and oral group differed significantly in terms of speech intelligibility ($X^2 = 8.67$; $df = 3$; $p = .034$) with the cueing group having significantly *lower* speech intelligibility ratings. This finding is interesting given the finding (discussed later) that although the oral group appears to have better speech skills, the cueing group appears to have a more reliable internal representation of traditionally spoken words. A one-way ANOVA, run with group (two levels: cueing and oral) and degree of deafness, revealed a significant effect of group ($F = 5.40$; $p < .05$), with the cueing group having a significantly greater degree of deafness than the oral group. This finding also is particularly interesting given the finding

(discussed later) that despite having less access than the oral group to the auditory signal required for the processing of spoken language, the cueing group appears to have a more reliable internal representation of traditionally spoken language. This relative independence from auditory information in the development of English and other traditionally spoken languages is likely attributable to the cuers' integration of available auditory information with the greater specificity of phonemes provided by the manual handshapes and placements of Cued Speech.

Question 1: Comparability of PA in Oral, Cueing, and Hearing Participants

To answer the question of whether comparable PA differs in developing readers who are deaf from oral and cueing backgrounds, percentages of total correct rhyming responses that were orthographically dissimilar (OD) from the target were computed. Correct OD responses indicated the presence of phonological awareness. That is, OD responses could not have been generated based orthographic comparison, but instead indicate the presence of an internal phonological representation for the printed form of the word. Table 14–2 reflects: (1) the numbers of correct responses, classified as orthographically-similar (OS) and OD, and their respective percentages of the total correct responses and (2) the number of errors and proportion of total responses for cueing, oral, and hearing participants. Although PA is observable in all three groups, the degree of PA differs as a function of group membership (hearing, cueing, oral). That is, correct OD responses make up approximately 50% of correct responses provided

Table 14–2. Percentages of Correct (OS and OD) and Incorrect Responses on Rhyming Test by Group

| Group | Correct OD and OS Responses and Percentage of Total Correct | | | | |
	Correct OS and % of Total Correct Responses	Correct OD and % of Total Correct Responses	Total OD + OS Responses and % of Total Responses	Errors and Percentage of Total Responses	Total Responses
Cued Speech	456 (40.5%)	670 (59.5%)	1126 (91.6%)	103 (8.4%)	1229
Oral	372 (49.3%)	383 (50.7%)	755 (82.6%)	159 (17.4%)*	914
Hearing	995 (30.4%)	2273 (69.6%)	3268 (96.5%)	120 (3.5%)	3388
Total	**1823 (35.4%)**	**3326 (64.6%)**	**5149 (93%)**	**382 (6.9%)**	**5531**

*significant

by the oral group, approximately 60% of correct responses provided by the cueing group, and approximately 70% of correct responses provided by the hearing group.

To determine whether the two groups of developing readers who are deaf and the hearing comparison group statistically differ in regard to PA, a one-way ANOVA with Group (3 levels: Hearing, Cueing, and Oral) was performed on the percentage of correct OD rhyming responses. The ANOVA revealed a significant effect of group, $F (2,27) = 4.570; p = .020$. A post hoc Tukey HSD test revealed that the hearing group differed from the oral group ($p = .015$), but not from the cueing group ($p = .333$), and the cueing group did not differ from the hearing group (.333) or the oral group ($p = .272$). In sum, the observed difference between the hearing and oral groups (with the hearing group obtaining a higher OD accuracy rate) reflected in Table 14–3 reached statistical significance. The observed difference between the hear-

ing and cueing groups did not reach statistical significance. The observed difference between the cueing and oral groups also did not reach statistical significance (although, as discussed in Question 2 Results) a difference in PA was observed when controlling for reading comprehension. The fact that hearing and cueing groups do not differ significantly on PA suggests that they share a more reliable phonological recoding strategy for rhyme generation than the oral group, which supports the conclusion of the LaSasso et al. (2003) study of the generative rhyming abilities of deaf adults from cueing and noncueing backgrounds. This finding is not surprising because hearing individuals and deaf individuals from Cued Speech backgrounds have more clear and complete access to the phonemes of English and other traditionally spoken languages than do deaf individuals from oral backgrounds. At the same time, the cueing and oral groups also do not differ significantly on this

Table 14–3. Correlations Between PA (OD Accuracy) and Degree of Deafness, Reading Comprehension, and Speech Intelligibility

Correlation Between PA and:	All Deaf Participants	Oral Group Only	Cueing Group Only
degree of deafness	No	Yes $p < .001$	No
reading comprehension	Yes $p = .008$	Yes	Yes
speech intelligibility	No	Yes $p = .01$	No

measure, and this may be due to the significantly higher hearing levels observed in the oral group.

Differences were observed in frequency and proportion of error responses given. Errors accounted for 17.4% of the 914 total responses provided by the oral group, and 8.4% of the 1229 responses provided by the cueing group. The one-way ANOVA revealed a significant effect of group, $F (2,27) = 4.57$; $p < .05$. A post-hoc Tukey HSD test revealed that the hearing group differed from the oral group ($p < .05$), but not from the cueing group ($p > .10$), and that the cueing group did not differ from the hearing group ($p > .10$) or the oral group ($p > .10$). Vowel-related errors constituted the majority of errors for each group of participants in this study. Interestingly, the proportion of vowel-related errors demonstrated by the oral group is 60.9% higher than that of the cueing group. This may be due to the visually discrete placement of vowels in cueing as opposed to the speechread similarity of certain vowels in speech. For example, PIN and PEN can be confused for one another on the lips of a speaker, but when the words are cued, the vowel is placed at the throat or at the chin, respectively (refer to the Cued Speech Chart in Chapter 1), thereby fully specifying, or distinguishing, the vowel.

Question 2: Relationship of PA to Degree of Deafness, SAT-9 Reading Comprehension, and/or Speech Intelligibility

In order to determine whether a relationship exists for PA and degree of deafness, a Spearman's *rho* correlation coefficient was computed for the entire group of deaf participants and for each group (oral, cueing) separately. As noted in Table 14–3, the correlation, when performed on the entire group of deaf participants, failed to reach statistical significance ($r = -.279$; $p = .234$). When calculated separately for the cueing and oral groups, the correlation coefficient also failed to reach statistical significance ($r = -.624$; $p > .05$) for the cueing group; however, it reached statistical significance ($r = -.710$; $p = < .01$) for the oral group. It appears that PA is more related to degree of deafness for the oral group than the cueing group. That is, in contrast with cueing participants, oral participants with greater degrees of hearing loss also had lower measured PA as indicated by the proportion of correct OD rhyming responses.

In order to determine whether a relationship exists between PA and SAT-9 performance for the all deaf group ($n = 20$), a Pearson's *rho* correlation coefficient was calculated. The proportion of correct OD rhyming responses correlated significantly to the SAT-9 scores ($r = 0.572$; $p = .008$, two-tailed). In sum, deaf participants with relatively higher proportions of correct OD rhyming responses also have relatively higher SAT-9 scores. Given the finding of a correlation between PA and SAT-9 Reading Comprehension for the combined groups of deaf participants (oral and cueing), it was necessary to examine whether the observed difference in proportion of correct OD responses could be explained by differences in SAT-9 scores. An ANCOVA was computed to analyze OD responses with communication modality as the between-subjects factor and SAT-9 Reading Comprehension as the covariate. When controlling for SAT-9 Reading Comprehension, a significant effect of group on PA ($F = 6.281$; $p = .0.23$) was found, with the cueing group demonstrating a higher degree of PA than the oral group, indicating that the higher scores demonstrated by the cueing group are not explained by their higher reading ability. This suggests that although PA and reading comprehension may have a reciprocal relationship, the individuals in the cueing group did not develop their superior PA skills through reading alone. Results suggest that for all participants in this study (hearing, cueing, and oral), those with relatively higher proportions of PA, as reflected in correct OD rhyming responses, also have relatively higher SAT-9 reading comprehension scores. This finding of a correlation between PA and reading comprehension

achievement are not surprising, and is in keeping with findings from previous studies of hearing and deaf adults (Hanson & McGarr, 1989; LaSasso et al., 2003), and previous studies of *hearing* (Bradley, 1988; Bradley & Bryant, 1983) and *deaf* children (Dyer et al., 2003).

In order to determine whether a relationship exists between PA and speech intelligibility, a Spearman's *rho* correlation coefficient was calculated for the proportion of correct OD rhyming responses and speech intelligibility. The correlation coefficient for the all deaf group failed to reach statistical significance ($r = -.049$; $p = .837$). It also failed to reach significance for the cueing group alone ($r = .063$; $p = .862$); however, it reached significance for the oral group alone ($r = .564$; $p = .01$). In sum, PA appears to be more related to speech intelligibility for the oral group than for the cueing group. That is, oral participants with relatively higher speech intelligibility ratings also had relatively higher proportions of correct OD rhyming responses, reflecting PA; however, cueing participants' PA was unrelated to speech intelligibility.

Although the relationship between speech intelligibility and SAT-9 scores of participants who are deaf was not originally a question to be addressed in this study, data collected in this study made it possible to address the question. A Spearman's *rho* correlation coefficient was computed to determine whether there was a relationship between speech intelligibility and SAT-9 scores. When computed for oral and cueing groups combined, the correlation coefficient failed to reach statistical significance ($r = -.006$; $p = .981$). It also failed to reach statistical significance for the cueing group alone ($r = -.253$; $p = .480$); however, it reached significance for the oral group ($r = .694$; $p = .001$). These findings suggest that reading ability may be more related to speech intelligibility for the oral group than the cueing group; that is, unlike cueing participants, oral participants with relatively higher ratings of speech intelligibility also have relatively higher scores on the SAT-9 reading test. This finding suggests that participants in the oral group depend more heavily on their own accurate speech production to provide auditory and/or tactile-kinesthetic feedback both for internal phonological recoding and to access printed material. In contrast, participants in the cueing group, despite lower levels of speech intelligibility, do not appear to rely as much on speech production as a self-monitoring system for either internal phonological recoding or decoding of text but, rather, might rely to a large degree on the cued representations of phonological structures that involve visual, speech-motor and/or manual kinesthetic information. It also could be that the participants in the oral group employ an *under*specified tactile-kinesthetic feedback loop (LaSasso, 1996), which necessarily relies more principally on articulators of the mouth than from multiple sources, whereas the participants in the cueing group may rely on a more fully-specified tactile-kinesthetic feedback loop that integrates speech-related mouth movements with the production of manual cues that serve to further specify phonemes and phonological structures (e.g., onsets, rimes, syllables).

Discussion

Our data clearly support a relationship between PA and exposure to Cued Speech in emerging readers of English. This study extends the findings obtained with deaf children from French-speaking families to those from English-speaking families. This study also provides a clear answer to the questioning raised by Spencer and Marschark (2006, p. 16) who urge caution when interpreting results of PA studies of French readers to English readers due to differences in the transparency of the two languages. The claim that PA has only been found in French (and not in English) can no longer be assumed.

Although the relationship between PA and reading comprehension for younger, emerging readers who are deaf from oral or cueing backgrounds has been supported by findings in this study, more research is needed to determine whether a *causal* connection exists between PA and reading comprehension for emerging readers who are deaf (see Colin et al., 2007 for such research on French deaf children exposed to Cued Speech). In addition, further research is needed to determine whether the higher reading achievement observed in the cueing group in this study is related chiefly to increased PA as a result of exposure to Cued Speech, or possibly to a combination of PA and additional language experience gained as a result of acquiring language via Cued Speech.

The Report of the National Reading Panel (NRP) *Teaching Children to Read* (2000) identified five critical abilities related to reading. These include: phonemic awareness, phonics, fluency, vocabulary, and comprehension strategies. A major conclusion of the NRP was that explicit instruction in phonemic awareness is essential for effective developmental reading programs. Findings from the study described here provide scientific evidence that 10 to 14-year-old developing readers who are deaf *are* capable of developing PA that is comparable to that of hearing peers.

Cued Speech has at least two types of instructional applications for improving deaf students' reading abilities. One instructional application is as *a communicative tool in schools for explicit and systematic instruction in phonemic awareness and phonics*. It should be noted that this is the same application provided by Visual Phonics (Friedman-Narr, 2006). Estimates of the time needed to learn Visual Phonics and gain fluency have not been found in the professional literature, though training workshops typically take two full days and consist of learning to recognize and produce the 46 gestures and 46 accompanying graphic symbols used to represent speech sounds. The eight handshapes and four placements of Cued Speech, which convey the phonemes of English and other traditionally spoken languages, can be acquired by a novice parent in less than 20 hours (Cornett & Daisey, 2001) and have been observed to provide a rich linguistic environment for deaf children in as short as three months (Torres, Moreno-Torres, & Santana, 2006). The major advantage of Cued Speech over fingerspelling, MCE sign communication systems, or lipreading is that Cued Speech is capable of clearly and completely conveying phonemic information in a visual manner in the absence of acoustic information (see LaSasso & Metzger, 1998).

The major advantage of Cued Speech over Visual Phonics is that besides its application for explicit phonics instruction, it can be used as a conversational mode for visually conveying and receiving English clearly and completely. Visual Phonics is solely an educational tool intended for explicit phonics instruction (the instruction being carried out via speaking, signing, or some combination of the two). Cued Speech, on the other hand, is a communication modality through which the deaf child can see both larger units of language (i.e., words, phrases, sentences) and smaller units of language (i.e., bound morphemes and phonemes) as they occur in natural language contexts. In this way, the child can *naturally* and *simultaneously* acquire the phonological structure of the language necessary for phonics-based decoding, and the vocabulary, syntax, and figurative language necessary for fluent independent reading.

The second and broader application of Cued Speech is for *the natural acquisition of English and other traditionally spoken languages in preparation for reading and academic instruction*. Findings from Leybaert and associates (Alegria & Lechat, 2005; Colin et al., 2007; Leybaert, 2000; Leybaert & Charlier, 1996; see Chapter 11 for a review) show unequivocally, that Cued Speech is most beneficial for the natural acquisition of traditionally spoken languages and skills associated with reading when Cued Speech is used *both* at home and at school. Research shows that deaf students who are exposed to clear and complete access to English and other traditionally spoken languages, at the phoneme level, and are given opportunities to interact with fluent language models, *can* and *do* acquire language milestones in keeping with those of hearing peers (Kyllo, 2003). This comparable language development facilitates the development of reading and academic achievement of deaf students.

Cued Speech also has applications for bilingual programs that focus on visual approaches to language development. A prototype ASL-Cued English instructional program for deaf children exists and is showing promising results for reading achievement of students who are deaf (Kyllo, 2003; see Chapter 10 in this volume).

One of the most important applications of Cued Speech is for the ever-increasing numbers of children with cochlear implants who are too young to respond behaviorally as to how much of the speech signal they are receiving via the implant, how clearly they are receiving it, and how they perceive it (see Chapter 6 in this volume). Cochlear implant technology has not advanced to the point where children with a cochlear implant are receiving clear, complete auditory signals; rather, to date, the signal is less than clear and is ambiguous (Fu & Shannon, 1999a, 1999b), requiring that the child augment auditory information with visual information, such as that provided to a certain extent by lipreading. Given the limitations of lipreading for providing visual information about speech (Nicholls & Ling, 1982), however, Cued Speech should be considered by parents, educators, and policy makers for augmenting and clarifying the visible portion of speechread phonological information about traditionally spoken languages.

References

Alegria, J., & Lechat, J. (2005). Phonological processing in deaf children: When lipreading and cues are incongruent. *Journal of Deaf Studies and Deaf Education, 10*, 122–133.

Bradley, L. (1988). Rhyme recognition, reading and spelling in young children. In R. Masland & M. Masland (Eds.), *Preschool prevention of reading failure* (pp. 143–162). Parkton, MD: York Press.

Bradley, L., & Bryant, P. (1978). Difficulties in auditory organization as a possible cause of reading backwardness. *Nature, 271,* 746–747.

Bradley, L., & Bryant, P. (1983). Categorizing sounds and learning to read: A causal connection. *Nature, 301,* 419–421.

Campbell, R., & Wright, H. (1988). Deafness, spelling, and rhyme: How spelling supports written words and picture rhyming skills in deaf subjects. *Quarterly Journal of Experimental Psychology, 40,* 771–778.

Charlier, B., & Leybaert, J. (2000). The rhyming skills of deaf children educated with phonetically augmented lipreading. *Quarterly Journal of Experimental Psychology, 53A,* 349–375.

Chomsky, N. (1975). *Reflections of language.* New York, NY: Pantheon Books.

Colin, S., Magnan, A., Ecalle, J., & Leybaert, J. (2007). Relation between deaf children's phonological skills in kindergarten and word recognition performance in first grade. *Journal of Child Psychology and Psychiatry and Allied Disciplines, 48,* 139–146.

Cornett, R. O., & Daisey, M. (2001). *The Cued Speech resource book for parents of deaf children.* Cleveland, OH: National Cued Speech Association.

Crain, K. L. (2003). *The development of phonological awareness in moderately-to-profound deaf developing readers: The effect of exposure to cued American English.* Unpublished doctoral dissertation, Gallaudet University, Washington DC.

Dodd, D., & Hermelin, B. (1977). Phonological coding by the prelinguistically deaf. *Perception and Psychophysics, 21,* 413–417.

Dyer, A., MacSweeney, M., Szczerbinski, M., Green, L., & Campbell, R. (2003). Predictors of reading delay in deaf adolescents: The relative contributions of rapid automatized naming speed and phonological awareness and decoding. *Journal of Deaf Studies and Deaf Education, 8,* 215–229.

Friedman-Narr, R. (2006). Teaching phonological awareness with deaf and hard of hearing students. *Teaching Exceptional Children, 38,* 53–58.

Fu, Q., & Shannon, R. (1999a). Effects of electrode location and spacing on speech recognition with the Nucleus-22 cochlear implant. *Ear & Hearing, 20,* 321–331.

Fu, Q., & Shannon, R. (1999b). Phoneme recognition as a function of signal-to-noise ratio under nonlinear amplitude mapping by cochlear implant users. *Journal of the Acoustical Society of America, 106,* L18–L23.

Hanson, V., & Fowler, C. (1987). Phonological coding in word reading: Evidence from hearing and deaf readers. *Memory and Cognition, 15*, 199–207.

Hanson, V., & McGarr, N. (1989). Rhyme generation in deaf adults. *Journal of Speech and Hearing Research, 32*, 2–11.

Harris, M., & Beech, J. (1998). Implicit phonological awareness and early reading development in prelingually deaf children. *Journal of Deaf Studies and Deaf Education, 3*, 205–216.

Individuals with Disabilities Education Improvement Act (IDEA) of 2004. (2004). Retrieved December 10, 2009, from http://idea.ed.gov/download/statute.html

Karchmer, M., & Mitchell, R. (2003). Demographic and achievement characteristics of deaf and hard-of-hearing students. In M. Marschark & P. Spencer (Eds.), *Handbook of deaf studies, language, and education* (pp. 21–37). New York, NY: Oxford University Press.

Koo, D. (2003). *On the nature of phonological representations and processing strategies in deaf cuers of English.* Unpublished doctoral dissertation, University of Rochester, New York, NY.

Kyllo, K. (2003). Phonemic awareness through emersion in cued American English. *Odyssey, 5*, 36–44.

LaSasso, C. (1985). Test-taking strategies used by deaf students in the U.S. and Greece. *Teaching English to Deaf and Second Language Students, 3*, 16–20.

LaSasso, C. (1996). Foniks for deff tshildrun? *Perspectives in Education and Deafness, 14*, 6–9.

LaSasso, C., Crain, K., & Leybaert, J. (2003). Rhyme generation in deaf adults: The effect of exposure to Cued Speech. *Journal of Deaf Studies and Deaf Education, 8*, 250–270.

LaSasso, C., & Metzger, M. (1998). An alternate route for preparing deaf children for BiBi programs: The home language as L1 and Cued Speech for conveying traditionally-spoken languages. *Journal of Deaf Studies and Deaf Education, 3*, 264–289.

Leybaert, J. (2000). Phonology acquired through the eyes and spelling in deaf children. *Journal of Experimental Child Psychology, 7*, 291–318.

Leybaert, J., Alegria, J., & Foncke, E. (1983). Automaticity in word recognition and word naming by the deaf. *Cahiers de Psychologie Cognitive, 3*, 255–272.

Leybaert, J., & Charlier, B. (1996). Visual speech in the head: The effect of Cued Speech on rhyming, remembering, and spelling. *Journal of Deaf Studies and Deaf Education, 1*, 234–248.

Leybaert, J., & Lechat, J. (2001). Phonological similarity effects in memory for serial order of Cued Speech. *Journal of Speech, Language, and Hearing Research, 44*, 949–963.

MacLean, M., Bryant, P., & Bradley, L. (1987). Rhymes, nursery rhymes, and reading in early childhood. *Merrill-Palmer Quarterly, 33*, 255–281.

Mitchell, R., & Karchmer, M. (2006). Demographics of deaf education: More students in more places. *American Annals of the Deaf, 151*, 95–104.

National Reading Panel. (2000). *Teaching children to read: An evidence-based assessment of the scientific literature on reading and its implications for reading instruction.* United States Department of Health and Human Services.

Nicholls, G., & Ling, D. (1982). Cued Speech and the reception of spoken language. *Journal of Speech and Hearing Research, 25*, 262–269.

Paul, P. (2001). *Language and deafness* (3rd ed.). San Diego, CA: Singular.

Paul, P. (2003). Processes and components of reading. In M. Marschark & P. Spencer (Eds), *Oxford handbook of deaf studies, language, and education* (pp. 97–109). New York, NY: Oxford University Press.

Paul, R., & Jennings, P. (1992). Phonological behavior in toddlers with slow expressive language development. *Journal of Speech and Hearing Research, 35*, 99–107.

Read, C. (1978). Children's awareness of language, with an emphasis on sound systems. In A. Sinclair, R. Jarvella, & W. Levelt (Eds.), *The child's conception of language* (pp. 65–92). New York, NY: Springer-Verlag.

Slobin, C. (1978). A case study of early language awareness. In A. Sinclair, R. Jarvella, & W.

Levelt (Eds.), *The child's conception of language* (pp. 45–54). New York, NY: Springer-Verlag.

Spencer, P., & Marscharck, M. (2006). Spoken language development of deaf and hard-of-hearing children: Historical and theoretical perspectives. In P. Spencer & M. Marschark (Eds.), *Advances in the spoken language development of deaf and hard of hearing children* (pp. 1–21). New York, NY: Oxford University Press.

Sterne, A., & Goswami, U. (2000). Phonological awareness of syllables, rhymes, and phonemes in deaf children. *Journal of Child Psychology and Psychiatry, 41,* 609–625.

Subtelny, J. (1977). Assessment of speech with implications for training. In F. Bess (Ed.), *Childhood deafness: Causation, assessment, and management* (pp. 183–194). New York, NY: Grune & Stratton.

Subtelny, J., Orlando, N., & Whitehead, R. (1981). *Speech and voice characteristics of the deaf.* Washington, DC: Alexander Graham Bell Association for the Deaf.

The Psychological Corporation. (1996). *The Stanford Achievement Test* (9th ed.). Houston, TX: Harcourt Brace Jovanovich.

Torres, S., Moreno-Torres, I., & Santana, R. (2006). Quantitative and qualitative evaluation of linguistic input support to a prelin-

gually deaf child with Cued Speech: A case study. *Journal of Deaf Studies and Deaf Education, 11,* 438–448.

Traxler, C. (2000). The Stanford Achievement Test, 9th Edition: National norming and performance standards for deaf and hard of hearing students. *Journal of Deaf Studies and Deaf Education, 5,* 337–348.

Velleman, S. (1988). The role of linguistic perception in later phonological development. *Applied Psycholinguistics, 9,* 221–236.

Wagner, R., Torgesen, J., & Rashotte, C. (1994). The development of reading-related phonological processing abilities: New evidence of bi-directional causality from a latent variable longitudinal study. *Developmental Psychology, 30,* 73–87.

Waters, G., & Doehring, G. (1990). Reading acquisition in congenitally deaf children who communicate orally: Insights from an analysis of component reading, language, and memory skills. In T. Carr & B. Levy (Eds.), *Reading and its development: Component skills approaches* (pp. 323–373). San Diego, CA: Academic Press.

Webster, P., & Plante, A. (1995). Productive phonology and phonological awareness in preschool children. *Applied Psycholinguistics, 16,* 43–57.

Section V:

CUED SPEECH FOR ATYPICAL POPULATIONS

Chapter 15

CHILDREN WITH AUDITORY NEUROPATHY/AUDITORY DYS-SYNCHRONY: THE VALUE OF CUED SPEECH IN THE FACE OF AN UNCERTAIN LANGUAGE DEVELOPMENT TRAJECTORY

Michelle L. Arnold and Charles I. Berlin

This chapter focuses on the special case of auditory neuropathy/auditory dys-synchrony (AN/AD), a hearing disorder unique among others in that the dimension of hearing affected is temporal (i.e., related to timing). We contrast AN/AD with the more commonly understood concept of deafness, and suggest procedures for appropriate differential diagnosis. We illustrate our recommendations with specific (and real) cases, and conclude the chapter with practical suggestions for the improved management of patients with AN/AD, including the early and consistent use of Cued Speech for disambiguating and corroborating the incoming acoustic signals experienced by patients with AN/AD.

The Special Case of Auditory Neuropathy/Auditory Dys-synchrony

There are three acoustic dimensions to speech: frequency (roughly analogous to pitch), intensity (roughly analogous to loudness), and time. However; the audiogram displays only the two dimensions of frequency and intensity to describe a patient's hearing loss. Because auditory neuropathy/dys-synchrony (AN/AD) is a disorder of timing, common rules of audiogram interpretation, including anticipated speech and hearing results with hearing aids, generally do not apply. The major consequence of AN/AD is not a lack of sensitivity to sound; instead, this disorder causes a disruption in the timing of incoming speech signals, resulting in a degraded and often unintelligible message, regardless of the amount of hearing loss suggested by the audiogram.

Individuals with AN/AD roughly may be categorized within the following three groupings: those with little/no difficulties hearing and understanding language, those with severe difficulties hearing and understanding language, and those that fall somewhere in between. Regardless of the severity of the disorder, using Cued Speech as a management tool for AN/AD has multiple benefits: it can serve as a noninvasive intervention that distinguishes spoken messages, thus allowing a diagnosed child to eavesdrop on the language cued in his home. It complements a wide variety of other interventions, including speech-language therapy, auditory-oral therapy, and cochlear implantation. It also "buys time," instilling language while the child is observed for the possibility of spontaneous recovery and while decisions are made regarding interventions that might be more invasive. Moreover, Cued Speech allows a fallback position that can help to produce a "literate taxpayer" in those cases where cochlear implantation is not recommended or fails to provide expected spoken language outcomes.

AN/AD is a condition in which some dysfunction in the auditory system interferes with the synchronous firing of auditory nerve fibers (a disorder of timing). Possible sites of lesion included are: lack

of or damage to the inner hair cells of the cochlea, damage to the spiral ganglia cell bodies, or degeneration of myelin along axons responsible for the transmission of auditory signals (Berlin, Hood, Morlet, Rose, & Brashears, 2003; Cone-Wesson, 2004; Rance, McKay, & Grayden, 2004; Rapin & Gravel, 2003; Starr, Picton, Sininger, Hood, Berlin, 1996). AN/AD commonly follows premature birth, hypoxia, or hyperbilirubinemia (Amatuzzi et al., 2001; Rance et al., 1999). There are also various genetic causes of AN/AD (Cheng et al., 2005; Starr et al., 2003; Varga et al., 2003). For more information on genetics and AN/AD, go to: http://gateway.nlm .nih.gov and enter "Auditory Neuropathy Genes." Research suggests that approximately 2 to 11% of hearing impairment in schools for the deaf results from AN/AD (Cheng et al., 2005). The exact time of onset for AN/AD is uncertain; the disorder can present at any age, although generally it is apparent at birth or in early childhood (Foerst et al., 2006; Rance et al., 2004; Rapin & Gravel, 2003). The condition is typically bilateral (affecting both ears), although a small percentage of affected individuals present with unilateral (affecting one ear) AN/AD (Cone-Wesson, 2004).

Diagnosis and Avoiding Misdiagnosis

A Brief Review of Conventional Approaches to Diagnosing Deafness and Hearing Impairment in Behaviorally Testable Children

Common audiologic evaluation without sedation often consists of: (1) otoscopic evaluation, (2) immittance testing, (3) otoacoustic emissions, (4) pure tone air and bone conduction audiometry, (5) speech audiometry, and (6) auditory brainstem response testing. *Otoscopy* is the visual inspection of the auditory canal, in which the audiologist looks for any abnormalities, obstructions, or damage to the canal or eardrum, which could affect test interpretation.

Immittance consists of two parts: tympanometry and middle ear muscle reflex (MEMR) testing. Tympanometry results indicate the physical condition and function of the middle ear (eardrum and connected ossicles). In order to elicit a MEMR, it is necessary to have the following: (1) a mechanically normal middle ear, which is presumably insured by a normal tympanogram, (2) use of a sufficiently "loud" sound to elicit the reflex contraction of the stapedius tendon (MEMR), usually 70 to 90 dB HL, and (3) the nerve pathways between the ears and the brainstem (the "reflex arc") must be intact—damage along the arc can result in absent or elevated MEMRs.

Otoacoustic emissions (OAEs) are actual sound signals created in the inner ear by the outer hair cells in response to various stimuli, and sometimes occur spontaneously. Two types of OAEs are assessed clinically: transient-evoked (TEOAEs) and distortion-product (DPOAEs). TEOAEs are evoked by a series of click stimuli. DPOAEs are evoked by a combination of two tones. Clinically, the presence of OAEs reflects the "active process" of the outer hair cells. This active process can be considered the amplification stage of sound transmission, with the outer hair cells providing about 40 to 60 dB of gain. If the outer hair cells are damaged, OAEs will be absent, or will not occur at all frequencies. Individuals with AN/AD are expected to have present OAEs (Berlin, Hood, & Rose, 2001; Cone-Wesson, 2004), however; they sometimes disappear spontaneously or are destroyed through the use of powerful hearing aids. Similar to noise-induced hearing loss, over-amplification may stimulate outer hair cells to the point of exhaustion, with degeneration and dysfunction often following the overexposure.

Pure-tone audiometry requires the active participation of the individual being tested in that the individual must respond to pure-tone stimuli (beeps) by raising a hand or signaling hearing in some other way (in the case of adults and older children). Infants and toddlers can be evaluated by visual reinforcement (a head turn toward a reinforcer when the stimulus is presented) or by performing a play task. Test results are plotted on an audiogram as pure tone thresholds. From these thresholds, pure-tone averages (PTAs) can be calculated.

Speech audiometry also requires active participation, in which the individual must respond to live or recorded voice stimuli by either turning the head toward the stimulus, pointing to a picture representing the stimulus, or repeating the stimulus. Speech audiometry provides speech detection and/or speech recognition results, which, when compared to PTAs, can provide vital information about an individual's perception of speech. The PTA (calculated at 500, 1,000, and 2,000 Hz) is the most common description of an individual's hearing status and usually agrees with the patient's ability to hear speech within ±6 dB. Thus, a 3-frequency average of 40 dB should be coupled with a speech reception threshold of 34 to 46 dB.

Auditory brainstem response (ABR) is a measure of VIIIth nerve and brainstem activity that does NOT require active participation of the individual being tested; in fact, it is preferable for an infant to be sleeping during ABR testing. Electrodes (similar to those used for EEG) are placed on three to four sites on the head, usually the forehead, the vertex, and behind each earlobe. The electrodes record synchronous discharges of nerve fibers which, when averaged, appear to be "waves" in response to auditory stimuli (usually clicks). The ABR concerns waves that are produced within the first 7 ms following the clicks. In the course of the ABR, the click stimuli can be presented in positive or negative polarity, meaning the initial phase of the click pushes the eardrum membrane *in* (positive), while the opposite phase of the click first pulls the eardrum membrane *out* (negative).

In patients with AN/AD, the ABR is absent or grossly abnormal (Berlin et al., 1998; Starr et al., 1996). For these individuals, however, the test result can *appear to be* normal ABRs if only one polarity of stimulus is used. If alternating polarity is used, the patient will appear to be "deaf" or severely hearing impaired. To make the correct diagnosis, the complete average in response to a positive polarity click must then be repeated using a negative polarity click, and the two tracings must be overlaid to reveal the true response.

AN/AD can be distinguished from other forms of sensorineural hearing loss (SNHL) when one looks at the results of ABR tests in conjunction with ART and OAE tests. Individuals with "garden variety" hearing impairment show an absence of OAEs, whereas individuals with AN/AD have OAEs that are (or were at one time) intact. Additionally, in individuals with SNHL that does not result from AN/AD, speech recognition abilities coincide with pure tone sensitivity, depending on the level of hearing dysfunction. In many AN/AD patients, auditory measures may show relatively normal sensitivity (Sininger, 2002).

Behavioral Indicators of AN/AD

AN/AD should be considered as occurring along a continuum, with behavioral audiograms ranging from "normal" peripheral hearing to a profound hearing loss. Certain children who exhibit little or no overt displays of hearing loss may perform well in a variety of listening situations, however; they will normally demonstrate marked difficulties in paying attention to speech in noise (Oba, 2005; Zeng, Oba, Garde, Sininger, & Starr, 1999, 2001). If they are categorized and labeled as having "normal" hearing solely by virtue of presence of otoacoustic emissions, these children run the risk of being misdiagnosed with a central auditory processing disorder (CAPD) or a number of pervasive developmental disorders, such as ADHD or mild autism. Children that fall somewhere along the middle of the continuum tend to display erratic auditory behaviors, which results in unpredictable responses to auditory stimuli, especially speech (Berlin et al., 2001; Berlin et al., 2002; Franck, Rainey, Montoya, & Gerdes, 2002). Children with total inner hair cell loss and AN/AD display a total lack of sound awareness, regardless of the listening situation (Berlin et al., 2002). These children may act and be treated as though they have "garden variety" SNHL and fitted with hearing aids or FM systems, which do not address the timing deficiencies associated with AN/AD.

Amplification and Cochlear Implantation Outcomes

Amplification Outcomes

Rance, Cone-Wesson, Wunderlich, and Dowell (2002) compared 15 children with AN/AD to children with SNHL ranging from 3 to 6 years of age. They reported that after at least 12 months of hearing aid use, open-set speech perception scores improved by as much as 50% in over half of the children with AN/AD. Although most of these children had access to the speech spectrum with amplification, only 4 had scores high enough to suggest they could comprehend speech (compared to 7 of the children with SNHL). These results were obtained after the children were aided for at least 12 months.

Controversy still exists as to whether or not children with AN/AD should be fit with conventional amplification. A review of 95 AN/AD patients who had tried hearing aids that had been fit properly (i.e., using real ear measurements and NAL targets, a common hearing aid fitting algorithm) revealed that only 5 of the 95 actually learned and used language auditorily, while the rest ultimately rejected hearing aids (Berlin et al., in press).

Berlin, Hood, Hurley, and Wen (1996), studying some of the same patients, demonstrated little to no perceived benefit in patients with AN/AD whom they attempted to fit with hearing aids. The amplification assisted the patients (including one who had a normal audiogram) in terms of speech awareness, but did not assist them in understanding the speech message. Berlin reports that prescribing conventional amplification to patients with AN/AD, in his experience, seemed rea-

sonable at the time of diagnosis. But when viewed over a 28-year perspective (see Berlin et al., 2008) these prescriptions are not cost-effective in this culture, given that parents (*not* insurance companies) must pay for hearing aids that do not alleviate the listening difficulties of individuals with AN/AD. Some insurance company guidelines require a trial amplification period before a person can be considered a candidate for cochlear implantation (which are, for the most part, covered under most policies). In these cases, recommended amplification might be a loaner hearing aid, one ear at a time, with wide dynamic range compression and a conservative maximum output so as not to destroy outer hair cells via noise exposure (Hood, 1998). This latter step is important in the event that the patient turns out to be one of the few who: (1) have delayed maturation of the auditory system or (2) will develop speech and language with little intervention

Cochlear Implantation Outcomes

Because AN/AD is a disorder of timing, the auditory nerve fibers do not react to sounds in synchrony. Temporal firing of auditory nerve fibers is necessary for speech to be understood. Cochlear implants (CIs) directly stimulate the auditory nerve with pulses of electricity, thus *forcing* the fibers to fire synchronously. If there are sufficient amounts of nerve fiber reserves, the benefits of implantation can be great. Research suggests these benefits are displayed in many implanted AN/AD patients.

Shallop, Peterson, Facer, Fabry, and Driscoll (2001) reported negative outcomes using conventional amplification in a group of 5 pediatric patients with AN/AD who subsequently received cochlear implants. These children, all of whom had severe to profound hearing loss in the presence of OAEs and cochlear microphonics, were followed for 4 years postimplantation. Preimplantation, these children's audiometric results demonstrated speech detection within their PTA hearing levels; however, speech recognition scores were not high enough to facilitate the understanding and acquisition of spoken language via "eavesdropping" (i.e., incidental exposure and/ or unintentional access to environmental spoken language input). Postimplantation, these children's speech recognition scores all improved, some within a few days of initial activation and mapping. Two of the five subjects (Case A and Case B, siblings) used Cued Speech as their main communication mode with varying results after mapping. Case A demonstrated appropriate skills using the telephone and was ultimately placed in a mainstreamed kindergarten class without a transliterator. Case B was found to be apraxic, and was not as successful in speech production post-mapping, but now with bilateral implantation reportedly has made significant language and speech improvements.

Cochlear implant studies now show increased cortical responses and improvement in speech and language acquisition and understanding, especially if the patient is implanted at an early age (Nicholas & Geers, 2006; Sharma, Dorman, & Kral, 2005). For prelingually deafened children, the most improvement is seen when implantation occurs before 3 years of age; however, marked improvements are also seen in older children (Nicholas & Geers, 2006). Buss, et al. (2002) administered the Paden Brown Phonological Kit (an assessment of spontaneous use of phonological patterns for use with children who are

deaf or hard of hearing) to measure speech outcomes in four children with AN/AD before implantation, and again one year after. The 4 children obtained scores comparable to the general population of implanted children, with 2 performing above these norms in all tested categories. Peterson et al. (2003) had similar findings in 10 children with AN/AD. These 10 were matched with 10 non-AN/AD children and compared on an extensive battery of speech perception tests. There were no significant differences between groups using before and after outcome measures regarding communication in the home. These findings suggest that for some children with AN/AD, cochlear implantation is a viable option to assist in development of speech understanding and production.

It should be noted that not all cochlear implant reports are positive with AN/AD. In a single case study involving a 4-year-old child diagnosed with Friedrich's ataxia, Miyamoto, Kirk, Renshaw, Hussain, and Seghal (1999) reported better vowel recognition postimplantation, but limited access to consonants and a 4% correct score on an open-set word recognition list. This 4% postscore was the same as the preimplantation score. The lack of benefit for this patient most likely reflects the damaging affects of Friedrich's ataxia on brainstem rather than the eighth nerve neurons per se. Thus, strictly speaking, Friedreich's ataxia in this patient may not have been AN/AD but a brainstem disorder.

Effects on Speech and Spoken Language Development

Research shows that in individuals diagnosed with AN/AD the level of speech understanding is unrelated to pure-tone audiometric thresholds, with the degree of understanding probably dependent on the temporal firing characteristics of the auditory nerve (Cone-Wesson, 2004; Rance et al., 2004). If temporal firing is disrupted to a large extent, a child with AN/AD who shows relatively normal audiometric sensitivity will not "eavesdrop" on environmental speech stimuli and will display a concomitant delay in language development (Rance et al., 2004).

Patients with either some residual hearing or later onset progressive AN/AD tend to rely heavily on speechreading to supplement whatever auditory information is available to them. Although reception of speech is difficult, many patients produce normal-sounding speech and vocal qualities, suggesting the presence of some level of internal monitoring (Hood, Berlin, Morlet, Brashears, Rose, & Tedesco, 2002). As stated earlier there are three general categories that individuals tend to fall into: those with little or no difficulty hearing and understanding speech, those with severe difficulties understanding speech, regardless of pure tone audiometric sensitivity, and those that fall in between. Individuals with AN/AD with little to no difficulty listening and engaging in conversational speech tend to display more difficulty when attempting to do the same in a noisy environment.

Case Study 1

ML was (mis-) diagnosed at birth as profoundly deaf as a result of an ABR screen and follow-up test using an alternating polarity click. Her mother was told that she had a profoundly deaf child who should go to the school for the Deaf and learn sign language. The mother noted many examples of auditory alerting and responsivity and could not accept the diagnosis. She reported being told that she was "in denial" of her daughter's diagnosis. When otoacoustic emissions were added to the battery, they were found to be normal and a corrected diagnosis of AN/AD was made. By age 2½ the child was showing normal speech, language, and hearing behaviors and ultimately produced the behavioral audiogram shown in Figure 15–1. At present she shows virtually perfect speech understanding in quiet, much poorer hearing in noise, but as of the age of 7, continues to present with no ABR. She is one of about 7% of the children in a large study soon to be published (Berlin et al., in press) who have needed no hearing aid or cochlear implant intervention, yet continue to show no ABRs throughout life.

Individuals who fall in the middle of the continuum are those who display unpredictable behaviors and responses to speech.

Case Study 2

KA, diagnosed at birth with AN/AD, has been raised entirely with Cued Speech. The family tried hearing aids for her, but at present (at the age of 8) does not continue to wear them. Her family does not at present see the need for cochlear implantation. She is described elsewhere (Berlin, Keats, Hood, Gregory, & Rance, 2007) as a positive example of Cued Speech in the management of AN/AD throughout the life of the child. At present, the family reports that they are still considering a cochlear implant but will not do so until or unless their child begins to fall behind her school mates in language or academic achievement. She is now doing well in a regular educational setting with a cued language transliterator (CLT).

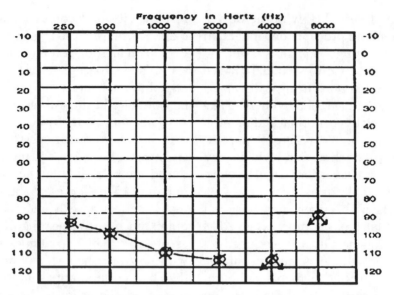

Figure 15–1. CHILD AG and her brother show no ABR but have normal otoacoustic emission (see Figure 15–2). She and her brother started with Cued Speech but no longer need it.

Individuals with severe difficulties understanding speech require intensive intervention, with the use of CIs in conjunction with Cued Speech resulting in the best outcomes, in the authors' experience. Those who do not receive intervention as soon as possible after diagnosis run the risk of never fully acquiring functional language abilities.

Case Study 3

AG and her brother both have an Otoferlin form of AN/AD in which the inner hair cells are nonfunctioning (Varga et al., 2003). They both produce behavioral audiograms as in Figure 15–1 but have normal otoacoustic emissions as in Figure 15–2.

In conventional terms, this would be considered a paradox because emissions are said to be absent when hearing loss exceeds 30 to 40 dB HL. Both children were raised with Cued Speech and acquired excellent receptive language skills compared to their deaf peers in an auditory-oral educational setting; however, their speech production lagged behind considerably. At their mother's insistence they were implanted, AG at age 4½ and her brother when he was 3, and have made remarkable progress in spoken language since then. Both subsequently received second implants, a recommendation that has been especially useful for AN/AD patients because it ostensibly prevents the second ear from sending distorted and desynchronized messages to the brain.

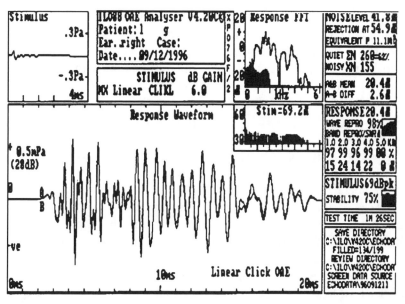

Figure 15–2. Normal otoacoustic emissions for child AG and her brother (see Figure 15–1).

Visual Supports for the Acquisition of Language

The acquisition of spoken language for hearing children is achieved by stimulating the brain with sounds and words in meaningful contexts. With constant exposure, the child comes to make associations between spoken words and the concrete or abstract concepts to which they refer. Hearing children typically learn language as a result of this auditory stimulation, by direct conversations with language models, by incidental "eavesdropping" of live conversations, television, radio, and other media messages, by imitating what they hear, by playing verbal games and singing songs, and so forth. Children with hearing impairments or disorders, by contrast, rely on direct conversations with language models, and cannot as readily acquire traditionally spoken language by incidental exposure. To the extent that they can "eavesdrop" on the language being produced around them, they can integrate what they can see with what they can hear. If the spoken message is accompanied by a visual correlate, language can be more easily learned and appreciated regardless of the presence, absence, or acoustic clarity of the speech signal.

The Case for Cued Speech

All concerned with AN/AD (e.g., parents, educators, clinicians, researchers) who wish to improve the lives of children with this condition must first appreciate the many differences between speech and language. Language is a means to conjure, organize, and store abstract concepts. Such concepts can be communicated between or among people in a number of ways. For example, concepts can be signed, spoken, or cued.

In the case of signed languages, such as American Sign Language (ASL), concepts are communicated via signing, with accompanying facial information. Signs are said to convey their own phonological information (behaviors that do not carry meaning, but can affect meaning) which build to create morphemes, words, and phrases (Brentari, 1998). Signed languages are, however, completely separate from spoken languages; signs from a signed language do not inherently convey phonological, morphological, or lexical information about spoken languages.

A common practice in the United States is to learn a form of manually coded English (MCE), by which an individual learns signs from ASL and additional invented signs (for specific words and for affixes such as *–er* and *dis–*) and produces those signs in English word order while speaking or mouthing English. To the extent that any phonological information specific to English is provided, it comes from the mouth movements and not the signs, and the level of efficacy of this approach would depend on a number of factors, including the level of importance placed on the accuracy and accessibility of this speech-related information, and the ability of the signer to make correct sign choices in synchrony with the spoken message.

In the case of traditionally spoken languages, concepts are generally communicated via speech, with accompanying visible facial information. Spoken words are comprised of phonemes (often mis-labeled "speech sounds," due to their close relationship to the audible phonetic speech signal), which are ordered to convey morphemes and subsequently provide meaning to those spoken words. Hearing users of a spoken language generally perceive phonemes (and the distinctions among them) primarily through listening to speech, with a certain amount of assistance from the visual information found on the lips of the speaker (Rosenblum, Johnson, & Saldaña, 1996). This is because certain mouthshapes are more closely associated with certain audible speech sounds, and the two come together to form a single phoneme percept (Rosenblum & Saldaña, 1998).

In the very special case of cued languages (traditionally spoken languages that are cued), concepts are communicated via the combination of visible mouthshape information (with or without accompanying audible speech) and the manual information of hand shape and placement (see Chapter 2 for a detailed description of Cued Speech). This integration of phonological information is similar to the case of spoken language, in that multiple sources converge to form a single percept. It is also unique in that the coupling of visible and audible information may or may not occur (depending on whether or not the sender is voicing or whether or not the receiver can hear), while the integration of two visible sources of phonological information does occur, even when auditory information is also accessed.

As stated previously, the signs of signed languages such as ASL carry no phonologic representation of the sounds of a spoken language. For example, the spoken words *baby* and *boy* have a particular relationship, in that they share an onset (i.e., they begin with the same initial phoneme, /b/). The ASL signs most commonly translated as *baby* and *boy*, whether used in ASL or MCE, do not convey this phonological information and thus cannot express this relationship. These same words, when properly cued, always begin with handshape 4 occurring in conjunction with the bilabial mouthshape associated with /b/ and thus express the feature of a /b/ onset (as would be the case for every English word beginning with /b/). Similarly, the words *boy* and *toy* have a particular relationship, in that they rhyme (i.e., they have different onsets and the same rime). Again, the ASL signs most commonly translated as *boy* and *toy* do not convey this phonological information, but when cued, this onset and rime relationship is visibly obvious (in this case, and in the case of every English word that rhymes with *boy* and *toy*).

Applications of Cued Speech for Children with AN/AD

Cued speech has been a valuable tool, allowing the AN/AD child to "eavesdrop" on the traditionally spoken language of the home regardless of whether invasive interventions, such as cochlear implants, are used. Its major advantages are that the family does not have to learn a new sign for each concept or word, and the phonological, morphological, lexical, and syntactic information of whichever traditionally spoken language is used in the home is conveyed simultaneously and without additional cognitive energy on the part of the cuer. Thus, English-speaking parents can model the English language for their child, Spanish-speaking parents can model Spanish, German-speaking parents, German, and so forth. Cued Speech is ideally suited for bilingual families or families

wishing to raise bilingual children, because it can be used to model and/or teach virtually any language. Cued Speech complements baby signs, signing and speaking, and cochlear implants ideally. Anecdotally, the fastest language growth and quickest transition to spoken language and literacy has been reported in the Kresge studies regarding children who have been implanted by one year of age and/or were exposed to Cued Speech and then implanted after age 2. Once acquired, Cued Speech remains a lifelong tool, useful when implants fail or are turned off (e.g., during bathing or swimming) or for adults in situations where ambiguity of spoken messages cannot be resolved by hearing alone.

If the child with AN/AD presents behaviorally similar to a profoundly deaf child and remains delayed in spoken language, a family has options to consider. On one end, they may consider learning a signed language (such as American Sign Language in the United States) and attempting to assimilate into the Deaf community. On the other end of the continuum, they may opt for a cochlear implant and pursue the path toward spoken language. In either case, the early use of Cued Speech will have facilitated early language acquisition and will have done no harm. If the child shows few, if any, indications of auditory problems, Cued Speech can help in noisy situations and situations where specificity is crucial. For a child such as this, the use of Cued Speech can be phased out, if and when it is no longer needed, and can be reintroduced later if the need arises.

If and when the child is implanted, Cued Speech can help disambiguate the new sounds and phonemes the child will access via the implant. A common and useful therapy technique for newly implanted children with exposure to Cued Speech is to bridge the familiar cued representation of a phoneme to the novel auditory information. For example, a child who already has an internalized representation of /d/ can learn to associate his new perception of the speech sounds associated with /d/, as opposed to working to develop a new phonological representation and contexts. For such a child as this, Cued Speech can also be retained as a tool for difficult listening situations or when the implant is off.

If a family opts to do nothing invasive other than use visual language, combining the use of Cued Speech for access to traditionally spoken language with ASL (or another signed language) will give the child with AN/AD entrée to Deaf culture while still having an additional language acquisition tool that supports literacy and English (or any other desired spoken language) word order and usage. Thus, the child can have the joys and benefits of belonging culturally and linguistically to the Deaf community with ASL, and to the larger hearing community of her family, while also having access to a tool that will make it unnecessary to learn English as a second language.

A Multidisciplinary Approach to AN/AD Management

Perhaps the single most important collaboration in a multidisciplinary approach to AN/AD management is the one between parent/child and a speech-language pathologist (SLP) or teacher of the deaf who is linguistically sophisticated enough to facilitate optimal progress for the child and the family. Because the time course will be unclear and the parents will have to make crucial decisions, a language baseline (e.g., a Rossetti scale by 6 months of age) should be established. Then this scale, or its equivalent, should be repeated every three months. Changes in management should be contingent on the results of those tests, with more invasive procedures (e.g., cochlear implants) considered at the parents' discretion and as a well-informed decision. An ideal team, in addition the above mentioned SLP might include:

- A parent educator/early interventionist (if the child is under the age of 3 years), who will make regular home visits to educate parents about hearing disorders, bonding, communication, and community resources;
- A knowledgeable educational audiologist who can answer parents' questions about the hearing status and language perception/understanding of their child; this professional would also be able to answer questions about the benefits and limitations of various interventions, such as hearing aids, cochlear implants, FM systems, or other options that may be especially useful in classroom environments;
- A pediatrician who is able to make appropriate referrals to various specialists, such as neurologists, otolaryngologists, or optometrists, contingent on the health status of the child. Regarding optometrists, as visual acuity is crucial to incorporating Cued Speech into AN/AD management, the child's eyesight should be evaluated immediately upon referral;

- A developmental psychologist who can track how the child is doing psychosocially and cognitively compared to children with normal hearing. It is particularly beneficial to find a psychologist who has experience working with children with hearing loss, who might also counsel and educate parents on child-rearing practices specific to special populations (see Chapter 16);
- A family counselor, who can assist family members in coping with stress, fears, and in communicating effectively with one another (not just with the child) to ensure continuity/ stability in the language/literacy, developmental, cognitive, and psychosocial upbringing of the child;
- A physical therapist, who can compare the child's fine and gross motor skill development with that of children with normal physical development, and can assist in developing and/or enhancing these skills (if they are impaired); and
- Educators and school staff, who will perform daily equipment (e.g., FM, CI) checks, will monitor the child's use of equipment and listening behaviors. Educators are crucial in helping the child with AN/AD and the other children in a class to socialize, play, and learn together. It is also the professionals in the classroom who will need to learn Cued Speech, or become familiar with it and may need to accommodate a Cued Language Transliterator (CLT) in the classroom.

Conclusion

AN/AD has been with us from the beginning, but is only now being recognized and commonly diagnosed. Many children previously implanted but not diagnosed with AN/AD likely have the disorder, as inner hair cell and neural loss are common to all patients who do not benefit greatly from hearing aid use, and who fail to acquire spoken language readily. AN/AD is characterized by temporal dysfunction of the auditory nerve, whether caused by a lesion on the nerve, demyelination of axons, spiral ganglion dysfunction, or lack of/damage to inner hair cells.

After compiling data on more than 260 cases of AN/AD of all ages, Berlin et al. (in press) report that approximately 7% of children with AN/AD who have histories of premature birth or hyperbilirubinemia learn speech and language around 14 to 16 months old despite absent auditory brainstem responses (ABRs) and with little intervention (see Case 1 [ML] in this chapter). For all but 5 of the children in the Kresge database, hearing aids and covering the mouth have not been useful. Cued Speech is a valid and noninvasive lifelong tool that can allow a child with AN/AD to eavesdrop on the home language in its full complexity and gain language and literacy skills. Cued Speech is simpler to learn than a signed language (such as ASL), thus reducing stress for families attempting to communicate with the child and model language. Cued Speech is capable of conveying all of the phonemes in many languages, allowing for the natural development of a spoken language's phonology, morphology, vocabulary, and syntax. Depending on the particular goals of parents, Cued Speech can be incorporated with baby signs or ASL, allowing a family, if they so desire, to raise a child with AN/AD to become bilingual and participate in both the Deaf and hearing communities.

References

Amatuzzi, M., Northrop, C., Liberman, M., Thornton, A., Halpin, C., Herrmann, B., . . . Eavey, R. D. (2001). Selective inner hair cell loss in premature infants and cochlea pathology patterns from neonatal intensive care unit autopsies. *Archives of Otolaryngology Head and Neck Surgery, 127*, 629–636.

Berlin, C., Bordelon, J., St. John, P., Wilensky, D., Hurley, A., Kluka, E., & Hood, L. (1998). Reversing click polarity may uncover auditory neuropathy in infants. *Ear and Hearing, 19*, 37–47.

Berlin, C., Hood, L., Hurley, A., & Wen, H. (1996). Hearing aids: Only for hearing-impaired patients with abnormal otoacoustic emissions. In C. Berlin (Ed.), *Hair cells and hearing aids* (pp. 99–111). San Diego, CA: Singular.

Berlin, C., Hood, L., Morlet, T., Rose, K., & Brashears, S. (2003). Auditory neuropathy/dys-synchrony: Diagnosis and management. *Mental Retardation and Developmental Disabilities Research Reviews, 9*, 225–231.

Berlin, C., Hood, L., Morlet, T., Wilensky, D., Li, L., Rose, K., . . . Frisch S. (in press). An analysis of 260 patients with confirmed diagnoses of auditory neuropathy dys-synchrony. *International Journal of Audiology.*

Berlin, C., Hood, L., & Rose, K. (2001). On renaming auditory neuropathy as auditory dys-synchrony. *Audiology Today, 13*, 15–17.

Berlin, C., Keats, B., Hood, L., Gregory, P., & Rance, G. (2007). Auditory neuropathy/dys-synchrony (AN/AD). In S. Schwartz (Ed.), *Choices in deafness* (pp. 49–78). Bethesda, MD: Woodbine House.

Berlin, C., Li, L. Hood, L., Morlet, T., Rose, K., & Brashears, S. (2002). Auditory neuropathy, dys-synchrony: After the diagnosis, then what? *Seminars in Hearing, 23*, 209–214.

Brentari, D. (1998). *A prosodic model of sign language phonology.* Cambridge, MA: MIT Press.

Buss, E., Labadie, R., Brown, C., Gross, A., Grose, J., & Pillsbury, H. (2002). Outcomes of cochlear implantation in pediatric auditory neuropathy. *Otology & Neurotology, 23*, 328–332.

Cheng, X., Li, L., Brashears, S., Morlet, T., Ng, S., Berlin, C., . . . Keats, B. (2005). Connexin 26 variants and auditory neuropathy/dys-synchrony among children in schools for the deaf. *American Journal of Medical Genetics, Part A, 139*, 13–18.

Cone-Wesson, B. (2004). Auditory neuropathy: Evaluation and habilitation of a hearing disability. *Infants and Young Children, 17*, 69–81.

Foerst, A. Beutner, D., Lang-Roth, R., Huttenbrink, K., von Wedel, H., & Walger, M. (2006). Prevalence of audiotory neuropathy/synaptopathy in a population of children with profound hearing loss. *International Journal of Pediatric Otolaryngology, 70*, 1415–1422.

Franck, K., Rainey, D., Montoya, L., & Gerdes, M. (2002). Developing a multidisciplinary protocol to manage pediatric patients with auditory neuropathy. *Seminars in Hearing, 23*, 225–237.

Hood, L. (1998). Auditory neuropathy: What is it and what can we do about it? *Hearing Journal, 51*, 10–18.

Hood, L., Berlin, C., Morlet, T., Brashears, S., Rose, K., & Tedesco, S. (2002). Considerations in the clinical evaluation of auditory neuropathy/auditory dys-synchrony. *Seminars in Hearing, 23*, 201–208.

Miyamoto, R., Kirk, K., Renshaw, J., Hussain, D., & Seghal, S. (1999). Cochlear implantation in auditory neuropathy. *Larygoscope, 109*, 181–185.

Nicholas, J., & Geers, A. (2006). Effects of early auditory experience on the spoken language of deaf children at 3 years of age. *Ear and Hearing, 27*, 286–298.

Oba, S. (2004). Young children with auditory neuropathy. In *SKI-HI curriculum: Family-*

centered programming for infants and young children with hearing loss. North Logan, UT: HOPE, Inc.

Peterson, A., Shallop, J., Driscoll, C., Breneman, A., Babb, J., Stoeckel, R., & Fabry, L. (2003). Outcomes of cochlear implantation in children with auditory neuropathy. *Journal of the American Academy of Audiology, 14,* 188–201.

Rance, G., Beer, D., Cone-Wesson, B., Shephard, R., Dowell, R., King, A., . . . Clark, G. (1999). Clinical findings for a group of infants and young children with auditory neuropathy. *Ear and Hearing, 20,* 238–252.

Rance, G., Cone-Wesson, B., Wunderlich, J., & Dowell, R. (2002). Speech perception in individuals with cortical event related potentials in children with auditory neuropathy. *Ear and Hearing, 23,* 239–253.

Rance, G., McKay, C., & Grayden, D. (2004). Perceptual characterization of children with auditory neuropathy. *Ear and Hearing, 25,* 34–46.

Rapin, I., & Gravel, J. (2003). Auditory neuropathy: Physiologic and pathologic evidence calls for more diagnostic specificity. *International Journal of Pediatric Otohinolaryngology, 67,* 707–728.

Rosenblum, L., Johnson, J., & Saldaña, H. (1996). Visual kinematic information for embellishing speech in noise. *Journal of Speech and Hearing Research, 39,* 1159–1170.

Rosenblum, L., & Saldaña, H. (1998). Time-varying information for visual speech perception. In R. Campbell, B. Dodd, & D. Burnham (Eds.), *Hearing by eye (Vol. II): The psychology of speechreading and audiovisual speech* (pp. 61–83). Hillsdale, NJ: Erlbaum.

Shallop, J., Peterson, A., Facer, G., Fabry, L., & Driscoll, C. (2001). Cochlear implantation in five cases of auditory neuropathy: postoperative findings and progress. *Laryngoscope, 111,* 555–562.

Sharma, A., Dorma, M., & Kral, A. (2005). The influence of a sensitive period on central auditory development in children with unilateral and bilateral cochlear implants. *Hearing Research, 203,* 134–143.

Sininger, Y. (2002). Identification of auditory neuropathy in infants and children. *Seminars in Hearing, 23,* 193–200.

Starr, A., Michalewski, H., Zeng, F., Fujikawa-Brooks, S., Linthicum, F., Kim, C., . . . Keats, B. (2003). Pathology and physiology of auditory neuropathy with a novel mutation in the MPZ gene (Tyr145→Ser). *Brain, 126* (Pt. 7), 1604–1619.

Starr, A., Picton, T., Sininger, Y., Hood, L., & Berlin, C. (1996). Auditory neuropathy. *Brain, 119,* 741–753.

Varga, R., Kelley, P., Keats, B., Starr, A., Leal, S., Cohn, E., & Kimberling, W. (2003). Nonsyndromic recessive auditory neuropathy is the result of mutations in the otoferlin (OTOF) gene. *Journal of Medical Genetics, 40,* 45–50.

Zeng, F., Oba S., Garde S., Sininger Y., & Starr, A. (1999). Temporal and speech processing deficits in auditory neuropathy. *Neuroreport, 10,* 3429–3435.

Zeng, F., Oba S., Garde S., Sininger Y., & Starr, A. (2001). Psychoacoustics and speech perception in auditory neuropathy. In Y. Sininger & A. Starr (Eds.), *Auditory neuropathy: A new perspective on hearing disorders* (pp. 141–164). San Diego, CA: Singular Press.

Chapter 16

APPLICATIONS OF CUED SPEECH WITH DEAF CHILDREN WITH ADDITIONAL DISABILITIES AFFECTING LANGUAGE DEVELOPMENT

Donna A. Morere

In the simplest terms, a deaf child with additional disabilities is a child with a hearing loss significant enough to impede natural spoken language development, co-occuring with one or more disabilities, creating a situation requiring interventions above and beyond that which would be appropriate for either disability category alone. For purposes of education, the deaf child with additional disabilities is often labeled with a hearing impairment as primary disability, with additional disabilities ranked as secondary, tertiary, and so forth, in respect to their relative contribution to the child's risk for academic failure. Each child presents a unique case due to great variability in onset of deafness and/or other disabilities, configura-

tions of hearing loss, attendant communication and language delays, and learning styles. Perhaps the one thing that these children can be said to have in common is that they require communication access and avenues for learning that are markedly different from deaf children without additional disabilities. Among the more common additional disability categories are primary language disorders (PLD), nonverbal learning disabilities (NLD), attention deficit/hyperactivity disorder (ADD/ADHD), and autism spectrum disorder. This chapter focuses on these disability categories, and applications for Cued Speech with deaf and hard of hearing children who present with these additional disabilities.

Deaf Children and Learning Disabilities

For many years, deaf or hard of hearing children[1] were not diagnosed with learning disabilities as many definitions of learning disabilities (LD) have specifically excluded children with primary conditions including hearing loss. Jones (1999) conducted a survey of educational programs providing services to deaf children and found that while most states acknowledge the possibility that children may suffer from both deafness and LD, many of the definitions were worded to exclude learning impacts that were secondary to deafness, and the differentiation of such fine distinctions was such that LDs in deaf children were simply not diagnosed. Despite the diagnostic difficulties, deaf children would certainly be at least as vulnerable as hearing children to the genetic, environmental, and social factors responsible for conditions such as LD, attention deficit hyperactivity disorder (ADHD), Autism, and primary language disorders (PLD). Additionally, research suggests that some etiologies of deafness, such as maternal rubella, meningitis, anoxia, prematurity, CHARGE syndrome, Rh incompatibility, and cytomegalovirus (CMV), place them at even greater risk for a range of additional conditions affecting learning (Mauk & Mauk, 1992, 1998; Samar, Parasnis, & Berent, 1998; Spreen, Risser & Edgell, 1995; Vernon & Andrews, 1990).

In addition to the environmental impacts common to all individuals, prelingually deaf individuals are subject to threats to language development due to their hearing loss, particularly in the case of the more than 90% of deaf children who are born to hearing parents. These threats include delayed diagnosis, delayed or inadequate intervention, a poor match of communication approach with the child's needs, and a lack of ongoing exposure to accessible language. However, there also are significant neurologically based challenges that interact synergistically with deafness resulting in serious impacts on language development. These include ADHD, nonverbal learning disabilities (NLD), PLD, pervasive developmental delays (PDD) and autism, mental retardation (MR), and vision disturbances. When the communication method used is Cued Speech, there also may be an impact of delayed or poor fine motor skills on expressive cueing. In some cases, an individual may be affected by the interaction of two or more of these conditions in addition to their deafness.

Due to the combined impact of these additional disabilities and deafness, early intervention is critical; however, based on the author's clinical experience, these diagnoses are often overlooked and even in severe cases of language disorders resulting in minimal language development a diagnosis is often not made until the child is 5 or 6 years old. The focus of the early intervention system is on the hearing loss. As the child confronts increasing frustration due to communication breakdown, secondary behavioral problems often develop and then become the focus of attention. Milder cases are often overlooked completely or not diagnosed until adolescence or adulthood. Thus, once the diagnosis has been made, rapid implementation of an effective communication and intervention strategy is critical to ensure optimal functioning of the child given his or her challenges.

---

[1]Deaf and hard of hearing children are referred to as deaf children in this chapter.

Primary Language Disorders (PLD)

Definition and Diagnosis

When a hearing child has delays in language development in the absence of other conditions, generally it is labeled a specific language impairment (SLI). Specific language impairments are typically defined as "delayed acquisition of language skills, occurring in conjunction with normal functioning in intellect, social-emotional, and auditory domains" (Watkins, 1994, p. 1), a definition that clearly excludes deaf individuals. Indeed, Fey, Long, and Cleave (1994) argue that because hearing loss directly affects language development, the exclusion of children with hearing loss is justified, while the requirement of an average IQ should be relaxed. Due to the additional impact of deafness, this author refers to these types of language disorders in deaf children as primary language disorders (PLD), rather than specific language impairments.

The diagnosis of PLD in deaf children is beyond the scope of this chapter. It requires both extensive assessment to rule out other potential causes of the language deficits and a careful history and evaluation of both the accessible language exposure of the child and the mode of communication used at home and at school. For a child to receive this diagnosis, all modes of communication should be affected. Thus, if a child has residual hearing or a cochlear implant (CI), auditory verbal language should be affected. Similarly, deficits in the development of sign skills and/or Cued Speech should be significantly greater than can be explained by delays in, or inadequacy of, exposure to that communication approach. Often

the child is able to identify individual signs, particularly those with minimal movement, or cues in isolation, but is unable to follow spoken, signed, or cued communication at a conversational rate. Those with milder forms of the disorder may be able to follow conversations if they are presented at a slow rate, using brief statements in simple language structure and using words/signs within the child's vocabulary. Frequent pauses for them to process what has been said will further support their comprehension. Deaf children with milder forms of PLD typically are overlooked or misdiagnosed. Those who are diagnosed with a PLD usually are otherwise bright children who present with the more severe forms of the disorder.

Social and Behavioral Characteristics

Although they are commonly excluded from definitions of specific language impairment, as previously noted, deaf individuals are at least as vulnerable to these disorders as hearing children. It should be noted that language disorders are commonly thought to exist on a continuum, with severe language disorders at one end and mild language impairments and even some types of developmental reading disorders on the other (Catts, 2004; McArthur et al., 2000). Additionally, children with severe language disorders, particularly when accompanied by reading deficits, often develop secondary behavior disorders (Tomblin & Zhang, 2000). Clinical observation and parent reports suggests that this may be secondary to social isolation and increasing frustration due an inability to communicate with others and make their needs known, a phenomenon commonly referred to as *communication frustration* (cf. Wolke & Giesen, 2000). Children often begin to act out and become aggressive, but they may also withdraw and become increasingly isolated. In older children and adults, this may be expressed in secondary depression or anxiety disorders (Cohen, 2001).

Peer relationships often suffer, and the deaf child with a PLD may be rejected by deaf peers, who expect other deaf children to have language skills comparable to their own. The child may also prefer to play alone as the difficulties of communication become frustrating and overwhelming. Unlike most deaf children, those with PLD may develop better relationships with hearing peers who have different expectations of their communication needs and abilities and who anticipate having to use alternative approaches to communication with a deaf child. The child with a PLD also may prefer the company of younger children or adults, again due to the differential communication demands.

Observed in settings in which language is required, such as the classroom, the child with a severe language disorder will often appear confused or "lost." He may be completely unable to understand information or answer questions, and at times may appear to be panicked or "frozen" or try to cover his confusion by acting out in an angry or otherwise inappropriate manner. When a child does try to respond, her answers may be unrelated to the topic, or be related, but off the point. Often, if a picture has been used in the lesson, her answer will relate to something about the picture, regardless of the question. If other children respond first, the child may get some idea about the task from them, but still may miss key ideas in the question. The child with a significant language disorder may not follow rules or instructions. Although this may be mistaken for misbehavior, the problem is often that he simply does not know what is expected of him. Furthermore, he may become frustrated and begin to act out behaviorally when his attempts to respond correctly repeatedly fail. This is compounded by negative feedback when parents and teachers express anger or frustration and peers show contempt or tease him due to his repeated errors or apparent misbehavior.

The child's difficulty with understanding information and instructions in both the classroom and at home may be mistaken for inattention. This impression is reinforced by the observation that when long or complicated information is being conveyed, she may "glaze over." Whereas this can be misidentified as an attention disorder, it is more like an overloaded circuit shutting down to avoid burnout; the child is simply giving herself a break from attempting to process an excess of information she cannot understand. In an effort to compensate for her inability to manage linguistic input, the child often depends on nonlinguistic visual cues for information. For example, he may look to peers to see what he should be doing or what materials he should have out, depend on established routines to know what to do, or attempt to use pictures or other visual cues to support any words he is able to understand. He may remember elaborate stories presented by video or pictures, and even be able to act them out, but be unable to answer simple questions about a story that is spoken, signed, or presented in Cued English.

Despite the range of difficulties these children have, they also present with some strengths, including counting and numerical skills; visual reasoning, perception, and analysis of static visual stimuli; and use of nonlinguistic cues (e.g., facial expression, gesture, and body language) to convey information. Additionally, while they often have difficulty with coordination and complex motor sequencing (Hill, 2001) and delays in fine motor skill development, many of these children develop artistic skills. As the focus typically is on the challenges these children face, it is important to keep in mind that all of these children have strengths which can be used both to help compensate for their weaknesses and to provide opportunities for building self-esteem.

Language Characteristics

Despite adequate residual hearing or a reasonable degree of exposure to visually accessible language, these children have minimal language comprehension and poor expressive skills. Educators may see these children as frustrating and puzzling, and may focus on the behavioral issues that arise secondary to communication frustration.

Receptive Conversational Language

These children, despite their best efforts and although they are clearly not cognitively impaired, do not seem to understand what is being said/signed/cued to them and do not retain or use vocabulary in the expected manner. Another aspect of the individuals with language impairment is that linguistic memory is often impaired (Montgomery, Windsor, & Stark, 1991). Thus, although they may be able to mimic vocabulary during lessons, they often do not retain the words or signs learned. Ongoing, intensive review and over-learning is necessary for any lan-

guage learning (Bebko & Metcalf-Haggert, 1992), and arguably, subsequent reading acquisition (Bebko, 1998) to occur.

Expressive Language

Expressive communication may be attempted via pointing, pantomime, acting, or gesturing, and use of facial expressions and body language may be used to compensate for the lack of linguistic content. This may be supported by isolated words or signs. Children's gestures and pantomime may be mistaken for American Sign Language (ASL) even if they have had minimal or no exposure to true ASL. Their static visual analysis may be well developed, and they may attempt to draw or locate pictures of the focus of their communicative intent. When they do attempt to use signs or cues, the expression typically is telegraphic, and includes errors in both grammar and production of individual words or signs. The child who has developed more expressive skills may try to control the conversation, talking incessantly about an area of interest. This way, they can control the language level and vocabulary involved and decrease the need to understand what others are saying.

Written Expressive Language

A consistent finding in children diagnosed with PLD, and one which is contrary to typical outcomes for deaf children, is that if the child is able to learn to read, even at a relatively low level, he or she may receive language best through print. Indeed, children raised with Cued Speech who have milder forms of this disorder have demonstrated reading comprehension only one to two years below grade level, while "listening" (via Cued Speech) comprehension may be five or more years below grade level. When information is spoken, cued, or signed, these children appear to be constantly guessing at what was said. This is comparable to trying to speechread a language one does not know. Using a very limited subset of the necessary information, they are trying to guess meaning based on an inadequate knowledge of the vocabulary and grammar of the language, and are thus heavily dependant on context for accurate analysis. The increased communication access in print observed even with very limited reading skills appears to relate to the typical presence of at least adequate visual skills when the target is static, but limited ability to process visual information quickly enough to manage moving targets. This is consistent with the findings of Samar and colleagues (2002, 2005) that deaf individuals with relative reading deficits have impairments in rapid visual processing and related visual abilities. They suggest that this deficit is seen in biologically-based reading disorders, but not in individuals with poor reading skills resulting from the impact of deafness. Studies of hearing dyslexics have also found deficits in visual-motion perception (Buchholz & McKone, 2004; Eden et al., 1996; Hansen, Stein, Orde, Winter, & Talcott, 2001; Hari, Renvall, & Tanskanen, 2001). These visual processing deficits affect the perception of moving, but not static, visual stimuli. Research with autism spectrum disorders also suggests that a key difference between those with relatively preserved language and those who have significant language impairments involves impaired rapid visual motion perception of the language impaired group (Gepner & Mestre, 2002). Although there are no data on deaf individuals with PLD, research with hearing children with SLI has indicated slowed auditory processing consistent with these results. Although still controversial, this research suggests that the primary disorder for language impairment in hearing children may be a processing deficit that affects rapid processing in the auditory system and which also may involve the visual system (Merzenich & Jenkins, 1995; Tallal, 1990).

If the child does present with slow visual processing, and this is consistent with observations of deaf children with PLD, he may be trying to learn language while being unable to process the entire sign or cued word, and in more severe cases, may in effect be perceiving different parts of the word or sign each time it is presented. When some receptive skills are developed, the child may be trying to understand what is said to him by trying to capture a few key words and use that information to try to understand what was said. He may try to hold in working memory what he has seen and "replay" it repeatedly in order to make sense of it. Research with hearing children with language impairments, however, indicates that these children also typically present with limited working memory, reducing the effectiveness of this approach (Montgomery, 1995). By the time the child with PLD has been able to process the information, the rest of the group may have moved on to a different topic.

Due to the combination of verbal memory limitations and difficulty with language input, these children require massed practice to develop basic language skills. In effect, teaching these children language can be likened to building a structure on quicksand; if they do not have massed practice with ongoing review, they quickly lose vocabulary and related skills that they may have appeared to master. They seem to require a foundation of basic, core vocabulary that is over learned through drill and ongoing review before language development can proceed. The foundation vocabulary must be learned to the point that it is analyzed automatically rather than requiring an active cognitive search ("Now, what does that mean?") for the child to access meaning. When using Cued Speech, this automaticity is critical for both decoding individual cues and single words. The cues must automatically be decoded before this can be successfully performed at the word level. Similarly, word decoding must be automatic before sentence level comprehension is consistently accurate. Once this foundation is developed, additional vocabulary and grammar skills must be presented in an organized structure, with new information related to that which the child has already mastered.

Applications of Cued Speech for Language Teaching with the PLD Child

Clearly, development of reading skills is important for optimal functioning of these children, since it may represent their best means of receptive communication. As noted elsewhere in this volume, Cued Speech is a well-documented method of making literacy accessible to children who are deaf or hard of hearing. In order for Cued Speech to be accessible for deaf children with PLD, a well-developed understanding of the phonology of the language used at home and at school will be required, yet these children may have difficulty accessing this information through receptive cueing in face-to-face communication. It should be noted that deaf children who do not have additional disabilities affecting language development, who receive consistent exposure to cued language are observed to learn these skills naturally though their cued interactions with family, peers and educators, and are thus not said to receive Cued Speech "instruction." The following strategies were developed to address the specific needs of deaf children with additional challenges to language development.

Serialized Digital Images for Phoneme Learning and Sequencing

One advantage that Cued Speech has over signing is the limited demand for analysis of spatial information and motion involved in reading cues. Unlike signs, individual cues can be represented via digital photographs, either singular or in short series. Figures 16–1 through 16–3 illustrate this technique by showing discrete digital images of the phonemes /k/, /æ/, and /t/, respectively.

As a result, the phonemes comprising individual words can be graphically presented in order, and bound into worksheets that the child can use for practice

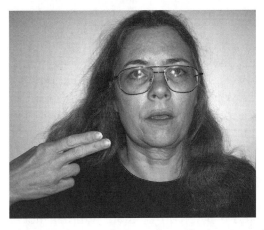

Figure 16–1. Image of cued phoneme /k/.

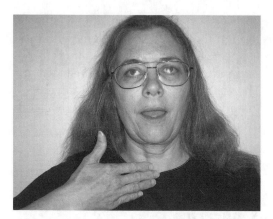

Figure 16–2. Image of cued phoneme /æ/.

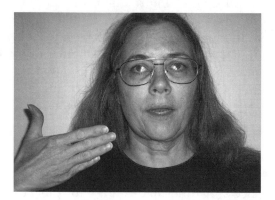

Figure 16–3. Image of cued phoneme /t/.

repeated practice using such worksheets, the child can develop automaticity with phoneme recognition, increasing the likelihood that she will be able to accurately decode what she is seeing in slow, simply presented cued communication. One additional benefit of Cued Speech is that speech information can be slowed or prolonged to a greater extent than oral speech is produced. Thus, even in face-to-face communication, comprehension can be enhanced by decreasing the speed of cued production until the child is able to demonstrate comprehension. Natural communication with typically developing deaf children is best achieved through cueing standard English at the rate of normal speech. Due to the language limitations experienced by the deaf child with PLD and the need for additional processing time, however, she will require this slowing of rate, simplification, and addition of pauses in order to access and process cued language.

For initial tasks focusing on phoneme awareness and discrimination, the child can be presented with phonemes that are similar in either hand or mouthshape. Ideally, in order to enhance literacy outcomes, these pictures could be paired with the printed letter and practice can be based on the child placing the appropriate letter with the cued phoneme. This can begin by having them tracing over the letters or writing next to the printed letter. Such an activity serves as exposure and practice of the individual phonemes and their legal sequences in the language, and also as a graphic display of phonics (i.e., phoneme-grapheme) relationships. Over time, the child should be offered worksheets with previously practiced cued phonemes that he will have to "read" (decode) and fill in with the appropriate letters.

at his own pace and with repetition as needed to ensure mastery. Such worksheets should use photographs and not drawings, as the child needs to learn to discriminate the same visual information that they would observe in face-to-face communication rather than a symbolic representation of the cues.

As the stimuli are static, the child with PLD can take her time to evaluate them and develop an accurate internal model of the phonology of the language. With

Serialized Digital Images for Phoneme Sequencing and Word Building

Once a basic set of consonants and vowels has been learned, the individual phonemes can be combined to produce words. This can be used to introduce the changes in placement of the consonants that occur with consonant-vowel pairs. Simultaneously, by pairing the cued words with pictures representing the meaning of the word, the child will be able to learn the core set of vocabulary required to provide the foundation for language learning. Figures 16–3 and 16–4 illustrate this by showing the cued segments /t/ and /kæ/, respectively. Using worksheets made from such images, the child can begin to associate the cued syllabic segments he produces with their associated graphemes.

In addition to worksheets, posters with word groups (again using a combination of cues, print, and pictures) and labels for objects around the house (cues and print) can be placed throughout the home and school to help support the development of printed and cued vocabulary with static access to phonological as well as orthographic information. These approaches can be used to teach basic sentence structure as well as individual words. Sight words, which are not readily decodable, should be presented only in the vowel-consonant pair form of Cued Speech and can be identified through color coding to help the child understand that they are words she will simply have to memorize.

Using this approach, basic language skills and literacy can be provided to these children by taking advantage of their strength in static visual analysis. Depending on the severity of the child's disorder and the age at which intervention is im-

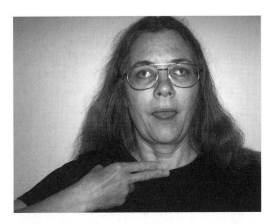

Figure 16–4. Image of cued syllable /kæ/.

plemented, he will likely continue to have significant language limitations, but this approach allows for the development of basic communication skills and an avenue for academic skill development. As such, children typically experience organizational difficulties and other challenges related to executive functioning, and most deaf children with PLD this author has worked with also qualify for a diagnosis of ADHD. Additional supports related to these needs, addressed in later sections, are also desirable.

Strategies to Support Effective Communication with the PLD Child

General practices that will support language comprehension when using Cued Speech with a child with a PLD include the following:

1. Cue slowly and allow time for language processing. It is important to remember that many children with

language disorders (including PLD) need more time to process linguistic information. Use short, simple phrases for important information. If you have a three-part instruction, break it down into three steps and work within the vocabulary you know they understand. This will allow for processing time, and provides the child with shorter sequences of more accessible information to commit to short-term memory. It is acceptable to elaborate for language and concept development, but recognize that information will be missed, and will need to be covered again later.

2. Present information in linguistic and nonlinguistic ways, preferably together. Nonlanguage visual cues might include: pictures, models, or diagrams. This allows the child to take advantage of other visual learning skills, and may be achieved by providing visual supports for comprehension, modeling task demands, and/or having "hands on" demonstrations.

3. In a classroom or other group situations, calling on other children first can allow additional information about the topic in question.

4. Provide a consistent approach to work. For example, when possible, have a standard format for classwork and homework or assignments: how information is arranged and how they are to place information on the paper. This provides context within which the child can work comfortably and decreases stress and task demands, as all she must learn is the new information, instead of having to determine the format required for each assignment.

5. Recognize that misbehavior may be the result of misunderstanding. Check to see if a communication problem has occurred when the child does not behave/perform as expected. Watch for signs of frustration that may reflect communication breakdown. If the child seems overwhelmed, allow him to take a break to clam down and catch up. When he is frustrated or overwhelmed, he is even less able than usual to process information. Keep in mind that the child is working harder than his peers just to understand what is being said and try to express himself.

6. Use visual means to gain the child's attention, and consistently monitor attention. A child with a language or learning disorder may become distracted or inattentive because she has become overwhelmed and "given up," due to her inability to understand what is being said. Alternatively, she may be taking a break due to the fatigue associated with attempting to process the class communication. Although this may be an appropriate response, she will then need any missed information to be provided later, so awareness of such episodes by the teacher is important. This is often compounded by a coexisting attention disorder, which should be managed appropriately. When recalling the child's attention, a subtle approach that will not single out the child is preferable. A system should be developed that the child understands, such as touching a picture or print-based chart on her desk while walking past or pointing to a symbol or sign at the front of the room, or using a previously agreed upon gesture. Ideally, the system used should be matched to the child.

7. In school settings, monitor the child for signs of stress and fatigue, and time tasks to optimize outcomes. When

possible, arrange class activities/requirements so that more demanding tasks are preformed when the child is less stressed and fatigued, and when his attention is better under control. At other times, physical activities, desk work, pull out, or work with a teaching assistant on alternative tasks may be more effective. Although some of these may seem equally taxing, academic tasks in larger group settings are the most problematic activities for these children and even individual language therapy may be seen as a break from such activities.

8. Encourage positive peer relationships. The deaf child with PLD is often rejected or ignored by peers due to her communication limitations. Due to the effort involved in communication attempts and limited success, she may prefer solitary activities. Peer relationships also suffer because the child does not know the rules of games, many social norms or cues, or information that is common knowledge. She may be better able to interact with hearing children who may adjust their communication due to her deafness. These children often need help developing adequate social interactions. With older children, it may be possible to explain the child's needs to her peers, and how they can help to meet them (e.g., slow speech/cueing). Teachers can model clear communication and encourage positive interactions through games, discussions, and other activities in small group settings with communication facilitated by a teacher or speech language therapist.

9. Cue, but allow a range of ways to communicate. Remember, this child wants to communicate, but may not be able to do so through Cued Speech or speech alone. He may try to cue, sign, gesture, pantomime or act out the object or character he wishes to discuss. He may also use a few words to try to give you the general idea either in isolation or in conjunction with pointing, drawing, or showing you pictures to complete the thought. If this is the case, a picture dictionary may be helpful to clarify information he does not understand and for him to support his expressive communication. Children with more severe language deficits may benefit from picture communication charts of words consistently needed to express their needs. These should be used to support communication while continuing to work on the development of cued language.

Case: Cued Speech for a Deaf Child with PLD

In the interests of full disclosure, it should be noted that this is the child of the author of this chapter. However, the assessments cited were performed by either a private speech-language therapist or staff in the child's school.

Diagnoses

Thomas is the deaf child of hearing parents, one of whom (the author) worked in the field of deafness at the time of his birth. He was diagnosed with a severe to profound sensorineural hearing loss at 8 months, with the residual primarily in the lower frequencies and no measurable response in the higher frequencies. He was immediately exposed to signs, with Cued Speech added at eleven months. He also was transferred to a signing deaf babysitter and then a daycare that included both deaf and hearing staff and peers. As a 2-year-old, he attended an early intervention classroom using ASL at the pre-college on the campus of Gallaudet University. At that time it was noted that he tended to use one or two signs and use gestures and body language to complete his thoughts.

Due to distractibility, inattention, impulsivity, and over activity both at home and school, Thomas was diagnosed with ADHD shortly before his fourth birthday, and started on stimulant medication. No other formal diagnoses were made until kindergarten, and attention by the school generally focused on his behavior. Despite the range of intensive interventions for his deafness, Thomas was essentially nonverbal at age 5½ despite nonverbal cognitive abilities measured in the high average range, with more purely visuospatial reasoning in the superior range, and a diagnosis of a mixed receptive language disorder was made. This reflected minimal language skills orally, via Cued Speech and signed communication.

Amplification and Cochlear Implantation

Thomas was fitted with hearing aids and a personal FM system at nine months. These provided a limited amount of hearing in the lower frequencies due to his corner audiogram, however, he responded well to the sound he received and wore his equipment consistently. Loss of his limited residual hearing was signaled by acting out behavior when he was about 2½ years old. Following the loss of his already minimal residual hearing, he was provided with a cochlear implant (CI) at 3 years old. He entered a Cued Speech classroom just after his third birthday.

Interventions

Following the diagnosis of a language disorder, Thomas was provided with alternative interventions, which included the previously described worksheets based on digital photographs of Cued Speech, print, and pictures. This allowed Thomas to learn the individual cued phonemes and their graphemic (letter) associations. He was able to learn some words cued in this static manner, but was not able to follow even slow cueing through the air for communication.

Concurrently, he was administered a computer based intervention developed for hearing children with specific language impairment (SLI), which was accessed through his cochlear implant with the support of Cued Speech. This latter was necessary as the program was not designed for children with the severity of impairment seen in Thomas. The typical hearing child using this program completed it in approximately eight weeks. Thomas required 18 weeks with additional practice outside of the standard program. As he began to progress on the program, he began to be able to process more language aurally through his implant and his auditory-oral vocabulary began to increase. Despite significant gains, he remained profoundly language impaired.

Schooling

In addition to the above interventions, Thomas was transferred out of the Deaf and Hard of Hearing Program and into an augmentative and alternative communication classroom. Although this decreased his stress, the focus of that class was on expressive language disorders and it did not adequately meet his needs. After two years in that program, he was transferred to a special school for children with complex or multiple disabilities, with a focus on disabilities affecting language and communication, where he has made slow, but continuous progress. He has developed advanced skills in art, but progress in most academic areas is hindered by his language limitations. He benefits from "hands on" activities and use of pictorial supports, and enjoys areas of study that involve maps. He often performs the function of classroom artist and currently draws a weekly cartoon that is distributed throughout the school. These latter activities have provided him with important supports for self-esteem as he has come to understand his areas of deficit relative to his peers and others around him.

Current Language Functioning

Over the past decade, Thomas has continued to demonstrate severe language impairment despite ongoing interventions; however, he is now able to manage basic communication with family, school staff, and friends receptively through listening and Cued Speech. Although he is able to understand some signs, he is heavily dependent on his hearing for sign comprehension and he manages signs best through simultaneous presentation of signs and speech. Recent observations suggest that while he is able to understand Cued Speech without auditory support, he may struggle unless there is context to support his comprehension. Expressively, Thomas prefers to talk. His speech is often supported through pantomime and gestures and some signs or sign equivalents. As his speech has improved, these supports have declined unless he is excited and does not know the words he needs or cannot retrieve the words he wants quickly enough. He prefers not to cue expressively, although he does so when necessary.

Recent Language Testing

Thomas demonstrates the typical strengths in math, although he has difficulty with word problems. His static visual analysis is advanced (performance on a recently administered measure of visual spatial reasoning was "very superior"), and he is considered a gifted artist by the staff at his school. As he progresses, his difficulties with word retrieval and verbal memory have become increasingly apparent. The best indication of the relative impacts of his language disorder and Cued Speech is seen in his reading assessment performed at his school when he was 13. His performance on Word Attack, a measure of letter-sound decoding skills was average (standard score [SS] 99, test mean 100, standard deviation 15; 48th percentile; grade equivalent 7.5) reflecting age-appropriate basic decoding skills. In contrast, his score on a measure of reading comprehension was significantly impaired (SS 52, 0.1 percentile, grade equivalent 1.4). Supplementary measures of reading comprehension estimated possible skills up to the mid-second grade level; however, in practice, Thomas continues to struggle with reading comprehension at the sentence level. Thus, although he can read aloud most materials placed in front of him, he has little understanding of what he is reading and generally uses compensatory strategies to glean meaning from text. Even so, his communication is often supported by having information presented through a combination of speech/ Cued Speech and print.

Discussion

One thing is clear: despite presenting with one of the most profound language disorders this author has seen among the two dozen or so deaf children with PLD with whom she has had direct contact, Thomas has developed age-appropriate decoding skills. This would be surprising in either a child with a language disorder or one with a congenital hearing loss, and professionals working with him are at a loss to explain it in a child with profound levels of both of these conditions. This unique skill is best explained by his massed practice to accessible phonemic information via the photographs of Cued Speech paired with graphemes. If the other interventions provided were responsible for his decoding skills, his reading comprehension would be expected to be at near comparable levels. In contrast, they continue to reflect his continued severely deficient language skills as reflected in his language assessment performed at the same time as the reading tests which yielded both receptive and expressive language SS of 50 (mean 100; standard deviation 15).

Nonverbal Learning Disability (NLD)

Definition and Diagnosis

NLD is a neurological disorder characterized by difficulties with visual and spatial information, motor skills deficits, social skills deficits, and learning difficulties related to math (Rourke, 1995). The difficulties with visual and spatial information include poor visuospatial organization, difficulty with visualization, tracking, and processing of visuospatial information, and deficits in receptive and expressive spatial relations (e.g., location and movement of signs). Additional signs seen with NLD include motor skills deficits, such as balance problems, poor coordination, and difficulty with fine and complex motor skills, the latter of which would affect both expressive cueing and writing in addition to signing. Additionally, children with NLD commonly demonstrate deficits in executive functioning, primarily characterized by difficulty managing novel stimuli and "shifting," making transitions difficult as it is hard for him to stop one activity and switch to another, inadequate planning and organizational skills, and difficulty learning from experience.

Contrasting NLD and PLD

In contrast to individuals with PLD, who generally do well on nonverbal measures, those with NLD tend to score poorly on nonverbal measures despite demonstrating adequate or better cognitive capacity in daily life in areas less affected by their disorder. Also in contrast to individuals with PLD, those with NLD may have difficulty with the emotional aspects of communication, which generally is intact compared to formal language in subjects with PLD. Those with NLD demonstrate a relative lack of emotional expression in their attempts at communication. In contrast, individuals with severe PLD may use facial expressions, posture, pantomime, and gesturing as their primary means of communication. Individuals with NLD have difficulty interpreting the emotional components of the communication of others, whereas those with PLD may depend on components such as facial expression, posture, and other nonverbal cues to grasp the intended message.

That is, although the individual with a PLD will have difficulty with all modes of linguistic communication (e.g., ASL and other types of signed communication, Cued Speech, and speech), they may have relatively preserved abilities to use the emotional aspects of communication and attempt to use gestures, pantomime, facial expression, and posture to try to convey their message (Morere, 1999; Trauner, Ballantyne, Chase, & Tallal, 1993). Individuals with PLD also may have enhanced awareness of these aspects of communication and try to use them to interpret incoming messages that they cannot understand based on the linguistic information. Additionally, while math skills are generally problematic for individuals with NLD, they may represent the best area of academic functioning for an individual with PLD.

Socialization and Peer Relationships

In addition to their sensory and motor difficulties, children with NLD generally present with social skills deficits. These appear to be secondary to difficulties understanding nonverbal communication, including facial expressions, posture, and tone of voice. The above noted need consistency also impacts social functioning, and these children generally demonstrate poor social judgment and difficulty with social interactions. Essentially, these children cannot "read" others and have little understanding of common social expectations. They do not learn these things naturally and must be taught the cues and expectations involved in social situations. This has a major impact on understanding of receptive language regardless of the modality involved.

Language Skills

Hearing children with NLD tend to excel on basic verbal skills, including basic reading and spelling. They tend to do well with rote learning and often develop high levels of specialized vocabulary. They typically depend on their verbal skills to explore and interact with the world. In contrast, they tend to have difficulty with reading comprehension; math, and particularly math reasoning; handwriting, although this may improve over time; and science.

NLD and the Deaf Child

While the hearing child may benefit from his relative verbal strengths, the wide-ranging impact on visual-spatial skills and nonverbal communication has significant implications for the deaf child. Due to the visual demands associated with language development in deaf children, rather than a strength in basic verbal skills, they generally present with a secondary language impairment. Ratner (1985, 1988, and as cited in Mauk & Mauk,1998), in her studies of visual spatial skills in deaf children found that in addition to the standard symptoms, deaf children with NLD demonstrate a range of communication deficits, including difficulty with reception of all forms of visual communication, including signs, Cued Speech, speechreading, and simultaneous signs and speech. She also reported that ratings of these children on a measure of psychosocial functioning resulted in elevated scores on scales reflecting symptoms of psychosis, impaired social skills, anxiety, withdrawal, and depression.

The diagnosis of NLD in a deaf individual is often missed as clinicians generally depend on a difference in verbal and nonverbal functioning, with better performance on verbal tasks to make the diagnosis. This is unlikely in deaf individuals, who may do equally poorly on both aspects of standard tests due to the

English loading on most verbal tasks and the secondary language impacts of their NLD on the verbal skills. Additionally, the typical accommodations made for deaf individuals when evaluating cognitive functioning involve a focus on nonverbal and visuospatial tasks. The result is that individuals with NLD may be inaccurately diagnosed as having low overall cognitive functioning.

Socialization

The aspects of NLD associated with the social skills deficits may have even more impact on deaf children than hearing children. The difficulty understanding nonverbal communication (e.g., facial expression, posture, emphasis of signs) would remove one of the main routes of receptive language for the deaf child. Facial expressions and posture are essential components of ASL. Thus, difficulty understanding these linguistic cues will impede the accurate understanding of signed communication. Although this would also affect the understanding of emotional messages through Cued Speech, speechreading, or oral communication, the literal message could be received through these routes.

Receptive and Expressive Language

It would be expected that the limitations in visuospatial functioning seen with NLD would have an impact on both the development of ASL skills and ongoing reading of signed messages. Although there also would be an impact on receptive Cued Speech due to the diminished visual analysis, since there are limited spatial demands for reading cues, the child would have a greater likelihood to be able to develop receptive language via

Cued Speech. Additionally, if the previously described worksheets using digital photographs are used in conjunction with print, skill development in cue reading as well as print analysis can be developed with no spatial demands. The motor skill deficits associated with NLD would be expected to impact writing, and expressive cueing as well as expressive sign skill development and accurate signing if ASL is learned. The fine motor skill demands of Cued Speech would mean that even if the child could cue expressively, he or she might have difficulty doing so in a fluent manner.

Deaf children with NLD may have difficulty learning sign language due to the visuospatial nature of signs, as well as the above noted postural and facial expression components of the language, all of which are impaired in children with NLD. Deaf children who are attempting to learn language using a dynamic visuospatial system, such as ASL, may demonstrate both the standard symptoms of NLD and secondary language and social skills deficits. Depending on the severity of the disorder, with intensive language stimulation, the child may develop adequate ASL skills, but may continue to be awkward in both receptive and expressive signing.

Cued Speech and NLD

Regardless of the interventions provided, deaf individuals with concurrent NLD are likely to continue to have difficulties in communication due to the problems with facial expression and emotional tone that are important for oral language as well as visual communication. However, they may develop better access to language if provided with a mode of communication that is less dependent on visuospatial skills and facial expressions, such as Cued Speech. Although they may have difficulty with the fine motor requirements of expressive cueing, they may be better able to perceive the formal language as Cued Speech has a minimal spatial component and a very limited set of formational components. Also, although the emotional message requires analysis and comprehension of facial expressions for Cued Speech as well as other forms of communication, the literal linguistic information is fully available via Cued Speech without such information.

The child's ability to use this Cued Speech access to language may be supported by taking advantage of their strength in rote learning though the use of massed practice with the previously described Cued Speech worksheets. Due to their limitations in visual analysis and tracking, such children may need this support to develop adequate skills with visual discrimination of the individual cued phonemes. Such skill development in the absence of the demands of attempting gaze shifts and the analysis of ongoing communication may allow for greater automaticity of phoneme discrimination and increased success with such analysis during face-to-face communication.

If these children are able to develop literacy skills, although they may continue to have difficulty with advanced reading comprehension due to their emotional analysis limitations, they may be able to develop the enhanced basic reading and spelling skills commonly reported as strengths in hearing children with NLD. Thus, they may be able to develop some of the typical strengths seen in hearing children with NLD. Again, Cued Speech provides enhanced opportunity for the development of literacy skills in deaf children. As children with NLD also generally demonstrate deficits in executive functioning, the supports for these skills noted in the section on ADHD also should be considered.

Case: Cued Speech for a Child with NLD

Diagnoses

"Robin" (a gender-neutral pseudonym) is a deaf young adult with hearing parents who had a diagnosis of CHARGE syndrome, a congenital disorder characterized by a cluster of birth defects including vision, cranial nerve, cardiac, nasal, genitourinary, ear and hearing, and growth and developmental disorders, and commonly accompanied by learning disabilities and social and emotional delays. Robin was referred for assessment related to college placement and planning, and presented with the symptoms typical of this disorder. In addition to a bilateral profound sensorineural hearing loss, there were cardiac and hormonal disorders, social and emotional delays, and documented learning disabilities, for which the school system had provided supports. The deafness was identified when Robin was about 15 months old. During kindergarten, a school evaluation indicated problems with visual acuity, gross and fine motor delays, slow psychomotor functioning, and oculomotor problems resulting in visual scanning and tracking difficulty and problems with binocular vision.

Amplification/Cochlear Implantation

Robin was fitted with hearing aids shortly after diagnosis and responded well to amplification, although the level of hearing loss was such that visual communication was required for language input. The hearing aids were worn consistently and Robin was aided during the assessment.

Interventions

The family consistently used Cued Speech with Robin beginning soon after the deafness was diagnosed, and within a few months of initiation of Cued Speech in the home Robin began to demonstrate language development, which had been absent prior to this intervention. Cued Speech services were also provided through the school system. Services for learning disabilities were also provided beginning early in elementary school. Robin learned to sign in middle school in order to communicate with signing deaf friends. The parents noted, and the examiner observed, that Robin preferred CS for receptive communication and signs for expressive communication. When signing, Robin tended to use "simultaneous communication" (the use of signs from American Sign Language and additional invented signs in English word order with accompanying speech or mouthing), but demonstrated the ability to use American Sign Language for communication. In school, in addition to intervention for the impacts of deafness, Robin consistently received support services for learning disabilities related to visual functioning and some academic coursework.

Schooling

Robin attended a preschool in a self-contained classroom with teachers of the deaf who were able to cue. Although most children using Cued Speech quickly move to the mainstream, the self-contained setting continued through much of the educational process due to the learning disabilities that hindered the Robin's ability to progress at the rate of the typical classroom. Mainstream experiences were accomplished through the support of a cued language transliterator (CLT) and academic support services, and this eventually became the primary educational setting. Although the impacts of the learning disabilities and psychosocial delays affected both social and academic functioning, Robin was able to complete high school and obtain a degree.

Testing

Cognitive testing over the years generally indicated average intellectual functioning, although the scores varied depending on the impact of difficulties with certain areas of visual functioning. School based academic testing generally indicated grade appropriate reading levels despite Robin's congenital deafness. This author, who is fluent both in Cued American English and signed communication, administered a neuropsychological evaluation. Robin was asked about the preferred mode of communication and indicated that the examiner should use Cued Speech, but that response preference was simultaneous communication. This was the manner in which the assessment was administered except when Robin needed to produce accurate phonemic information, at which times the examiner asked Robin to cue. One memory task, which was designed and normed for signing adults, was administered via simultaneous communication. The assessment was performed in a quiet, distraction free environment. The examiner wore plain, dark colored clothes and only a watch, glasses, and wedding ring for jewelry in order to minimize distractions and optimize the contrast between the clothing and cueing hands. The results of the assessment indicated average intellectual abilities based on the Performance Scales of the Wechsler Adult Intelligence Scale, Revised, Neuropsychological Instrument administration (WAIS-R-NI) and the Raven's Progressive Matrices. It was noted that responses tended to be slow, but accurate. Cognitive processing and academic, visual, motor, memory, and executive functioning were further evaluated using a wide range of tests, including subtests of the Woodcock-Johnson-Revised, Tests of Cognitive Abilities and Tests of Achievement, the Boston-Rochester Neuropsychological Screening Test, Colorado Neuropsychology Tests, the Developmental Test of Visual-Motor Integration, Benton Form Discrimination, the Rey-Osterreith Complex Figure, the Rey Visual Design Learning Test, UCCD Signed Paired Associates Test, Ruff Figural Fluency, Alternate Uses Test, the Wisconsin Card Sorting Test, Porteus Mazes, and several tasks evaluating motor strength and control. Psychosocial and emotional functioning were evaluated using interviews, the Incomplete Sentences Blank, Human Figure Drawings, and the Patient's Behavior Checklist and Self-Rating Symptom Checklist for ADHD.

In general, Robin demonstrated the pattern consistent with a diagnosis of a nonverbal learning disability. Despite congenital deafness, performance on cognitive tasks tended to be weaker on those that relied on more visuospatial processes and stronger on those more amenable to verbal mediation. Mild deficits were observed on all tasks measuring visual scanning and visuo-spatial perception and organization. In addition to these difficulties, there was evidence of inconsistent attention and deficits in executive functioning. These latter were reflected in difficulty with planning and organization,

somewhat concrete thinking and difficulty with the generation of unique responses, and a tendency to revert back to previous strategies even they were no longer effective. Despite demonstrating the ability to perform adequately on reasoning and problem solving tasks, Robin was not always able to consistently apply these skills or the strategies that had been developed. Additionally, there were mild to moderate difficulties both visual and verbal memory, although verbal memory strategies and the use of English grammar and syntax appeared to optimize recall.

Despite the history of well-documented LDs and the above noted deficits, Robin demonstrated college level word attack skills in conjunction with weaker, but still average to low average sight word reading. These data suggest that Robin's most successful reading strategy involves "sounding out" words, a strategy based on the well-known phonemic access afforded via Cued Speech. As is common with individuals with NLD, reading comprehension was lower than expectations based on the average basic reading skills, but still within the low average range. Even so, the grade equivalent of 6.9 was well above the standard expectations for deaf students of third to fourth grade reading even without the challenges of learning disabilities. Somewhat slowed cognitive processing combined with some memory limitations hindered development of more complex grammatical structures, and lack of sophistication and creative thinking resulted in more low average scores on writing tasks despite accuracy of written output. Some reading and writing organization difficulties were also noted. These types of difficulties are typical of individuals with NLD, as are the mild to moderate fine motor skills deficits and a relative weakness in math demonstrated by the subject.

Although it is difficult to distinguish the impacts of CHARGE syndrome, which typically produces social skills deficits, and the impact of the NLD, Robin did demonstrate ongoing social skills deficits.

Discussion

The above noted preference for receptive cueing appeared to reflect the verbose-quential nature and decreased visuospatial demands of Cued Speech, while use of expressive signing appeared to relate to the lower level of fine motor sequencing demands in that modality. Despite the atypical communication preferences, this case demonstrates that language skills and literacy can develop in a deaf child with a NLD when early, consistent use of Cued Speech is implemented. This contrasts sharply to a range of cases of NLD in deaf children in signing environments that produced significant secondary language deficits. Due to the impacts of NLD on sign skill development, deaf children with NLD typically demonstrate significant language and communication deficits (Ratner, 1988). Often these children are diagnosed as cognitively impaired, as the tests typically used to evaluate cognitive functioning in deaf children depend on heavily visuospatial skills, as language-based tests are considered unfair to most deaf children. Even when there is a general consensus that the child has adequate cognitive functioning, there are generally significant language delays. Indeed, even relatively mild and specific deficits in visual perception, such as impairments in figure-ground discrimination and visual closure, produce significant delays in sign skill development. In the absence of adequate language development, these children also have limited development of literacy. In contrast, the above case demonstrates that a deaf child with clear, well-documented learning disabilities diagnosable as a NLD who has had early, consistent exposure to Cued Speech can develop optimal language and literacy skills when the effects of the learning disabilities are taken into consideration.

Attention Deficit Hyperactivity Disorder (ADHD)

Definition and Diagnosis

Attention deficit hyperactivity disorder (ADHD) is one of the most commonly diagnosed disabilities in children. According to the National Center for Health Statistics, in 1997–1998 approximately 11 percent of children between the ages of six and eleven had a current or previous diagnosis of either ADHD or a LD (Pastor & Ruben, 2002). Of those, 3% were reported to have only ADHD, while 4% were reported to have some type of LD and another 4% to have both ADHD and a LD. Thus, within this sample, approximately 7% of children surveyed were reported to have a diagnosis of ADHD. Estimates within the deaf population are highly variable, ranging from 3.5 to over 38% (Kelly, Forney, Parker-Fisher, & Jones, 1993). Although there are methodological difficulties with the surveys producing those estimates, the higher estimates were generally associated with acquired deafness and etiologies typically associated with increased risk of additional disabilities rather than hereditary deafness. "Nevertheless, regardless of its exact incidence, ADHD is widely believed to be one of the most frequent secondary disabilities among deaf children and adults" (Kelly et al., 1993, p. 1167). Although the higher estimates likely overreport ADHD, it is generally believed to be one of the most common secondary disabilities in deaf populations.

The diagnosis of ADHD is made based on the presence of inattention, impulsivity, and/or overactivity (American Psychiatric Association, 2000; NIMH, 1996). In addition to these commonly recognized symptoms, individuals with ADHD generally demonstrate deficits in executive functioning, resulting in poor organizational skills, difficulty learning from feedback, deficient working memory and mental computation, difficulty developing and implementing effective strategies, and difficulty altering approaches to tasks and with motor coordination and sequencing (Barkley, 2005). ADHD typically is addressed by a variety of approaches including parent training, behavior modification, organizational and social skills training, management of dietary, nutritional and sleeping habits, and medication.

Impacts of ADHD on the Language Development of Deaf Children

Prelingually deaf children with ADHD may have an added impact on learning and developing language in any modality. In order for a deaf or hard of hearing child to receive information from the environment, he or she must be attending to the stimulus. Although the hearing child can passively receive language input while he is playing, running around the room, or otherwise act in a hyperactive or distracted manner, language input is inaccessible to the deaf child at these times. Thus, language reception will be diminished compared to other deaf children for the deaf child with ADHD regardless of the modality or com-munication method used. Even the deaf child relying on residual hearing, wearing hearing aids, or using a cochlear implant must actively attend in order to process incoming language stimuli. Thus, in the presence of ADHD, lack of attention may result in delays in learning language. They also may experience increased incidents of miscommunication once language is learned, as the child may not receive complete information if they are unable to maintain attention throughout the message. To compound the problem, delays in language development may make standard approaches to behavior management of ADHD more difficult, as they generally involve teaching the person to use language to help manage his behavior. When this occurs in a deaf child of hearing parents, the combination of ADHD and deafness may further strain the coping resources of the parents, causing secondary impacts on language modeling and attachment.

In the absence of additional conditions affecting language development, the impact of ADHD should be relatively mild and should affect all modes of communication. However, as noted above, there is a high level of comorbidity between ADHD and learning disabilities. Indeed, most deaf children with PLD seen by the author have also qualified for a diagnosis of ADHD. When ADHD combines with conditions such as NLD and PLD, the resultant impacts tend to be synergistic rather than additive, resulting in significant increases in the language impacts of the primary disorders. In addition to the effects of impulsivity and inattention, the deficits in executive functioning can have major impacts on language development. Children with impaired organizational skills may have such poor organization of the language input that is received that they have difficulty retrieving information.

It is comparable to having to search through a pile for a specific card after the entire card catalogue of a library has been dumped on the floor. This results in difficulty with both word and information retrieval and the organization of both visual and linguistic output. It is not uncommon for these children to recall many of the details of a story, but to recount them in such a disorganized manner that the "listener" may have significant difficulty determining what the child is intending to convey unless they are already familiar with the content. Thus, even in the absence of formal language deficits, communication difficulties may be observed. When this is combined with a PLD or a secondary language deficit due to a NLD, the resultant communicative attempt may be completely unintelligible.

Using Cued Speech with Deaf Children with ADHD

While language development and communication via Cued Speech will be affected in a manner comparable to signed communication, there are some potential benefits of Cued Speech for these children. As in the case of PLD and NLD, the affect of AHDH on language development is greatest when communication is through the air. If the child's attention drifts or is distracted while he is observing signs, cues, or speech, he may miss all or part of the incoming information. Unfortunately, signed, spoken, or cued information is ephemeral, and by the time the child's attention returns to the speaker, if they are still talking, a different set of language stimuli will be occurring. If the information is repeated the child may be able to fill in some of the information, but it may still not be complete.

Print Materials

While the child's attention may also be inconsistent for printed information, information on paper is consistent over time. Thus, even if it occurs in a fragmented manner, the child can benefit from language stimuli presented in print as it remains available in the original form whenever she is able to attend to it. Thus, development of literacy skills is important for the deaf child with ADHD, and this again may be significantly supported through Cued Speech worksheets, such as those described in the section on PLD, which are also available whenever the child is able to focus her attention.

Graphic Materials

In addition to the use of Cued Speech worksheets and labels, organizational skills can be supported using Cued Speech charts displaying categories of objects (e.g., birds, vehicles, etc.) to support the development of internalized organization of information. For example, a chart with the category "birds" could be created on a poster board with pictures of various birds, with the common name of the bird in print and with digital photographs of a person cueing the name presented below each picture. Such posters are available in educational supply stores on which the cued representations of the labels can simply be added. Additionally, digital pictures of Cued Speech can be used to support any of the academic and intervention materials typically used with children with ADHD. One simple manner of implementing this is to print digital photographs of the cues on commercially available labels, which then can be peeled off and added to the commercial products. This will both make the information more available to the child with weak reading skills but adequate Cued Speech comprehension, and expand the child's reading vocabulary and comprehension. Similarly, behavior contracts and charts, and home and classroom rules, which need to be available to be pointed out to the child on a regular basis to provide external structure to support his self management, could be provided through Cued Speech supported print as long as the child has weak reading skills.

Communication Strategies and Techniques

Maintain Visual Attention. When cueing with a deaf child with ADHD, work to maintain visual attention. Set up gentle visual signals to recall attention. For example, in a classroom, have a sign or symbol on the front of the room that can be touched to call the child's attention. If the teacher tends to walk around the room, he or the CLT can gently touch the child's desk within the range of the child's gaze. A parent or caregiver can gently touch the child's shoulder or arm or wave their hand in front of their own face briefly before starting to cue to signal that they are about to begin talking. The latter techniques may also be appropriate for transliterators to use in the classroom.

Set up a behavioral contract targeting attention. While the child's attention is not fully under his control, the use of external structure in the form of behavioral contracts can help the child with ADHD to learn to attend optimally.

Target very specific behaviors, such as watching the CLT. Start with brief periods of time in order to allow the child to succeed and earn reinforcement. As the child is able to earn high levels of reinforcement, the length of time he or she must sustain his attention can be increased. Be

alert and catch the child paying attention. Negative behaviors can be managed in a similar manner, but each behavior must be very specific, and alternative, positive behaviors should be taught to replace those that are targeted for extinction.

Start important information with the child's name. Both children and adults tend to respond and automatically attend better in response to hearing (seeing) their name. Starting important information with a brief, well-practiced standard phrase, such as, "Listen, Joey, news flash!" will both naturally attract his attention and alert him to the fact that important information is coming.

Repeat Before Rephrasing. Repeat what you said the same way the first time the child asks what you said. The child may not have seen the whole message and needs more information to be able to make sense of what was said. If the child still doesn't get it, *then* rephrase. If you rephrase what you said the first time the child asks, he or she will have to start from scratch, trying to watch and take in the complete message. However, if you first repeat as closely as possible what was initially presented, the child will have the opportunity to fill in the blanks of what was missed and increase the likelihood of comprehension.

Autism

Definition and Diagnosis

The DSM IV-TR defines autism spectrum disorder as being characterized by impairment in social interaction and communication, and atypical patterns of behavior with a focus on having a limited range of behaviors and interests and inadequacies of social behaviors (American Psychiatric Association, 2000). Unlike children with PLD, those with autism generally demonstrate little interest in communication or sharing information. They often make little eye contact and research suggests that they have deficits in facial recognition (Klin, Sparrow, de Bildt, Cicchetti, Cohen, & Volkmar, 1999) and abnormalities in processing of faces (Pierce, Müller, Ambrose, Allen, & Courchesne, 2001) and the analysis of emotional content of faces (Wang, Dapretto, Hariri, Sigman, & Bookheimer, 2004).

In many ways, children with autism, particularly those described as having high functioning autism or Asperger syndrome, are similar to those with NLD. They demonstrate a similar profile of neuropsychological deficits (Klin, Volkmar, Sparrow, Cicchetti, & Rourke, 1995). These limitations include deficits in fine and gross motor skills, visual-motor integration, visual-spatial perception, ability to manage novel material, visual memory, concept formation for both verbal and nonverbal material, prosody and other social and emotional aspects of communication, and basic math skills. Additionally, despite often large quantities of verbal output, they demonstrate a paucity of content. Similarly, despite strengths in basic reading skills, reading comprehension generally is poor. Overall, these individuals demonstrate limited social and emotional functioning. In contrast to the general strengths or preserved functioning related to auditory perception in those with NLD and Asperger syndrome, those with autism generally have deficits in these areas as well. In their 1995 study, Klin's team noted that while those with Asperger syndrome are most similar to the presentation of NLD, those diagnosed with autism, even when described as "high functioning,"

generally demonstrated additional weaknesses in auditory perception and auditory-verbal memory, vocabulary, and basic reading skills. In contrast, whereas those with Asperger syndrome consistently demonstrated the visual memory deficits seen with NLD, those with autism often had preserved visual memory.

These latter factors may relate to the previously mentioned research involving Autism spectrum disorders (ASD) which found that ASD individuals who have significant language impairments have impaired rapid visual motion perception whereas those with relatively preserved language do not (Gepner & Mestre, 2002). This suggests that there may be an overlap in the processes involved in language deficits of individuals with autism and those with PLD/SLI.

Klin and colleagues (2002) studied the visual aspects of social behavior in individuals with autism, and found that although control subjects tended to focus on the eyes of people even when observing them in film clips, those with autism tended to focus their gaze on the mouth and neck area. Additionally, when viewing scenes with multiple players and objects in the environment to which they referred, control subjects would repeatedly shift their gaze between the players and use cues from the actors to direct their gaze to specific environmental targets. In contrast, those with autism would rarely shift their gaze, tending to remain with one person, or if their gaze shifted to another player, they would persist in viewing that person over time. Additionally, when prompted by comments in the scene to look at an object in the background, they appeared to perform more random perusal of environmental stimuli rather than directing their gaze based on gestures of the actors.

As individuals with autism demonstrate relative strengths in rote memory, massed practice with ongoing review is often used to support their language and social skills development. Additionally, their focus on the mouth region may provide insights into avenues for supporting their language development.

Using Cued Speech with the Deaf Child with Autism

A fact sheet located on the Web site of the National Cued Speech Association describes the use of Cued Speech with children with autism to compensate for auditory language reception deficits common with these disorders, and can be accessed at http://www.cuedspeech.org/sub/cued/cs_autism_pdd.asp (retrieved November 19, 2009). The theory behind its use is to access the visual strengths to compensate for the difficulties these children have using auditory stimuli. An additional target is to use Cued Speech to help children with autism to focus on faces. As noted above, children with autism generally have deficits in facial recognition and analysis. The use of Cued Speech may support the focusing of the child's visual attention on the face. The use of expressive Cued Speech would then provide motoric feedback to support the internal model of phonology provided through the visual-auditory information provided by receptive cueing.

Cued Speech for Visual Attention

Research (see above) suggests that individuals with autism may tend to focus their gaze on the mouth and neck area when viewing speakers. Thus, their visual attention appears to be naturally drawn to the region of the face most critical for language reception via Cued Speech. While most listeners focus attention on the eyes, which provide information about the emotional aspects of language, effective reception of literal language via Cued Speech is supported by attention to the mouth and neck, where cueing occurs. Furthermore, when Cued Speech is used with a child with autism in face-to-face communication, this would appear to be best accomplished by a single speaker (e.g., a CLT), as individuals with autism apparently tend to maintain their gaze on a single speaker even when that person has ceased to speak and other individuals have begun to do so. This likely would result in significant loss of information for the autistic child if multiple speakers were involved in turn taking even if all speakers were cueing. However, with the use of a CLT, the information from each speaker could be conveyed through a single person, and the use of Cued Speech would take advantage of the inclination of the individual with autism to focus his attention on the mouth and neck area of a single speaker.

Cued Speech for Receptive Language

Based on the above data, it appears likely that the core deficit in language development in autism may be similar to that in children with PLD. Thus, slow presentation of CS may help compensate for some of the problems with auditory language reception and development. The slowness of the cueing is important as, similar to those with PLD, these children appear to have slowed visual as well as auditory processing. Although some degree of slowing of speech is possible, in practice, language presentation via Cued Speech can be slowed much more than simple slowing of speech, which begins to distort the phonemes as the speech is slowed excessively. With slowed Cued Speech, the child with autism can be provided with extended time for processing of the incoming language stimuli and at the same time take advantage of the relative strength in visual perception and memory while compensating for the auditory processing and memory limitations.

Cued Speech for Literacy and Language Development

As rote learning based on massed practice is a consistently reported relative strength in autism, it appears likely that children with autism may benefit from massed practice with Cued Speech worksheets. This would take advantage of their relative strengths in visual memory and rote learning while limiting the auditory and social demands typically associated with language learning, but which represent areas of difficulty for individuals with autism. This can provide simultaneous access to development of language through ongoing practice with language presented though digital photographs of Cued Speech and literacy through the concurrent pairing of the cued words with print. Labels for everything in the house can be made with both cued and printed words to develop vocabulary in addition to worksheets. As children with autism often enjoy interacting with the computer, they may enjoy playing with any of a number of games (available from www.cuedspeech.com) developed to teach Cued Speech and which use print in conjunction with cueing avatars or videoclips, many of which can have the cueing slowed down, thus accommodating their need for slowed

cueing. Although it will not compensate for social and emotional deficits observed in this population, the access to language development available through these techniques may help some of those who would not otherwise achieve the label "high functioning" to do so.

Cued Speech for Expressive Language

Although individuals with autism may struggle with expressive cueing due to the complex fine motor demands of cueing, if they are able to do so, the multimodal aspect of CS may support their expressive language when it is possible. The tactile and kinesthetic (muscle) feedback intrinsic in expressive cueing would support word retrieval and has been found to support speech production in many deaf children. If expressive cueing is not possible, the access to language and literacy provided by Cued Speech would facilitate the use of text based expressive communication through typing or communication boards, decreasing the need for picture communication systems and increasing the opportunities for independence.

Conclusion

Cued Speech was invented to support the literacy development of deaf children. However, it has proved to have much more widespread applications. It has been used to support the language development of children, both deaf and hearing, who have challenges, such as auditory processing and language disorders, to the development of language skills. This chapter focused on the application of Cued Speech with children who are deaf and have additional challenges to language development. The patterns of strengths and deficits associated with primary language disorders, nonverbal learning disabilities, attention deficit hyperactivity disorder, and autism, were reviewed. The ways in which these strengths and weaknesses were suited to the use of Cued Speech to support the development of language, communication, and literacy were discussed. For example, the fact that phonemes represented by cues can be photographed and presented in a static manner was found to be particularly helpful for some of these children, while the fact that the need for gaze shifts or visual spatial analysis is limited in the reception of Cued Speech was helpful for others. Specific recommendations were made for ways to implement the use of Cued Speech to support the access to language and literacy for these children and examples of two children whose functioning and quality of life were dramatically enhanced through the use of Cued Speech were presented.

Although this chapter focuses on a specific subset of deaf children with additional disabilities, Cued Speech is a tool that can be applied to a range of children, both deaf and hearing, who have a wide range of disabilities. In addition to the disabilities discussed in this chapter, this author has been involved with deaf children with vision impairments, motor skill limitations, and cognitive and developmental disabilities who have benefited from the use of Cued Speech to provide language access. The Web site of the National Cued Speech Association contains articles describing adaptations of the use of Cued Speech to benefit children with a range of needs and disabilities, such as deaf-blindness, apraxia or aphasia, motor deficits, Down syndrome, and developmental delays. Parents of children with multiple challenges have often reported that they have been discouraged from using Cued Speech with their children as it is thought to be too difficult for such children to learn or because it is intended only for high functioning deaf children. Although as yet there is little research on the use of Cued Speech with children with multiple challenges, there are research based rationales, such as those described in this chapter, that support its use. There also are case studies and anecdotal reports that strongly support the continued use of Cued Speech with a wide range of deaf children. At this time, these efforts are guided by a combination of common sense and trial and error. It is important that in the future a program of research be implemented in order to clarify the optimal application of Cued Speech with each of the unique areas of need seen in deaf children with additional disabilities.

References

American Psychiatric Association (2000). *Diagnostic and statistical manual of mental disorders* (4th ed., text revision). Washington, DC: Author.

Barkley, R. (2005). *Attention-deficit hyperactivity disorder (3rd Edition): A handbook for diagnosis and treatment*. New York, NY: Guilford.

Bebko, J. (1998). Learning, language, memory, and reading: The role of language automatization and its impact on complex cognitive activities. *Journal of Deaf Studies and Deaf Education, 3,* 4–14.

Bebko, J., & Metcalf-Haggert, A. (1992). Deafness, language skills, and rehearsal: A model for the development of a memory strategy. *Journal of Deaf Studies and Deaf Education, 2,* 131–139.

Buchholz, J., & McKone, E. (2004). Adults with dyslexia show deficits on spatial frequency doubling and visual attention tasks. *Dyslexia, 10*, 24–43.

Catts, H. (2004). Language impairment and reading disability. In R. Kent (Ed.), *The MIT Encyclopedia of Communication Disorders.* Cambridge, MA: MIT.

Cohen, N, (2001). *Language Impairment and psychopathology in infants, children, and adolescents.* Thousand Oaks, CA: Sage.

Eden, G., VanMeter, J., Rumsey, J., Maisog, J., Woods, R., & Zeffiro, T. (1996). Abnormal processing of visual motion in dyslexia revealed by functional brain imaging. *Nature, 382*, 66–69.

Fey, M., Long, S., & Cleave, P. (1994). A reconsideration of IQ criteria in the definition of specific language impairment. In R. Watkins & M. Rice (Eds.), *Specific language impairment in children* (pp. 161–178). Baltimore, MD: Paul H. Brookes.

Gepner, B., & Mestre, D. (2002). Postural reactivity to fast visual motion differentiates autistic from children with Asperger syndrome. *Journal of Autism and Developmental Disorders, 32*, 231–238.

Hansen, P., Stein, J., Orde, S., Winter, J., & Talcott, J. (2001). Are dyslexics visual deficits limited to measures of dorsal stream function? *Neuroreport, 12*, 1527–1530.

Hari, R., Renvall, H., & Tanskanen, T. (2001) Left minineglect in dyslexic adults. *Brain, 124*, 1373–1380.

Hill, E. (2001). Non-specific nature of specific language impairment: A review of the literature with regard to concomitant motor impairments. *International Journal of Language & Communication Disorders, 36*, 149–171.

Jones, T. (1999). Can a deaf student have a learning disability? The exclusion clause and state special education guidelines. In H. Markowicz & C. Berdichevsky (Eds.), *Bridging the gap between research and practice in the fields of learning disabilities and deafness conference proceedings* (pp. 113–118). Washington, DC: Gallaudet University.

Kelly, D., Forney, J., Parker-Fisher, S., & Jones, M. (1993). Evaluating and managing attention deficit disorder in children who are deaf or hard of hearing. American *Annals of the Deaf, 138*, 349–357.

Klin, A., Jones, W., Schultz, R., Volkmar, F., & Cohen, D. (2002). Defining and quantifying the social phenotype in autism. *American Journal of Psychiatry, 159*, 895–908.

Klin, A., Sparrow, S., de Bildt A., Cicchetti, D., Cohen, D., & Volkmar, F. (1999). A normed study of face recognition in autism and related disorders. *Journal of Autism and Developmental Disorders, 296*, 499–508

Klin, A., Volkmar, F., Sparrow, S., Cicchetti, D., & Rourke, B. (1995). A validity and neuropsychological characterization of Asperger syndrome: Convergence with nonverbal learning disabilities syndrome. *Journal of Child Psychology and Psychiatry and Related Disciplines, 36*, 1127–1140.

Mauk, G., & Mauk, P. (1992). Somewhere, out there: Preschool children with hearing impairment and learning disabilities. *Topics in early childhood special education: Hearing-impaired preschoolers, 12*, 174–195.

Mauk, G., & Mauk, P. (1998). Considerations, conceptualizations, and challenges in the study of concomitant learning disabilities among children and adolescents who are deaf or hard of hearing. *Journal of Deaf Studies and Deaf Education, 3*, 15–34.

McArthur, G., Hogben, J., Edwards, V., Heath, S., & Mengler, E. (2000). On the "specifics" of specific reading disability and specific language impairment. *Journal of Child Psychology and Psychiatry, 41*, 869–874.

Merzenich, M., & Jenkins, W. (1995). Cortical plasticity, learning, and learning dysfunction. In B. Julesz & I. Dovacs (Eds.), *Maturational windows and adult cortical plasticity* (pp. 247–272). New York, NY: Addison-Welsey.

Montgomery, J. (1995). Sentence comprehension in children with specific language impairment: The role of phonological working memory. *Journal of Speech and Hearing Research, 38*, 187–199.

Montgomery, J., Windsor, J., & Stark, R. (1991). Specific speech and language disorders. In J. Orzbut & G.Hynd (Eds.), *Neuropsychological foundations of learning disabilities: A hand-*

book of issues, methods, and practice (pp. 573–601). New York, NY: Academic Press.

Morere, D. (1999). Diagnosis and management of language learning impairments in deaf children. In H. Markowicz & C. Berdichevsky (Eds.), *Bridging the gap between research and practice in the fields of learning disabilities and deafness conference proceedings* (pp. 73–80). Washington, DC: Gallaudet University Press.

National Institute of Mental Health. (1996). *Attention deficit hyperactivity disorder.* Retrieved November 18, 2006, from http://www.nimh.nih.gov/publicat/NIMHadhdpub.pdf. Bethesda, MD: National Institute of Mental Health, National Institutes of Health, U.S. Department of Health and Human Services.

Pastor P., & Reuben C. (2002). Attention deficit disorder and learning disability: United States, 1997–98. National Center for Health Statistics. *Vital Health Statistics, 10, 206.*

Pierce, K., Müller, R., Ambrose, J., Allen, G., & Courchesne, E. (2001). Face processing occurs outside the fusiform 'face area' in autism: Evidence from functional MRI. *Brain, 124,* 2059–2073.

Ratner, V. (1985). Spatial-relationship deficits in deaf children: The effect on communication and classroom performance. *American Annals of the Deaf, 130,* 250–254.

Ratner, V. (1988). New tests for identifying hearing-impaired students with visual perceptual deficits. Relationship between deficits and ability to comprehend sign language. *American Annals of the Deaf, 133,* 336–343.

Rourke, B. (Ed.). (1995). *Syndrome of nonverbal learning disabilities: Neurodevelopmental manifestations.* New York, NY: Guilford.

Samar, V., & Parasnis, I. (2005). Dorsal stream deficits suggest hidden dyslexia among deaf poor readers: Correlated evidence from reduced perceptual speed and elevated coherent notion detection thresholds. *Brain and Cognition, 58,* 300–311.

Samar, V., Parasnis, I., & Berent, G. (1998). Learning disabilities, attention deficit disorders, and deafness. In M. Marschark & M. Clark (Eds.), *Psychological perspectives on deafness* (Vol. 2, pp. 199–242). Mahwah, NJ: Lawrence Erlbaum Associates.

Samar, V., Parasnis I., & Berent G. (2002). Deaf poor readers' pattern reversal visual evoked potentials suggest magnocellular system deficits: implications for diagnostic neuroimaging of dyslexia in deaf individuals. *Brain and Language, 80,* 21–44.

Spreen, O., Risser, A., & Edgell, D. (1995). *Developmental neuropsychology.* New York, NY: Oxford University.

Tallal, P. (1990). Fine-grained discrimination deficits in language-learning impaired children are specific neither to the auditory modality nor to speech perception. *Journal of Speech and Hearing Research, 33,* 616–617.

Tomblin, J., & Zhang, X. (2000). The association of reading disability, behavioral disorders, and language impairment among second-grade children. *Journal of Child Psychology, 41,* 473–482.

Trauner, D., Ballantyne, A., Chase, C., & Tallal, P. (1993). Comprehension and expression of affect in language-impaired children. *Journal of Psycholinguistic Research, 22,* 445–452.

Vernon, M., & Andrews, J. (1990). *The psychology of deafness: Understanding deaf and hard-of-hearing people.* New York, NY: Longman.

Wang, A., Dapretto, M., Hariri, A., Sigman, M., & Bookheimer, S. (2004). Neural correlates of facial affect processing in children and adolescents with autism spectrum disorder. *Journal of the American Academy of Child and Adolescent Psychiatry, 43,* 481–490.

Watkins, R. (1994). Specific Language Impairment in children: An introduction. In R. Zatkins & M. Rice (Eds.), *Specific language impairment in children* (pp. 1–15). Baltimore, MD: Paul H. Brookes.

Wolke, L., & Giesen, J. (2000). A phonological investigation of four siblings with childhood autism. *Journal of Communication Disorders, 33,* 371–389.

Chapter 17

CUED SPANISH AS L1: TEACHING LA PALABRA COMPLEMENTADA TO SPANISH-SPEAKING PARENTS OF DEAF CHILDREN IN THE UNITED STATES

Claire Klossner and Kelly Lamar Crain

Introduction

This chapter addresses the issue of whether the home language can be L1 for deaf children of hearing parents (see Chapter 12), and whether such a model of language acquisition can apply to families in the United States for whom neither ASL nor English is the home language. We consider the situation of a growing segment of American society: Spanish monolingual parents of children educated in English-only school programs, and more specifically, parents who are raising deaf children. We describe a school system attempting to serve the needs of these very special families, not by attempting to teach the parents a language that is *new* to them (e.g., English or American Sign Language), but by teaching the parents to visually communicate via Cued Speech the language in which they are already fluent (i.e., Spanish). Such an approach builds on parents' strengths as primary language models and conveyors of culture and serves to approximate the situation of hearing Spanish speaking children who arrive at school with a spoken language base on which to build English language fluency and literacy. This chapter is of particular interest to school or educational program administrators seeking an innovative approach to meeting the needs of this underserved, at-risk, and growing segment of American society.

Background

Language Development of Hearing and Deaf Children

The language acquisition process in hearing children is extensively studied and well documented. Hearing children, who do not experience sensory deficits or other impairments, will attain predictable receptive and expressive spoken language development milestones according to nearly universal timelines (Berko, 1958; Brown, 1973) irrespective of the language studied (de Boysson-Bardies & Vihman, 1991; Dromi & Berman, 1982; Luinge, Post, Wit, & Goorhuis-Brouwer, 2007; Oller & Eilers, 1982).

Researchers have documented language development trajectories observed in oral (see Spencer & Marschark, 2006) and signing deaf children of deaf and hearing parents (see Schick, Marscharck, & Spencer, 2006; Volterra & Erting, 1994, for summaries). Although findings are mixed, when taken collectively, they suggest a variety of factors affecting whether or not deaf children acquire language typically. Among the factors most often implicated concerning oral language development are *parental stress*, *parental involvement*, and *cochlear implantation* (Blamey et al., 2001a, 2001b; Geers, 2002; Lederberg & Everhart, 2000; Lichtert & Loncke, 2006). Among the factors most often implicated concerning signed language development

are *parental hearing status* and *communication ability* (Kantor, 1982; Loots & Devisé, 2003; Meadow, Greenberg, Erting, & Carmichael, 1981; Meadow-Orlans, 1997; Mitchell & Karchmer, 2004; Nicholas & Geers, 2003; Spencer, 1993; Waxman & Spencer, 1997), with an overall trend in conclusions that hearing parents are less equipped than deaf parents to serve as fluent signed language models for deaf infants, which leads to the observed gap in language abilities between deaf children of deaf parents and deaf children of hearing parents. Regardless of the communication modalities used by parents of deaf and hard of hearing children, however, the age of identification and commencement of early intervention services have been found to be the most important factors in early language acquisition and development (Yoshinaga-Itano, Sedey, Coulter, & Mehl, 1998).

The Home Language as L1

As discussed by LaSasso and Metzger (1998), it is unusual for a child, anywhere in the world, who has full and unambiguous access to a language and consistent opportunities to interact with competent models of that language not to develop the phonology, morphology, semantics, syntax, and pragmatics of that language naturally and in accordance with widely known developmental milestones. LaSasso and Metzger recommend that a deaf child's *home* language (whether it be a spoken or signed language) serve as L1, and that Cued Speech be used to convey traditionally spoken languages such as English and Spanish. Their rationale for this position is that parents/primary caregivers are typically the people in the best position to serve as language models for their children, as they are: (1) present at or soon after the birth of the child; (2) constantly and consistently in the child's immediate environment and field of perception; and (3) fluent in the language of the home at the time of the child's birth. For hearing parents raising hearing children, these qualifications are largely taken for granted.

Hearing parents who realize that their child is deaf are faced with a number of important decisions to make, including which communication modalities and language(s) the child will be exposed to. Regarding communication modalities, these parents can choose oral/aural (spoken), signed (including fingerspelling) or cued modalities, or any combination thereof. Regarding language choices, hearing parents typically choose the language spoken in their home and/or the signed language of the local Deaf community.

When making communication and language decisions for their deaf child, hearing parents (as much as 95% of the parents of deaf children; Mitchell & Karchmer, 2004) must consider: (1) the importance they place on their home language and culture; (2) their fluency in that language and capacity as a language/culture model; (3) the importance they place on a signed language and Deaf culture; and (4) their potential for acquiring fluency in a timely manner in that language (oral or signed) and their capacity as a language/culture model in a new language. In the majority of cases in the United States, the home language is English, and it is spoken. In a rapidly growing number of cases, however, the parents' home language is not English, but Spanish. Latinos and Hispanics are the fastest growing ethnic group in the United States (Zuniga, 1998). Hispanic and Latino parents face the same

number of potential communication modality choices (i.e., oral, signed, cued), but the number of potential languages expands to: (1) the home language (i.e., Spanish); (2) the dominant language (i.e., English); and/or (3) American Sign Language.

La Palabra Complementada and Cued Spanish

Cornett invented Cued Speech specifically for the English language but soon realized that Cued Speech could be adapted for nearly any spoken language (Cornett, 1994). Before his death, he collaborated on the adaptation of Cued Speech to over 50 languages and dialects. As of this writing, Cued Speech has been adapted to 63 languages and dialects (http://www .cuedspeech.org/sub/cued/language .asp#dialects), including such tonal languages such as Igbo, Thai, and Cantonese (see Chapter 2).

Among the first languages to which Cornett adapted Cued Speech is Spanish, which he adapted in collaboration with Santiago Torres in 1970 and named la Palabra Complementada (LPC) (Torres, 1988). Torres, a native of Spain, is largely responsible for introducing Cued Speech to the country, where it continues to be used for speech, language, and literacy development in deaf and hard of hearing children (Torres, Moreno-Torres, & Santana, 2006).

For the adaptation of Cued Speech for Spanish, consonant phonemes considered comparable across English and Spanish remain associated with their original handshapes. For example, /m/, /f/, and /t/ are assigned to handshape 5 in both systems. It was necessary, however, to remove from the LPC Cued Speech chart certain phonemes that do not occur in

Spanish (e.g., /z/ was removed from handshape 2) and to insert certain phonemes that do not occur in English (e.g., /ñ/ [as in the Spanish word *baño*] was assigned to handshape 2). The greater difference between Spanish and English, however, lies in the number of vowels; it was necessary to consider the mouthshapes of the five vowels of spoken Spanish, and assign them to placements, irrespective of the placements for the 15 vowels and diphthongs in the American English Cued Speech system.

The product of the expressive use of LPC is referred to as *Cued Spanish*, in the same way that the product of the expressive use of Cued Speech (in the United States) is referred to as *Cued American English* (in contrast to *Cued British English*). LPC is used principally in Spain, but it has been used in Mexico and is applicable to the Spanish spoken in Central and South America, Cuba, and Puerto Rico. If the use of LPC were to gain in popularity and become more widely used in different Spanish-speaking countries, it could very well begin to mirror specific linguistic differences related to those locations (e.g., the appearance of /θ/ in Castilian Spanish, the appearance of /ʒ/ in Argentine Spanish). If this were to occur, populations might one day refer to Cued Castilian Spanish and Cued Mexican Spanish, in much the same way as we now refer to Cued American English and Cued British English.

Bilingual Theory Applied to Cued L1 and Cued L2

In 1989, Jim Cummins first proposed his theory of bilingual development (Cummins, 1989), the linguistic interdependence theory. The linguistic interdependence theory suggests a common underlying language proficiency, in which proficiency in a first language (L1) can lead to proficiency in a second language (L2). Cummins details prerequisites for pairs of languages in order for his theory to be applicable. Most importantly, he requires that the following assumptions be satisfied regarding the two languages: (1) both L1 and L2 have conversational and written forms; (2) a person has the opportunity to acquire the conversational form of L1; (3) the individual has the opportunity to learn the written form of L1; and (4) the person has opportunities to participate in a linguistic community that uses L2 in both spoken and written forms (Cummins, 1989). Cummins' theory is commonly cited to support bilingual education in the United States (Baker, 2001).

Cummins' theory has also been cited in support of ASL/English bilingual programs for deaf children (cf. Haptonstall-Nykaza & Schick, 2007; Israelite, Ewoldt, & Hoffmeister, 1992; Mason, 1997; Singleton, Morgan, DiGello, Wiles, & Rivers, 2004; Strong & Prinz, 1997), though Mayer and Wells (1996, 1997) discuss in detail how none of the aforementioned assumptions required to apply Cummins' theory is satisfied, calling into question the appropriateness of applying this theory to the case of ASL and English, despite its being cited more often than any other as support for bilingual-bicultural education in the United States (LaSasso & Lollis, 2003).

When discussing the most common application of Cued Speech in the United States (i.e., the cueing of American English), the application of a theory of bilingualism is a moot point; English-speaking parents learn to *cue* English (as opposed to only *speaking* English) for the direct purpose of English language development and the indirect purpose of subsequent literacy development. Although there are multiple forms of the English language (i.e., spoken, cued, written), English-speaking parents need to concern themselves with only one language.

Non-English speaking parents of deaf children in the United States, however, present a unique application of Cued Speech. In the case of Spanish-speaking parents, Spanish would be considered L1 (i.e., the language of the home) for a deaf child, and English (primarily or initially acquired by their children at school) would be L2. The cueing of both English and Spanish satisfies the assumptions of Cummins' theory of an underlying language proficiency leading to conversational and written fluency in L1 and L2: (1) cued Spanish (L1) and cued English (L2) indeed have both conversational and written forms; (2) a deaf individual can have the opportunity to naturally acquire the conversational form of L1 from parents and/or other family members who learn to cue; (3) the individual who is deaf has the opportunity to apply knowledge of the conversational form of L1 to learning its written form; and (4) the individual who is deaf has the opportunity to participate in a linguistic community (the school community) that uses L2 in both spoken and written forms.

Educationally, the end goal of the early language acquisition process for traditionally spoken languages is for deaf children to become fluent users of their home language and to be able to use that conversational language base to continue to develop language proficiency (conversational and written) at school. Following is a description of a school system that has chosen to employ a novel approach to Cummins' linguistic interdependence theory to the case of deaf students whose parents speak a language other than that of the public education system.

Program in Action: Fairfax County Public Schools, Virginia

Description of Fairfax County Public Schools

Fairfax County Virginia covers over 400 square miles in Northern Virginia, and is one of the counties comprising the Washington, DC metropolitan area. Fairfax County is home to a number of linguistic and cultural groups, including large Salvadoran, Guatemalan, and Colombian communities. As of the 2000 census, 12.9% of the population of Fairfax County was Hispanic/Latino in origin (United States Census Bureau, 2008). Fairfax County Public Schools (FCPS) is the 12th largest school system in the United States, with 239 elementary, middle, high, and alternative schools and a projected student body for the 2009-2010 school year of over 173,000 students. The county provides special education services (including deaf and hard of hearing) to over 23,000 students. FCPS serves students representing 150 countries of origin and over 100 different home languages. As of 1999 (the most recent figures publicly available), 12.6% of elementary students and 9.9% of students in special education centers in the county were of Hispanic origin (Fairfax County Public Schools, 2008a). These figures represent increases of 3% or more for each of the two most recently reported 5-year periods (Fairfax County Public Schools, 2008b).

Approximately 500 deaf and hard of hearing students in the county receive services along a continuum, from the provision of assistive technologies, to itinerant supports, to self-contained classes at site-based programs. Of the site-based programs, FCPS provides instruction and support services in three communication modalities: oral/aural, total communication (including sign communication) and Cued Speech. Canterbury Woods Elementary School (CWES) serves as the base for the Cued Speech program, with approximately 25 deaf and hard of hearing students from preschool through the 6th grade.

FCPS Cued Speech Program

The Cued Speech program in Fairfax County represents the most common approach to educating deaf and hard of hearing children with Cued Speech in the United States. That is, in FCPS and similar programs in other states such as Maryland, North Carolina, and Louisiana, students in early elementary grades are educated by teachers of deaf students who cue and/or in mainstream classes with the aid of cued language transliterators (CLTs). By the late elementary or middle school grades, the majority of instruction is received in mainstream classes, and by high school, virtually all instruction is received in the mainstream with the aid of CLTs and/or assistive technologies (see Chapter 9 in this volume).

The program described in this chapter, of a monolingual public school system striving to provide services for deaf and hard of hearing children from non-English-speaking families, does *not* present itself as a bilingual program, in that it offers and supports only one language of curricular instruction (i.e., English) for enrolled students. Refer to Chapter 10 for a description of an ASL-cued American English bilingual program for deaf students.

A *Cued Speech Culture* in FCPS

The FCPS Cued Speech program for deaf students is unique among the programs educating deaf and hard of hearing students in the county, regarding the focus on visible access to English, via Cued Speech, throughout every level of the program. Undergirding the Cued Speech program is the philosophy that to the extent that the educational environment offers the maximum possible visible (and auditory, if applicable) exposure to the continuous phoneme stream of English from fluent language models, deaf children will acquire English (first conversational and then written) in comparable ways and rates as hearing peers. To this end, FCPS Cued Speech program staff members strive to create an environment where the students are exposed to accessible English as much as possible, regardless of their hearing level and in as many contexts as possible, including: direct instruction, transliterated instruction, environmental print, intentional communication among deaf, hard of hearing, and hearing peers, and incidental exposure to conversations between adults in the hallways. With that goal in mind, the staff consists of teachers of deaf students, instructional assistants, speech clinicians, and audiologists who cue directly with students, and cued language transliterators (CLTs), whose job it is to cue the spoken language being produced by hearing individuals. The main goal of the FCPS program, in keeping with Ramsey's (1997) caution against the "mascot principle" is to be able to include deaf children to the utmost extent possible, not just in name only but in a way mindful of actual participation and interaction with the rest of the school. To that end, the FCPS Cued Speech program actively involves the entire school in the awareness of and active use of Cued Speech. General education teachers of all grade levels take Cued Speech classes. Therefore, classroom teachers, teachers of art, music and physical education, instructional assistants, and administrative and clerical staff have a basic knowledge of Cued Speech and can incorporate it at some level into their interactions with deaf and hard of hearing students.

A "cue club" is an optional extracurricular activity for deaf and hard of hearing, and hearing students at the school. In it, general education students from kindergarten through 6th grade are taught how to cue to and with their deaf and hard of hearing classmates. The goal is not for Cued Speech to replace all other forms of communication, but instead, for hearing peers to simultaneously cue and speak English and be better able to understand the cueing and speech of deaf peers, to make natural and normal communication accessible to students of all hearing levels. It is not unusual to see groups of hearing and deaf students at the school cueing a poem on the news, cueing songs during assemblies, or cueing to each other in the hall.

Cueing at Home and at School

While focusing on access to cued English as much as possible during the school day, the Cued Speech program staff recognizes that communication and learning opportunities at home are equally if not more important that those at school. Soon after the Cued Speech program was initiated, an active campaign was undertaken to teach parents how to cue, to support them in building their communication skills, and to show them how to integrate cueing into their families' lives at home. Parents and staff formed the Northern Virginia Cued Speech Association (NVCSA) to support parents in this process. "Cued Speech Coffees" are held monthly at the elementary school, as are regular Cued

Speech evening events with guest speakers, games, food, and childcare. The NVCSA initiated an annual "Cue Camp," a full learning weekend for any and all stakeholders, including parents, deaf and hearing children, extended family, and friends. The highest priority for all school-based, community-based, and camp activities is to make sure parents of children in the program learn how to cue. The lead cued language transliterator (lead CLT) is responsible for holding evening cueing classes back-to-back at the elementary school. Each class lasts eight weeks, and when one class is completed, the next begins. When parents "graduate" from the beginner class, they are able to join the Cued Speech practice class held at the same time. The lead CLT holds sibling cueing classes for the brothers and sisters of deaf students attending the program. If a parent cannot attend the evening classes, he or she can make one-on-one appointments with the lead CLT at a mutually convenient time. If parents, caregivers, or family members cannot attend the 8-week class, they have the opportunity every year to take the class in 2 solid days at Cue Camp Virginia. The lead CLT also keeps a lending library, and will lend materials to those who think that workbooks or videotapes would suit them better. The most important goal for any of the learning opportunities is for individuals to: (1) learn how to cue, and (2) learn how to integrate cueing into their family's routines at home.

Another responsibility of the Cued Speech program staff is to meet families of children in the county who are diagnosed with a hearing loss, describe the program, and help them understand what Cued Speech is and how it is implemented throughout the school. This responsibility presents a unique challenge: although most parents in the United States have a basic understanding of the concept of signing and/or the concept of spoken communication for deaf children (i.e., oralism), most parents visiting the Cued Speech program have never heard the term *Cued Speech*, much less have an understanding of what it is or its applications. In addition, when a visit is scheduled with a family whose native language is one other than English, the challenge grows. Often, such a tour of the program involves interpreters or translators for any of a variety of spoken languages (e.g., Arabic, Farsi, Korean, or Spanish). These interpreters or transliterators must work to understand the finer points of Cued Speech, cued language, and audiologic terms being presented by Cued Speech staff members, and then attempt to convey that information to parents in a coherent manner. Following such a visit to the school, Cued Speech staff members often report a sense that these parents fluent in a language other than English might be interested or curious about Cued Speech, but might have left the tour feeling afraid to be the first or only ones to try something new, presented in a language that they themselves did not understand.

From Cued American English to Cued Languages

Years into its existence, a paradigm shift occurred within the program, from viewing Cued Speech as a means of developing *English* to viewing Cued Speech as a means of developing *multiple languages*. The paradigm shift began when a family from Peru scheduled a tour with a Spanish interpreter. Previous tours conducted for non-English speaking families had not resulted in new enrollments to the program, but this family expressed an understanding of the potential benefits of Cued

Speech for their 3-year-old profoundly deaf son, and an interest in learning more about Cued Speech. After the parents had a chance to also visit the oral and Total Communication sites, they contacted the Cued Speech program to enroll their son.

Within months, a second and third Spanish-speaking family had toured the three programs (i.e., oral, total communication, and Cued Speech) and had ultimately chosen to enroll their children in the Cued Speech program. This could only be seen as a coincidence, in that the families came from different countries, and reported not knowing one another prior to joining the school "community." Nonetheless, within a short period of time the Cued Speech program had enrolled 3 deaf preschool students whose parents spoke fluent Spanish, and little or no English.

American Cues Versus Spanish Cues. When the three preschoolers with Spanish-speaking parents enrolled in the FCPS Cued Speech program, it entered a new phase of its existence. The staff, subscribing to the belief that the power of Cued Speech resides in the accessibility to natural language it affords families, had previously explained to dozens of English-speaking families how they could memorize the finite system and apply it to their own language, and could thus erase the most significant communication barriers often experienced between deaf children and their hearing parents. The Cued Speech team taught parents that they could quickly become expert language role models for their deaf children by learning how to communicate visually the language they already knew: English. Further, they were told that with Cued Speech, parents could practice and further develop their skills independently, without the need to find native or fluent users of another language. They could use this communication tool to convey their own vocabulary choices, expressions particular to their family and region, and the various ways in which words can be ordered to express ideas. Up until this time, Cued Speech program staff had only discussed cueing in the context of the English language. The Cued Speech program had always been a monolingual deaf education program: staff members spoke and/or cued English with children and parents who spoke and/or cued English.

Prior to the admission of preschoolers of Spanish-speaking parents, the only application of Cued Speech to other languages occurred when deaf cueing high school students took foreign language classes with CLTs. In order to transliterate foreign language classes, CLTs receive specialized training, where they learn to listen to unfamiliar words (from another language) and cue syllable-by-syllable, using cues from the Cued American English system in which they are already trained (Fleetwood & Metzger, 1990). In the county, Deaf cueing students often take French, Spanish, and Latin this way. For example, a deaf cueing student, after years of using Cued Speech for English language reception, can take a Spanish class with a CLT who will cue, for example, *gato* (cat) by producing the cued syllables /ga/ and /to/. The deaf cueing student, who has been exposed to these two syllables individually innumerable times in many English words now sees them applied in this novel combination, to represent a word in Spanish. In this way, the student who is deaf can learn a second language in a manner equivalent to hearing students: by receiving familiar consonants and vowels in novel combinations, in meaningful contexts. This practice, however, relies on at least two assumptions: (1) both the transliterator

and the student who is deaf are already fluent users of English and the cueing system for English; and (2) an *approximation* of Spanish consonants and vowels is sufficient for learning and using the language. For example, the Spanish vowel in the first syllable of the word *peso* sounds similar to (but is not actually the same as) the English vowel in the word *play*. Therefore, the transliterator would cue the word as though cueing the English words/syllables *pay* and *so*. Deaf cueing students in FCPS and other school systems have learned Spanish, French, and other languages this way. As is explained to transliterators in the *Cued Language Transliterator Professional Education Series* (Language Matters, Inc., 2008), using American English cues in a Spanish class is similar to speaking Spanish with an American accent; the consonants and vowels are similar, but not exactly the same. As English-speaking hearing students in such a class will hear the Spanish through their own American English phonological filter, the deaf cueing student receives as approximate an experience as possible. Transliterators learn in their training that, if a deaf cueing student wishes to travel abroad or engage in advanced study of a language, it would be advantageous for the student to learn that Cued Speech system, to gain access to any phonemes specific to that language.

Although the use of the Cued American English system for second language learning remains a common practice among CLTs in public school systems, the enrollment into the Cued Speech program of three deaf children of Spanish-speaking parents presented a different set of circumstances. Like all preschoolers in the program, these three boys entered an English immersion self-contained classroom with a teacher of deaf students who cues.

The next step would have normally been to provide their parents with Cued Speech instruction and support as similar as possible to that provided to English-speaking parents. Staff members, including the cueing preschool teacher, the audiologist (a native Spanish speaker), and the lead CLT (a linguist), considered their options: (1) arrange for a Spanish interpreter for the regularly scheduled evening parent class in order to teach the Spanish-speaking parents the American English system; or (2) teach the parents to cue in their own language, using the Spanish version of Cued Speech, la Palabra Complementada, in order to allow the parents to develop cued fluency in the language they could already speak.

The staff members expressed immediate concerns regarding the first option. Cued Speech is taught as discrete segments that new learners can immediately arrange into words that they already know. This is often cited by new learners as an exciting feature of learning to cue; every time they learn a new handshape or placement, they can figure out independently how to cue more and more words. If an English speaker learns how to cue *see/sea*, for example, she can easily figure out how to cue *sir, sue, saw*, and so forth, by experimenting with vowel placements. Similarly, upon learning to cue *to/too/two*, she can figure out how to cue *moo, sue, who*, and so forth, by experimenting with consonant handshapes. The Spanish-speaking parents of these three preschoolers could not share in that benefit if the words used to teach them were English words. They would need to learn English vocabulary, and memorize how to cue each word individually. The ability of Spanish-speaking parents to model English words in context at home would be severely limited, as well. Alternatively, they could attempt to apply the American English cues to Spanish words, resulting in an "American accent" that they did not really have. Staff members were concerned that, faced with such a daunting task, the Spanish-speaking parents would be unlikely to feel successful enough to continue cueing.

A second concern of staff members related to the shared belief that more communication and language learning happens at home than at school. The staff members knew that these children would develop some English language abilities through immersion at school, but they would spend more time interacting with their parents, siblings, and family members speaking Spanish. Without a way to make the natural language of the home visibly accessible to these deaf boys, the boys would be at serious risk of falling behind in language development, the very problem that Cued Speech had proven itself so useful in avoiding.

Ultimately, the program staff elected to pursue their second, albeit novel, option: to teach the new parents to cue in Spanish, using la Palabra Complementada. This cueing system for Spanish has been used in Mexico and Spain (see Chapter 2 in this volume), with communication and language outcomes similar to those observed in English-speaking countries such as the United States and England (Torres, Moreno-Torres, & Santana, 2006). It was felt by FCPS Cued Speech staff that if this could be accomplished, these deaf children from Spanish-speaking homes could experience a language learning situation more comparable to that of hearing children from Spanish-speaking homes: accessing and acquiring Spanish at home from fluent language models, and English at school from fluent language models.

Creation, Adaptation, and Trial of Materials. In order to begin teaching LPC, the lead CLT would need materials similar to those used in traditional Cued Speech classes offered at the school. A simple chart showing handshapes and placements is readily available for download off of the internet, but this was viewed as insufficient for thorough, systematic instruction; the goal must be to teach LPC to Spanish-speaking parents in a fashion as similar as possible to the teaching of Cued Speech to English-speaking parents: not by simply handing them a chart, but by teaching them handshapes and placements in the most logical sequence to maximize retention and minimize overload.

The lead CLT located Spanish-English dictionaries for adults and for children and children's books in Spanish, while the audiologist requested and received an instructional CD from a Cued Speech center in Spain. The books provided a source for simple Spanish words that could be used to teach only those handshapes being targeted for instruction (i.e., to include only phonemes that had been covered to that point), and the CD from Spain provided guidance regarding the best order in which to teach the placements and handshapes, which was different than the order most often used for Cued American English. Realizing that there can be differences in pronunciation or meaning of words across different Latin American countries, the staff members chose words such as *rojo* (red) and *leche* (milk) that are consistent across countries, and avoided words such as *tortilla* and *llama*, which are less consistent in pronunciation or meaning.

With the help of a Spanish-speaking linguist who had previous Cued Speech experience, the lead CLT constructed word lists for the teaching of each handshape. The linguist provided feedback regarding possible confusions, clarifications, and challenges, as well as insight into syllabication of Spanish words (e.g., the Spanish word *bien* is perceived as monosyllabic to a native Spanish speaker, whereas it would likely be perceived as bisyllabic to a native English speaker). Table 17–1 provides examples from three such lists.

The linguist assisted in generating simple Spanish sentences specific to each handshape or groups of handshapes, for purposes of mnemonics and practice. Table 17–2 provides examples of such sentences. The linguist also provided the lead CLT opportunities to cue read LPC, so that she would be able to provide feedback and correction to new learners.

The lead CLT created multiple word lists and sentences, settled on the order of presentation for handshapes and vowel

Table 17–1. Examples of Word Lists for Cued Spanish Instruction

All Vowels, Plus Handshape 5		
Me	Tu	Fe
Mi	Tia	Fea
Mama	Tio	Feo
All Vowels, Plus Handshapes 5 & 3		
Aseo	Frio	Hija
Asar	Frisa	Ahora
Ser	Frutas	Oreja
All Vowels, Plus Handshapes 5, 3, & 4		
Abajo	Mano	Nariz
Beber	Mono	Venir
Saber	Uno	Verano

Table 17–2. Examples of Sentences by Handshape

Cues	Sentences
All Vowels, Handshape 5 (/m/, /f/, /t/)	Mi mama me mima. (My mother spoils me.) Mi mama me amo. (My mother loves me.)
All Vowels, Handshape 5 & 3 (/m/, /f/, /t/) (/h/, /s/, /r/)	Este es mi hijo. (This is my son.) Esta es mi hija. (This is my daughter.)
All Vowels, Handshapes 5, 3, & 4 (/m/, /f/, /t/) (/h/, /s/, /r/) (/b/, /n/)	Jose ve una mono. (Jose sees a monkey.) Jose ve su brazo. (Jose sees his arm.)

placements, and assembled a master LPC workbook. Each parent would receive a copy of the workbook to refer to in class and take home for reinforcement and practice.

Teaching Spanish-Speaking Parents

Upon completing and testing the new Spanish-language materials, the lead CLT held the first beginner LPC parent class. As with all of the Cued American English parent classes, the lead CLT served as the instructor, and for this class, the Spanish-fluent program audiologist served as the interpreter. The class consisted of six new learners (i.e., both parents of each new preschooler). In preparation for teaching this class, the lead CLT had listened to Spanish language tapes as much as possible, in order to: (1) pronounce Spanish words correctly; (2) speak directly to the new learners as much as possible; and (3) lessen the anxiety of new learners by attempting to making them equals in the learning process (e.g., learning something new, trying and accepting correction).

As the class got underway, the parents were observed to progress through stages similar to new parents in Cued American English classes. The first stage typically is one of apprehension, followed by the physical (and often emotional) awkwardness of making the handshapes for the first time, then comprehension, followed by trial and error, and finally, being able to cue newly presented words before being shown how. Toward the end of the first class, these parents were engaged in conversations (in Spanish) about differences in dialect and how different people in the class pronounce words differently. At this point, the staff members conferred and agreed that they could see clearly that the power of Cued Speech for hearing parents is not limited to the English language itself, but in the ability to apply it to one's own language, and use that language at home with one's children.

Additional Parent and Family Support

Taking an introductory class and learning the "mechanics" of Cued Speech system is only an early step for parents, regardless of the language they speak. In keeping with the "Cued Speech culture" philosophy of the program, staff members concern themselves not only with language learning in the classroom, but with learning opportunities for the children and their families at home and in the community. In addition to home visits available to all parents, the program staff needed to consider supports specific to Spanish-speaking families at risk of being excluded.

In addition to the school system's provision of all countywide printed materials in multiple languages (including Spanish), the elementary school added resources to receive phone calls from Spanish-speaking parents, and provided direct communication with a Spanish-native educational audiologist. Special attention was paid to maximizing the program's outreach to the families, as well as the families' opportunities to access the school community.

Home Visits. Regular visits to families' homes are provided by Cued Speech program staff as part of FCPS preschool services; special education services begin for families at the point of an infants' diagnosis, and at the age of 2 years, K to 12 instructional and support services (as determined by a given students' individualized education program, or IEP) are provided in the classroom, with supplemental home visits at least twice per month. In addition to teaching the self-contained preschool class (in the morning), the cueing preschool teacher conducts regular home visits with each family (in the afternoon).

The major goal of home visits is to facilitate communication and language at home, so the program staff incorporates Cued Speech practice into each visit. The cueing preschool teacher typically brings teaching manipulatives or toys from the classroom and shows the parents what the class had been working on subsequent to the last visit (e.g., skills, vocabulary). The teacher and parents talk about suc-

cesses and challenges related to communication at home and discuss strategies and suggestions for progress. Prior to the enrollment of these three students, the cueing preschool teacher had been able to manage these visits without assistance. Though home visits are not included in the job description for either the lead CLT or the Spanish-native educational audiologist, they both decided to dedicate time to the home visits for these families. The Spanish-native audiologist made herself available for direct communication regarding anything related to the child's hearing, assistive devices, and aural communication. The audiologist then shifted roles, serving as a Spanish-English translator, with whom the lead CLT (who had also been the parents' LPC instructor) answered questions about accurate cueing, and offered teaching and practice opportunities related to phrases requested by the parents, as well as familiar family routines and household objects.

Increased Accessibility of School Services. The Cued Speech program, along with the NVCSA, regularly hosts events for cueing children and their families. It became especially important for the program staff to host events for which it would be more likely that as many Spanish-speaking families as possible would be able to attend (i.e., by being mindful of families' work schedules, trips out of town, etc.). It was hoped that these families would form an internal support network, encouraging one another to attend events and to practice cueing. Program staff immediately involved with these Spanish-speaking families began participating in more preschool classroom and field trip activities, to establish a constant presence that the families could come to depend on and predict.

Program staff also responded with encouragement and support when Spanish-speaking parents expressed interest in learning to speak, cue, and/or write English words and phrases. All parents indicated that they believed it was important that their children learn English. Parents who had taken the beginner LPC class and felt that they had sufficient spoken English skills, were encouraged to join the regular English-language Cued Speech parent class (taught by the same lead CLT who had designed the LPC class). Other parents, who did not feel they could benefit from English-language Cued Speech instruction, expressed eagerness to learn relevant English words as individual tokens (i.e., memorized as entire spoken/cued segments). Feedback from parents who took advantage of both of these opportunities was positive and instructive.

Outcomes

In judging the effectiveness of its pilot project for LPC instruction to Spanish-speaking parents, the FCPS Cued Speech program staff recognized significant challenges to progress, as well as encouraging signs from various vantage points. Challenges related to the sometimes transient nature of families moving into and out of the county, transportation limitations expressed by most of these families, and the ever possible presence of additional disabilities affecting language development and/or academic progress. Encouraging signs of initial success came from observed child language and educational growth, increased parental involvement in school activities, additional families joining or considering the Cued Speech program based on site visits or recommendations from parents, and a request

for similar access to Cued Speech instruction in yet another language common in the FCPS system.

Challenges

The process of tailoring FCPS support to the special group of Spanish-speaking families was not without its disappointments and challenges. Of the original three boys enrolled, one left the program when his family moved outside of the county. This was especially disappointing for the program staff, because the boy's mother had learned the Cued Speech system quickly and well, and had proven to be among the most consistent cuers, by her own report and by observations made at home visits. The child, coincidentally or not, was making age-appropriate progress through the grade levels of his attendance. With their departure, the preschool class lost a communication peer, and the other Spanish-speaking parents lost a peer mentor and role-model.

The family of another of the original students made moves *within* the county, remaining connected to the FCPS Cued Speech program, but experiencing work- and family-related disruptions associated with the moves. Unfortunately, but not surprisingly, the parents did not show signs of maintaining their expressive cueing at home. This student, at the time of publication, has not experienced age-appropriate language gains (in either Spanish or English), nor grade-level progress in school. There are many possible reasons for this outcome aside from the supposed home-school connection, and it is possible the child may be referred for testing to determine whether additional disabilities may be contributing to his situation.

Transportation issues proved to be almost universal among these six parents, contributing to the overall challenge faced by the program staff to provide accessible, inclusive support activities. Aside from a lack of personal transportation on the part of families, the school is located in a part of the county that is not heavily canvassed by public transportation, making trips to and from various Cued Speech and regular school events difficult for these families.

Successes

Despite challenges and disappointments on the part of program staff or parents, there are clear indications of the potential of programs such as the one described in this chapter. Particularly, the program staff report encouraging language and educational outcomes for the third child (described in the next paragraph), and both staff and parents report increased parental involvement in visual communication at home and at school. Additional Spanish-speaking families have inquired about Cued Speech or the Cued Speech program, in addition to one request from a Korean-speaking family for similar supports for their deaf child.

Child Language Development and Educational Progress. As noted above, one student left the county and a second moved multiple times while in FCPS. The third boy presents the most encouraging outcomes for this pilot project. Specifically, program staff report that the student has experienced rapid gains in receptive and expressive language during his two years in the preschool classroom, but that his spoken and cued English "exploded" during his kindergarten year. His parents report cueing inconsistently, although they report and have been observed to cue in Spanish at home, but they report

feeling as though the outreach efforts have made them feel more a part of the school and feel that they benefitted by the outreach efforts. The student's father reported that his own English language skills have improved, and that he began to use English primarily around his child. The cueing preschool teacher reports that the student developed good expressive cueing skills. Both the cueing preschool teacher and the kindergarten CLT report that he is developing excellent receptive cueing skills, and quickly learned to appropriately work with his CLT in mainstream kindergarten classroom to communicate with noncueing teachers and students, in addition to cueing expressively with other deaf classmates.

Parent Involvement Outcomes. Comments from Spanish-speaking parents of deaf children enrolled in the Cued Speech program indicate that they feel as though they have a greater understanding of the school and its activities, as a result of the concerted efforts of program staff, and that they feel confident that they can receive answers to questions when they arise. Comments also indicate that they feel confident in their knowledge of the communication system used with their children, and have a greater understanding of language development in general.

The preschool teacher, who also conducts home visits, reported an increase in the frequency of transactions using the daily "communication journal" between teacher and parents. Perhaps because of the increased use of, and apparent respect paid to, the Spanish language by program staff members found that these parents became more likely to include notes to school staff. Program staff members also reported a phenomenon among the Spanish-speaking parents very similar to that of the English-speaking parents: given that parents are new to cueing, they are generally not proficient cue readers. Parents often report that their children come home every day, cueing new words they had learned at school, and expecting a reaction from their parents. Unless the child's speech is also fairly intelligible, parents are not likely to recognize the new cued word, and specifically will ask cueing staff members for help. This "daily vocabulary" has become part of the preschool teacher's home visits, as well as being included on daily notes sent home (translated by staff members, as necessary).

Additional Spanish-Language Families Expressing Interest. By the time the third boy had made the transition from cueing preschool to mainstream kindergarten, another Spanish-speaking parent had enrolled her child in the Cued Speech program, in the third grade. The mother reported at initial meetings that her child requests that she cue, and expressed motivation to learn. As of this writing, plans are underway to initiate a beginner LPC class for her, and the staff hopes to find other interested individuals to take the class with her. Additionally, "older" parents will be contacted regarding support meetings and/or practice sessions.

In addition to the Spanish-native educational audiologist, the Cued Speech program staff now includes a native Spanish-speaking CLT. It is possible that, with the materials and instructions in place, the Spanish-speaking CLT can be trained to teach the beginner LPC class to future groups of parents, without the need for a Spanish-language translator.

Request for Cued Korean. Perhaps the most unexpected outcome, positive or negative, was the request for information regarding Cued Speech instruction in yet another language other than English. A couple who speaks both English and Korean, had enrolled their child in the Cued Speech preschool, after deciding that Cued Speech was the best route for their family to take toward English-language fluency for their child. Both parents had taken the beginner Cued Speech parent class, and soon, the mother was observed to be the more proficient cuer of the two parents.

The Korean parents reported that, in keeping with their strong Korean roots and traditions, they typically spoke Korean to each other at home, not English. They reported that one of the reasons they had been attracted to Cued Speech was the potential opportunity it afforded their child to learn Korean, as well as English; this was an exciting prospect, as the family regularly travels to Korea. Eventually, having seen and heard about the Spanish-speaking families learning to cue in Spanish, these parents inquired about how to go about learning Cued Speech in Korean. In similar fashion to the advent of the Spanish project, the staff began by locating a Korean Cued Speech chart. The available chart contained no English translations or English-language alphabetic symbols, so the staff members were at a greater disadvantage than they had been previously. The parents reported a high level of motivation to cue both English and Korean, so the program staff members have pledged to assist them however they can.

As of this writing, the Korean-speaking parents have continued to cue in English at home (the father being observed to cue more consistently than at first), and have begun to teach themselves the Korean Cued Speech system and incorporate cued Korean words and phrases in order to expose their child to both languages. The child has demonstrated comprehension of cued messages in English at school, and has begun to expressively cue one- and two-word utterances.

Conclusion

This chapter describes what we believe to be the only Cued Speech program that is actively supporting the view that the home language is the optimum L1 for non-English-speaking parents of a deaf child to foster communication and language development in the home in a way that both the home and school can contribute the development of language proficiency as described by Cummins (1989). Parents, practitioners, and educational policy makers need to realize the challenges in setting up and implementing such a program. These challenges include: (1) the likelihood of parents relocating to and from the United States or to different locations within the county, state, or United States, (2) having the resources needed to provide Spanish-speaking professionals (e.g., audiologists, speech-language pathologists, instructional staff, support staff), and (3) the time and effort to replicate the process for a new language. As daunting as these challenges are, as the diversity of students in public school systems increases, schools need to find resources to adapt programs designed for the dominant language populations to other language populations. Hopefully, this chapter has provided some examples of how to do this. It also might be noted that challenging as it is to adapt curricular materials to Spanish-speaking parents, in the case of Cued Speech, it is a finite task, and in the views of these authors, based on parent and student outcomes, it is well worth the effort.

The most positive outcome of the efforts described in this chapter were the documented English language development and school readiness gains made by the one boy whose parents most consistently cued at home. Other positive outcomes included: (1) Spanish-speaking parents reporting feeling valued and included in the school community (which is unusual even for Spanish-speaking parents of hearing children) and (2) interest expressed by other non-English-speaking families in the Cued Speech program. The educational attainment of these Spanish-speaking children should continue to be documented. We hope other programs will consider adapting this program to their own so that it can be verified whether this is a viable program for other programs besides the one described in this chapter.

The application of Cued Speech for cued Spanish in the United States described in this chapter represents a significant shift in our schema related to bilingual education for deaf students, and perhaps comes closest to approximating the bilingual educational experience of hearing children educated in English language schools while living in Spanish (or other) language households. Although the data we have clearly are preliminary, they appear to support the view that hearing parents of deaf children *can* be models of their home language for their deaf children, and the language *does not* need to be English in order for language proficiency to develop and contribute to academic achievement of deaf children.

References

Baker, C. (2001). *Foundations of bilingual education and bilingualism* (3rd ed). Clevedon, UK: Multilingual Matters.

Berko, J. (1958). The child's learning of English morphology. *Word, 14,* 150–177.

Blamey, P., Barry, J., Bow, C., Sarant, J., Paatsch, L., & Wales, R. (2001a). The development of speech production following cochlear implantation. *Clinical Linguistics & Phonetics, 15,* 353–382.

Blamey, P., Sarant, J., Paatsch, L., Barry, J., Bow, C., Wales, R., . . . Tooher, R. (2001b). Relationships among speech perception, production, language, hearing loss, and age in children with impaired hearing. *Journal of Speech Language and Hearing Research, 44,* 264–285.

Bodner-Johnson, B. (2003). The deaf child in the family. In B. Bodner-Johnson & M. Sass-Lehrer (Eds.), *The young deaf or hard of hearing child: A family-centered approach to early intervention* (pp. 3–37). Baltimore, MD: Brookes.

de Boysson-Bardies, B., & Vihman, M. (1991). Adaptation to language: Evidence from babbling and first words in four languages. *Language, 67,* 297–319.

Brown, R. (1973). *A first language.* Cambridge, MA: Harvard University Press.

Cornett, R. O. (1994). Adapting Cued Speech to additional languages. *Cued Speech Journal, 5,* 19–29.

Cummins, J. (1989). *Empowering minority students.* Sacramento, CA: California Association for Bilingual Education.

Dromi, E., & Berman, R. (1982). A morphemic measure of early language development: Data from modern Hebrew. *Journal of Child Language, 2,* 403–424.

Fairfax County Public Schools, Virginia (2008a). Monthly membership figures for June 2008. Retrieved July 1, 2008, from http://www.fcps.edu/Reporting/historical/pdfs/ethnic/eth99.pdf

Fairfax County Public Schools, Virginia (2008b). Report of student membership by ethnic groups. Retrieved July 1, 2008, from http://www.fcps.edu/Reporting/historical/pdfs/ethnic/eth99.pdf

Fleetwood, E., & Metzger, M. (1990). *Cued Speech transliteration: Theory and application.* Silver Spring, MD: Calliope Press.

Geers, A. (2002). Factors affecting the development of speech, language, and literacy in children with cochlear implantation. *Journal of Language, Speech, and Hearing Services in Schools, 33,* 172–183.

Haptonstall-Nykaza, T., & Schick, B. (2007). The transition from fingerspelling to English print: Facilitating English decoding. *Journal of Deaf Studies and Deaf Education, 12,* 172–183.

Hatfield, N. (1990). *Unlocking the curriculum: One parent-infant program's search for keys.* American Society for Deaf Children Convention proceedings, Vancouver, British Columbia.

Isreaelite, N., Ewoldt, C., & Hoffmeister, R. (1992). *Bilingual/bicultural education for deaf and hard-of-hearing students.* Toronto, Ontario: MGS Publication Services.

Kantor, R. (1982). Communicative interaction: Mother modification and child acquisition of American Sign Language. *Sign Language Studies, 36,* 233–282.

Language Matters, Inc. (2008). Cued Language Transliterator Professional Education Series Downloaded April 28, 2008, from http://www.language-matters.com/preface.php3

LaSasso, C., & Lollis, J. (2003). National survey of residential and day schools that identify themselves as bilingual-bicultural programs. *Journal of Deaf Studies and Deaf Education, 8,* 79–91.

LaSasso, C., & Metzger, M. (1998). An alternate route for preparing deaf children for bi-bi programs: The home language as L1 and Cued Speech for conveying traditionally-spoken languages. *Journal of Deaf Studies and Deaf Education, 3,* 265–289.

Lederberg, A., & Everhart, V. (2000). Conversations between deaf children and their hearing mothers: Pragmatic and dialogic characteristics. *Journal of Deaf Studies and Deaf Education, 5,* 302–322.

Lichtert, G., & Loncke, F. (2006). The development of proto-performative utterances in deaf toddlers. *Journal of Speech, Language, and Hearing Research, 49,* 486–499.

Loots, G., & Devisé, I. (2003). The use of visual-tactile communication strategies by deaf and hearing fathers and mothers of deaf infants. *Journal of Deaf Studies and Deaf Education, 8,* 31–42.

Luinge, M., Post, W., Wit, H., & Goorhuis-Brouwer, S. (2007). The ordering in milestones of language development for children from 1 to 6 years of age. *Journal of Speech, Language, and Hearing Research, 49,* 923–940.

Mason, D. (1997). Response to Mayer and Wells: The answer should be affirmative. *Journal of Deaf Studies and Deaf Education, 2,* 277–279.

Mayer, C., & Wells, G. (1996). Can the linguistic interdependence theory support a bilingual-bicultural model of literacy education for deaf students? *Journal of Deaf Studies and Deaf Education, 1,* 93–107.

Mayer, C., & Wells, G. (1997). The question remains: A rejoinder to Mason. *Journal of Deaf Studies and Deaf Education, 2,* 280–282.

Meadow, K., Greenberg, M., Erting, C., & Carmichael, H. (1981). Interactions of deaf mothers and deaf preschool children: Comparisons with three other groups of deaf and hearing dyads. *American Annals of the Deaf, 126,* 454–468.

Meadow-Orlans, K. (1997). Effects of mother and infant hearing status on interactions and twelve and eighteen months. *Journal of Deaf Studies and Deaf Education, 2,* 26–36.

Mitchell, R., & Karchmer, M. (2004). Chasing the mythical ten percent: Parental hearing status of deaf and hard of hearing students in the United States. *Sign Language Studies, 4,* 138–163.

Nicholas, J., & Geers, A. (2003). Hearing status, language modality, and young children's communicative and linguistic. *Journal of Deaf Studies and Deaf Education, 8,* 422–437.

Oller, D., & Eilers, R. (1982). Similarity of babbling in Spanish- and English-learning babies. *Journal of Child Language, 2,* 565–577.

Ramsey, C. (1997). *Deaf children in publics Schools: Placement, context, and consequences.* Washington, DC: Gallaudet University Press.

Schick, B., Marscharck, M., & Spencer, P. (2006). *Advances in the sign language develop-ment of deaf children.* New York, NY: Oxford University Press.

Singleton, J., Morgan, D., DiGello, E., Wiles, J., & Rivers, R. (2004). Vocabulary use by low, moderate, and high ASL-proficient writers compared to hearing ESL and monolingual speakers. *Journal of Deaf Studies and Deaf Education, 9,* 86–103.

Spencer, P. (1993). The expressive communication of hearing mothers and deaf infants. *American Annals of the Deaf, 138,* 275–283.

Spencer, P., & Marschark, M. (2006). *Advances in the spoken language development of deaf and hard-of-hearing children.* New York, NY: Oxford University Press.

Strong, M., & Prinz, P. (1997). A study of the relationship between American Sign Language and English literacy. *Journal of Deaf Studies and Deaf Education, 2,* 37–46.

Torres, S. (Ed.). (1988). *La Palabra Complementada.* Madrid, Spain: CEPE.

Torres, S., Moreno-Torres, I., & Santana, R. (2006). Quantitative and qualitative evaluation of linguistic input support to a prelingually deaf child with Cued Speech: A case study. *Journal of Deaf Studies and Deaf Education, 11,* 438–448.

United States Census Bureau. (2008). *State & County Quickfacts: Fairfax County, Virginia.* Downloaded July 1, 2008. from http://quickfacts.census.gov/qfd/states/51/51059.html

Volterra, V., & Erting, C. (1994). *From gesture to language in hearing and deaf children.* Washington, DC: Gallaudet University Press.

Waxman, R., & Spencer, P. (1997). What mothers do to support infant visual attention: Sensitivities to age and hearing status. *Journal of Deaf Studies and Deaf Education, 2,* 104–114.

Yoshinaga-Itano, C., Sedey, A., Coulter, D., & Mehl, A. (1998). Language of early- and later-identified children with hearing loss. *Pediatrics, 102,* 1161–1171.

Zuniga, M. (1998). Families with Latino roots. In E. Lynch & M. Hanson (Eds.), *Developing cross-cultural competencies: 1044-01A guide for working with young children and their families* (pp. 209–249). Baltimore, MD: Brookes.

Section VI

CUED SPEECH/
CUED LANGUAGE
ON THE HORIZON

Chapter 18

LIPREADING, THE LEXICON, AND CUED SPEECH

Lynne E. Bernstein, Edward T. Auer, Jr., and Jintao Jiang

Introduction

When people lipread (speechread), they are using the visible motions and face configurations that the talker produces in order to recognize the segmental/phonemic (consonant and vowel), prosodic, and lexical distinctions that encode the words of the talker's language. As far as we know, beyond the level of recognizing words, the structure of the spoken language processing system is similar for lipread and heard speech, or combinations of the two. That is, the processing system(s) responsible for semantics, syntax, and pragmatics is (are) not specific to the source of the speech information, be it auditory, visual, and/or in some cases somatosensory (Chomsky, 1986). Cued Speech was developed in order to ameliorate deficiencies in visual phonetic information (see Chapter 2 in this volume) due to hearing loss. Specifically, the logic of Cued Speech is that it augments visible spoken phonetic (consonant and vowel)

information, so that psycholinguistic processes beyond the levels of the phoneme and the word can proceed normally.

This chapter discusses lipreading and how spoken word intelligibility for the lipreader is determined in part by the forms of words in the lexicon as a whole. We demonstrate how word forms can interact with cues in determining visual spoken word intelligibility. We introduce a computer-based Cued Speech synthesis system that can assist in training and practicing Cued Speech, as well as assist in training for vocabulary development, and we suggest how knowledge about the lexicon and cues can inform training and usage.

Lipreading in Deaf Versus Hearing Adults

Because Cued Speech was designed to augment lipreading, a detailed understanding of the latter is needed to understand fully

Cued Speech itself. The most detailed studies of lipreading have been with adults rather than children. Here, we describe a study carried out at Gallaudet University and the University of Maryland Baltimore County (UMBC) on 72 deaf and 96 hearing undergraduate students. The study was designed to obtain lipreading scores for nonsense syllables, isolated monosyllabic words, and isolated sentences (Bernstein, Demorest, & Tucker, 2000).

The selection criteria for the UMBC students were English as a native language, normal hearing, normal vision, and age between 18 and 45 years. The selection criteria for the Gallaudet (henceforth *deaf*) students were developed with the goal to recruit participants for whom lipreading is a socially important and well-practiced skill and to exclude participants whose native language was American Sign Language or another manual communication system other than English. The additional screening characteristics were: (1) between 18 and 45 years of age; (2) sensorineural hearing impairments greater than 60 dB HL better average across the frequencies 500, 1,000, and 2,000 Hz; (3) no self-report of disability other than hearing loss and university records reporting no disability other than hearing loss; (4) self-reported use of spoken English as the primary language of the participant's family; (5) self-report of English (including a manually coded form) as the participant's native language; (6) education in a mainstream and/or oral program for eight or more years; and (7) vision at least 20/30 in each eye, as determined with a standard Snellen chart.

Participants in the study identified the 22 initial consonants of English in a 22-alternative forced-choice task. The consonants were in consonant-vowel (CV) syllables with the vowel /ɑ/, and there were sets spoken by a male and female talker.

Participants identified, in an open-set task, isolated monosyllabic words spoken by the male talker. Also identified in an open-set task were isolated sentences spoken by both the male and female talkers.

Results were analyzed in terms of (1) phonemes correct in nonsense syllables, (2) whole words and phonemes correct for isolated monosyllabic words, and (3) whole words and phonemes correct for sentences. A sequence comparator (Bernstein, Demorest, & Eberhardt, 1994) was used to align the open-set sentence responses with the stimuli and extract the correct and incorrect phonemes. Deaf undergraduates' mean performance levels exceeded (statistically significant) those of the hearing students on nearly every measure.

Mean phonemes correct in nonsense syllables was 32.5% for the deaf and 30.5% for the hearing participants. Mean phonemes correct in isolated words was 52% for the deaf and 41% for the hearing participants. Mean whole words correct for isolated words was 19% for the deaf and 11% for the hearing participants. However, the distributions of the scores were highly skewed. The upper quartile scores for the deaf participants were 25 to 42% words correct. The comparable scores for the hearing participants were 15 to 24% words correct.

Phonemes correct scores on isolated sentence lipreading varied depending on the talker and the sentence list (Demorest & Bernstein, 1992). An example of the overall pattern of results, based on the male talker and the more difficult sentence set, was mean phonemes correct in sentences 53% for the deaf participants and 33% for the hearing participants. The comparable scoring for whole words correct was 47% for the deaf and 28% for the hearing. Again, the distribution of the scores was highly skewed. The upper quartile scores for the deaf participants were 61 to 80% words correct and for the hearing participants were 36 to 57% words correct. To be noted also, both groups included individuals whose scores were very low.

The results of the study suggested that the necessity to rely on vision resulted in substantial lipreading differences between the deaf and the hearing participants. Among those with the highest lipreading scores were individuals with profound and congenital hearing loss. Although individual differences in lipreading accuracy were shown to be large among adults with normal hearing, they were approximately twice as large among adults with hearing loss. One possible explanation for differences between groups in the study could be that hearing adults are unused to attempting to understand speech by vision alone. To investigate this possibility, in another study (Bernstein, Auer, & Tucker, 2001), deaf and hearing adults participated in a lipreading training study. The results showed that the lipreading advantage for deaf versus hearing participants was stable, even after extensive practice/training was given, suggesting that small gains could be made by individual deaf and hearing participants based on the laboratory lipreading training, but at the same time, the deaf individuals maintained their superiority.

Recently, we (Auer & Bernstein, 2007) examined sentence lipreading scores with a new set of 112 early-onset deaf and 220 normal hearing adults. Deaf participants' accuracy (M = 43.6% words correct; SD = 17.5%) greatly exceeded that of the normal hearing adults (M = 18.6% words correct; SD = 13.2%). The effect size was 1.7 (Cohen's d) (Cohen, 1988), suggesting that the average prelingually deaf lipreader will score above 95% of normal hearing

lipreaders. The results replicated the previous results with the Gallaudet students (Bernstein et al., 2000).

Another study carried out with deaf adults in England also found similar results (Mohammed et al., 2005). Thus, the finding that the deaf adults are more accurate lipreaders has been shown to generalize across studies when the sample sizes are reasonably large. Given the huge range in scores for both deaf and hearing lipreaders, there should be little surprise that small-sample studies of lipreading can produce quite different estimates of lipreading in each group. The statistical mean, which is often the descriptive statistic used to represent results, is highly influenced by the most extreme scores. A few low scoring or a few high scoring deaf or hearing participants in a small study can very much influence conclusions. Generalizations concerning lipreading should be based on relatively large sample sizes.

Normative data showing differences across groups raise the question, what makes a good lipreader? Educational practice and studies from the 20th century seemed to indicate that training programs were not effective in ameliorating effects of deafness through lipreading training (Jeffers & Barley, 1971). Therefore, the traditional answer has been that good lipreaders are born and not made (Hall, Fussell, & Summerfield, 2005; Summerfield, 1991). The results reported above suggest, however, that factors associated with deafness do result in enhanced lipreading for a large proportion of prelingually deaf lipreaders.

One *caveat* is that our results were obtained using a set of selection criteria that might have been biased toward obtaining enhanced lipreading in the deaf group. Similar data have not been obtained, to our knowledge, for deaf adults with quite different lifelong histories, for example, those without postsecondary education. Studies of deaf adults across a spectrum of education and jobs, for example, need to be carried out.

Our results also do not provide insight into the developmental course of lipreading proficiency. One possibility is that proficient lipreaders in our studies were always proficient, relative to others in their age cohort. A different possibility is that gradually over their lifetime into adulthood they achieved their relative level of expertise. Longitudinal studies of lipreading have suggested that ability is fairly stable (Jeffers & Barley, 1971), but the studies have not extended across childhood into adulthood, leaving open the possibility that experience later in life was a key factor in the differences we observed in our studies.

Phonetic Information and the Lexicon

Even under the clearest viewing conditions, certain types of phonetic information are invisible to the person who relies on vision alone for perceiving speech. The term *phonetic* refers to the physical stimulus information in speech signals. Speech production activities are partially occluded from view by the lips, cheeks, and neck. Hidden from view is vocal fold vibration, related to the phonological voicing distinction (e.g., /b/ vs. /p/ or /f/ vs. /v/); partially hidden is the type of vocal tract posture made by the tongue, related to phonological manner distinctions (e.g., /d/ vs. /r/); and hidden is the state of the velum, related to nasality (e.g., /n/ vs. /d/).

Because the phonological system used by language relies on multiple features (encoded by multiple phonetic cues), the invisibility of some features does not preclude speech perception but results in fewer segmental (vowel and consonant) distinctions. Several studies, including our own, have documented lipreading of isolated nonsense syllables and have shown the patterns of reduced segmental distinctions for the lipreader (Auer & Bernstein, 1997; Fisher, 1968; Iverson, Bernstein, & Auer, 1998; Montgomery & Jackson, 1983; Owens & Blazek, 1985). Table 18–1 shows a typical result for which there are a relatively small number of segment groups that are different from each other. The consonants within the group are similar to each other and might not be distinguishable to a particular lipreader. The standard set in the table approximates the distinctions available to the average hearing lipreader. The difficult set approximates the distinctions available to the expert deaf lipreader.

Because phoneme distinctions are reduced from the perspective of the lipreader, a logical question is how this reduction affects the distinctiveness of words. Auer and Bernstein (1997) developed a method to investigate what the lipreader's perceptual lexicon might comprise. The method used phoneme groupings derived by obtaining isolated nonsense syllable identifications from lipreaders (in this example, hearing individuals). The *phoneme equivalence class* (PEC) was defined to be a set of phonemes that are grouped together due to their perceptual similarity. This method uses hierarchical clustering of data from nonsense syllable perceptual confusion matrices to obtain the PECs.

The *lexical equivalence class* (LEC) was defined to be a set of words rendered notationally identical by re-transcribing words

Table 18–1. Phoneme Equivalence Classes

Level	Phoneme Equivalence Classes
Difficult	{p} {b m} {f v} {θ ð} {w} {r}
	{tʃ dʒ ʃ ʒ} {t} {d} {s z} {k} {g}
	{n} {l} {h} {i ɪ} {ɛ e æ} {aⁱ} {ɚ}
	{a ɔ} {o} {aʊ} {oⁱ} {ʌ} {ʊ u}
Standard	{p b m} {f v} {θ ð} {w} {r}
	{tʃ dʒ ʃ ʒ d} {t s z} {k g h} {n l}
	{i ɪ ɛ aɪ æ ʌ} {ɚ o oⁱ ʊ u} {a ɔ}
	{aʊ}
Easy	{p b m w} {f v} {θ ð t s z}
	{r tʃ dʒ ʃ ʒ d} {k g n l h}
	{i ɪ ɛ aɪ e æ a ɔ aʊ ʌ} {ɚ o oⁱ ʊ u}

Source: Bernstein, 2006.

in an online lexicon with only notations that stand for each of the PECs. The notation "{}" defines a set. For example, if the following three PECs are given,

$$B = \{b, p, m\},$$
$$T = \{t, s, z\}, \text{ and}$$
$$A = \{i, ɪ, ɛ, aɪ, e, æ, ʌ\},$$

then, "bat," "mat," and "pat," would be in the same LEC, BAT = {bat, mat, pat, mass, bate, . . . }.

After deriving the PECs, the method then follows these steps:

1. Rules are developed to re-transcribe the words in a computer-readable lexicon so that the transcriptions comprise only the single-character expressions standing for PECs at a particular level of phoneme confusability.
2. The rules are applied to the words in the PhLex database (Seitz, Bernstein, Auer, & MacEachern, 1998) of approx-imately 35,000 phonemically transcribed words.
3. The re-transcribed words are sorted so that words rendered identical (no longer notationally distinct) are placed in the same lexical equivalence classes (LECs).
4. Optionally, quantitative measures are applied to estimate the effects of the re-transcription process on the lexicon and on word recognition.

Software tools were developed to carry out the lexical modeling, and the PhLEX (Seitz et al., 1998) online lexical database was created for such studies.

Application of this method (Auer & Bernstein, 1997) showed that when only the 12 visual PECs—i.e., {u, ʊ, ɚr}, {o, aʊ}, {ɪ, i, e, ɛ, æ}, {ɔɪ}, {ɔ, aɪ, ə, a, ʌ, j}, {b, p, m}, {f, v}, {l, n, k, ŋ, g, h}, {d, t, s, z}, {w, r}, {ð, θ}, and {ʃ, tʃ, ʒ, dʒ}—were used to transcribe the lexicon, 54% of words (frequency weighted) were still notationally distinct. Theoretically, lipreaders could identify those words uniquely without resorting to context or guessing. Twelve PECs corresponds approximately to phoneme identification by average hearing lipreaders. When 19 PECs—i.e., {u, ʊ, ər}, {o, aʊ}, {ɪ, i} {e, ɛ},{æ}, {ɔɪ}, {ɔ}, {aɪ, ə, a, ʌ, j}, {b, p, m}, {f, v}, {l,}, {n, k}, {ŋ, g}, {h}, {d}, {t, s, z}, {w, r}, {ð, θ}, and {ʃ, tʃ, ʒ, dʒ}—were used, closer to expert deaf lipreading, approximately 90% of words (frequency weighted) were distinct.

As suggested earlier, the English lexicon does not use all of the possible combinations of strings of consonants and vowels (MacEachern, 2000). Thus, even when the information in the visible speech is reduced, the structure of the lexicon reduces the possibility for confusion among words. For example, although the phonemes, /b, p, m/ are visually similar, the English lexicon contains only the word "bought," and not "mought" or "pought." Thus, knowledge of the language can assist in recognizing words when the information in the stimulus is incomplete. Expert lipreaders could be relying on a combination of ability to extract phonetic information from the visual stimulus and implicit knowledge of the phonological forms of words in the lexicon.

To confirm that phoneme patterns in words are a factor in lipreading, Mattys, Bernstein, and Auer (2002) conducted a study in which deaf and hearing adults performed open-set identification with monosyllabic and disyllabic words that varied in word frequency of occurrence (high vs. low) and size of the word's lexical equivalence class (unique, medium, large) based on the type of lexical modeling described above. Words in unique-size LECs were predicted to be visually distinct and most intelligible. Stimulus words from medium LECs had 1 to 5 possible words

that were highly similar to them, and therefore predicted to be less intelligible. Words from large LECs had 9 to 59 possible words that were highly similar to them, and therefore predicted to be least intelligible. Deaf and hearing adults who were all above-average lipreaders relative to their group viewed, in isolation, 150 monosyllabic and 130 disyllabic spoken words presented randomly, and following each word, typed their identification response.

Whole words correct and phonemes correct were scored. Statistical analyses showed significant effects of LEC size, word frequency of occurrence, and word length. Words were identified more accurately when their LEC size was low (i.e., there were relatively few similar words), when their frequency of occurrence was high, and when they were monosyllables versus disyllables (with mixed evidence for the superiority of monosyllables). When participants *incorrectly* identified a word, their response came from the same LEC as that of the stimulus far more often than would be predicted by chance.

An index of phoneme intelligibility was computed for each word by determining its mean PEC size $[(\Sigma\ PECsize_i)/n$, where i indexes each phoneme, and n is the total number of phonemes in the word], that is, the mean confusability of its phonemes. In order to isolate the effect of LEC size on identification accuracy independent of phoneme intelligibility (because stimulus generation did not control for PEC size), a partial correlation was calculated between LEC size and response accuracy, statistically controlling for mean PEC size and word frequency. The significant correlation confirmed that lexical distinctiveness alone is reliably related to visual spoken word recognition.

A similar analysis examining the correlation between word frequency and response accuracy, controlling for LEC size and mean PEC size, revealed that word frequency of occurrence per se, too, correlated with recognition accuracy. Finally, mean PEC size by itself, with LEC size and frequency controlled, correlated with accuracy. Thus, phoneme intelligibility, lexical similarity, and word frequency each contributed to visual spoken word recognition. The results suggest that visual spoken word recognition is strongly influenced by the number of words in the lexicon visually similar to the stimulus word. This result implies that as phonetic perception improves in accuracy, the number of words that can be recognized accurately will increase, because they will be more dissimilar from each other.

Auer (2002) adapted the Neighborhood Activation Model (NAM) of auditory spoken word recognition (Luce, 1986; Luce & Pisoni, 1998) to model visual spoken word recognition. The NAM defines similarity among words on the basis of confusion matrices obtained from perceptual identifications of auditory nonsense syllable stimuli. The confusion data are used to compute probabilities for identifying each of the words in the lexicon, given the presentation of a specific stimulus word. Identification probabilities are computed with a frequency biased, activation-based version of Luce's (1959) choice rule,

$$p(ID) = \frac{p(S \mid S) * freq_s}{\{p(S \mid S) * freq_s\} + \sum_{j=1}^{n} \{p(N_j \mid S) * freq_{N_j}\}}$$

(Equation 1)

where $p(ID)$ is the probability of correctly identifying the stimulus word, $p(S \mid S)$ is the probability of identifying the stimulus word given the stimulus word, $freq_s$ is the stimulus word's frequency of occurrence,

$p(N_j \mid S)$ is the probability of identifying neighbor word j given the stimulus word, and $freq_{N_j}$ is neighbor word j's frequency of occurrence. In Auer's study, confusion matrices were from perceptual identifications of visual nonsense syllable stimuli. The NAM predicts that the ease with which a word can be recognized is a function of its perceptual similarity to other words in the lexicon. That is, words similar to many other words (dense neighborhoods) should be harder to recognize than words similar to few other words (sparse neighborhoods).

Twelve deaf and 12 hearing adults identified visible spoken words presented in isolation. Words in dense neighborhoods were more difficult to recognize than words in sparse neighborhoods. More specifically, $p(ID)$ values generated with Equation 1 were significantly correlated with word item percent correct scores (hearing: $r = .44$, $p < .05$; deaf: $r = .48$, $p < .05$). Luce and Pisoni (1998) reported correlations that ranged between .23 and .47 for comparable Equation 1 values correlated with auditory word identification scores. Thus, the NAM accounts for comparable variance in word recognition accuracy in both auditory and visual modalities. Words with many neighbors were more difficult to identify than words with few neighbors.

An implication of the PEC and LEC terminology is that items in those classes are perceptually so similar that they cannot be discriminated. But note that the definitions for PECs depend on numerical cluster analysis performed on confusion matrices and on operationally defining boundaries for when to group phonemes into a class. Bernstein (2006) questioned the notion that the PECs function as unitary perceptual categories (Massaro, 1998). An experiment was carried out to test explicitly several different clustering levels for defining PECs.

Hearing and deaf adult participants performed a target identification task: On each trial, they were presented with a visual orthographic word (the target word), followed by a spoken target-distracter pair, with the order of the spoken words counterbalanced and the sets of target-distracter pairs randomized for each participant. Participants indicated which of the spoken words best matched the orthographic target. Feedback was given during practice but not during experimental trials. Performance at chance would suggest that target-distracter pairs were visually ambiguous. Word pairs were generated based on the PECs in Table 18–1, so that there were easy, standard, or difficult distinctions to be made. When given a choice between two words that were theoretically within an LEC, perceivers were actually very accurate at selecting the target word. Some deaf participants were between 80% and 100% accurate for words predicted to comprise the same visemes. The results showed that phonetic information can be available even within the same LEC at a *difficult* level of resolution for which there were 25 PECs (as opposed to a *standard* level with 13 PECs). An implication of these results is that the need for Cued Speech cues might vary depending on the phonemic content of the words that are used and on the lipreading ability of the perceiver.

Lexical Modeling of Cued Speech

For this volume, we conducted a series of computational investigations to estimate the information in Cued Speech as a standalone sequence of gestures in relation-ship to the English lexicon, and we looked at individual cues in relationship to information that can be obtained via lipreading. First, we compared the results of our previous studies of lexical uniqueness during lipreading with the lexical uniqueness available from cues given in isolation from the articulating face. That is, we looked at Cued Speech without lipreading. Then, we investigated the percent of words rendered visually distinct when lipreading is combined with single Cued Speech cues. That is, what happens to word uniqueness if the cuer learns just one cue?

Similar to the lexical modeling described above, the method here was: First, a phonemically transcribed machine-readable lexical database was selected to serve as a representative sample of the words in the language. The lexical database was the PhLex database (Seitz et al., 1998). PhLex's entries have transcriptions that include stress and syllabification markers, and estimates of frequency of occurrence. When word frequency information was not available for an entry, frequency was set to 1.

Second, transcription rules were defined on the basis of measures of visual phonemically available distinctiveness. In the modeling reported below lipreading performance was simulated using the following PECs: {u, ʊ, ɚ}, {o, aʊ}, {ɪ, i, e, ɛ, æ}, {ɔɪ}, {ɔ, aɪ, ə, a, ʌ, j}, {b, p, m}, {f, v}, {l, n, k, ŋ, g, h}, {d, t, s, z}, {w, r}, {ð, θ}, and {ʃ, tʃ, ʒ, dʒ} (Auer & Bernstein, 1997). Transcription rules were generated in the form of single symbol substitutions for all phonemes in the phonemic equivalence classes.

Third, the lexical database was transcribed by applying the transcription rules. Lexical equivalence classes were formed by collapsing across identically transcribed words. For example, under the phoneme equivalence class definitions, "pat" and "bat" would both fall into the same lexical equivalence class. Finally, metrics were computed to compare the distribution of patterns in the newly transcribed lexicon with the distribution of patterns in the original lexicon.

To model the lexical uniqueness associated with viewing cues, sets of transcription rules were developed based on the phonemes sets assigned to each cue. To investigate the extent to which cues alone would render words uniquely in the lexicon, a set of PECs was used to represent the segmental distinctiveness provided by the cues alone, that is, without the articulating face. This set of PECs was: {u, ʊ} {a, o}, {aɪ, aʊ}, {ər, i}, {ɛ, ɔ, u},{æ}, {ɪ, ʊ, æ}, {ɔɪ, e}, {ʒ, p, d}, {θ, k, v, z}, {h, r, s}, {b, n}, {f, m, t}, {ʃ, l, w}, {ð, g, dʒ}, {tʃ, ŋ, j}.

Finally, to investigate the effectiveness of using a single Cued Speech cue in combination with lipreading, we modified the PECs for lipreading based on the distinctions added for each consonant cue. For example, the addition of the consonant handshape 1 would place each of the consonants {ʒ, d, p} into their own unique PEC. The cues in this analysis were: 1 = {ʒ, p, d}; 2 = {θ, k, v, z}; 3 = {h, r, s}; 4 = {b, n}; 5 = {f, m, t}; 6 = {ʃ, l, w}; 7 = {ð, g, dʒ}; and 8 = {tʃ, ŋ, j}. Each of these cues was used to model word distinctiveness, assuming no additional vowel information and then assuming complete vowel distinctiveness.

To assess the outcome of the modeling, two commonly employed metrics were computed to analyze the distributions of patterns in the transcribed lexicon (Auer & Bernstein, 1997). Log-frequency-weighted percent words unique was computed as:

$$\% \, WU = \frac{FU}{FL} \times 100$$

(Equation 2)

where FU is the sum of the frequencies of occurrence for unique words in the transcribed lexicon, and FL is the sum of frequencies of occurrence of words in the original lexicon. The log-frequency-weighted metric estimates the extent to which unique words are encountered in everyday language.

Log-frequency-weighted expected class size is computed as:

$$ECS = \sum_{a=1}^{n_E} Ia \, \frac{Fa}{FL}$$

(Equation 3)

where n_E is the total number of lexical equivalence classes, Ia is the number of words in equivalence class a, Fa is the sum of frequencies of occurrence of words in equivalence class a, and FL is the sum of the frequencies of occurrence of words in the lexicon. The log-frequency-weighted metric estimates the average size of the equivalence classes encountered in everyday language.

In Figure 18–1, comparison of lexical distinctiveness in the lipreading-alone versus cues-alone model shows a striking difference in the available information for these two channels of information. Overall, cues by themselves deliver more information than visible speech, when the latter is modeled using an average hearing lipreader. A higher percentage of the words remain unique, and on average, words fall into smaller LECs under the cues-alone transcription than under the lipreading transcription (Figure 18–2). In addition, the results suggest that communication could be conducted using cues only, no lipreading at all, if the words were selected to be unique in terms of cues. Comparison of each cue singly, with (filled bars in Figure 18–2) and without (open bars in Figure 18–2) the vowels considered to be

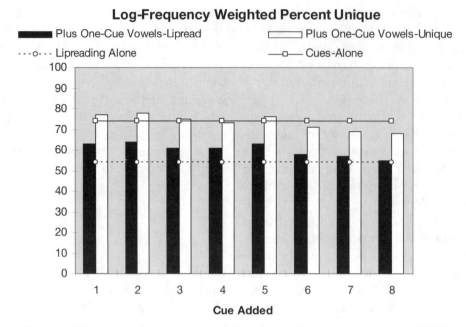

Figure 18–1. Log-frequency weighted words percent unique (fWPU) is plotted as a function of cue hand shape added to the lipreading model. The dashed line represents the lipreading-alone and the solid line represents cues-alone. The black bars represent modeled fWPU where vowel intelligibility was equivalent to the information available from lipreading. The white bars represent modeled fWPU where vowel intelligibility was perfect.

accurately perceived, suggests that the predicted level of performance with cues-alone is comparable to the mere addition of vowel information and a single consonant cue. That is, the combination of lipreading with all the vowels disambiguated and the use of one Cued Speech cue is roughly equivalent to using only cues (no lipreading). Thus, cues are highly informative.

The specific consonant cue added does seem to influence the predicted level of lexical distinctiveness for this English example. The addition of cue handshapes 1 through 5 increased modeled distinctiveness more than the addition of cue handshapes 6 through 8 (see Figure 18–1). This result suggests that cues, similar to

consonants, do not all carry the same informational load within English. Overall, the results are consistent with the conclusion that learning to cue the vowels and a few consonants would substantially increase the intelligibility of lipread words. Thus, even relatively novice cuers would, with a limited productive cue inventory, be expected to significantly increase the intelligibility of the visible speech signal.

Cued Speech Training

Lexical modeling techniques of the type described in this chapter can contribute to

Log-Frequency Weighted Expected Class Size

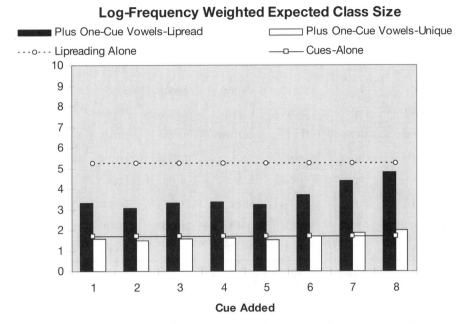

Figure 18–2. Log-frequency weighted expected class size (fECS) is plotted as a function of cue handshape added to the lipreading model. The dashed line represents the lipreading-alone and the solid line represents cues-alone. The black bars represent modeled fECS where vowel intelligibility was equivalent to the information available from lipreading. The white bars represent modeled fECS where vowel intelligibility was perfect.

the development of Cued Speech training materials that can be flexible and possibly more effective and efficient than traditional materials. Toward this end, an information analysis can be applied to the list of words that are to be learned. For example, Table 18–2 is a small set of words (68) from Ling and Ling (1977) recommended for training deaf children.

A lexical equivalence class analysis, using 12 phoneme equivalence classes, indicates that by lipreading alone, 63 of the 68 words are unique from one another. That is, these words would be predicted to be discriminable by an adult lipreader with average ability. For this set of words, the addition of only handshapes 1 or 3

renders the closed set completely visually unique. Clearly, children's phoneme confusions are needed to develop appropriate lists for them.

However, a general question is whether Cued Speech training should employ a more or less visually challenging set of words for lipreading. Possibly, at early training stages, a word set that is not particularly challenging would be more motivating for Cued Speech learners. Being able to lipread a distinct set of words might serve as a context to enhance Cued Speech training and integration with visible speech cues. As a closed set, the discriminability of these words might assist the learner to perceive cues. Alternatively,

Table 18–2. A List of 68 Training Words

cloud	pocket	rock	turtle	walk	call	listen
drink	yard	dot	cold	dig	blue	touch
toad	tent	clean	dance	wash	sky	turn
number	cry	blow	glass	fence	lake	rabbit
round	sleep	flies	clothes	party	push	jump
paint	ride	wood	bite	garage	snow	bench
climb	throw	cook	store	night	laugh	hunt
mail	pull	work	sing	cut	ocean	leaves
fight	drop	color	river	child	swim	
shot	write	feed	mirror	cross	jacket	

Source: selected from Ling and Ling (1977).

the distinctiveness of the words in terms of lipreading might reduce attention to the Cued Speech cues. Perhaps Cued Speech learning is easier if cues are critical to word identification. With lexical modeling methods of this type, methods can be developed to optimize training. However, research is needed to determine what are the optimal training methods.

Future Technical Aids to Training and Using Cued Speech

Technical aids to training Cued Speech are highly feasible at this time. One possible Cued Speech training method would use prerecorded video materials. However, early and extensive exposure to Cued Speech would exhaust prerecordings (e.g., Beck, 2000; Metzger & Fleetwood, 1992; Mills, 1999). Language is generative and productive. What is needed is an unlimited supply of Cued Speech materials, that is, a system that can synthesize materials.

Technical Cued Speech devices have long been a goal. An early one, the auto-cuer system (Cornett, Beadles, & Wilson, 1977), used a portable microprocessor to analyze acoustic inputs (zero crossing rates, pitch, etc.) and then display cues projected from eyeglasses with seven-segment LED (light-emitting diode) patterns (with nine distinct shapes and at four positions). Another system used automatic speech recognition (ASR) from acoustics to generate cues automatically (Bratakos, Duchnowski, & Braida, 1998; Duchnowski et al., 2000) This ASR-cuer system assigned pre-recorded static hand images to cues that were obtained using automatic speech recognition. The recorded images were superimposed on the simultaneously recorded talker video with consideration of the synchronization of hand and face. Performance of the autocuer (Cornett et al., 1977) and ASR-cuer (Bratakos et al., 1998; Duchnowski et al., 2000), was highly dependent on acoustic processing accuracy (Uchanski et al., 1994), which is still considered difficult with current state-of-the-art speech technologies. Also, the cues generated by these two systems were not at all natural. For example, the autocuer used a few LED patterns, and the ASR-cuer (Bratakos et al., 1998; Duchnowski et al., 2000) used static handshapes concatenated without transitions.

Another system, synFMCS (synthetic French Manual Cued Speech), used concatenative methods to synthesize hand and facial motion (Gibert, Bailly, & Elisei, 2004). Recordings were made using a Vicon motion capture system with 12 cameras that recorded the three-dimensional trajectories of 50 hand and 63 facial flesh points, which were used to control hand and face models. Speech articulators (including the hand for Cued Speech) cannot move instantaneously from one articulatory posture to another, and thus at any moment, one or more articulators may be simultaneously (and nonsynchronously) adjusting as they move to another position. The perceptual significance of coarticulation has been demonstrated in lipreading (Benguerel & Pichora-Fuller, 1982) and in auditory perception (Martin & Bunnell, 1981, 1982). The French Cued Speech synthesis system, synFMCS (Gibert et al., 2004), used concatenative methods to obtain natural coarticulation. That is, di-keys, which comprised naturally recorded hand movements between two successive keys (hand gesture and position combinations), were concatenated.

We are developing an English Cued Speech training system. A focus of the project is the naturalness of the hand and finger motions, under the hypothesis that unnatural motion could impede learning and perception. Visible speech coarticulation contains time-varying information that is important for visual speech perception (Rosenblum & Saldana, 1998). Synthesis of Cued Speech without coarticulation results in disjointed hand gestures that could not

only interrupt perceptual processing but also fail to integrate with ongoing visual (and auditory) speech information.

Our system, catDi-Cuer (Concatenative Di-Cue System), is designed to synthesize Cued Speech coarticulation, that is, the natural flow of motion from one cue to the next. As a first approximation to Cued Speech coarticulation, concatenative methods are used. The basis for the coarticulatory synthesis is in the technology of acoustic speech synthesis. The *di-cue* here is analogous to the *diphone* in acoustic speech synthesis (Peterson, Wang, & Sivertsen, 1958). The di-cue begins and terminates in the middle of manual cues. These segments, whose temporal boundaries are located in the most stable regions of hand gestures, are edited by an experimenter for use by the synthesizer, in order to guarantee accuracy. Fortunately, the number of di-cues is much smaller than that of acoustic diphones, significantly alleviating system design complexity.

For concatenative methods, a key undertaking is to extract hand motion from video images, especially when the hand is near the mouth, resulting in similar pixel values for hand and mouth. In our data recording system, the video bluescreen technique is used to segment hand and face automatically, using image processing techniques (e.g., color classification).

The synthesis process involves superimposing Cued Speech images on visible speech. This requires examining the synchronization of hand and face (Duchnowski et al., 2000; Leybaert, 2003) in English (cf. Attina, Beautemps, Cathiard, & Odisio, 2004). We have videorecorded a female talker, a native speaker of American English, who is highly visually intelligible and an expert in Cued Speech. We have recorded several databases produced by this individual. One comprises Cued

Speech alone for developing a di-cue inventory. In order to sample hand motions appropriately for developing the di-cue inventory, the required sequences were: 320 CCVs (consonant-consonant-vowel; 8 handshapes in a neutral position × 8 handshapes × 5 hand positions) and 320 CVCs (consonant-vowel-consonant; 8 handshapes × 5 hand positions × 8 handshapes at a neutral position). This set was initially recorded in 1999 (by Auer and Bernstein). Subsequently, to model the English diphthongs, a set of 66 words were more recently recorded. The Cued Speech-only data also include 260 nonsense CVCVC words (consonant-vowel-consonant-vowel-consonant), 150 monosyllable words used previously (Mattys et al., 2002), 50 words from the Northwestern University-Children's Perception of Speech (NU-CHIPS) (Elliot & Katz, 1980), 100 words from the Word Intelligibility by Picture Identification (WIPI) (Ross & Lerman, 1970), 68 words from Ling and Ling (1977), and 162 words from Nicholls (1979). Another database comprises visible speech (lipreading) test materials. Yet another comprises Cued Speech and visible speech materials for providing reference (synchronization and hand position) for use in synthesis.

The data were recorded with a Sony video recorder and digital video camera (frame rate = 29.97 Hz). The female talker produced Cued Speech while speaking and viewing a teleprompter that was mounted below the camera. She looked directly into the camera through the teleprompter, and her face and hand (during speech) filled the video monitor. Lighting and positioning were carefully adjusted. A blue background and blue hood on the talker were used to facilitate later extracting hand motion from the video images. A 3-D optical recording system (Qualisys

MCU120/240-Hz CCD Imager) was used to digitally record the positions of passive retro-reflectors on the face and hand during infrared flashes (Bernstein, Auer, Chaney, Alwan, & Keating, 2000). The 3-D motion data were recorded for future development of a synthetic 3-D face and hand.

Figure 18–3 illustrates the synthesis technique, for which CCV and CVC represent consonant-consonant-vowel and consonant-vowel-consonant syllables, respectively. Video data are first manually segmented and digitized. Image processing is applied to generate hand and head images. For each token, hand di-cue and visual diphone boundaries are manually selected at the time points where the gesture is typical and stable. For synthesis, each test word is transcribed with a string of di-cues. The constituent di-cues are extracted from the di-cue inventory and are then concatenated. Image processing (e.g., translation, rotation, and scaling) is applied to smooth between di-cues. The concatenated di-cues are superimposed onto the corresponding visual spoken words. Figure 18–4 shows how the videos are processed to generate synthetic Cued Speech.

The full capability to synthesize an unlimited vocabulary will probably require a synthetic talking face. Visual speech synthesis systems have been developed (Cole et al., 2003; Massaro & Light, 2004; Xue, Borgstrom, Jiang, Bernstein, & Alwan, 2006). We have been working on a visible speech synthesis system (Bernstein & Jiang, 2009; Xue et al., 2006) that can be integrated with the Cued Speech synthesis system.

A future Cued Speech training system, based on a flexible computer-based Cued Speech synthesizer, lexical modeling as illustrated in this chapter that can be performed online, and adaptive software that responds to users, seems a feasible

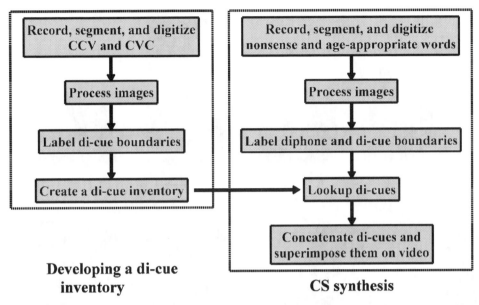

Developing a di-cue
inventory

CS synthesis

Figure 18–3. An overview of the di-cue based synthesis system. CCV and CVC refer to the consonant-consonant-vowel and consonant-vowel-consonant syllables, respectively. The system comprises a di-cue inventory and Cued Speech synthesis. Speech materials were recorded, segmented, digitized, image-processed, and appropriately labeled with boundaries for di-cues and diphones. The Cued Speech synthesis component then retrieves di-cues from the precreated di-cue inventory, contenates them, and superimposes them onto corresponding video images.

product for the not too distant future. Words can be selected for their visual and Cued Speech properties. Other properties can be incorporated, such as word frequency of occurrence. By combining lexical analyses and a Cued Speech synthesizer, training can potentially be more efficient and less repetitive, compared to training with video or other predefined materials.

Discussion

In Chapters 12 and 14 in this book, the relationship between reading comprehension and Cued Speech is discussed, sug-

gesting that learning Cued Speech can greatly benefit deaf children to achieve higher levels of literacy. Children who use hearing aids and/or cochlear implants could also benefit from Cued Speech. Hearing aids and cochlear implants are imperfect in delivering auditory information, individuals vary in the benefit they receive, and the benefits depend on many factors (e.g., pre- or postlingual deafness, survival of auditory nerve fibers, and communication mode) (American Speech-Language-Hearing Association, 2004; Eisenberg, Kirk, Martinez, Ying, & Miyamoto, 2004; Kirk, Pisoni, & Miyamoto, 2000; Osberger, 1997; Pisoni, Cleary, Geers, & Tobey, 2000). Computer-based systems

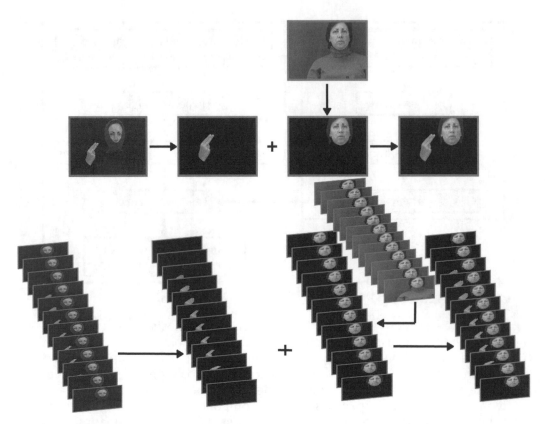

Figure 18–4. An example of the Cued Speech synthesis. Di-cue images were processed to remove the blue background and face. Face images were processed to remove the blue background. The processed di-cue images were superimposed onto the processed face images.

can be designed that integrate Cued Speech training with development of vocabulary and literacy. Specific information about a child's lipreading ability and vocabulary knowledge could be incorporated into training, using the types of modeling approaches discussed in this chapter.

The magnitude of the improvement in speech perception and literacy associated with use of Cued Speech depends on the age at which Cued Speech is initiated and the extent of exposure or use: Effects appear to be greater in "early" Cued Speech groups than in "late" groups, for sentences (Perier, Charlier, Hage, & Alegria, 1987), pseudowords (Alegria, Charlier, & Mattys, 1999), rhyme judgments (Charlier & Leybaert, 2000), new written words (Leybaert, 2003), and spelling ability (Leybaert, 2000; Leybaert & Lechat, 2001). The finding that knowledge and use of even one cue might benefit a deaf child learning a spoken language could encourage more widespread use of Cued Speech with very young children.

Our recent work focuses on implementing a computer-based Cued Speech synthesis system and integrating it with a lexical analysis tool. This training system would effectively provide early and extensive Cued Speech experience, assist children with hearing loss to achieve phonological representations of spoken words, provide cochlear implant recipients with visible and augmented inputs in the format of spoken language to facilitate their auditory habilitation, and adequately and efficiently train teachers and parents to use Cued Speech. Parents could have an effective, efficient, and affordable method to assist their children during the critical period of language development. The use of a technical system could potentially contribute to development of children's reading proficiency.

References

Alegria, J., Charlier, B., & Mattys, S. (1999). The role of lipreading and Cued Speech in the processing of phonological information in French-educated deaf children. *European Journal of Cognitive Psychology, 11*, 451–471.

American Speech-Language-Hearing Association. (2004). Technical report: Cochlear implants. *ASHA Supplement, 24.*

Attina, V., Beautemps, D., Cathiard, M.-A., & Odisio, M. (2004). A pilot study of temporal organization in cued speech production of French syllables: Rules for a Cued Speech synthesizer. *Speech Communication, 44,* 197–214.

Auer, E. (2002). The influence of the lexicon on speech read word recognition: Contrasting segmental and lexical distinctiveness. *Psychonomic Bulletin and Review, 9,* 341–347.

Auer, E., & Bernstein, L (1997). Speechreading and the structure of the lexicon: Computationally modeling the effects of reduced phonetic distinctiveness on lexical uniqueness. *Journal of the Acoustical Society of America, 102,* 3704–3710.

Auer, E., & Bernstein, L.(2007). Enhanced visual speech perception in individuals with early onset hearing impairment. *Journal of Speech, Hearing, and Language Research, 50,* 1157–1165.

Beck, P. (2000). *Discovering Cued Speech* [Videorecording]. Cleveland, OH: Cued Speech for Integrated Communication.

Benguerel, A., & Pichora-Fuller, M. (1982). Coarticulation effects in lipreading. *Journal of Speech and Hearing Research, 25,* 600–607.

Bernstein, L. (2006). Visual speech perception. In E. Vatikiotis-Bateson, G. Bailly, & P. Perrier. (Eds.), *Audio-visual speech processing.* Cambridge, MA: MIT.

Bernstein, L., Auer, E., Chaney, B., Alwan, A., & Keating, P. (2000). Development of a facility for simultaneous recordings of acoustic, optical 3-D motion and video, and physiological speech data. *Journal of the Acoustical Society of America, 107,* 2887.

Bernstein, L., Auer, E., & Tucker, P. (2001). Enhanced speechreading in deaf adults: Can short-term training/practice close the gap for hearing adults? *Journal of Speech, Language, and Hearing Research, 44,* 5–18.

Bernstein, L., Demorest, M., & Eberhardt, S. (1994). A computational approach to analyzing sentential speech perception: Phoneme-to-phoneme stimulus-response alignment. *Journal of the Acoustical Society of America, 95,* 3617–3622.

Bernstein, L., Demorest, M., & Tucker, P. (2000). Speech perception without hearing. *Perception and Psychophysics, 62,* 233–252.

Bernstein, L., & Jiang, J. (2009). Visual speech perception, optical phonetics, and synthetic speech. In A. Liew & S. Wang. (Eds.), *Visual speech recognition: Lip segmentation and mapping* (pp. 439–461). Hershey, PA: Medical Information Science Reference.

Bratakos, M., Duchnowski, P., & Braida, L. (1998). Toward the automatic generation of Cued Speech. *Cued Speech Journal, 6,* 1–37.

Charlier, B., & Leybaert, J. (2000). The rhyming skills of deaf children educated with phonetically augmented speechreading. *Quarterly Journal of Experimental Psychology, 53A,* 349–375.

Chomsky, C. (1986). Analytic study of the Tadoma method: Language abilities of three deaf-blind subjects. *Journal of Speech and Hearing Research, 29,* 332–347.

Cohen, J. (1988). *Statistical power analysis for the behavioral sciences* (2nd ed.). Hillsdale, NJ: Erlbaum.

Cole, R., Van Vuuren, S., Pellom, B., Hacioglu, K., Ma, J., Movellan, J., Schwartz, S., Wade-Stein, D., Ward, W., & Yan, J. (2003). Perceptive animated interfaces: First steps toward a new paradigm for human-computer interaction. *Proceedings of the IEEE, 91,* 1391–1405.

Cornett, R., Beadles, R., & Wilson, B. (1977). *Automatic Cued Speech.* Paper presented at the Research Conference on Speech-Processing Aids for the Deaf, Washington, DC.

Demorest, M., & Bernstein, L. (1992). Sources of variability in speechreading sentences: A generalizability analysis. *Journal of Speech and Hearing Research, 35,* 876–891.

Duchnowski, P., Lum, D., Krause, J., Sexton, M., Bratakos, M., & Braida, L. (2000). Development of speechreading supplements based on automatic speech recognition. *IEEE Transactions on Biomedical Engineering, 47,* 487–496.

Eisenberg, L., Kirk, K., Martinez, A., Ying, E., & Miyamoto, R. (2004). Communication abilities of children with aided residual hearing: Comparison with cochlear implant users. *Archives of Otolaryngology, Head and Neck Surgery, 130,* 563–569.

Elliot, L., & Katz, D. (1980). *The Northwestern University-children's perception of speech test.* St. Louis, MO: Auditec.

Fisher, C. (1968). Confusions among visually perceived consonants. *Journal of Speech and Hearing Research, 11,* 796–804.

Gibert, G., Bailly, G., & Elisei, F. (2004). *Audiovisual text-to-cued speech synthesis.* Paper presented at the 5th ISCA Speech Synthesis Workshop, Pittsburgh, PA.

Hall, D., Fussell, C., & Summerfield, A. (2005). Reading fluent speech from talking faces: Typical brain networks and individual differences. *Journal of Cognitive Neuroscience, 17,* 939–953.

Iverson, P., Bernstein, L., & Auer, E. T., Jr. (1998). Modeling the interaction of phonemic intelligibility and lexical structure in audiovisual word recognition. *Speech Communication, 26,* 45–63.

Jeffers, J., & Barley, M. (1971). *Speechreading (Lipreading).* Springfield, IL: Charles C. Thomas.

Kirk, K., Pisoni, D., & Miyamoto, R. (2000). Lexical discrimination by children with cochlear implants: Effects of age at implantation and communication mode. In S. Waltzman & N. Cohen (Eds.), *Cochlear implants* (pp. 252–253). New York, NY: Thieme Medical Publishers.

Leybaert, J. (2000). Phonology acquired through the eyes and spelling in deaf children. *Journal of Experimental Child Psychology, 75,* 291–318.

Leybaert, J. (2003). *The role of Cued Speech in language processing by deaf children: An overview.* Paper presented at the AVSP, St. Jorioz, France.

Leybaert, J., & Lechat, J. (2001). Variability in deaf children's spelling: The effect of language experience. *Journal of Educational Psychology, 93,* 554–562.

Ling, D., & Ling, A. (1977). *Basic vocabulary and language thesaurus for hearing impaired children.* Washington, DC: A.G. Bell Association for the Deaf.

Luce, R. (1959). *Individual choice behavior.* New York, NY: Wiley.

Luce, P. (1986). *Neighborhoods of words in the mental lexicon* (Technical Report No. 6). Bloomington, IN: Indiana University, Department of Psychology, Speech Research Laboratory.

Luce, P., & Pisoni, D. (1998). Recognizing spoken words: The neighborhood activation model. *Ear and Hearing, 19,* 1–36.

MacEachern, E. (2000). On the visual distinctiveness of words in the English lexicon. *Journal of Phonetics, 28,* 367–376.

Martin, J., & Bunnell, H. (1981). Perception of anticipatory coarticulation effects. *Journal of the Acoustical Society of America, 69,* 559–567.

Martin, J., & Bunnell, H. (1982). Perception of anticipatory coarticulation effects in vowel-stop consonant-vowel sequences. *Journal of Experimental Psychology: Human Perception and Performance, 8,* 473–488.

Massaro, D. (1998). *Perceiving talking faces: From speech perception to a behavioral principle*. Cambridge, MA: MIT Press.

Massaro, D., & Light, J. (2004). Improving the vocabulary of children with hearing loss. *Volta Review, 104,* 141–174.

Mattys, S., Bernstein, L., & Auer, E. (2002). Stimulus-based lexical distinctiveness as a general word-recognition mechanism. *Perception and Psychophysics, 64,* 667–679.

Metzger, M., & Fleetwood, E. (1992). *Becoming a proficient cuer* [Videorecording]. Silver Spring, MD: Metzger and Fleetwood.

Mills, A. (1999). *An adventure in Cued Speech* [Videorecording]. Boise, ID: A. Mills.

Mohammed, T., Campbell, R., MacSweeney, M., Milne, E., Hansen, P., & Coleman, M. (2005). Speechreading skill and visual movement sensitivity are related in deaf speechreaders. *Perception, 34,* 205–216.

Montgomery, A., & Jackson, P. (1983). Physical characteristics of the lips underlying vowel lipreading performance. *Journal of the Acoustical Society of America, 73,* 2134–2144.

Nicholls, G. (1979). *Cued Speech and the reception of spoken language*. Montreal, Canada: McGill University.

Osberger, M. (1997). Current issues in cochlear implants in children. *Hearing Review,* 28–31.

Owens, E., & Blazek, B. (1985). Visemes observed by hearing-impaired and normal hearing adult viewers. *Journal of Speech and Hearing Research, 28,* 381–393.

Perier, O., Charlier, B., Hage, C., & Alegria, J. (1987). Evaluation of the effects of prolonged Cued Speech practice upon the reception of spoken language. In I.G. Taylor. (Ed.), *The education of the deaf—Current perspectives* (pp. 616–628). Kent, UK: Croom Helm.

Peterson, G., Wang, H., & Sivertsen, E. (1958). Segmentation techniques in speech synthesis. *Journal of the Acoustical Society of America, 30,* 739–742.

Pisoni, D., Cleary, M., Geers, A., & Tobey, E. (2000). Individual differences in effectiveness of cochlear implants in prelingually deaf children: Some new process measures of performance. *Volta Review, 101,* 111–164.

Rosenblum, L., & Saldana, H. (1998). Time-varying information for visual speech perception. In R. Campbell, B. Dodd, & D. Burnham. (Eds.), *Hearing by eye (Vol. II): Advances in the psychology of speechreading and auditory-visual speech* (pp. 61–81). East Sussex, Hove, UK: Psychology Press Ltd.

Ross, M., & Lerman, J. (1970). A picture identification test for hearing impaired children. *Journal of Speech and Hearing Research, 13,* 44–53.

Seitz, P., Bernstein, L., Auer, E., & MacEachern, M. (1998). *PhLex (Phonologically Transformable Lexicon): A 35,000-word computer readable pronouncing American English lexicon on structural principles, with accompanying phonological transformations, and word frequencies*. Los Angeles, CA: House Ear Institute.

Summerfield, Q. (1991). Visual perception of phonetic gestures. In I. G. Mattingly & M. Studdert-Kennedy (Eds.), *Modularity and the motor theory of speech perception* (pp. 117–137). Hillsdale, NJ: Lawrence Erlbaum Associates.

Uchanski, R., Delhorne, L., Dix, A., Braida, L., Reed, C., & Durlach, N. (1994). Automatic speech recognition to aid the hearing impaired: Prospects for the automatic generation of Cued Speech. *Journal of Rehabilitation Research and Development, 31,* 20–41.

Xue, J., Borgstrom, J., Jiang, J., Bernstein, L., & Alwan, A. (2006). *Acoustically-driven talking face animations using dynamic Bayesian networks*. Paper presented at the IEEE ICME, Toronto, Canada.

Chapter 19

ANALYSIS OF FRENCH CUED SPEECH PRODUCTION AND PERCEPTION: TOWARD A COMPLETE TEXT-TO-CUED SPEECH SYNTHESIZER

Virginie Attina, Guillaume Gibert, Marie-Agnès Cathiard, Gérard Bailly, and Denis Beautemps

Background for the Study

Our research, conducted at the Institut de la Communication Parlée (ICP, Institute of Speech Communication, Grenoble, France) focuses on understanding the temporal relationship between the manual components of Cued Speech and the nonmanual mouth movements in order to produce a virtual cueing head/hand for text-to-Cued Speech processing. In the first part of the chapter, we describe our research findings related to: (1) the temporal relationship between the production of the manual components of Cued Speech and the nonmanual components of Cued Speech and (2) how deaf users of Cued Speech predict the next syllable or word. This is discussed in the context of a perceptual and cogni-tive control approach. In the second part of the chapter, we describe our findings related to our complete system of text-to-Cued Speech audiovisual synthesis based on the temporal relationship principles described in Part I of this chapter together with preliminary evaluation of the intelligi-bility of the output of the synthesizer, which has applications to televised productions.

Part I: Temporal Relationship in the Production and Perception of Cued Speech

The fact that manual cues in Cued Speech must be associated with lip shapes to be effective for speech perception probably reveals a real link in the production of the hand movement and the speech; however, as yet, no fundamental study has been devoted to the analysis of the production of Cued Speech gestures (i.e., the temporal organization existing between lip movements and hand gestures in relation with speech sound). The research related in this first part focuses on how the components (i.e., manual handshapes and hand placements of cues, mouth movements, and speech sounds) of this communication system are linked together, in the time course of speech production.

In the literature related to Cued Speech, especially that which focuses on the practical aspects of Cued Speech for parents, speech therapists, and others who work with deaf children, several definitions and recommendations can be found on how hand cues should be provided relative to time course of speech. For example, Cornett (1994), noted that it was important to completely synchronize hand movements with speech sounds, since he defined Cued Speech as "A time-locked system; that is, the cues must synchronize with the spoken sounds. Every cue is essentially a hand movement that is timed relative to the sound" (p. 26). In his handbook, Beaupré (1997) provides numerous recommendations and practice exercises for synchronizing manual cues with speech. Hence, in the case of consonant-vowel (CV) syllables cueing, Beaupré indicates that the hand gesture towards the corresponding target hand position should start with the beginning of the syllable vocalization, thereby defining the onset as the synchronization instant. Most professionals who use Cued Speech seem to agree that particular attention should be paid to the synchronization of hand and speech movements (see the recommendations from the National Cued Speech Association of America [NCSA], 1994). Indeed, the correct synchronization of manual cues with visible speech (i.e., nonmanual mouth movements) is one of the criteria of evaluation for Cued Speech proficiency rating in the United States (see the basic Cued Speech proficiency rating in Beaupré, 1997). The term "synchronization," however, requires clarifications because to date, no one has really studied how manual cues, lip movements, and speech sounds are coordinated in time during Cued Speech production.

Synchronization of cues with speech has been an implicit issue with researchers who have applied technology to Cued Speech (Bratakos, Duchnowski, & Braida, 1998; Cornett, Beadles, & Wilson, 1977; Duchnowski et al., 2000). The first technologic adaptation of Cued Speech was the Autocuer (Cornett, 1982; Cornett et al., 1977), which displays cues as virtual images of a pair of seven-segment LED elements projected near the face of the talker in the viewing field of an eyeglass lens. Nine distinct symbol shapes, cueing consonant distinctions, can appear at each of four positions, cueing vowel distinctions. The phoneme identification results from audio speech recognizer processing. In their most advanced implementation of the Gallaudet-R.T.I. Autocuer (Cornett et al., 1977), Duchnowski et al. (2000) found that the speech recognizer required roughly 150 ms to derive and display a cue after the corresponding syllable was spoken. Note that the speech recognizer was based on the processing of the speech sound; thus the delay of the display was in reference to the audio part. Identification scores on isolated word tasks attained 84 versus 63% with lipreading alone. The effect of the 150 ms of delay was not discussed, however.

Bratakos and colleagues (1998) evaluated the effect of a delay of the cue appearance. They used an automatic cuer display coupled with an audio speech recognizer. In this system, cues consisting of images of hands were dubbed at appropriate locations onto recordings of the faces of talkers who spoke sentences. The authors found deleterious effects of recognizer delays on the effectiveness of these cues for speech perception: a delay of 165 ms (relative to the indicated beginning of the phone derived from the speech recognizer) in the cue display could reduce the score of 38 points with respect to the score due to a 10% error rate of speech recognizer alone.

As noted in Chapter 20, Duchnowski and colleagues (2000, p. 491) noticed an anticipation of the cue gesture with respect to the speech sound, noting that cuers often begin to form cues well before producing audible sound. Accordingly, Duchnowski et al. (2000) used this observation to enhance the performances of their automatic cuer generator. As in Bratakos et al. (1998), the cues were superimposed to the video recording of the talker face but the result was displayed continuously to the cue receiver (a delay of two seconds relative to the real talker was required for the whole process). To achieve a similar effect as observed with human cuers, the time at which cues were displayed at the right location was advanced by 100 ms relative to the start time determined by the audio-speech recognizer. This condition allowed for the best performances for the system.

To summarize, a review of the literature reflects that, surprisingly, at the turn of this 21st century, apart from the rule-of-thumb of the Duchnowski et al. (2000) system, the time course of the "natural" coordination in Cued Speech production has not been extensively studied.

Research Questions Related to Temporal Processing of Cued Speech

Our research focuses on the temporal relationship between the hand cues and mouth movements. Specifically, we are interested in the following questions:

1. Do the manual components of Cued Speech (i.e., handshape and placement) anticipate the nonmanual mouth movement of Cued Speech? If so, how much?
2. Do Cued Speech readers take advantage of this anticipatory phenomenon?
3. What explains this anticipatory production-perception behavior?

We hypothesize that it is the outcome of a basic compatibility between two similar controls, that is, one control related to the nonmanual mouth movement of Cued Speech associated with the vocal-tract and the second control related to the manual components of Cued Speech. If this is found to be true, it could be an argument for an integration of the Cued Speech manual components with the nonmanual mouth movement and the production of speech into a common motor mode. The originality of our approach lies in considering production and perception of Cued Speech as a linked perceptuomotor system within the Perception-for-Action-Control framework (Schwartz, Abry, Boë, & Cathiard, 2002).

An Original Method for Cued Speech Production Analysis

We studied Cued Speech production in order to describe for the first time the precise temporal relationships between hand movements and mouth movements with respect to sound units produced during CV syllabic sequences (Attina, Beautemps, Cathiard, & Odisio, 2004; Attina, Cathiard, & Beautemps, 2006). Our methodology was based on an audio-visual recording of four professional French Cued Speech transliterators simultaneously pronouncing and cueing sequences of CV syllables (Figure 19–1). The originality of the ICP Lip-Shape-Tracking System (Lallouache, 1991) is to deliver the whole lip configurations, which, in addition to visual cue measurements, is crucial for computing the acoustics of the output of the vocal-tract. To this end, the lips of the speaker are painted in blue, and colored marks are put on the back of the hand in order to automatically extract the parameters that convey the information from the videos. Data processing revealed: (1) the temporal evolution of the area between the lips; (2) the x and y positions of the colored hand markers in the two dimensional plane; (3) joint-angle measurements representing finger gestures for handshape formation (in case of additional use of a data glove); and (4) the corresponding synchronized acoustic signal. All of these time functions were labeled at different times, such as beginning and end of transitions or onset and offset of acoustic consonants and vowels (see Figure 19–1). This labeling allowed determining the temporal organization of the coordination between the different articulators involved.

Hand Anticipation: How Long Ahead of the Mouth Movements?

Using the method described above, we conducted several studies. The first was performed with one professional transliterator, referred to as GB here, who was recorded twice (Attina et al., 2004) while producing CV sequences simultaneously with cues and speech. In the data analysis, we focused first on hand transitions for one hand placement (corresponding to /ma/) to the next, such as /mi/. In a second experiment, with the same transliterator, we focused on transition from one handshape, such as /mi/ to the next, such as /pi/ using a data glove (CyberGlove®) illustrated in Figure 19–1.

The major result of both experiments was that the hand anticipated the corresponding mouth movements. Regarding hand placement, when cueing a CV syllable, the hand begins to move (M1, Figure 19–1) toward the appropriate placement (corresponding to the vowel) well in advance (200 ms) of the acoustic onset (A1) of the syllable (see Figure 19–1 and Table 19–1) (i.e., an anticipatory gain as long as the duration of a fairly long syllable). The hand reaches the Cued Speech target vowel placement (M2) during the first part of the acoustic consonant (after the beginning of its hold, A1), that is, well before the vocalic lip, or mouth target (L2). Thus, the anticipatory time span of the hand-vowel is clearly longer than the current anticipation of vocalic coarticulation in a CV speech sequence. A major finding related to the Cued Speech handshape, which corresponds to the consonant, is that the handshape starts to be formed (D1) during the hand placement transition and is completely shaped (D2) synchronously with the acoustic onset (A1) of the speech consonant (see Figure 19–1 and Table 19–1). In another series of experiments, we tested three other proficient French Cued Speech transliterators with a larger corpus of CV syllabic sequences (Attina et al., 2006).

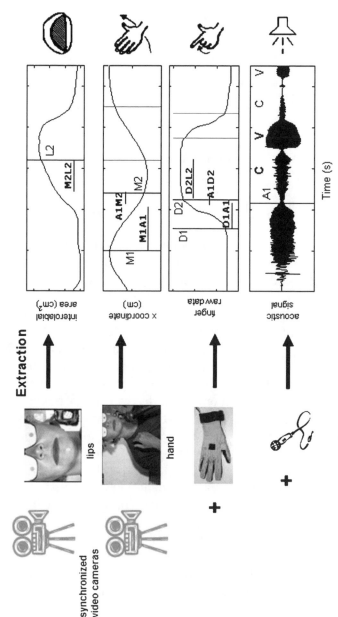

Figure 19–1. On the left, the general design for data acquisition. On the right, signal extraction. From top to bottom: temporal evolution of lip area (cm²); trajectory of the hand mark (cm); trajectory of the raw data from the glove sensor; and acoustic signal(s). On each signal, labeled events used for the analysis are indicated by vertical lines and temporal intervals are indicated. For the 1st CV syllable, L2 is the beginning of the labial vocalic target; M1 is the onset, and M2 the offset of the hand transition toward the vocalic position; D1 and D2 correspond to the phase of the handshape formation; and A1 represents the onset of the acoustic hold of the consonant.

453

Table 19–1. Mean Values and Standard Deviations of the Temporal Intervals (Obtained From Experiment With a Data Glove)

Temporal Intervals	Mean (ms)	Standard Deviation (ms)
M1A1	205	54
A1M2	33	50
M2L2	172	67
D1A1	171	48
A1D2	–3	45
D2L2	208	64

The same temporal pattern of coordination was found consistently for these three transliterators, thus confirming the anticipation of manual components as a general feature of French Cued Speech temporal organization.

Our observed temporal coordination between Cued Speech manual components and speech sound confirms the advance of the beginning of the hand gesture over the acoustics of sound, as implemented by Duchnowski et al. (2000) for their automatic Cued Speech display. Our findings contradict the standard view of Cued Speech, that is, the manual movements of Cued Speech disambiguate the simultaneously received nonmanual mouth movements related to speech. Our findings suggest the opposite (i.e., that hand placement precedes the mouth movement), thereby giving a set of possibilities for the vowel, and it is the mouth movements that disambiguate among these possibilities.

Is the Manual Anticipation Perceptively Efficient for Deaf Individuals?

We next examined how profoundly deaf receivers of French Cued Speech process this specific temporally related manual, nonmanual mouth information (Attina, Cathiard, & Beautemps, 2007; Cathiard, Attina, Abry, & Beautemps, 2004). We hypothesized that deaf individuals process the manual movement information prior to processing the mouth information. We concluded that we would confirm our hypothesis if we were able to observe: (1) for the vowel information, a correct identification score of the manual placement earlier than for the vowel mouth information; and (2) for the consonant, a quasisimultaneous identification of consonant handshape and mouth information.

The "gating" paradigm (Grosjean, 1980) was used for our perception experiment. It allows us to test specifically the temporal integration of both manual and mouth information by truncating video sequences of cued syllables at different moments, indeed six critical points such as when the hand placement or the vocalic lip target is reached. In the experiment, the syllables were made of CV sequences with C = [k,v,p,d] and V = [ɛ̃, ø, ɛ, ɔ]. The CVs to be identified were presented inside the /mytymaCVma/ nonsense logatome, such as /mytymadema/, to avoid the possibility of being predicted by the semantic context. For each of the truncated videos (presented in a random order), the 16 deaf participants were asked to identify both the consonant and the vowel from a list of possibilities. The results showed that the deaf participants used the manual information to anticipate the information on the mouth in order to predict the correct vowel, since the Cued Speech hand placement was correctly identified before the mouth target (the mean advance in this study was 155 ms). Moreover, the results showed a progressive identification of the stimuli, illustrating first a perceptual selection of a subset of consonant and vowel alternatives from the manual information, and then selection of the correct alternative when the mouth information finally was available.

Cornett's "Time Locked" Issue and the Compatibility of Controls in Cued Speech

We have found that the temporal organization of French Cued Speech as well as in perception by deaf individuals leads to a more complex view of Cued Speech than that held by Cornett (1994). Indeed, perception and production seem more tightly linked than was conceptualized by Cornett. What explains this anticipatory production-perception behavior? As we mentioned above, Cornett (1994) conceived Cued Speech to be a "time-locked system" (p. 26). To evaluate Cornett's conceptualization, we needed to consider how the coordination pattern varies within the syllabic domain.

First, our data showed that the manual transition movement duration (M1M2 in Figures 19-1 and Table 19–1) was relatively stable and did not vary with syllable duration (Attina, 2005). For that, we tested whether within the gesture duration (M1M2), there was a constant sum when adding the first phase (i.e., from gesture beginning [M1]) to the acoustic onset (A1), to the second phase (i.e., from this acoustic onset to the reaching point of the hand [M2]). A negative M1A1/A1M2

significant correlation was found (varying according to the subjects between −0.77 and −0.85, $p < .01$) in the linear relation between M1A1 and A1M2, characterized by a slope near −1, thus revealing that the total duration M1M2 of the manual transition is quasiconstant.

Second, we observed that for short syllable realizations, the hand gesture begins with a large advance on the acoustic onset (i.e., up to more than a syllable, reaching its final placement quite in synchrony with the consonant acoustic onset). For longer syllables, however, the hand gesture was less anticipated and could be completed quite after this consonant acoustic onset. Thus, it appears that the coordination between hand and speech varies according to the syllable duration. In our understanding, it seems that the cuer is less tightly constrained by the rather longer consonant of a long syllable and can thus delay more the hand gesture initiation in order to reach the Cued Speech placement during the consonant hold. However, this result reveals the link of the hand rhythm to the speech rhythm and thus confirms Cornett's (1994) intuitive formula of a "time-locked" phasing or a phase-locked hand/mouth control.

This phase-locking remains a topsy-turvy view of the Cued Speech organization that is opposed to the traditional one, in which the lips convey the core phonological information, the hand being secondarily considered (see, for example, Alegria, Charlier, & Mattys, 1999). Our data on production and perception showed that the deaf people take into account the hand information as soon as it is available. But, in this topsy-turvy view, the phase-locking is not synonymous with a general synchronicity: We clearly evidenced an articulated story (i.e., a common motor mode for the control of the Cued Speech hand and speech), in which the phase-locking of the hand to the speech consonantal hold can explain the asynchronicity of the hand, anticipating on the speech vowel, largely in advance on the mouth.

To demonstrate this hypothesis, we now consider the three types of control classically met in speech. One is proximal (the carrier) and the other two are distal controls (the carried ones). In this framework, the control of the mandibular open–close oscillation can be considered as the carrier of speech (following Abry, Stefanuto, Vilain, & Laboissière, 2002; MacNeilage, 1998), that is, the proximal control which produces the syllabic rhythm. The carried articulators (i.e., the tongue and the lower lip) together with their coordinated partners (i.e., upper lip, velum, and larynx) are involved in the distal control. Following Öhman (1967) (see also Vilain, Abry, & Badin, 2000), the consonant gesture is produced by the local control of contact and pressure performed on local parts along the vocal tract; while the vowel gesture is produced by a global control of the whole vocal tract—from the glottis to the lips (i.e., a figural or postural motor control type).

Let us now consider the two Cued Speech components in terms of control. For transmitting the Cued Speech *consonant* information, the control type is a figural one, that is, the postural control of the Cued Speech hand configuration. The type of control for transmitting the Cued Speech *vowel* information is a goal-directed (aiming) movement, placing the finger configuration at a defined position respectively to the face. In doing this, the hand is carried by the wrist, which is carried by the arm. Thus, once speech rhythm has been converted into Cued Speech rhythm, that is, a general CV syllabification, the two

carriers, the mandible and the wrist, operate within their temporal coordination in a coupled entrainment.

The control type of the Cued Speech vowel carried gesture corresponds to the one of a goal-directed movement, which aims at a local placement of the hand on/around the face; whereas the Cued Speech consonant carried gesture needs a postural (figural) control. Thus, the two types of control in Cued Speech are inversely distributed: In comparison to speech, the "configurational" global control of the speech vowel corresponds to a local control in Cued Speech, whereas the local control for the speech consonant corresponds to a global control in Cued Speech.

So far, the Cued Speech code represents a unique system closely binding the hand and the speech. In our view, it is the outcome of a basic compatibility between the two similar controls: the one for approximating the articulators in the production of the speech consonant, and the one for aiming at different placements of the hand around the face. This reveals a phasing of the two local components (the Cued Speech hand position on/around the face in synchrony with the articulatory realization of the consonant) explaining the anticipation of the hand.

Since our answer is definitely "yes" to this compatibility in control issue, an argument can be made for an integration of the Cued Speech hand within speech into a common motor mode. This preserves the cognitive compatibility of controls in learning Cued Speech, in spite of the claims of a postlipreading disambiguation or a global synchronization stated by its promoters and defenders. This view accounts for the exploitation of the time unfolding of the coordination pattern for its perception. Such a production-perception organization favors that the deaf, via the visual modality, can recover the hand-mouth controls. This control retrieval, in order to master perception, typically is one of the principles of the perception-for-action-control theory (Schwartz et al., 2002), which adds to the classical motor theory of speech perception (Liberman & Mattingly, 1985), perceptual constraints, offering an integrated perceptuomotor version of speech —here, Cued Speech—processing.

Part II: From Recording the 3-D Movements of the Head, Face, and Hand of a Speaker Using Cued Speech to a Virtual Cued Speech Cuer

Taking advantage of the work that has been devoted to Cued Speech in our lab has allowed us to create a Cued Speech synthesis system, a domain in which very few realizations have been achieved (see first attempts by Attina et al., 2004; Duchnowski et al., 2000, and Chapter 20 in this volume). In this section, we describe a multimodal text-to-speech system for broadcast television, which drives a virtual Cued Speech speaker and its first evaluation by deaf users. This system was developed at the Institut de la Communication Parlée in the framework of the ARTUS project (Bailly et al., 2007). The technologic and scientific challenge addressed by ARTUS is to build a virtual talking agent (VTA), similar to Baldi that conveys spoken language (see Chapter 22 by Massaro, Carreira-Perpiñán, & Merrill). ARTUS is able to produce French Cued Speech from an unconstrained textual input. This VTA (Figure 19–2) can then be superimposed—on demand and at the reception—in the original broadcast as an

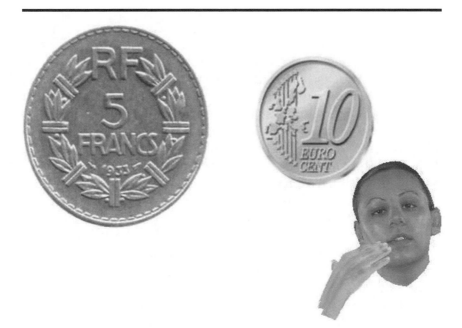

Figure 19–2. Superimposition of the ARTUS virtual speech cuer in a program of the French/German TV channel ARTE.

alternative to subtitling. ARTUS further proposes solutions to embed computed hand, head, and face gestures of the VTA in the broadcasted audiovisual sequence (watermarking). The real-time transparent transmission of animation parameters permits the online control of the VTA by movements captured on a human French Cued Speech transliterator (for news or live talk shows). Other uses of the virtual speech cuer include computer-assisted telecommunication and French Cued Speech learning.

The VTA is parameterized using analysis results of real 3-D hand, head, and face movements captured on a human speaker. We first describe the main features of this experimental work, and then present the components of the complete text-to-Cued Speech synthesizer that are based on the production study and the results of its formal evaluation.

Data Recording

Our female target speaker is a nonprofessional hearing French Cued Speech talker with a dozen years of intensive everyday practice in her home environment. The postexperimental evaluation of her cueing performance (less than 1% of cueing errors and high intelligibility scores) demonstrates that she can compete with professional transliterators. We recorded the 3-D positions of 113 markers glued on the hand and face of our subject using a Vicon© motion capture system with 12 cameras (Figure 19–3). 3-D positions of candidate markers are recorded at 120 Hz. Two different settings of the cameras enabled us to record three corpora: (1) handshapes transitions produced in free space, (2) visemes with no complementary French Cued Speech gestures, and (3) a corpus of sentences uttered with French Cued Speech. The two first corpora were used to build statistical models of the hand and face movements separately. These models were then used to characterize and regularize noisy data from the third corpus as Cued Speech gestures may occlude parts of the face and the fingers to surrounding cameras.

Data Modeling

Statistical shape models of the hand and face built from raw motion capture give access to a detailed analysis of French Cued Speech production. If the positions of markers are reliable and precise enough, we have access to the kinematics of the articulation, of the fingertips and fingers/face constrictions and to the laws governing the coordination between acoustics, face, and hand movements during Cued Speech production.

Face

The basic methodology developed at ICP for cloning facial articulation consists of an iterative linear analysis (Badin et al., 2002; Revéret, Bailly, & Badin, 2000) using the first principal component of different subsets of flesh points. We subtract iteratively the contribution of the jaw rotation, the lips rounding/spreading gesture, the proper vertical movements of upper and lower lips, of the lip corners as well as the movement of the throat to the residual data obtained by iteratively subtracting their contributions to the original motion capture data. These operations are performed using the motion capture data of the face from the second and third corpora where all markers are visible.

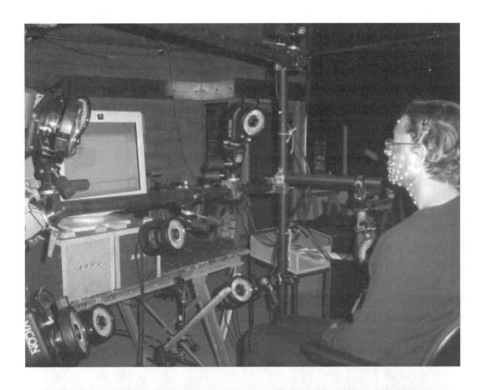

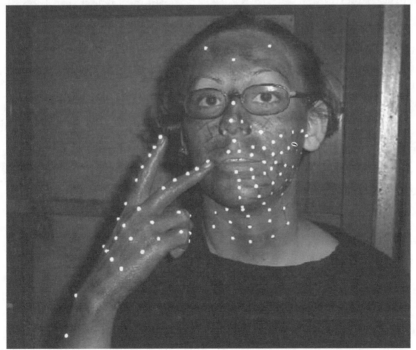

Figure 19–3. Motion capture using a Vicon© system with 12 cameras (*top*) and 63 beads glued on the face and 50 on the hand (*bottom*).

Hand

Building a statistical model of the hand formations is a more complex task. We hypothesize that the forearm is the carrier of the hand: the 50 markers undergo a rigid motion that will be considered as the forearm motion. Therefore, the movements of the wrist, the palm, and the phalanges of the fingers have a quite complex nonlinear influence on the 3-D positions of the markers. The underlying rotations of the joints are poorly reflected by these positions: skin deformation induced by the muscle and skin tissues produces very large variations of the distances between markers glued on the same phalange. To resolve these constraints, a two-stage nonlinear model was built. All possible angles between hand segment and the forearm and between successive phalanges (rotation, twisting, spreading) were first computed and the first principal components of this set of data were retained as control parameters. A simple linear regression is performed that predicts x, y, z coordinates of all hand points from sinuses and cosines of all angles.

Results

We retained nine handshape parameters and seven face parameters. The resulting average absolute modeling error for the position of the visible markers is equal to 1.2 mm for the hand and 1 mm for the face (Gibert, Bailly, Beautemps, Elisei, & Brun, 2005).

Motion Capture Data Analysis

Before implementing the multimodal text-to-speech, we needed to segment the ges-tural scores produced by our speaker into elementary gestural units and characterize the phasing relations between hand movements and speech for that particular speaker.

Automatic Recognition of Handshape

We selected a target frame for each of the eight hand gestures of French Cued Speech and assigned them with the appropriate key value (i.e., a number between 0 and 8: 0 is dedicated to the rest position chosen by the cuer with a closed knuckle). These target frames were carefully chosen by plotting the values of seven parameters against time:

- The absolute distance between the flesh points of the first phalange closest to the palm and that closest to the fingertip for each finger: an extension corresponds to a maximal value whereas retraction corresponds to a minimal value.
- The absolute distance between the tips of the index and middle finger in order to differentiate between handshape 2 (coding [k, v, z]) versus 8 (coding [j, ŋ]).
- The absolute distance between the tip of the thumb and the palm in order to differentiate between handshapes 1 ([p, b, m]) versus 6 ([l, ʃ, ɲ, w]), and 2 ([k, v, z]) versus 7 ([g]).

In total, 4,114 handshapes were identified and labeled. Simple Gaussian models are estimated for each handshape using the seven characteristic parameters associated with these targets.

Automatic Recognition of Hand Placement

The labels of nine handshape targets were added—set by the procedure described above—a key value for the hand placement (between 0 and 5: 0 corresponds to the rest position). Handshape and placement targets were added for single vowels and labeled with handshape 5 while the rest position (closed knuckle far from the face) was labeled with hand placement 0. Simple Gaussian models were estimated for each hand placement using the hand placement for these target configurations in a 3-D referential linked to the head. This hand placement was defined by the 3-D position of the longest finger (index for handshape 1 and 6 and middle finger for the others).

The a posteriori probability for each frame to belong to each of the nine handshape and six hand placement models was then estimated. Despite application of single Gaussian models, recognition scores were very high: the channels that had the highest probability at target frames did correspond to the manually labeled handshapes and positions (4,114 frames) respectively 98.14 and 95.52% of the cases. True errors (not due to simplistic modeling but to wrong cues provided by our speaker) mainly concern mid-open vowels.

We show in Figure 19–4 the time course of these probability functions over one utterance of the corpus together with the acoustic signal. We further analyzed and characterized the profile of handshape and hand placement gestures in reference to the acoustic realization of the accompanying speech segment. The extension of a gesture is defined as the time interval where the probability of the appropriate key (shape or placement) dominates the other competing keys. We excluded from the analysis adjacent segments with two identical keys.

Our data gathered valuable information on phasing relations between speech and hand gestures and confirmed the advance of the hand onset gesture with reference to lip movements and sound already shown by Attina et al. (2004, 2006; see also Part I of this chapter) on other subjects. Not only did the maximal extension/retraction of the fingers coincide most of the time with the acoustic onset of the consonant, but also the hand placement: Cued Speech provided both cues for the upcoming vowel and the consonant together, far ahead of the actual realization of the segments. As also noted in Part I, we observed important variability around this prototypical behavior. Our text-to-Cued Speech synthesis system, however, adopts the average phasing relation that synchronizes gestural targets (full extension of the handshape and placement) with the consonantal acoustic onset in CV and C-schwas and with vocalic acoustic onset for isolated vowels.

Multimodal Generation

The corpus of 238 sentences offers an extensive coverage of the movements implied by French Cued Speech, and we have designed the first audiovisual text-to-Cued Speech synthesis system using concatenation of various multimodal speech segments. This system, to our knowledge, is the first that generates hand and face movements and deformations together with speech using the concatenation of gestural and acoustic units. Two units are considered: polysounds for the generation of the acoustic signal and the facial

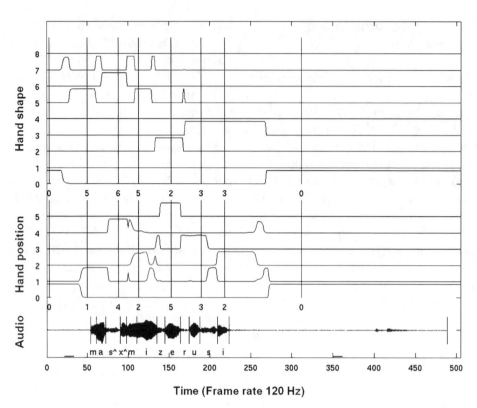

Figure 19–4. Recognition of the handshape (*top*) and the hand placement (*bottom*) by simple Gaussian models.

movements (a polysound is the part of speech from one stable part of a sound to the next; sounds such as semivowels and glides are not considered as having a sufficiently stable part and are included into larger segments) and di-keys for the generation of head and hand movements (a di-key is the part of gesture from one gestural target to the next).

Multimodal generation from phonetic input is thus accomplished in two steps: (1) sound and facial movements are generated by a concatenative synthesis using polysounds as basic units while (2) the head and hand movements are generated by a second concatenative synthesis using di-keys as basic units. Note that head

movements do entirely contribute to the realization of hand-face constrictions; that is, on average, 16% of the constriction gesture is done by the head.

Once selected, these di-keys are further aligned with the middle of the consonant for a full CV realization, vocalic onsets for isolated vowels and consonantal onsets for isolated consonants. If the full di-key does not exist, we seek for replacement di-keys by replacing the second hand placement of the di-key by the closest one that exists in the di-key dictionary. The proper di-key will still be realized by VTA because an anticipatory smoothing procedure (Bailly, Gibert, & Odisio, 2002) is applied that considers the onset of each di-key as the intended target: a linear interpolation of hand placement applied gradually within each di-key copes thus easily with a small (or even larger) change of the final target imposed by the onset target frame of the next concatenated di-key.

Videorealistic Animation

The text-to-Cued Speech synthesis system sketched above delivers trajectories of a few flesh points placed on the surface of the right hand and face. High definition models of these organs are then mapped onto the existing face and hand parameter space. A further appearance model using video-realistic textures is then added (Figure 19–5).

The Text-to-French Cued Speech System

We have described above the modules responsible for synthesis and parameter generation. The system, of course, performs a complete structural linguistic analysis of the input text in order to provide the generation module with the proper string of phonemes, syllabic organization, and prosodic information. This front end does not really differ from a standard text-to-speech system with the exception of the prosodic module that has to be adapted to the particular rhythmical organization of French Cued Speech that superimposes a basic CV structuring to usual suprasegmental beats such as the syllable, the word, or the foot. Prosody includes the organization of phoneme durations, audible cues such as pauses or melody, and visible cues such as head movements. Even though experienced speech cuers can minimize the impact of hand gestures on speech rate, the inertia of the arm imposes a slower articulation especially for complex syllables. A trainable prosodic generator (Bailly & Holm, 2005) has been fed with Cued Speech data. In the three TV programs we have processed so far, only four sentences could not be pronounced in the time interval devoted to their initial subtitling. The average delay for these sentences was 120 ms (corresponding roughly

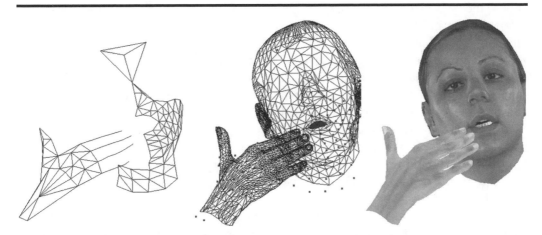

Figure 19–5. The virtual cuer from motion capture data to a video-realistic animation.

to one syllable); note however that the generation of these time-stamps is performed without any automatic procedure that verifies that viewers have sufficient time to effectively read—and thus pronounce—the subtitles.

Evaluation

A first series of experiments have been conducted to evaluate the intelligibility of this virtual cuer with skilled deaf users of the French Cued Speech (Gibert, 2006). The first evaluation campaign was dedicated to segmental intelligibility. This test was conducted to assess the contribution of the cueing gestures in comparison with lipreading alone.

Minimal Pairs

The test mirrors the Modified Diagnostic Rime Test developed for French by Peckels and Rossi (1973): the minimal pairs here not testing acoustic *phonetic* features but *gestural* ones. We developed a list of CVC word pairs to test systematically pairs of consonants in initial positions that differ almost only in handshapes: we choose the consonants in all pairs of eight subsets of consonants that are highly visually confusable (Odisio & Bailly, 2004 for French; Summerfield, 1991). The vocalic substrate was chosen so as to cover all potential hand positions, whereas the final consonant was chosen to avoid rarely used French words or proper names and test our ability to handle coarticulation effects. Due to the fact that minimal pairs cannot be found in all vocalic substrates, we end up with a list of 196 word pairs.

In order to avoid a completely still head, head movements of the lipreading-only condition are those produced by the text-to-Cued Speech synthesizer divided by a factor 10. No attempt is made to modify segmental or suprasegmental settings that could have enhance articulation.

Minimal pairs are presented randomly and in both orders. The lipreading-only condition is tested first. The Cued Speech condition is then presented in order to be able to summon up cognitive resources for the most difficult task first. Eight adult subjects were tested. They are all individuals with hearing impairment who have used French Cued Speech since the age of three years.

Results

Mean intelligibility rate for "lipreading" condition is 52.36%. It is not different from random distribution of responses: minimal pairs are not distinguishable using lipreading only. Mean intelligibility rate for French Cued Speech is 94.26%. The difference in terms of intelligibility rate between these two conditions shows that our virtual cuer gives significant information in terms of hand movements. In terms of cognitive efforts, the "Cued Speech" task is easier: the response time is also significantly different (Kruskall-Wallis test, $p < 0.01$) and lower than for the "lipreading" one.

Conclusion

The observation and recordings of Cued Speech in action have allowed us to implement a complete text-to-French Cued Speech synthesizer. The results of the preliminary perceptive tests show that significant linguistic information with minimal cognitive effort is transmitted by our system. This new technology may provide a valuable aid to deaf users for accessing numeric content and services.

Several technologic and scientific challenges still have to be overcome to widely distribute this innovative system: If high-quality segmental generation is obtained, suprasegmental organization of the synthetic French Cued Speech should be improved. Gestural strategies that ease discourse segmentation, identification of hierarchy between constituents as well as emphasis of parts-of-speech have to be identified and modeled. These aspects are of most importance for discourse processing and comprehension since cognitive resources already highly solicited by French Cued Speech phonetic decoding should not only be devoted to linguistic processing.

References

Abry, C., Stefanuto, M., Vilain, A., & Laboissière, R. (2002). What can the utterance "tan, tan" of Broca's patient Leborgne tell us about the hypothesis of an emergent "babble-syllable" downloaded by SMA? In J. Durand & B. Laks (Eds.), *Phonetics, phonology, and cognition* (pp. 226–243). Oxford, UK: Oxford University Press.

Alegria, J., Charlier, B., & Mattys, S. (1999). The role of lip-reading and Cued Speech in the processing of phonological information in French-educated deaf children. *European Journal of Cognitive Psychology, 11*, 451–472.

Attina, V. (2005). *La Langue Française Parlée Complétée (LPC): Production et perception.* Unpublished Ph.D. thesis, Institut National Polytechnique de Grenoble, Grenoble, France.

Attina, V., Beautemps, D., Cathiard, M.-A., & Odisio, M. (2004). A pilot study of temporal organization in Cued Speech production of French syllables: Rules for a Cued Speech synthesizer. *Speech Communication, 44*, 197–214.

Attina, V., Cathiard, M.-A., & Beautemps, D. (2006). Temporal measures of hand and speech coordination during French Cued Speech production. In S. Gibet, N. Courty, & J.-F. Kamp (Eds.), *Gesture in human-computer interaction and simulation, Vol. 3881* (pp. 13–24). Berlin Heidelberg, Germany: Springer-Verlag.

Attina, V., Cathiard, M.-A., & Beautemps, D. (2007). French Cued Speech: From production to perception and vice-versa. *AMSE-Advances in Modeling, 67*, 188–197.

Badin, P., Bailly, G., Reveret, L., Baciu, M., Segebarth, C., & Savariaux, C. (2002). Three-dimensional linear articulatory modeling of tongue, lips and face, based on MRI and video images. *Journal of Phonetics, 30*, 533–553.

Bailly, G., Attina, V., Baras, C., Bas, P., Baudry, S., Beautemps, D., . . . Nguyen, P. (2007). ARTUS: Synthesis and audiovisual watermarking of the movements of a virtual agent interpreting subtitling using Cued Speech for deaf televiewers. *AMSE-Advances in Modelling, 67*, 177–187.

Bailly, G., Gibert, G., & Odisio, M. (2002). Evaluation of movement generation systems using the point-light technique. *Proceedings of 2002 IEEE Workshop on Speech Synthesis*, Santa Monica, CA, pp. 27–30.

Bailly, G., & Holm, B. (2005). SFC: A trainable prosodic model. *Speech Communication, 46*, 348–364.

Beaupré, W. (1997). *Gaining Cued Speech proficiency. A manual for parents, teachers, and clinicians.* Web Edition. Retrieved September 4, 2006, from http://www.uri.edu/comm_service/cued_speech/gcsphome.html

Bratakos, M., Duchnowski, P., & Braida, L. (1998). Toward the automatic generation of Cued Speech. *Cued Speech Journal, 6*, 1–37.

Cathiard, M.-A., Attina, V., Abry, C., & Beautemps, D. (2004). La Langue Française Parlée Complétée (LPC): Sa coproduction avec la parole et l'organisation temporelle de sa perception. In J.-L. Nespoulous & J. Virbel (Eds.), *Handicap langagier et recherches cognitives: Apports mutuels (II)* (Vol. 31–32, pp. 255–280). Mons, Belgique: Université de Mons-Hainaut.

Cornett, R. O. (1982). Le Cued Speech. In F. Destombes (Ed.), *Aides Manuelles à la Lecture*

Labiale et perspectives d'aides automatiques (pp. 5–15). Paris: Centre Scientifique IBM-France.

Cornett, R. O. (1994). Adapting Cued Speech to additional languages. *Cued Speech Journal, 5*, 19–29.

Cornett, R., Beadles, R., & Wilson, B. (1977). Automatic Cued Speech. *Research Conference on Speech Processing Aids for the Deaf*, 224–239.

Duchnowski, P., Lum, D., Krause, J., Sexton, M., Bratakos, M., & Braida, L. (2000). Development of speechreading supplements based on automatic speech recognition. *IEEE Transactions on Biomedical Engineering, 47*, 487–496.

Gibert, G. (2006). *Conception et évaluation d'un système de synthèse 3-D de Langue française Parlée Complétée (LPC) à partir du texte.* Unpublished Ph.D. thesis, Institut National Polytechnique de Grenoble, Grenoble, France.

Gibert, G., Bailly, G., Beautemps, D., Elisei, F., & Brun, R. (2005). Analysis and synthesis of the three-dimensional movements of the head, face, and hand of a speaker using Cued Speech. *Journal of the Acoustical Society of America, 118*, 1144–1153.

Grosjean, F. (1980). Spoken word recognition processes and the gating paradigm. *Perception and Psychophysics, 28*, 267–283.

Lallouache, M.-T. (1991). *Un poste visage-parole couleur. Acquisition et traitement automatique des contours des lèvres.* Unpublished Ph.D. thesis, Institut National Polytechnique de Grenoble, Grenoble, France.

Liberman, A., & Mattingly, I. (1985). The motor theory of speech perception revised. *Cognition, 21*, 1–36.

MacNeilage, P. (1998). The frame/content theory of evolution of speech production. *Behavioral and Brain Sciences, 21*, 499–548.

National Cued Speech Association. (NCSA). (1994). Guidelines on the mechanics of cueing. *Cued Speech Journal, 5*, 73–80.

Odisio, M., & Bailly, G. (2004). Tracking talking faces with shape and appearance models. *Speech Communication, 44*, 63–82.

Öhman, S. (1967). Numerical model of coarticulation. *Journal of the Acoustical Society of America, 41*, 310–320.

Peckels, J., & Rossi, M. (1973). Le test de diagnostic par paires minimales. Adaptation au francais du 'Diagnostic Rhyme Test' de W.D. Voiers. *Revue d'Acoustique, 27*, 245–262.

Revéret, L., Bailly, G., & Badin, P. (2000). MOTHER: A new generation of talking heads providing a flexible articulatory control for video-realistic speech animation. *Proceedings of the International Conference on Speech and Language Processing*, Beijing, China, 755–758.

Schwartz, J., Abry, C., Boë, L., & Cathiard, M. (2002). Phonology in a theory of perception-for-action-control. In J. Durand & B. Laks (Eds.), *Phonetics, phonology and cognition* (pp. 254–280). Oxford, UK: Oxford University Press.

Summerfield, Q. (1991). Visual perception of phonetic gestures. In I. G. Mattingly & M. Studdert-Kennedy (Eds.), *Modularity and the motor theory of speech perception* (pp. 117–138). Hillsdale, NJ: Lawrence Erlbaum Associates.

Vilain, A., Abry, C., & Badin, P. (2000). Coproduction strategies in French VCVs: Confronting Öhman's model with adult and developmental articulatory data. *Proceedings of the 5th seminar on speech production. Models and data*. Kloster Seon, Bavaria, 81–84.

Chapter 20

DEVELOPMENT OF SPEECHREADING SUPPLEMENTS BASED ON AUTOMATIC SPEECH RECOGNITION[1]

Paul Duchnowski, David S. Lum, Jean C. Krause,
Matthew G. Sexton, Maroula S. Bratakos, and
Louis D. Braida,* *Member, IEEE*

Abstract

In manual-cued speech (MCS) a speaker produces hand gestures to resolve ambiguities among speech elements that are often confused by speechreaders. The shape of the hand distinguishes among consonants; the position of the hand relative to the face distinguishes among vowels. Experienced receivers of MCS achieve nearly perfect reception of everyday connected speech. MCS has been taught to very young deaf children and greatly facilitates language learning, communication, and general education.

[1]© 2000 IEEE. Reprinted, with permission, from *IEEE Transactions on Biomedical Engineering*, Vol. 47, No. 4, April 2000, pp. 487–496.

*Manuscript received December 30, 1997; revised January 4, 2000. This work was supported by the National Institute on Deafness and Other Communication Disorders, the H. E. Warren Professorship at Massachusetts Institute of Technology (M.I.T.), and the Motorola Corporation. Asterisk indicates corresponding author. P. Duchnowski is with the Research Laboratory of Electronics, Massachusetts Institute of Technology, Cambridge, MA 012139 USA. D. S Lum, J. C. Krause, M. G. Sexton, and M. S. Bratakos are with the Research Laboratory of Electronics, Massachusetts Institute of Technology, Cambridge, MA 02139 USA. L. D. Braida is with the Research Laboratory of Electronics, 36-747, Massachusetts Institute of Technology, Cambridge, MA, 02139, USA (e-mail: braida@mit.edu). Publisher Item Identifier S 0018-9294(00)02640-9.

This manuscript describes a system that can produce a form of cued speech automatically in real time and reports on its evaluation by trained receivers of MCS. Cues are derived by a hidden markov models (HMM)-based speaker-dependent phonetic speech recognizer that uses context-dependent phone models and are presented visually by superimposing animated hand shapes on the face of the talker. The benefit provided by these cues strongly depends on articulation of hand movements and on precise synchronization of the actions of the hands and the face. Using the system reported here, experienced cue receivers can recognize roughly two-thirds of the keywords in cued low-context sentences correctly, compared to roughly one-third by speechreading alone (SA). The practical significance of these improvements is to support fairly normal rates of reception of conversational speech, a task that is often difficult via SA.

Introduction

The ability to see and interpret the facial actions that accompany speech production can enhance communication in difficult listening conditions substantially (Grant & Braida, 1991). Although listeners with normal hearing can benefit from integrating cues derived from speechreading with those conveyed by the speech waveform, for many listeners with severe hearing impairments, speechreading is the principal mode of communication. However, speechreading alone (SA) typically provides only a minimal basis for communication because many distinctions between speech elements are not manifest visually. While some of the resulting ambiguity can be overcome if the receiver makes use of

contextual redundancy, the concomitant demands on attention and memory are often daunting (Douglas-Cowie, 1988). Even when dealing with easy material that is spoken slowly, with repetitions, and that is viewed under optimal reception conditions, speechreaders typically miss more than one-third of the words spoken.

Although several means are available to help persons who are deaf overcome the limitations associated with speechreading, none are without limitations. One approach, the use of sign language (Klima & Bellugi, 1979) supports high levels of communication, linguistic development, and general education, but is based on a language other than English, so that reading skills are not always well developed (Wandel, 1989). A second approach, electrical stimulation of the peripheral auditory system, can evoke auditory sensations that are highly effective speechreading supplements for many deaf adults, and enables many to communicate without the use of speechreading (Osberger, Fisher, Zimmerman-Phillips, Geier, & Baker, 1998; Clark, 1998). However, not all deaf adults are helped by this approach, perhaps because the benefits provided by cochlear implants depend on the number of peripheral auditory neurons surviving. In addition, in current medical practice the implantation of deaf infants is restricted to those beyond the age of two years, well beyond the point at which deafness can be detected and well after normal-hearing infants begin to acquire speech and language skills. A third approach is based on the presentation of speechreading supplements via the visual or tactile senses. These supplements are intended to enable the speechreader to make distinctions between elements or patterns of speech that are not possible via SA.

Although there are many types of such supplements, it is useful to distinguish between two different types. One type uses signal processing techniques to derive parameters or waveforms from acoustic speech (e.g., voice pitch, the speech amplitude envelope contour, etc.), and codes them for presentation to the speechreader. The other type uses automatic speech recognition (ASR) techniques to derive a sequence of discrete symbols from the speech waveform. Many examples of the former type have been evaluated, including those that present the supplements to the visual (Upton, 1968; Ebrahimi and Kunov, 1991), and tactile (Oller, 1995) senses and several tactile speechreading aids are currently in use by deaf individuals. No supplements based on speech recognition, such as those related to the system of cued speech developed for the education of deaf persons, appear to be in use at the present time. In Section II [Cued Speech], we describe cued speech and review previous attempts to develop speechreading supplements based on cued speech. In Section III [Automatic Cue Generating Systems], we outline the operation of the automatic cueing systems evaluated in the current study. In Section IV [Evaluation Methods], we describe the methods used to evaluate the reception of automatically cued speech (ACS). In Section V [Results], we report the results of these evaluations. In Section VI [Discussion], we compare the results obtained in this study with those reported for other aids for the deaf and identify problems to be addressed in future research.

Cued Speech

In cued speech, communication relies on a combination of speechreading and a synchronous sequence of discrete symbols. The symbols attempt to help the receiver distinguish between speech elements with similar facial articulations. Several different systems of cued speech that have been developed share several common elements. Each symbol in the sequence is typically displayed while a CV syllable is articulated. The symbol typically consists of two components or indicators, one for the consonant and the other for the vowel. Each consonant indicator represents a group of consonants that are readily distinguished by SA. Similarly, each vowel indicator represents a group of vowels that are readily distinguished by SA. For ease of reception, the consonant and vowel indicators are typically displayed by perceptually independent elements.

Within these constraints, a wide variety of cued speech systems can be defined. In manual-cued speech (MCS), developed more than 30 years ago by Cornett (Cornett, 1967), the indicator for vowels is the position of the hand relative to the face of the talker. The vowels are divided into four groups, each having the property that its members can be distinguished by speechreading. Similarly, the indicator for consonants, which are divided into eight groups, is the shape of the hand. An alternative system, *Q-codes*, was proposed (Fant, 1970), for Swedish and subsequently adapted to Japanese (Hiki & Fukuda, 1981). In these systems, the assignment of consonants and vowels to groups was based on acoustic-phonetic dimensions that were thought to be easy to detect automatically in the acoustic speech waveform. The set of hand shapes used to represent the consonant groups differ from those of MCS, with specific aspects of shape conveying phonemic distinctions. For example, the spread of the thumb is used to distinguish voiced from unvoiced consonants.

There is no general agreement on the optimal number or constitution of cue groups, either for consonants or vowels. Recent research at Massachusetts Institute of Technology (M.I.T.) has explored methods for constructing such groups automatically (Uchanski, Delhorne, Dix, Reed, Braida, & Durlach, 1994), based on the accuracy with which the speech elements can be recognized by an automatic recognizer and the perceptual confusions made by speechreaders. The recognizers available at that time were estimated to aid speech reception maximally when only a relatively small number of groups was used.

Parents and educators have taught the MCS system successfully to very young deaf children, who have subsequently used the system to facilitate communication, language learning, and general education. Several studies have documented the benefits MCS can provide to speech reception (Kaplan, 1974; Ling & Clarke, 1975; Clarke & Ling, 1976; Nicholls & Ling, 1982). For example, after seven years of MCS use, 18 teenagers were able to identify words in low-context sentences with an accuracy of 26% by SA versus 97% via MCS (Nicholls & Ling, 1982). Studies of highly experienced users of MCS conducted at our laboratory have found similar gains for keywords in low-context IEEE sentences (IEEE, 1969) with scores improving from 25% to 31% for SA to 84% for MCS (Uchanski et al., 1994; Bratakos, Duchnowski, & Braida, 1997). Comparable evaluations of alternative cueing systems are not available.

To derive real benefit from cued speech in everyday communication, the talker, or a transliterator, must produce cues for the receiver. However, the number of individuals who are proficient at producing MCS is relatively small, perhaps several thousand, so that cued speech is not widely used by the deaf. To overcome this limitation, Cornett and his colleagues at Gallaudet University and the Research Triangle Institute (R.T.I.) attempted to develop an "Autocuer," a system that would derive cues similar to those of MCS automatically, by electronic analysis of the acoustic speech signal, and display them visually to the cue receiver.

The Gallaudet-R.T.I. Autocuer

The most advanced implementation of the Gallaudet-R.T.I. Autocuer (Cornett, Beadles, & Wilson, 1977) displays cues as virtual images of a pair of seven-segment LED elements projected near the face of the talker in the viewing field of an eyeglass lens. Nine distinct symbol shapes, cueing consonant distinctions, can appear at each of four positions, cueing vowel distinctions.

The operation of the speech analysis subsystem used in the wearable version of the Autocuer has not been described publicly. A published block diagram of the system suggests that speech sounds would be assigned to cue groups on the basis of estimates of the voice pitch as well as the zero crossing rates and peak-to-peak amplitudes in low- and high-frequency bands of speech. Evaluations of the performance of the most recent implementation of the Autocuer (R. Beadles, personal communication, August 31, 1989) indicate that the phoneme identification score is roughly 54%, with a 33% deletion rate and a 13% substitution rate.

The Gallaudet-R.T.I. development effort used simulation techniques to estimate the level of recognition performance that would be required for a successful Autocuer system. Speech reception tests were conducted both with "ideal" cues derived manually from spectrograms, and with cues derived automatically by the analyzer. Both normal- and impaired-hearing listeners were tested. They were provided with 40 h of training since many had no experience with MCS. Early tests of a simulation of the Autocuer system (Cornett et al., 1977) used spectrogram-derived cues. Scores for the reception of common words spoken in isolation improved from 63% (SA) to 84% when cues were presented. However, the subjects do not appear to have been trained sufficiently to use the cues when the words were embedded in short phrases. More recent simulation studies (R. Beadles, personal communication, August 31, 1989) indicated that considerably less benefit would be obtained with recognizer-produced cues: scores on isolated words improved from 59% (SA) to 67% with the automatically produced cues.

Unfortunately the results of the Gallaudet-R.T.I. studies make very limited contributions to the general development of automatic cueing systems. The participants in these studies were not sufficiently trained on the cues that were produced and displayed to derive much benefit when using the cues to supplement the speechreading of connected discourse, even when the cues were perfectly matched to what was said. In addition, the simulation studies assumed that the recognizer would require roughly 150 ms to derive and display a cue after the corresponding syllable was spoken. The effect of this delay was not explored, although it arguably could have different effects when test materials consist of running speech rather than isolated words.

The M.I.T. Simulation Study

To evaluate potential automatic cueing systems under more realistic conditions,

new studies of the effects of imperfections in the recognition and display of cues were recently conducted at M.I.T. (Bratakos et al., 1997). To avoid the problems posed by inadequate training, six highly trained receivers of MCS were tested. The reception of words in low-context sentences (IEEE, 1969) was evaluated under conditions that simulated the recognition errors and delays expected of current ASR systems. Cues consisting of images of hands were dubbed at appropriate locations onto recordings of the faces of talkers who spoke sentences.

The test protocol included three reference conditions [SA; MCS; and perfect synthetic cues, (PSC)], in which the cues were specified by phonetic transcriptions of the sentences) and ten test conditions. In the test conditions, errors were introduced into the phonetic transcriptions and/or the appearance of cues was delayed relative to the indicated beginning of the phone. Several combinations of errors and delays were evaluated. In the reference conditions, the lowest scores were obtained with SA (30%); and the highest with MCS (83%). With PSC, scores were slightly lower than in MCS (77%) perhaps reflecting differences in speaking rates (100 wpm for MCS, 140 for PSC), cue display (articulated versus static), and cue timing (in the PSC condition, the time reference for the display of cues was derived from the acoustic waveform; in MCS the shapes and positions of the cuer's hands often change before there is detectable sound).

Both simulated recognizer errors and delays in the display of cues reduced scores. When 10% of the phones were in error, scores decreased by 14 percentage points; a 20% rate of errors reduced scores by 24 points. In combination with a delay of 165 ms, the effect of a 10% error rate was even larger, reducing scores by 38 points. The effect of a 20% error rate was also increased by a delay of 100 ms (from a 24- to a 36-point reduction in scores). When cues were derived by a state of the art phonetic recognizer that produced 20% phone errors when operated off-line, scores were roughly the same as for the simulated recognizer that produced 10% errors. Apparently the errors produced by the real recognizer tended to cluster in words, so that, for the same error rate, more words in a sentence were likely to be free of errors for the real than for the simulated recognizer.

These results suggest that state of the art recognizers can produce cues that aid speechreading substantially. On the other hand, they also underscore the deleterious effects of recognizer delays on the effectiveness of these cues. The MCS system is based on presenting cues corresponding to CV pairs. While the manual cuer can produce the cue at the start of the initial consonant, an automatic system cannot determine what cue to produce until after the final vowel is spoken and recognized. Typically this would impose a delay in the display of the cue that is well in excess of 165 ms, whose effect was found to be highly deleterious. One approach to minimizing the effect of such delays is discussed in the following sections.

Automatic Cue Generating Systems

The automatic cue generator investigated here performed three principal functions: (1) capture and parameterization of the acoustic speech input (the recognizer front end); (2) cue identification via speech recognition; (3) presentation of the identified cues to the cue receiver. Fig. 1 [Figure 20–1] shows the block diagram of this system, which, for convenience, was implemented on two computers.

Parameterization

The first two functions were tightly coupled, the recognition algorithm determining the type of speech preprocessing. The speech waveform was captured using a standard lapel-type omni-directional microphone, sampled at 10-kHz, high-frequency pre-emphasized by a first-order filter with a cutoff frequency of 150 Hz (to flatten the spectrum; e.g., O'Shaugnessy, 1990), and divided into 20-ms-long frames with 10-ms overlap. For each frame a vector of 25 parameters was derived from the samples including 12-mel-frequency cepstral coefficients, 12 differences of cepstral coefficients across frames, and the difference between frame energies. Differences were computed over a four frame span so that the difference parameters of the nth frame were computed from the static parameters of frames $n+2$ and $n-2$. RASTA processing (Hermansky & Morgan, 1994) was applied to the parameter vectors to improve robustness.

Signal acquisition and parameterization was performed on a Motorola DSP96000 board running on PC1, a Pentium Pro class computer. The same parameterization was used in all experiments. Parameter vectors were time-stamped to allow for subsequent synchronization with the video and sent over the local Ethernet to the recognition program.

Phone/Cue Recognition

The second subsystem recognized the phones corresponding to the acoustic in-

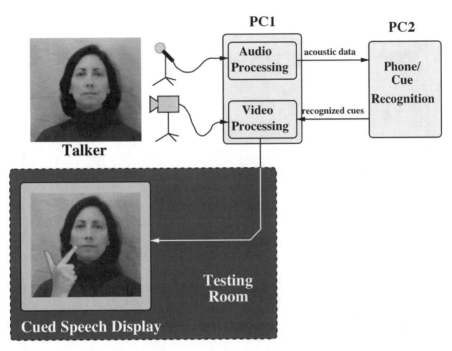

Figure 20–1. Block diagram of the automatic cue generator.

put and converted them to a time-marked stream of cue codes which was sent to the display subsystem. Speech was recognized as phones by PC2, a DEC AlphaStation. This software implemented hidden markov models (HMM), (Rabiner, 1989), based on routines in the HTK suite of programs (Woodland & Byrne, 1993; Woodland, Leggetter, Odell, Valtchev, & Young, 1995), and operated in speaker-dependent mode.

Three phonetic recognizers were studied. The recognizers differed primarily in the number of separate models trained for each phone and the method of assignment of a subclass of the given phone to each of the available models. In all cases, three-state left-right models were used. Output probability densities were described by mixtures of six diagonal-covariance Gaussian distributions. Static and dynamic parameters formed distinct "streams"

with different probability densities, under the implicit assumption that static and dynamic parameters were statistically independent (Furui, 1986). Pilot studies showed that this was the broadly optimal configuration for this application. For each speaker, models were trained on roughly 60 min (1,000 sentences) of speech data using the forward-backward algorithm (Baum, 1972; Bahl, Jelinek, Mercer, 1983; Rabiner, 1989). Recognition was performed using the HTK Viterbi beam search modified to accept continuously arriving data vectors and to decode the corresponding phone sequence in real time.

The first recognizer, C1, used context-independent models of 46 phones (Table I [Table 20–1]) similar to the simplified phone set used in the TIMIT database (Lamel, Kassel, & Seneff, 1986; Fisher, Zue, Bernstein, & Pallett, 1987), but with some

Table 20–1. Phones Modeled by the Recognition Software

Phone	Example	Phone	Example	Phone	Example
iy	beet	l	lay	t	tea
ih	it	r	ray	p	pea
eh	bet	y	yacht	k	key
ae	bat	w	way	dd	udder
ax	about	er	bird	dt	utter
ah	but	m	man	z	zone
uw	boot	n	man	zh	usual
uh	book	en	button	v	van
ao	bought	ng	sing	f	fin
aa	cot	ch	choke	th	thin
ey	bait	jh	joke	s	sea
ay	bite	dh	then	sh	she
oy	boy	b	bee	h	hay
aw	bout	d	day	cl	*Unvoiced closure*
ow	boat	g	gay	vcl	*Voiced closure*
				sil	*silence*

Note. A closure refers to the brief period immediately preceding a plosive burst when the vocal tract is completely closed and no sound is emitted from the mouth.

minor modifications.[2] The sentences used in our simulation studies were transcribed using this set by trained phoneticians. This recognizer operated in real time with virtually no restrictions on the search beam and achieved a phone recognition accuracy[3] of 71% in off-line experiments and 65% for live speech. Poor recognizer accuracy, relative to off-line recognition, was likely due to differences between the speaking style, microphones, recording conditions, etc. of the prerecorded and real-time speech.

The second recognizer, C2, used right-context-dependent models, i.e., separate models were trained for a given phone for each possible following phone. This resulted in a significant increase in the number of models, from 46 to 2116, and con-

---

[2]For example, we used separate models for the flapped "d" and the flapped "t" because in MCS the cue would reflect the underlying phoneme. Using the separate models, the recognizer was able to distinguish between them at a level that was well above chance, even though they are acoustically very similar.

[3]Accuracy = 100 (total phones-substitutions-deletions-insertions)/(total phones).

sequently required much greater amounts of computation during recognition. To achieve real-time operation we implemented a modified decoding procedure, similar to the Forward-Backward search (Austin, Schwartz, & Placeway, 1991). In our approach context-independent models were used in the first (backward) pass to identify a subset of phone hypotheses that exceed a likelihood threshold. This reduced drastically the number of phone models (the "beam width") whose match to the acoustic data was then evaluated in the second (forward) pass using the more accurate context-dependent models. This method of reducing the number of the context-dependent models generally resulted in higher accuracy than the simpler beam search (Rabiner, 1989), which constrained the number of phone hypotheses based only on one pass.

In practice the number of phone models that exceed the likelihood threshold varied significantly. For example, steady portions of vowels and strong fricatives tended to be matched well to only a few models while nasals and phone transitions initially produced fairly good matches to many models. Consequently, the time required to process a given vector of acoustic parameters varied as well. To make good use of computational resources, we imposed additional, dynamically adapted, constraints on the beam width. The accuracy of C2 was 79% in off-line conditions but only 66%–70%[4] for live speech. Apparently some correct phone hypotheses were erroneously pruned, nullifying the gains from improved modeling.

Recognizer C3 used phone models that depended on both the preceding and subsequent phones. To limit the number of models, generalized contexts were used. Thirteen context classes, each containing between two and six phones, were constructed. Thus the same phone model was used for an "ah" when followed by a "b" as when followed by a "p" but a different model was used when "ah" was followed by a "d." The phone context classes generally group consonant phones with similar manner and place of articulation and vowel phones with similar tongue position (Table II [Table 20–2]). Of the 7,774 possible models we used only roughly half—those most frequently occurring in training data. The accuracy of the C3 recognizer was 80% off-line and 74% for live speech. The live speech accuracy was higher than that of the C2 recognizer when implemented on the same processor (70%). All recognizers produced running estimates of the sequences of spoken phones together with estimated start and end times. The recognized phones were converted into a sequence of codes for cues via a finite-state grammar. These codes and start/stop times were then sent to the cue display subsystem.

Cue Display

The cue display subsystem (1) captured images of the speaker's face, (2) overlayed the appropriate cues on these images, and (3) displayed the sequence of overlayed images to the cue receiver. As discussed above, the simulation study had underscored the importance of synchronizing the presence of cues to the talker's speech. Since cues cannot be identified and displayed before the speaker has uttered the corresponding syllable, the video image

---

[4]Differences between recognizer scores of 1.5 percentage points are significant at the 0.05 level.

Table 20–2. Assignment of Phones to Context Classes

Class Code	Class Description	Phones in Class
FH	front/high vowels	iy ih y
FL	front/low vowels	ae ey eh
BH	back/high vowels	uh uw w
BL	back/low,mid vowels	ao aa ow ay oy aw
NR	neutral, retroflex vowels	ah ax er
N	nasals	m n ng en
LS	labial stops	p b
AS	alveolar stops	t d ch jh dd dt
VS	velar stops	k g
DF	dental fricatives	f v dh th
AF	alveolar fricatives	s z sh zh
L	liquids	l r
S	silence, etc.	sil h

Note that, for purposes of context forming, closures were considered to be part of the stop that followed them.

of the talker's face was stored for delayed playback while the cue to be displayed was recognized. An Oculus TCi frame-grabber card (Coreco Inc.), running on PC1 digitized the output of a video camera recording the speaker's face at 30 frames/s. The digital images were stored in memory for 2 s, a period that was more than adequate to allow the cue to be identified by the recognizer, and delivered to the display program. Each stored frame was then retrieved, one of the hand shapes was overlayed at the appropriate location, and the overlayed image was displayed on a monitor. The eight hand shapes of MCS were available in memory as digitized still images of an actual hand (not neces-sarily the speaker's). The artificially cued talker, as seen by the cue receiver, was thus delayed by 2 s relative to the real talker, but was displayed continuously, using smooth, full-motion video.

Since some of the cue receivers who had participated in the simulation study (Bratakos et al., 1997) reacted negatively to the discrete motion of the hand shapes from position to position, several alter-nate styles of cue display[5] were studied. In the "smooth" display, the hand image was moved at a uniform rate along a straight line path between target positions, without pausing at these positions. The display computer interpolated the inter-mediate locations from the cue endpoints

---

[5]Examples of these styles are available on CD-ROM (Duchnowski, Braida, Bratakos, Lum, Sexton, Krause, 1998).

specified by the recognizer (Sexton, 1997). The "dynamic" display used heuristic rules to apportion cue display time between time paused at target positions and time spent in transition between these positions. Typically, 150 ms was allocated to the transition provided the hand could pause at the target position for at least 100 ms. The movement between target positions was, thus, smooth unless the cue was short, in which case it would tend to resemble the original "static" display.

Comparison of the output of the system with the hand motions of human cuers suggested further modifications to the cue display. In particular, human cuers often begin to form cues well before producing audible sound. To achieve a similar effect, in our "synchronous" display, the time at which cues were displayed was advanced by 100 ms relative to the start time determined by the recognizer. We also changed the timing of the transition from one hand shape to the next so that cues changed halfway through a transition rather than at the end (as in the "dynamic" display). Special rules were used for cues corresponding to diphthongs. In particular, a minimum of 200 ms was allocated to the diphthong motion and 150 ms was allocated for the transition

from the diphthong final position to the next cue position. Any remaining time was added to the diphthong motion and any shortfall was first subtracted from the transition to the next cue. MCS specifies that during the diphthong motion the hand shape must change from the shape associated with the consonant to the "open" shape. We selected that point at 75% of the diphthong motion.

Evaluation Methods

To assess the benefit of ACS, we conducted speech reception experiments with experienced users of MCS. The goal was to compare the subjects' performance under SA, MCS, and ACS. These experiments also guided the development of the automatic cueing system and allowed us to evaluate its various versions.

Subjects

A total of five subjects, ranging in age from 19–24 yrs, were tested in the experiments (Table III [Table 20–3]). All were highly skilled receivers of MCS and native speak-

Table 20–3. Histories of Subjects Experienced in Receiving MCS

Subject	Age (years)	Deafness Onset (months)	Etiology	Past MCS Use (years)	Current MCS Use (hours/day)
S1	23	Birth	Unknown	14	0–1
S2	24	18	Unknown	20	0–1
S3	21	42	Meningitis	18	0–1
S4	19	Birth	Unknown	14	4
S5	21	Birth	Unknown	19	3–4

ers of English. While all of the subjects used MCS extensively in primary school, at the time of the study they used MCS for 1–4 h/day, usually with a relative or transliterator.

Subjects S1 and S3 had participated in our simulation study (Bratakos et al., 1997). The others had no previous exposure to ACS.

Talkers

Cued and uncued sentences were produced by three female talkers with normal hearing. Two teachers of the deaf who use MCS, T1 and T2, produced all the sentences used in Experiment I. Talker T3, certified by the National Cued Speech Association as an Instructor of Cued Speech, produced all sentences in the remaining experiments.

Materials

Three types of test materials were used to measure speech reception. The CUNY sentences (Boothroyd Hnath-Chisolm, Hanin, 1985) exhibit relatively high context (e.g., "The football field is right next to the baseball field."). They are organized in lists of 12, each sentence containing from three to fourteen words, for a total of 102 words per list. The IEEE sentences (IEEE, 1969) are more difficult and provide fewer contextual cues (e.g., "Glue the sheet to the dark blue background."). They are divided into lists of ten sentences with each sentence containing five *keywords* for a total of 50 keywords/list. Additional IEEE-like sentences were specially created for these experiments to extend the number of low-context test materials. They used the same keywords

and sentence structure as the IEEE sentences, but used different phrasing. The resulting sentences (e.g., "Cars left outside are prone to rust.") are, thus, believed to be of comparable difficulty.

Procedures

Live, rather than recorded, sentence productions were used. The talker sat in a sound-proof booth, faced a video camera and monitor and wore a lapel-style, omnidirectional microphone. A monitor displayed the text to be spoken. The cue receiver, who sat in a separate booth, observed the video of the talker on another monitor. The video was delayed by 2 s whether or not artificial cues were superimposed. No audio signal was provided to the receiver. In some experiments, several subjects were tested simultaneously. No communication was allowed among the subjects.

A typical experiment lasted 3–4 h and was divided into sessions comprising reception of four or five sentence lists. Subjects were given 10–20-minute breaks between sessions. A single session included a list in the speechreading-alone mode, a list cued manually by the speaker, and two or three lists cued automatically. The order of conditions was randomized from session to session. Over the course of an experiment at least 50 sentences were presented in each of the conditions. Each sentence was presented to a given subject only once.

Subjects wrote as much of each observed sentence as they understood on prepared answer sheets. Guessing at imperfectly perceived words was encouraged. A single training session was conducted at the beginning of the experiment. In general, the subjects had little difficulty understanding the task and the procedure.

Results

The receivers' responses were scored as the percentage of keywords recognized correctly. Strict scoring rules were used: responses considered correct had to agree in tense, number, and form with the sentence text. Homophonic responses were scored as correct. For the CUNY sentences all 102 words in a list were considered keywords. The IEEE and IEEE-like sentences had 50 designated keywords per list.

Table IV [Table 20–4] summarizes the results[6] of the four experiments tests using the recognizers and displays described in Section III [Automatic Cue Generating Systems]. Scheduling constraints made it impractical to test each subject on a wide variety of systems.

Analysis of variance indicated that in no experiment was there significant interaction (at the 0.01 level) between subject and the pattern of scores across presentation conditions. The Mann-Whitney test indicated that scores for MCS were significantly greater than for SA and for ACS in all experiments. ACS scores were significantly greater than SA scores in Experiments III and IV. The difference scores between ACS display types was not significant in Experiment III, but was significant in Experiment IV.

The scores shown in Table IV [Table 20–4] and the statistical analyses indicate the following. First, the better automatic cueing systems improved word reception relative to SA, although the improvement was less than when MCS was used. Second, while improving performance of the cue recognizer (from C1 and C2 to C3)

clearly improved scores, the changes in the display style (from "dynamic" to "synchronous") produced a greater improvement in scores. All three subjects (S3, S4, and S5) commented positively on the final system tested (C3-"synchronous"), indicating that it provided them with appreciable aid relative to SA.

Discussion

The outcome of our experiments with the automatic cue generation systems largely confirms the results of our earlier simulation studies: speechreaders can derive a significant improvement in speech reception from artificial cues produced by an ASR system. Cues produced by the C3 recognizer and presented in the synchronous mode gave our subjects over 57% of the benefit that would accrue from MCS. Keyword scores increased from 35% via unaided speechreading to 66% when speechreading was supplemented by automatically produced cues. Since these results were obtained using low-context sentences, they show an unambiguous potential for improving speech comprehension by the deaf in realistic, full discourse situations.

Other Aids Based on ASR

Although the automatic production of cued speech is not the only way ASR technology can be used to aid communication by the deaf, it offers certain advantages that make it an attractive approach. One alternative would be simply to display the

---

[6]Percentage benefit, B, reports the proportion of the increase in MCS score (S_{MCS}) relative to the speechreading score (S_{SA}) that is achieved by a given automatic cueing system, i.e., $B = 100(S_{ACS} - S_{SA}) / (S_{MCS} - S_{SA})$.

Table 20–4. Results of Speech Reception Experiments With Various Cue Systems

Experiment	Automatic System		Subject	Talker	Material	Keyword Score			Percentage Benefit
	Recognizer	Display				SA	MCS	ACS	
I	C1	smooth	S1	T1	CUNY	70.1	98.4	73.8	13.1
				T2		54.6	93.9	61.0	16.3
			S2	T3	IEEE	28.0	89.2	43.8	25.8
II	C2	smooth	S3	T3	IEEE	15.5	87.8	26.9	15.8
III	C3	discrete	S3	T3	IEEE-like	24.5	91.0	34.7	15.3
		dynamic						43.3	28.3
		discrete	S4	T3	IEEE	29.5	92.0	47.0	28.0
		dynamic						48.7	30.7
		discrete	S5	T3	IEEE	22.5	92.0	51.0	41.0
		dynamic						49.0	38.1
IV	C3	dynamic synchronous	S3	T3	IEEE-like	21.7	92.7	48.8	38.2
								63.2	58.5
		dynamic synchronous	S4	T3	IEEE	42.4	86.0	53.6	25.7
								67.2	56.9
		dynamic synchronous	S5	T3	IEEE	40.7	90.0	52.4	23.7
								68.4	56.2

recognized phones, perhaps as a running stream of phonetic symbols. This technique was investigated in the VIDVOX project (Huggins, Houde, & Colwell, 1986). However, it was found that a phone recognition accuracy of roughly 95% would be required to provide significant benefit to the receiver. This level of recognizer performance is well in excess of the capabilities of currently existing systems.

Another approach would use ASR to caption the speech with words. However, such a display would only benefit those with good reading skills. It would not be appropriate for young children or adults with inadequate reading abilities. The technical feasibility of such a system is also questionable. The most advanced continuous speech recognition systems achieve word accuracies of 90%–95% (Young, 1996; Dragon Systems, 1997), but only after significant adaptation to a given speaker and with heavy reliance on language models. Moreover such high levels of performance are typically achieved only under relatively benign conditions: low ambient noise, constant acoustic transmission characteristics, grammatically correct utterances, and careful speaking style. Relaxation of any of these constraints typically increases the error rate substantially (Young, 1996). For example, when such systems are applied to spontaneous speech, as found in everyday conversations, error rates often exceed 30% (Young, Odell, & Woodland, 1994).

Spontaneous speech is less of a problem for an automatic system that produces cues for all of the phones uttered by the speaker, including hesitation sounds (e.g., "umm"), repeated words, even stutter. Since phonetic recognizers do not rely on word-level language models, they can deal with unusual or ungrammatical utterances. The performance of all ASR systems is degraded by disturbances in the acoustic environment. Trained receivers appear to ignore cues when they are produced by unreliable phonetic recognizers and to rely on speechreading (e.g., Table IV [Table 20–4] and Bratakos et al., 1997). How well speechreading would be integrated with an unreliable word-based display is not known.

Alternate Visual Speechreading Aids

The approach to developing visual speechreading supplements proposed in this paper is based on the presentation of a small set of discrete symbols that are abstracted from the acoustic speech signal via speech recognition. Visual supplements that do not identify discrete linguistic units have also been studied (Upton, 1968; Gengel, 1976; Ebrahimi & Kunov, 1991). These approaches estimate parameters of the acoustic speech signal (e.g., energy in low- and high-frequency bands), and quantize the parameters. The results of logical computations performed on the quantized parameters control the illumination of light-emitting elements in the field of view or visual periphery of the speechreader. For example, Upton's original system (Upton, 1968) used five lamps to indicate the presence of five types of speech sounds. Evaluations of such supplements (Gengel, 1976) indicated that they had potential for aiding speech reception. After only 6 h of training, college students with moderate to severe hearing losses achieved 14%–19% higher scores for monosyllabic words when the aid was used as a supplement to speechreading. Upton himself was documented as achieving a 20% improvement using the device.

Demonstrating benefits to the reception of connected discourse proved more difficult: there was no carryover for the college student group. However, one subject with a severe hearing loss achieved 19% higher word scores on IEEE sentences after using the device for a period of 6 mo, and Upton himself achieved 27% higher scores for words in more contextual sentences using a colored-light version of the display. These improvements are noticeably smaller than those achieved by our subjects in Experiment IV.

More recently, Ebrahimi and Kunov (1991) presented an extensive rationale for the design of a speechreading supplement. They concluded that it would be beneficial to represent voicing (vocal fold activity) and voice onset time, intonation patterns such as fundamental frequency contours, formant frequencies, and the levels of high frequency sounds. To allow the supplementary cues to be integrated with speechreading without increasing the visual workload, they advocated presenting the supplements via peripheral rather than foveal vision. Their display was based on a 5×7 LED matrix that presented three parameters derived from the acoustic waveform: voice fundamental frequency, the speech waveform envelope, and speech power above 3 kHz. Ideally, the display would present five distinct spatio-temporal patterns to distinguish among consonants that differ in voicing and manner of articulation. Eight young adults (3 normal-hearing and five profoundly deaf) evaluated this device in a 12-consonant ($/a/$-C-$/a/$ context) identification task. Scores improved from 41% for SA to 76% for aided speechreading. In particular, distinctions between voiced and unvoiced consonants, which were made with only 55% accuracy with SA, were made with greater than 88% accuracy with the aid.

In spite of the encouraging results reported for these systems, the development of these speechreading supplements is incomplete. Both approaches are highly empirical, and necessarily confound the effects of parameter selection and parameter display with those of training. Even if the benefit can be fairly evaluated after only 6 months of experience with the supplement, it would be extremely time consuming to compare the benefits provided by different parameter sets and/or different displays. Note that although several variants of Upton's aid were developed, no two variants were ever compared in a formal study. Although the use of closed-set identification tests might seem to minimize this problem, this conclusion is highly suspect. Greater amounts of practice would be required to evaluate reception of the complete set of English consonants, particularly if the presentation conditions included a wider set of vowel contexts. Additional tests would be needed to evaluate the reception of vowels. Thus, while this approach might serve to eliminate some parameter sets and/or displays, it is not capable of proving the adequacy of a given system.

Our approach circumvents many of these difficulties. Since the supplements consist of sequences of discrete symbols, it is possible to evaluate the adequacy of the recognition stage of the system separately from the adequacy of the display stage. Furthermore, analytical models can be used to predict how well speech segments can be recognized based on the error patterns made by the speech recognizer (Uchanski et al., 1994). Additional advantages accrue from the fact that the supplement is closely related to MCS. As we have shown, highly trained cue receivers are sensitive to differences in display strategies without the need for months of training. Perhaps more importantly, it is possible to incorporate many of the desirable properties of MCS in the system. For example, MCS displays the cues for consonants over the duration of the CV segment rather than for the duration of the consonant itself. This is likely to improve the reception of consonant cues since many English consonants are of relatively short duration. Similarly, it is unnecessary to speculate whether supplements should use peripheral vision for the display: MCS

provides high levels of speech reception via foveal vision.

Tactile Aids and Implants

Fig. 2 [Figure 20–2] compares word reception scores obtained by the subjects who evaluated our most advanced system with those obtained with comparable test materials by a sample of users of the Ineraid cochlear implant and the tactile aids (Tactaid 2 and Tactaid 7; Reed &

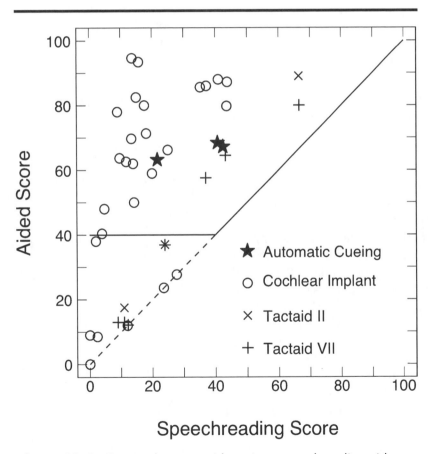

Figure 20–2. Keyword scores with various speechreading aids versus unaided scores. Solid line delineates the region of significant benefit (speech reception allowing for reasonable conversation).

Delhorne, 1995). As can be seen, scores obtained by users of ACS exceed those obtained by roughly one-third of the users of the cochlear implant and by roughly two-thirds of the users of the tactile aids. Note that the only superior scores for tactile aids were obtained by a single subject with exceptional speechreading skills.

Practical Applications

The development of the cue generating system has progressed rapidly; less than a year elapsed between the first and final versions tested. Additional research directed towards the improvement of recognition and display technology seems likely to increase the benefit that the system provides to the cue receiver. It should be possible to reduce the 2-s delay incorporated in the current system substantially, to facilitate face to face communication, and to provide a delayed acoustic output for users with partial hearing. In addition, the cost of providing the recognition and display functions required by automatic cueing systems is decreasing rapidly.

Nonetheless the computational requirements of ASR and the complexity of the display make it unlikely that a truly portable cueing system, as envisioned by the developers of the Autocuer, can be realized soon. Rather, we expect that initial deployments of the system will be in relatively static and controlled settings such as lecture halls, classrooms, or the homes of deaf children. A camera, controlled automatically to track the face of the speaker (Yang & Waibel, 1995; Oliver, Pentland, Berard, Coutaz, 1996) would be required in some applications. Cues would be generated and displayed on a laptop computers. In the home environment, the system could be used to produce cues for television broadcasts or to help train family members to produce MCS. Because the system produces a supplement that is compatible with MCS, it could be used immediately by skilled cue receivers with little need for additional training.

Acknowledgment. The authors would like to thank the experienced producers and receivers of MCS who participated in the studies reported. They would also like to thank A. K. Dix, who helped develop the IEEE-like sentences. Finally, they would like to thank C. M. Reed and L. A. Delhorne, who allowed them to use their data on the reception of speech via cochlear implants and tactile aids.

References

Austin, S., Schwartz, R., & Placeway, P. (1991). The forward-backward search algorithm. In *Proceedings of ICASSP-91, Toronto*, 697–700.

Bahl, L., Jelinek, F., & Mercer, R. (1983). A maximum likelihood approach to continuous speech recognition. *IEEE Transactions on Pattern Analysis and Machine Intelligence, (PAMI)*, 5(2), 179–190.

Baum, L. (1972). An inequality and associated maximization technique in statistical estimation of probabilistic functions of Markov processes. *Inequalities*, 3, 1–8.

Boothroyd, A., Hnath-Chisolm, T., & Hanin, L. (1985). *A sentence test of speech perception: reliability, set-equivalence, and short-term learning.* (Report RCI10). New York, NY: City University of New York.

Bratakos, M., Duchnowski, P., & Braida, L. (1997). Toward the automatic generation of cued speech. *The Cued Speech Journal*, 6, 1–37.

Clark, G. (1998). Cochlear implants in the second and third millennia. In *Proceedings of ICSLP-98, Sydney*, 1–6.

Clarke, B., & Ling, D. (1976). The effects of using cued speech: A follow up study. *Volta Review, 78*, 23–34.

Cornett, R. O. (1967). Cued Speech. *American Annals of the Deaf, 112*, 3–13.

Cornett, R. O., Beadles, R., & Wilson, B. (1977). Automatic Cued Speech. *Processing Aids for the Deaf, 224*–239.

Douglas-Cowie, E. (1988). Acquired deafness and communication. In R. Cowie (Ed.), *Coping with acquired hearing loss* (pp. 13–22). Belfast, Ireland: Social Services Inspectorate DHSS.

Dragon Systems. (1997). Product information for NaturallySpeaking speech recognition software available over the Internet at http://www.dragonsystems.com .

Duchnowski, P., Braida, L., Lum, D., Sexton, M., Krause, J., & Banthia, S. (1998). Automatic generation of Cued Speech for the deaf: Status and outlook. *Proceedings of ICSLP-1998, Sydney, Australia*, 3289–3293.

Ebrahimi D., & Kunov, H. (1991). Peripheral vision lipreading aid. *IEEE Transactions on Biomedical Engineering, 38*, 944–952.

Fant, G. (1970). Q-codes. In G. Fant (Ed.), *Proceedings of the International Symposium on Speech Communication Ability and Profound Deafness*, (pp. 261–299). Washington, DC: A. G. Bell Association for the Deaf.

Fisher, W., Zue, V., Bernstein, J., & Pallett, D. (1987). An acoustic-phonetic data base. *Journal of the Acoustical Society of America, 81*, S1, 92.

Furui, S. (1986). Speaker-independent isolated word recognition using dynamic features of the speech spectrum. *IEEE Transactions on Acoustics Speech and Signal Processing, ASSP-34*, 52–59.

Gengel, R. (1976). Upton's wearable eyeglass speechreading aid: History and current status. In S. Hirsh, D. Eldridge, I. Hirsh, & S. Silverman (Eds.), *Hearing and Davis: Essays Honoring Hallowell Davis*, (pp. 291–299). St. Louis, MO: Washington University Press.

Grant, K., & Braida, L. (1991). Evaluating the articulation index for audiovisual input.

Journal of the Acoustical Society of America, 89, 2952–2960.

Hermansky, H., & Morgan, N. (1994). RASTA processing of speech. *IEEE Transactions on Acoustics Speech and Signal Processing, 24*, 52–59.

Hiki, S., & Fukuda, Y. (1981). Proposal of a system of manual signs as an aid for Japanese lipreading. *Journal of the Acoustical Society of Japan, 2*(2), 127–129.

Huggins, A., Houde, R., & Colwell, E. (1986). *Vidvox human factors investigation* (Tech. Rep. 6187). Cambridge, MA: BBN Laboratories.

IEEE. (1969). IEEE recommended practice for speech quality measurements. *IEEE Transactions on Audio and Electroacoustics, AU-17*(3), 225–246. Standards Publication No. 297, available from IEEE.

Kaplan, H. (1974). *The effects of cued speech on the speechreading ability of the deaf.* Unpublished doctoral dissertation, University of Maryland.

Klima, E., & Bellugi, U. (1979). *The signs of language.* Cambridge MA: Harvard University Press.

Lamel, L., Kassel, R., & Seneff, S., (1986). Speech database development: Design and analysis of the acoustic-phonetic corpus. In L. Baumann (Ed.), *Proceedings of the DARPA Speech Recognition Workshop* (pp. 100–109). California: DARPA Speech Recognition Workshop, SAIC-86/1546.

Ling, D., & Clarke, B. (1975). Cued speech: An evaluative study. *American Annals of the Deaf, 120*, 480–488.

Nicholls, G., & Ling, D. (1976). The effects of using cued speech: A follow-up study. *Volta Review, 78*, 23–34.

Oliver, N., Pentland, A., Berard, F., & Coutaz, J. (1996). *LAFTER: lips and face tracker* (Tech. Rep. 396). Cambridge, MA: M.I.T. Media Laboratory.

Oller, D. (1995). Tactile aids for the hearing impaired [Special issue]. *Seminars in Hearing, 16*(1).

Osberger, M., Fisher, L., Zimmerman-Phillips, S., Geier, L., & Baker, M. (1998). Speech recognition performance of older children with cochlear implants. *American Journal of Otology, 19,* 152–157.

O'Shaughnessy, D. (1990). *Speech communication, human and machine.* Reading, MA: Addison-Wesley.

Rabiner, L. (1989). A tutorial on hidden Markov models and selected applications in speech recognition. *Proceedings of the IEEE, 77*(2), 257–286.

Reed, C., & Delhorne, L. (1995). Current results of a field study of adult users of tactile aids. *Seminars in Hearing, 16*(4), 305–315.

Sexton, M. (1997). *A video display system for an automatic cue generator.* Unpublished master's thesis, M.I.T., Cambridge, MA.

Uchanski, R., Delhorne, L., Dix, A., Reed, C., Braida, L., & Durlach, N. (1994). Automatic speech recognition to aid the hearing impaired: Prospects for the automatic generation of Cued Speech. *Journal of Rehabilitation Research and Development, 31*(1), 20–41.

Upton, H. (1968). Wearable eyeglass speech-reading aid. *American Annals of the Deaf, 113,* 222–229.

Wandel, J. (1989). *Use of internal speech in reading by hearing and hearing impaired students in oral, total communication, and Cued Speech programs.* Unpublished doctoral dissertation, Teacher's College, Columbia University, New York.

Woodland, P., & Byrne, W. (1993). *HTK: hidden Markov model toolkit version 1.5 user's manual.* Washington, DC.

Woodland, P., Leggetter, C., Odell, J., Valtchev, V., & Young, S. (1995). The 1994 HTK large vocabulary speech recognition system. *Proceedings of the 1995 International Conference on Acoustics, Speech, and Signal Processing, ICASSP-95,* 73–76.

Yang, J., & Waibel, A. (1995). *Tracking human faces in real time (Tech. Rep. CMU-CS-95-210).* Pittsburgh, PA: Carnegie Mellon University, School of Computer Science.

Young, S. (1996). A review of large-vocabulary continuous-speech recognition. *IEEE Signal Processing Magazine, 13,* 45–57.

Young, S., Odell, J., & Woodland, P. (1994). Tree-based state tying for high accuracy acoustic modeling. *Proceedings ARPA Workshop on Human Language Technology, Plainsboro, NJ,* pp. 307–312.

Chapter 21

AUTOMATIC CUED SPEECH

Jean C. Krause, Paul Duchnowski, and
Louis D. Braida

Introduction

Although initial work on Cued Speech was exclusively concerned with its presentation manually (Cornett, 1967), by 1971, studies related to the automatic generation of the cues were already underway at the Research Triangle Institute (Cornett, Beadles, & Wilson, 1977). Unfortunately, it was not possible to develop the RTI-Autocuer into a successful system during the 1970s, primarily due to two technological limitations. First, the accuracy of automatic speech recognition (ASR) systems was not adequate. Specifically, the Autocuer would generate many incorrect cues as a result of errors made by the speech recognizer. Moreover, the frequency of these errors increased when the naturalness of the setting was increased. In other words, the Autocuer would generate a higher proportion of erroneous cues for running speech than for isolated words. Second, the computational demands of processing video in real-time far outweighed the computing resources that were available in the 1970s. Consequently,

it was necessary for the cues to be coded and displayed as patterns of illuminated LED segments projected for the receiver onto his or her eyeglasses. Not only were the LED patterns initially unfamiliar to Cued Speech receivers, but the phonemes that each cue represented also differed from Manual Cued Speech (MCS). Therefore, the RTI-Autocuer system could not be used by Cued Speech receivers without considerable training. In addition, unlike Manual Cued Speech, the display of the cue was delayed relative to the mouth movements of the talker, because the cue's identity could not be determined until after the vowel component of the CV segment was recognized.

By the 1990s, however, technology had improved to a point where the prospects for the automatic generation of Cued Speech were much improved (Uchanski et al., 1994), and an Autocuer system was developed at Massachusetts Institute of Technology (MIT). With technology available at the time, the MIT-Autocuer achieved fairly good ASR performance for running speech and generated artificial cues that closely resembled manual cues. As a result, the system was considerably more successful than the RTI-Autocuer in improving the reception of sentences (compared to speechreading alone) for users of Manual Cued Speech. The research done on the MIT-Autocuer prior to 1998 is summarized in a paper by Duchnowski, Lum, Krause, Sexton, Bratakos, and Braida (2000) reprinted in Chapter 20 of this volume. The work described in this paper suggests that modifications to the display could substantially improve sentence reception, even if ASR performance remains unchanged. Subsequent work has therefore focused primarily on optimizing the display.

The goal for this chapter is to update the Duchnowski et al. (2000) paper with reports on work done since that paper was written. We begin by discussing the current state of ASR technology and implications for automatic cue systems and then describe three experiments aimed at optimizing the cue display used by the MIT-Autocuer. Experiment 1 examines the optimal timing of the cue display relative to mouth movements, and Experiments 2 and 3 explore the potential for enhancing cue saliency by modifying the appearance of the handshapes. Finally, the results of these experiments are considered alongside other plans for developing automated ways to improve speechreading discussed in Chapters 18 and 19 of this volume.

Recognition System Accuracy

Perhaps the most important component of an automatic cueing system is the automatic speech recognition system used to identify the phonemes spoken and thus to determine the cues to be presented. The speech recognition component of the RTI-Autocuer has been found (Beadles, personal communication, 1989) to identify phonemes in isolated words with an accuracy of roughly 54%, with a 33% deletion rate and a 13% substitution rate. With this level of recognition performance, it is not surprising (e.g., Bratakos, Duchnowski, & Braida, 1998) that the RTI-Autocuer system provided so little benefit that it was not evaluated as an aid to the speechreading of sentences. Despite the fact that the RTI-Autocuer was not tested with sentence materials, it is unlikely that good sentence reception could be achieved with cues that were unreliable and often missing. Although a wearable prototype of the RTI-Autocuer was produced, it does not appear to be in use at the present time.

The MIT-Autocuer (Duchnowski et al., 1998; Duchnowski et al., 2000) implemented speaker-dependent phonetic level speech recognition using Hidden Markov Models (Rabiner, 1989) based on routines in the Hidden Markov Model Tool Kit (HTK; Woodland, Leggetter, Odell, Valtchev, & Young, 1995) suite of programs. As a speaker-dependent system, recognition was optimized for specific speakers that the system had been "trained" to recognize. We studied three implementations that differed primarily in the number of separate phone models. The most advanced system used 3,887 generalized triphone models (i.e., one model for each 3-phoneme sequence that can occur in English). This recognizer achieved off-line phonetic accuracy of roughly 80% on the TIMIT corpus (a database of read speech from over 600 speakers, designed for the evaluation of speech recognition systems; see Lamel, Kassel, & Seneff, 1986, and Fisher, Zue, Bernstein, & Pallett, 1987) counting substitutions, insertions, and deletions as errors. Accuracy dropped to roughly 74%

in experiments on live speech, at least partly because of the need to operate in real time on 1997 computer hardware.

In the 10 years since this work was completed, there have been some advances in the state of the art of phonetic speech recognition that could further improve autocuers. The top accuracy currently attained on speaker-independent phonetic recognition of the TIMIT corpus by a variety of research ASR systems is roughly 80% (e.g., Chakrabartty & Cauwenberghs, 2002; Siniscalchi, Schwarz, & Lee, 2007). Adapting speaker-independent models to a particular speaker typically reduces word error rates by 20 to 30% (Gauvain & Lamel, 2003; Thelen, Aubert, & Beyerlein, 1997), so it is plausible that speaker-dependent recognition accuracy would be in the 85 to 87% range. Were one to attempt to construct an autocuer using today's faster computer and improved recognition technology, it would be reasonable to expect only half the rate of recognition errors on the speaker-dependent task (i.e., 87% accuracy) as seen in the recognizer used in live experiments with the MIT-Autocuer. This is a major improvement and would probably result in greatly increased aid to speechreading.

Recently, Pelley, Husaim, Tessler, Lindsay and Krause (2006) have shown that even experienced transliterators make errors when producing cues: their best transliterator made roughly 30% errors (including both substitutions and omissions) on slowly articulated speech and 40% on speech produced at normal rates. Although the effect of these errors on the reception of the Cued Speech has not yet been documented, and the similarities between the effects of these errors and those of the errors made by the MIT-Autocuer have yet to be established, it seems clear that it may not be necessary for the recognition component of an automatic cueing system to produce completely accurate cues in order to provide substantial benefit as an aid to speechreading.

Relative Timing of the Cues

In Cued Speech, communication relies on a combination of speechreading and a sequence of discrete symbols. Cornett envisioned Cued Speech as a time-locked system in which the cues are synchronized with the spoken sounds. The importance of synchrony is underscored by the results of Bratakos et al. (1998). They studied the reception of words in IEEE (1969) sentences (low-context, phonetically balanced sentences developed for standardized testing of speech systems; IEEE, 1969) in which 20% of the cues were in error and random delays were introduced into the timing of two-thirds of the cues, relative to the onset of the corresponding speech signal. They found that although introducing random delays of ±30 ms did not affect reception of sentences (percentage correct scores 48.8% without delays versus 49.0% with random delays), random delays of ±100 ms reduced scores to 37.2%. This underscores the need for displaying cues in fair synchrony with the speech signal (and corresponding mouth movements).

Comparison of the output of our automatic cueing system with the hand motions of human cuers indicated that human cuers often begin to form cues well before producing audible sound. To achieve a similar effect, the time at which cues were displayed was advanced by 100 ms relative to the start time determined by the speech recognizer in the MIT-Autocuer display. This was possible because the images of the artificially cued talker, as seen by the cue receiver, were delayed by two seconds relative to the real talker. It was thus a simple matter to arrange for simultaneous, delayed, or advanced presentation of the cues relative to images of the face. Although the choice of a 100 ms advance was based on informal observations, its optimality was demonstrated in an experiment (Experiment 1) conducted in 2000 (Braida & Duchnowski, 2000).

Experiment 1

Three experienced receivers of Cued Speech were tested on the reception of words in low-context sentences. In addition to speechreading alone and manually Cued Speech, tests included synthetic perfectly cued sentences that were delayed and advanced by 0, 100, 200, and 300 ms relative to the start times determined by the speech recognizer. A "static" cue display, in which the hand image is fixed in both shape and position for the duration of a cue and changes instantaneously at the beginning of the next cue, was used. Each cue receiver practiced on 3 to 4 lists of the CID everyday sentences (Davis & Silverman, 1970) and IEEE (low-context) sentences and tested on six lists of IEEE-like sentences[1] having delays/advances of each magnitude. Different sentences were used for the conditions for each subject.

Averaged across the three subjects, the highest scores (95.8% correct) were achieved with Manual Cued Speech and the poorest (30.3%) were achieved for

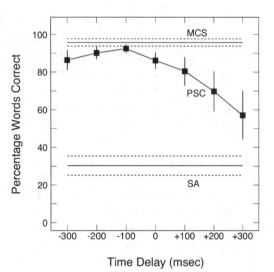

Figure 21–1. Effect of altering the presentation timing of the cues. The horizontal bars give the mean (and ±1 standard deviation) results for Manual Cued Speech (MCS) and Speechreading Alone (SA). The squares give the results for perfect synthetic cues (PSC) that are delayed (+) or advanced (–) relative to the start of vocal speech.

speechreading alone (Figure 21–1). As expected, scores with the synthetic cues fell off at large delays and advances of the presentation of the cue relative to the start of vocal speech as determined by the recognizer. Maximum scores with synthetic cues (92.4%) occurred when the cues were advanced by 100 ms relative to this point rather than simultaneously (86.1%). Note that in this test, average scores with the discrete cues presented with an advance of 100 ms are very nearly equal to the scores for Manual Cued Speech.

---

[1]To increase the number of low-context sentences IEEE-like sentences were specially created using the same keywords and structure as the IEEE sentences, but different phrasing (e.g., "Cars left outside are prone to rust.").

Results suggesting that some human transliterators may do this as well have been obtained by Attina, Beautemps, Cathiard, & Odisio (2004) who measured the timing of cued polysyllabic words produced by one transliterator. The speech was spoken at a slower rate (2.5–3.4 syllables/sec) than the sentences (3–5 syllables/sec) used by Duchnowski et al. (2000). They found that the displacement of the hand towards its final position began more than 200 ms before the consonant was spoken, and reached its target position an average of 172 to 276 ms before the vowel. The results of Experiment 1 underscore the need for properly timing cue presentation relative to the actions of the lips and jaw. It is possible that even greater benefits could be provided if the amount of advance were cue-dependent, as revealed by the study of Attina et al. (2004), rather than fixed at 100 ms.

Modifying the Appearance of the Handshapes

In theory, the combination of information conveyed by the speaker's visible facial actions and the information conveyed by manually produced cues should result in near perfect speech reception. This is, in fact, the case for conversational sentences with relatively easy vocabulary (Uchanski et al., 1994). Nevertheless, even highly experienced MCS receivers make errors on more difficult materials: reception of perfectly cued low-context sentences spoken at 100 wpm suggests that at least 10 to 20% of the segments are perceived incorrectly (Uchanski et al., 1994). These errors may be due to: (1) difficulty in distinguishing between similar handshapes or positions, (2) difficulty in accurately perceiving facial actions of the speaker (i.e., speechreading), (3) inability to integrate the cues with speechreading.

Preliminary analysis of the responses of cue receivers suggests that more than one-quarter of the word errors in sentences can be attributed to incorrect reception of cues for segments in words (Uchanski et al., 1994). One way to reduce the number of such errors in Cued Speech produced by artificial means may be to alter the appearance of the surface or the outline of the hand. Two easily confused shapes, for example, could be displayed differing in brightness, size, or color. In further experiments we focused on the use of cue coloration to improve discrimination.

Experimental Design

Experiments 2 and 3 tested the identification of handshapes before and after some of the hand images were digitally colored (Duchnowski et al., 1998). We used prerecorded consonant-vowel-consonant (CVC) syllables spoken by one female talker. There were 24 initial consonants with eight tokens of each for a total of 192 distinct syllable recordings. The vowel was always /a/ whereas the final consonant was drawn at random from a pool of eight and did not play a role in these experiments.

Our subjects were normal-hearing adults who had no familiarity with MCS. Prior to the experiments they were given about 10 hours of training in identifying the eight MCS handshapes and in speechreading CVCs (trained separately). They learned to identify handshapes shown for as little as 66 ms almost perfectly and scored 50 to 60% on initial consonant identification via speechreading alone. Two additional experiments were then conducted.

Experiment 2

A single handshape was superimposed on a CVC recording for the duration of one video frame (33 ms). This frame was temporally located about 100 ms after the start of the initial consonant. Four distinct versions of the handshape were overlaid on each token, one each in a different but random MCS position. A distinct handshape was associated with each CVC token in such a way that every initial consonant was paired equal number of times with each handshape, resulting in 768 distinct stimuli.

During an experimental session, 192 randomized tokens were presented to the subjects who were asked to identify both the handshape and the initial consonant. No audio was presented. Subjects were not required to identify the position of the cue.

After several practice sessions, we analyzed the responses of the subjects and identified the three handshapes with the lowest average identification scores, hand-

shapes 3, 6, and 7 (Figure 21–2). These three hand images were digitally colorized blue, red, and green respectively, while texture and contrast of the image were preserved to the extent possible. New stimuli were made using these and the five uncolored hand images using the procedure above.

Five subjects participated in Experiment 2. The experiment consisted of four sessions of uncolored (U) stimuli, followed by two sessions of colored (C) ones, then two U, and two C. Table 21–1 shows the average consonant and handshape identification scores. Results are given separately for each U and C session block chronologically. Note that since these subjects were ignorant of Cued Speech, their improvement in handshape identification did not produce improvement in consonant identification: they identified the consonants by speechreading alone.

We performed an ANOVA to evaluate the significance of the differences in scores. At the 0.01 level, we found no significant changes in the consonant recogni-

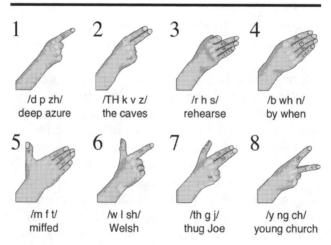

Figure 21–2. Assignment of consonant sounds to handshapes in Manual Cued Speech and as used in Experiments 2 and 3.

Table 21–1. Average Percent Correct Scores for Five Subjects in Experiment 2

	U (4)	C (2)	U (2)	C (2)
Consonants	43.2	45.0	43.4	44.5
Handshapes	83.6	91.6	88.3	94.1

tion between U and C stimuli or session blocks. On the other hand, the improvement in handshape recognition when color was added was significant. There also were differences in scores across subjects but no significant differences in the pattern of results across subjects.

Confusion Patterns

We analyzed confusion matrices obtained by pooling all of the responses made by the subjects over all experimental sessions for a given condition, forming two confusion matrices. These matrices were fit by a metric multidimensional scaling procedure (Braida, 1991). For each confusion matrix, this procedure was used to derive the coordinates of a set of points that represent the means of two-dimensional Gaussian distributions that characterize the perceptual properties of the perceptual cues used to identify the handshapes. Distances between points are inversely related to the rate at which the handshapes were confused, with the unit of distance corresponding to the common standard deviation of the Gaussian distributions.

The configurations derived from the confusions are shown in Figure 21–3. For the uncolored handshapes, as shown in the left panel of Figure 21–3, confusions are generally determined by the number of extended fingers (e.g., handshapes 1, 2, 3, and 4; 5, 6, and 7) and by the extension of

the thumb (e.g., handshapes 1 and 6, 2 and 7, and 4 and 5). The effect of coloration is shown in the right panel of Figure 21–3. First note that the general structure of configuration of the means for handshapes 1, 2, 4, 5, and 8 is relatively unchanged from that seen in the left panel, indicating that coloration did not affect the pattern of confusions between these stimuli. On the other hand, the occurrence of confusions between handshape 3 (blue) and handshapes 2 and 4, are reduced, as seen in the increased separation between the corresponding points. Similarly, the increased separation between the points corresponding to handshape 7 (red) and handshapes 5 and 6 (green) indicates that confusions between these stimuli were reduced by coloration.

Experiment 3

In Experiment 3, sequences of three handshapes were superimposed on the CVC images. The middle handshape, the *target*, lasted 6 video frames (198 ms) beginning at the same frame as the single handshape in Experiment 2. The same strategy of assigning four target handshape positions to each CVC token was followed although different combinations were used. The surrounding cues were chosen randomly with the restriction that they had to be of different shape and appear in positions distinct from the target. Each surrounding cue was shown for 2 video frames (66 ms).

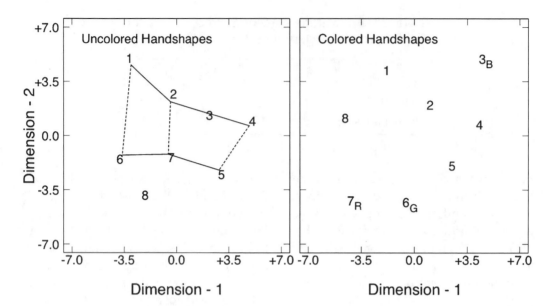

Figure 21–3. Means of two-dimensional distributions characterizing confusions among the eight handshapes in Experiment 2. The configuration in the left panel applies to uncolored handshapes, that in the right panel applies to handshapes in which handshapes 3, 6, and 7 were colored blue, green, and red, respectively. The solid curves in the left panel connect handshapes differing mainly in the number of outstretched fingers. The dashed lines connect handshapes differing only by the presence of the thumb. Subscripts in the right panel correspond to the color assigned to the particular handshape.

The subjects only had to identify the target handshape, not the position at which the shape was displayed.

Again, after several sessions, we identified the most frequently confused handshapes. In an attempt to reduce identification errors further, in addition to the three hand images of Experiment 1 (handshapes 3, 6, and 7), we colorized two more images using violet (handshape 1) and yellow (handshape 2). When re-recording the stimuli, we used this new set of hand images for the target as well as the surrounding images in the three-cue sequence.

Three of the subjects who participated in Experiment 2 completed the entire Experiment 3. A fourth subject completed part of Experiment 3—her scores are not reported here although they are consistent with the others. In this experiment two U sessions were followed by two C sessions, then one U, and one C. Table 21–2 shows the average scores. As in Experiment 2, an ANOVA showed no significant effects of conditions, sessions, or subjects on consonant scores. On the other hand, all three variables had an effect significant at the 0.01 level on handshape identification scores.

The patterns of errors made for the uncolored handshapes in Experiments 2 and 3 were fairly similar. As seen is the left panel of Figure 21–4, distances between points for these configurations were gen-

Table 21–2. Average Percent Correct Scores for Three Subjects in Experiment 3

	U (2)	C (2)	U (1)	C (1)
Consonants	43.0	43.7	43.3	42.7
Handshapes	65.2	75.5	73.3	79.3

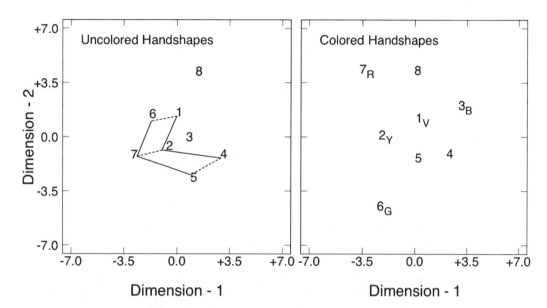

Figure 21–4. Means of two-dimensional distributions characterizing confusions among the eight handshapes in Experiment 3. The configuration in the left panel applies to uncolored handshapes, that in the right panel applies to handshapes in which handshapes 1, 2, 3, 6, and 7 were colored violet, yellow, blue, green, and red, respectively. See also the caption of Figure 21–3.

erally smaller than the corresponding distances in the left panel of Figure 21–3, consistent with the reduced identification accuracy caused by the more difficult stimulus configurations used in Experiment 3. On the other hand, handshape mean positions showed configurations similar to those of the left panel of Figure 21–3. The similarity in the structure of the configurations for the uncolored handshapes in the single-cue-single-frame and triple-cue

experiments suggests that the subjects used roughly the same visual cues (number of fingers extended and thumb extension) in both experiments. In contrast, the pattern of identification errors made for the colored handshapes was very different from that of the uncolored handshapes. Not only is the distance between points in the configuration of the right panel generally greater than that of the left panel (corresponding to the increased accuracy with which colored handshapes are identified) but also the shape of the configurations are very different (corresponding to a change in confusion patterns due to the coloration).

Taken together, Experiments 2 and 3 show that, with relatively little practice, color can be integrated by human observers to improve discrimination of confusable handshapes. The improvement, while not large, is statistically significant. It is encouraging that consonant scores for receivers unfamiliar with MCS do not change when the handshapes are colored. This suggests that coloration of handshapes is likely to increase the recognition of syllables for MCS users because attending to the color and shape of hands imposes no degradation on the ability to speechread.

The analysis of confusion matrices agrees with intuitive prediction of likely misidentifications and demonstrates how colorization can resolve many of these. We are planning to conduct experiments with artificially cued sentences to determine how well users of Manual Cued Speech can be trained to make use of the colored cues in connected speech.

Discussion

An early attempt to develop the RTI-Autocuer (Cornett et al., 1977) used a portable microprocessor-based device to analyze the acoustic input and used heuristic rules to identify speech sounds and assign them to cues. The cues were then coded as patterns of illuminated LED segments projected for the receiver onto his or her eyeglasses. No adjustments were made to correct for the time required to recognize the cue—the cues were always delayed somewhat relative to the start times of the corresponding phonemes. It did not prove possible to develop an effective system that worked in real time.

We believe that artificial cues whose appearance resembles manual cues fairly closely have a better chance of success, at least for those trained in the reception of manually Cued Speech. While improved speech recognition accuracy generally leads to higher cue accuracy and increases the benefit provided by the cues, the results of the experiments described in this chapter indicate that another significant contribution to the effectiveness of the MIT-Autocuer comes from the characteristics of the display. Notably, the issue of cue synchronization to the talker's visible facial actions seems crucial and was not considered for the RTI-Autocuer.

It is also worth noting that the flexibility of our cue display offers potential improvements in cue reception not possible with either MCS or the RTI-Autocuer's display. Yet, any changes in cue appearance designed to enhance their discriminability should retain the basic compatibility with MCS. Maintaining the similarity of the artificial cue display to natural MCS cues not only improves speech reception but also greatly alleviates the problem of training. Users of our system trained in MCS needed minimal practice to understand the display. It is also possible that those trained on naturally colored handshapes (the caregivers of the users of the system) could adapt relatively quickly to the enhanced colored display.

When we began our research on the development of an autocuer more than 20 years ago, cochlear implants were relatively novel devices whose potential was just beginning to be explored. Now, with more than 100,000 individuals implanted worldwide (Chertok, 2007), including many children, it is clear that cochlear implants are the treatment of choice for most deafened individuals. Despite the possible future advances in automatic cueing systems, the use of autocuers as transliteration devices, as we originally envisioned, is perhaps most appropriate for a relatively small group of users: those individuals who do not benefit from cochlear implants and/or who do not wish to rely exclusively on signing for communication.

Nonetheless, individuals with cochlear implants can still derive benefits from other applications of autocuers. For example, portable autocuers could be used to provide a rich auditory training environment, as individuals could use the device at home with unlimited speech materials of personal interest to the individual. Given the flexibility of the MIT-Autocuer's display, the cues in auditory training devices could progress over time from maximally redundant, with handshapes modified in appearance to enhance saliency (e.g., colors to reduce confusions, cues for fast syllables displayed longer, etc.), to no cues at all. With only minor modifications, the system could be set such that either all cues would gradually fade away (literally, with transluscent handshapes), or that cues for specific phonemes would be removed in succession as identification of those phonemes was mastered.

Another group who would benefit from an autocuer is those interested in learning to produce Manual Cued Speech, either to communicate more easily with a family member or friend or for a job (e.g., transliterators, teachers of individuals who are deaf). To use the device, learners would present words or phrases to the autocuer in order to determine how to cue them. The device would then generate a video of the learner speaking the utterance, with artificial cues superimposed on the learner's face. The learner could then view the video repeatedly and in slow-motion, as needed to produce the cues appropriately. In this manner, personalized utterances could be learned quickly, and utterances could be double-checked as needed to raise cueing confidence. Thus, an autocuer that provides feedback on cue production has the potential to increase both the rate at which these individuals learn to cue and their motivation for learning.

Implications for Other Research

Approaches of Attina et al. and Bernstein et al.

Both Attina et al. (Chapter 19) and Bernstein et al. (Chapter 18) are developing audio-visual text-to-Cued Speech synthesis systems. The Attina et al. system appears designed to exploit the careful timing measurements of Attina et al. (2004) initially in an effort to provide displays of cued facial actions as an alternative to signing for television applications. Bernstein et al. plan to use an extensive set of recordings of Cued Speech to develop a Cued Speech training system that is to feature a highly "natural" hand and finger motions. A major concern of these investigators is that synthesis of Cued Speech that does not include coarticulation, as in the discrete display of Duchnowski et al. (2000), could interfere with the integration of facial actions and cues. But the most realistic display of the hands need not be the most effective aid to speechreading. As shown in the results of Experiments 2 and 3, realistic handshapes may be poorly discriminated, and this failing can be compensated by coloring the displayed handshapes. It also seems plausible that cue receivers trained on colored handshapes could easily adapt to Manual Cued Speech.

The results of our research suggest that there is no obligation to maintain natural timing and appearance of the hands in an artificial visual display, and it cannot be assumed that doing so is always optimal. Whereas the hand is attached to the arm and as the result of inertia, cannot change position or shape instantaneously, the image of the hand in a synthetic display can move from one position to the next and change shape in as little as one video frame (33 ms), as in the "discrete" display studied by Duchnowski et al. (2000) which achieved an accuracy of 92.4% in Experiment 1. Such a display may be a more effective supplement to speechreading because it allows the full cue to be displayed for a greater amount of time and at a fixed location. Similarly, other "unnatural" adjustments in the display may also increase its efficacy (e.g., short cues could be lengthened to increase perceptibility, the relative timing of cues could be optimized for individual receivers, the locations of hand positions could be emphasized with highlighting, etc.). Given that the average cue receiver typically scores well below 100% on low-context materials (e.g., Uchanski et al., 1994), it is certainly worth exploring the utility of these display enhancements and any others that remain compatible with the Manual Cued Speech system.

Approach of Massaro et al.

An alternative approach to an automatic cueing system is to display not cues but rather acoustic parameters extracted from the speech waveform as an aid to speech-reading. Such systems typically display a stream of processed acoustic data more or less in synchrony with the speech waveform and they superimpose the display on the face of the talker. In the display described in Chapter 22 (Massaro et al.), for example, colored bars are used to display three aspects of consonant articulation: voicing, nasality, and frication. The bars differ with respect to two redundant display aspects: color and position. While the intensity of the illumination may be varied in future work, the colored bars appear currently to be operated in a simple off-on mode. Although initial results appear promising, it remains to be seen whether they will stand up to more rigorous speech reception tests, particularly in running speech.

One advantage of such systems over an automatic cueing system is that there is no need for delaying the image of the speaker's face, as the acoustic parameters usually can be extracted much more rapidly than cues can be identified. The output of an automatic cueing system must be delayed by roughly 300 to 500 ms relative to the spoken speech stream in order to produce the greatest benefit to speechreading. This delay is necessary to accommodate: (1) the need to recognize the vowel portion of the CV diphone before displaying the cue, and (2) the need to advance the cue display by roughly 100 ms relative to what is being said. Such delays (9–15 video frames) make automatic cueing systems relatively cumbersome (though no more so than transliterators, who must also hear/recognize the CV diphone before cueing it): the receiver of the cues must watch a delayed image of the face of the talker, rather than the talker's face itself. The seriousness of this objection depends on the situation: more so in interactive situations, less so in a lecture format.

Although the Massaro et al. system requires no delay of the talker's face, it is worth noting that users of the system were not able to receive isolated words with 100% accuracy. One possible reason for this deficit is that the three bars represent information that aids in the speechreading of consonants only. Ultimately, it may be necessary to supplement this information about consonants with information that assists in discrimination of vowels in order to improve user performance. However, another issue is that some consonants are very brief events relative to vowels, so that the display of parameters for consonants is generally much briefer than the display of parameters for vowels would be. This is unlike the strategy used in Cued Speech in which the handshape, which provides information about the consonant, is displayed for the duration of the CV syllable.

Like Massaro, both Upton (1968) and Ebrahimi and Kunov (1991) have advocated displaying parameters descriptive of speech features as supplements to speechreading. Upton's eventual system used a seven-segment display to convey the presence of high- and low-frequency fricatives, nasals, and voiced- and unvoiced-stops. Ebrahimi and Kunov's system used a 5×7 dot matrix subsystem to display fundamental frequency, high-frequency energy, and the total energy of the speech signal. Both of these supplements aided the reception of consonants. Upton's system (Pickett, Gengel, Quinn, & Upton, 1974) improved the reception of initial consonants from 52.3% by speechreading alone to 61.6% by aided speechreading and final consonants from 56.3 to 61.0%. Ebrahimi and Kunov's system improved the reception of 12 consonants in VCV format from 41 to 76%. Pickett et al. noted that Upton's aid was more effective for poor lipreaders

than good lipreaders. Gengel (1976) reported the performance of one subject with a severe hearing loss who trained on and used the Upton device for 6 months. She was tested on the fairly difficult PAL S-1 sentences (Egan, 1944) and scored on key words. She achieved scores of 42% by speechreading alone and 61% with the aid. She also benefited when speechreading was combined with amplified speech: 57 versus 70% correct. According to Gengel, these scores probably indicate the limits of the benefits that can be provided by the Upton device. To the best of our knowledge, the Ebrahimi and Kunov system has not been evaluated as an aid to sentence reception by highly trained subjects. Neither system appears to be in use at the present time.

Of course, the developers of autocuers have an important advantage over the developers of abstract displays of speech parameters: the existence of Manual Cued Speech and of users trained in its reception. Manual Cued Speech is a system whose capabilities are relatively well understood. It provides a criterion against which the performance of autocuers can be compared. Cued Speech receivers, having trained on Cued Speech since a young age, can explore variants of the cue display with relatively minimal training. This is in contrast to the problem faced by developers of abstract displays, who must expend effort to train the users of their baseline system and then retrain them on variants of the systems. The long period of training required to evaluate even baseline systems, makes this an activity not to be undertaken by the casual experimenter or the faint of heart.

The systems of Upton (1968), Ebrahimi and Kunov (1991), and Massaro et al. (Chapter 22) all face substantial disadvantages relative to autocuers with respect to training. Since an autocuer attempts to mimic a "natural" system on which training can be provided on an essentially full-time basis from a very young age, users are in effect "pretrained" on autocuer derived materials. This would be expected to lead to larger gains and to minimize the amount of training that would be required to use an automated system.

Conclusions

Duchnowski et al. (2000) successfully demonstrated a prototype automatic cueing system that provides a significant benefit to the cue receivers. Low-context keyword scores almost double relative to speechreading alone. The system's development suggests that appropriate cue display can be as important as the accuracy of the automatic cue recognition in determining the effectiveness of the system. In particular, we have found that the characteristics of cue transitions and synchronization to the visible facial actions of the speaker play a significant role.

Our preliminary investigation of cue identification suggests that cue receivers may make errors in handshape identification that could be reduced by enhancing the contrast among synthetic cues. Selectively coloring the hand images improves their discrimination by subjects untrained in MCS. We plan to test the effect of colored cues on the reception of sentences by experienced MCS users. We also intend to refine and test the timing of the cue display.

It is becoming increasingly apparent that an effective automatic cueing system can be developed in the next five years. Improved phonetic speech recognizers are now available and they are only likely to get better as time goes on. Similarly, the techniques for improving the effectiveness of the cue display are likely to improve as the result of research like that done by Attina et al. (Chapter 19), Bernstein et al. (Chapter 18), and Pelley et al. (2006). With these advances in science and technology, numerous applications for automatic cueing systems can be explored: CS instruction and training for new cuers, real-time transliteration for adults (at least in some settings), automatic generation of accessible materials for pre-readers, just to name a few. In research, the availability of automatic cueing systems would allow for controlled, systematic tests of Cued Speech perception that could advance our understanding of how Cued Speech is processed by those who use it for communication.

Acknowledgments. This work was supported by Grants DC-00117 and DC-002032 from the National Institute of Deafness and other Communication Disorders, by the Henry Ellis Warren Professorship at M. I. T., and by the Motorola Corporation. The authors would like to thank Ms. Ann K. Dix, who helped develop the IEEE-like sentences and Mr. Joseph Frisbie for providing the chart of handshapes reproduced in Figure 21–2.

References

Attina, V., Beautemps, D., Cathiard, M., & Odisio, M. (2004). A pilot study of temporal organization in Cued Speech production of French syllables: Rules for a Cued Speech synthesizer. *Speech Communication*, 44, 197–214.

Braida, L. (1991). Crossmodal integration in the identification of consonant segments.

Quarterly Journal of Experimental Psychology, 43A, 647–677.

Braida, L., & Duchnowski, P. (2000). *Automatic production of Cued Speech.* Paper presented at the IEEE Signal Processing Society DSP Workshop, Hunt, TX.

Bratakos, M., Duchnowski, P., & Braida, L. (1998). Toward the automatic generation of cued speech. *Cued Speech Journal, 6*, 1–37.

Chakrabartty, S., & Cauwenberghs, G. (2002). Forward-decoding kernel-based phone sequence recognition. *Proceedings of NIPS, Vancouver, 15*, 1165–1172.

Chertok, B. (2007). Rebuilding a life through new technology. *Hearing Loss Magazine, 28*, 18–22.

Cornett, R. O. (1967). Cued Speech. *American Annals of the Deaf, 112*, 3–13.

Cornett, R., Beadles, R., & Wilson, B. (1977). Automatic Cued Speech. In *Research Conference on Speech-Processing Processing Aids for the Deaf* (pp. 224–239) Washington, DC: Gallaudet University.

Davis, H., & Silverman, S. (1970). *Hearing and deafness.* New York, NY: Holt, Rinehart and Winston.

Duchnowski, P., Braida, L., Bratakos, M., Lum, D., Sexton, M., & Krause J. (1998). Automatic generation of Cued Speech for the deaf: Status and outlook. *Proceedings of the Audio-Visual Speech Proceedings Conference (AVSP-1998)* (pp. 161–166), Terrigal, Australia.

Duchnowski, P., Braida, L., Lum, D., Sexton, M., Krause, J., & Banthia, S. (1998). Automatic generation of Cued Speech for the deaf: Status and outlook. *Proceedings of ICSLP-1998*, pp. 3289–3293, Sydney, Australia.

Duchnowski, P., Lum, D., Krause, J., Sexton, M., Bratakos, M., & Braida, L. (2000). Development of speechreading supplements based on automatic speech recognition. *IEEE Transactions on Biomedical Engineering, 47*, 487–496.

Ebrahimi D., & Kunov, H. (1991). Peripheral vision lipreading aid. *IEEE Transactions on Biomedical Engineering, 38*, 944–952.

Egan, J. (1944). *Articulation Testing Methods II.* (NDRC: OSRD Rep. No. 3802). Washington, DC: Applied Psychology Panel.

Fisher, W., Zue, V., Bernstein, J., & Pallett, D. (1987). An acoustic-phonetic data base. *Journal of the Acoustical Society of America, 81*, S1, 92.

Gauvain J.–L., & Lamel, L. (2003). Large vocabulary speech recognition based on statistical methods. In W. Chou & B. Juang (Eds.), *Pattern recognition in speech and language processing* (pp. 149–190). Boca Raton, FL: CRC Press.

Gengel, R. (1976). Upton's wearable eyeglass speechreading aid: History and current status. In S. Hirsh, D. Eldridge, I. Hirsh, & S. Silverman (Eds.), *Hearing and Davis: Essays honoring Hallowell Davis* (pp. 291–299). St. Louis, MO: Washington University Press.

IEEE (1969). IEEE recommended practice for speech quality measurements. *IEEE Transactions on Audio and Electroacoustics, AU-17(3)*, 225–246. Standards Publication No. 297, available from IEEE.

Kunov, H., & Ebrahimi D. (1991). Measurement of performance of a peripheral vision lipreading aid. *Scandinavian Audiology, 20*, 131–137.

Lamel, L., Kassel, R., & Seneff, S. (1986). Speech database development: Design and analysis of the acoustic-phonetic corpus. In L. Baumann (Ed.), *Proceedings of the DARPA Speech Recognition Workshop* (pp. 100–109). San Diego, CA: DARPA Speech Recognition Workshop, SAIC-86/1546.

Pelley, K., Husaim, D., Tessler, M., Lindsay, J., & Krause, J. (2006). *The effect of speaking rate and experience on Cued Speech transliterator accuracy.* Poster session presented at the ASHA Convention (Session 0665, Poster 45), Miami, FL.

Pickett, J., Gengel, R., Quinn, R., & Upton, H. (1974). Research with the Upton eyeglass speechreader. In G. Fant (Ed.), *Speech communication: Vol. 4. Speech and hearing defects and aids.* Language Acquisition. Proceedings of the Seminar (pp. 324–328). Stockholm, Sweden.

Rabiner, L. (1989). A tutorial on hidden Markov models and selected applications in speech recognition. *Proceedings of the IEEE, 77*, 257–286.

Siniscalchi, S., Schwarz, P., & Lee, C. (2007). High accuracy phone recognition by combining high-performance lattice generation and knowledge based rescoring. *Proceedings of ICASSP 2007, Honolulu, IV*, 869–872.

Thelen, E., Aubert, X., & Beyerlein, P. (1997). Speaker adaptation in the Philips system for large vocabulary continuous speech recognition. *Proceedings of ICASSP-97, Munich, 2*, 1035–1038.

Uchanski, R., Delhorne, L., Dix, A., Reed, C. M., Braida, L., & Durlach, N. (1994). Automatic speech recognition to aid the hearing impaired: Prospects for the automatic generation of Cued Speech. *Journal of Rehabilitation Research and Development, 31*, 20–41.

Upton, H. (1968). Wearable eyeglass speech-reading aid. *American Annals of the Deaf, 113*, 222–229.

Woodland, P., Leggetter, C., Odell, J., Valtchev, V., & Young, S. (1995). The 1994 HTK large vocabulary speech recognition system. *Proceedings of the 1995 International Conference on Acoustics, Speech, and Signal Processing, ICASSP-95*, 73–76.

Chapter 22

AN AUTOMATIC WEARABLE SPEECH SUPPLEMENT FOR INDIVIDUALS' SPEECH COMPREHENSION IN FACE-TO-FACE AND CLASSROOM SITUATIONS

Dominic W. Massaro, Miguel A. Carreira-Perpiñán,
and David J. Merrill

This book on Cued Speech is representative of a fairly recent paradigm shift in spoken language processing. Traditionally, speech was viewed as solely an auditory phenomenon. Research manipulating multiple sources of potential information, however, indicates that speech perception is most productively viewed as *multimodal* and sensitive to a variety of inputs from the spoken input. This ability to exploit multiple modalities and multiple sources of information is a godsend to almost all individuals at some time in their lives.

Although the auditory input alone is insufficient for adequate communication for many individuals and/or in many situations, lipreading (more accurately referred to as *speechreading* because it involves more than just the lips) allows deaf and hard-of-hearing individuals to perceive and understand oral language and even to speak. Speechreading seldom disambiguates all of the spoken input, however, and other techniques have been used to allow a richer input. Cued Speech, the topic of this book, is a solution to having a limited auditory input, and consists of hand gestures while speaking that provide the perceiver with potentially disambiguating information to what is seen on the face. Before addressing the needs for language aids and the challenges they provide, we summarize evidence for viewing speech perception as a pattern recognition problem involving multiple sources of information from multiple modalities.

People Exploit Multiple Sources of Information in Speech Perception

Speech science evolved as the study of a unimodal auditory channel of communication because speech was viewed as primarily auditory (e.g., Denes & Pinson, 1963). There is no doubt that the voice alone usually is adequate for understanding for many individuals and, given the popularity of mobile phones, might be the most frequent medium for today's communication. However, there are many deaf and hard-of-hearing individuals who must have other sources of language input. The face is valuable even for normal hearing individuals because many communication environments involve a noisy auditory channel, which degrades speech perception and recognition. Speech should be viewed as a multimodal phenomenon because the human face presents visual information during speaking that is critically important for effective communication. Experiments indicate that our perception and understanding are influenced by a speaker's face, as well as the actual sound of speech (Bernstein, 2005; Massaro, 1987, 1998; Summerfield, 1987).

There are several reasons why the use of auditory and visual information in face-to-face interactions is so successful, and why it holds so much promise for language communication (Massaro, 1998). These include: (a) the information value of visible speech, (b) the robustness of visual speech, (c) the complementarity of auditory and visual speech, and (d) the optimal integration of these two sources of information. We review evidence for each of these properties and begin by describing an experiment illustrating how facial information improves recognition and memory for linguistic input.

Information Value of Visible Speech

The value of visible speech is demonstrated by the results of a series of experiments in which 71 typical college students reported the words of sentences presented in noise (Jesse, Vrignaud, & Massaro, 2000/2001). On some trials, only the acoustic sentence was presented (unimodal condition). On some other trials, the acoustic sentence was appropriately aligned with a highly realistic computer-animated face known as "Baldi" (bimodal condition). Baldi's presence facilitated performance for everyone. Accurate performance was more than doubled for those participants performing particularly poorly when given acoustic speech alone. Although a unimodal visual condition was not included in the experiment, we know that participants would have performed much more poorly than in the unimodal acoustic condition (Massaro, 2004). Thus, the combination of acoustic and visual speech is often described as synergistic because their combination can lead to a level of performance significantly higher than using either modality alone.

Similar results are found when noise-free speech is presented to persons with limited hearing (Erber, 1972). Adolescents and young adults who were either profoundly deaf or had severely impaired hearing benefited from face-to-face speech relative to just acoustic speech. The severely impaired perceivers (having a hearing loss between 75 and 90 dB) experienced the largest performance gain with nearly perfect performance in the bimodal condition relative to either of the unimodal conditions (Massaro, 1998, p. 159; Massaro & Cohen, 1999).

Robustness of Visual Speech

Empirical findings indicate that the ability to obtain speech information from the face is robust; that is, perceivers are fairly good at speechreading in a broad range of viewing conditions. To obtain information from the face, the perceiver does not have to fixate directly on the talker's lips but can be looking at other parts of the face or even somewhat away from the face (Smeele, Massaro, Cohen, & Sittig, 1998). Furthermore, accuracy is not dramatically reduced when the facial image is blurred (because of poor vision, for example), when the face is viewed from above, below, or in profile, or when there is a large distance between the talker and the viewer (Massaro, 1998, Munhall & Vatikiotis-Bateson, 2004; Munhall, Kroos, Jozan, & Vatikiotis-Bateson, 2004). These findings indicate that speechreading is highly functional in a variety of suboptimal situations. The robustness of visible speech is particularly important in the context of our research and development because perceivers will be combining speechread information with additional visual cues.

Complementary Auditory and Visual Speech

Complementary sources of information occur in circumstances where one source of information is most informative when the other source is weakest. In auditory/visual speech, two segments that are easily distinguished in one modality are relatively ambiguous in the other modality (Massaro & Cohen, 1999). For example, the difference between /ba/ and /va/ is easy to see but relatively difficult to hear. On the other hand, the difference between /ba/ and /pa/ is relatively easy to hear but very difficult to discriminate visually. The fact that two sources of information are complementary makes their combined use much more informative than would be the case if the two sources were redundant (Massaro, 1998, pp. 424–427). In our application for deaf and hard-of-hearing individuals, our goal is to optimize complementarity by making visible the linguistic information that is particularly difficult to see on the face.

Optimal Integration of Sources of Information

The final advantage afforded by having both auditory and visual sources of information is that perceivers tend to combine or integrate them in an optimally efficient manner (Massaro, 1987; Massaro & Cohen, 1999; Massaro & Stork, 1998). There are many possible ways to treat two sources of information: use only the most informative source; average the two sources together; or integrate them in such a fashion that both sources are used but that the least ambiguous source has the most influence. In fact, perceivers integrate the information available from each modality extremely efficiently, a pattern described by the Fuzzy Logical Model of Perception (FLMP) (Massaro, 1998). The FLMP assumes that the visible and audible speech signals are each evaluated (independently of the other source) to determine how much that source supports each alternative. The integration process optimally combines these support values to determine how much their combination supports the various alternatives. The perceptual outcome for the perceiver will be a function of the relative degree of support among the competing alternatives. As demonstrated elsewhere, the FLMP is mathematically equivalent to Bayes's theorem (Massaro, 1998), which is an optimal method for combining two sources of evidence to test among alternative hypotheses.

The best evidence for the FLMP comes from an important experimental manipulation that systematically varies the ambiguity of each source of information (Massaro, 1998). We have also found that, like adults, typically developing children integrate information from both the face and the voice (Massaro, 1984, 1987, 1998) as well as do deaf and hard-of-hearing children (Massaro, 1999, 2004, 2006; Massaro & Cohen, 1999) and autistic children (Massaro & Bosseler, 2003; Williams, Massaro, Peel, Bosseler, & Suddendorf, 2004). Critical for the requirements of our work is that this optimal integration occurs even if the auditory and visual speech are not perfectly synchronous (up to at least 100 ms). Finally, the pilot results described below indicate that individuals can easily learn to benefit from supplementary visual features when combined with facial information.

We now discuss the challenging need for supplementing spoken language and how our approach to speech perception can motivate the development of technology to provide additional sources of information in language processing.

Need for Language Supplements

There are millions of individuals with language and speech challenges who require additional support for language understanding and learning. An alarming statistic is that about 10% of the population in the United States is hearing-impaired (Better Hearing Institute, 2009). As an example of a specific need, it is well known that deaf and hard-of-hearing children have significant deficits in both spoken and written vocabulary knowledge (Breslaw, Griffiths, Wood, & Howarth, 1981; Holt, Traxler, & Allen, 1997). A similar situation exists for autistic children, who lag behind their typically developing cohort in language acquisition (Tager-Flusberg, 2000). Currently, however, these needs are not being met. One problem that the people with these disabilities face is that there are not enough skilled teachers, interpreters, and professionals to give them the one-on-one attention that they need.

In fact, humans can learn and use language successfully without adequate auditory input. Sign language parallels spoken language in acquisition, use, and communication. But even spoken language can serve communication when the auditory input is degraded or even absent. Lipreading (called speechreading because it involves more than just the lips) allows these individuals to perceive and understand oral language and even to speak

(Bernstein, Demorest, & Tucker, 2000; Kisor, 1990; Mirrelles, 1947). Speechreading seldom disambiguates all of the spoken input, however, and other techniques have been used to allow a richer input. Cued Speech, for example, is a deliberate solution to having a limited auditory input, and consists of hand gestures while speaking that provide the perceiver with information that potentially disambiguates what is seen on the face. However, very few people know Cued Speech or have the motivation to learn it, and therefore, individuals with limited auditory speech input are faced with insufficient input in many face-to-face and classroom-like environments.

Building on the innovative idea of Upton (1968), a solution Michael Cohen and Dominic Massaro proposed (Massaro, 1998) was to establish the technology required to design a device, which performs acoustic analysis of speech and transforms several acoustic features into visual features, which the speechreader would use in conjunction with watching the speaker's face. The acoustic features associated with important linguistic information not directly observed on the face will be transformed into *visual* cues intended to enhance intelligibility and ease of comprehension. A significant body of research supports the idea that people can easily learn to integrate such linguistic features with the incomplete visual information to achieve productive outcomes (Massaro, 1998, Chapter 14). Furthermore, similar to Cued Speech, the users of this device will have the advantage of gaining additional phonological awareness through the use of the linguistic features. We now discuss research that illustrates the value of providing additional visual cues to supplement the speech input.

Supporting Research on Supplementing Visible Speech

As illustrated throughout this book, Cued Speech has become an accepted form of communication for deaf and hard-of-hearing individuals. Cued Speech was designed as a means for supplementing lipreading by providing manual cues to phoneme identity to replace information not normally seen on the talker's face. Properties of Cued Speech include the following: (1) its hand gestures can be learned, (2) it is based on the phonemes of the spoken language, and (3) it can be used at the earliest stages of language acquisition. One drawback to Cued Speech, however, is that both communicating parties need to know the system of cues for it to be effective. Although being deaf or hard of hearing, or family and friends of the deaf or hard of hearing, might be motivation enough to learn a system of cues, we cannot expect other individuals to be similarly motivated. Thus, a solution for supplementing communication that does not depend on any special skills of the talker would be ideal.

Cornett (1967)'s idea was based on the realization that speechreading does not provide sufficient detail to distinguish all of the phonemes but only different subsets of phonemes, such as /b, p, m/ versus /f, v/ in a language. Different Cued Speech hand gestures were therefore designed to denote different subsets of phonemes so that both subsets together would indicate just a single phoneme. For example, the hand gesture with the index finger extended would signal the subset of phonemes /d, p, zh/ which when combined with the speechread /b, p, m/ would denote /p/. There is no linguistic or psychophysical structure within a Cued Speech category (e.g., /d, p, zh/), which most likely makes learning and understanding of the categories more difficult than necessary. Meaningful categories such as birds, fish, and chairs share perceptual and conceptual properties (Rosch & Lloyd, 1978). In contrast, the supplementary feature solution we propose is perceptually and conceptually based, and also provides continuous information indicating the degree to which a feature is present.

In the seminal patent description and demonstration by Upton (1968), relatively simple circuitry extracted three features from the acoustic signal: voicing, frication, and stop. These three simple features, plus two combination features: voiced fricative and voiced stop, were conveyed to the user via five tiny lamps, which were cemented to the lens of a pair of glasses so as to appear near the mouth of the talker being viewed. With a "considerable" training period, the user (Upton) was able to use the transformed acoustic cues to distinguish speechread information. Although Upton's initial paper gives only his subjective report, later papers (Gengel, 1976; Pickett, Gengel, Quinn, & Upton, 1974) documented positive results (with somewhat modified versions of the original device). Supporting research with laryngeal, nasal, and total intensity feature information presented tactilely (Miller, Engebretson, & DeFillipo, 1974) and voicing and stop features presented in visual and tactile modalities (Martony, 1974) were reported at about the same time.

Two other attempts have been made to design an automatic cueing system that accomplishes the same outcome as Cued Speech. The first attempt began in 1969 and was termed the Autocuer (Cornett, 1977). The Autocuer consists of a pair of eyeglasses through which a virtual image of seven light emitting diode (LED) elements is projected. Cues are presented to the user in the form of patterns in the LED array. Evaluation of the Autocuer was performed with normal-hearing as well as deaf and hard-of-hearing listeners. Recognition of isolated words was tested after a considerable training period of 40 hours, and was shown to increase from 63% with speechreading alone to 84% when using the Autocuer (Cornett, 1977). This result was obtained using ideal (hand-extracted) acoustic cues. Later evaluations of the original Autocuer report a less impressive increase (8%) when the cues were generated by a real-time recognizer (Duchnowski et al., 2000). This weaker result most likely was due to poor accuracy (54%) of the cue recognizer.

The second attempt at an automatic cueing system used a sophisticated, speaker-dependent speech recognizer to derive individual phones for conversion into a time-aligned set of cues for display (Duchnowski et al., 2000). There was a 2-second delay in the cue output, however, which is outside the window for fusing information from different inputs (Massaro, 1998). The cues were designed to look identical to Cued Speech so that those already familiar with it would have no trouble interpreting its display. Keyword scores for low-context sentences increased by 31% over speechreading alone (Duchnowski et al., 2000) although the scores fell well below Cued Speech controls. (Keyword scores using Upton's device for 6 months yielded an increase of 18% relative to sentences in the speechreading alone case.) Despite this achievement, Duchnowski et al. (2000) expressed doubt that a portable version of this device was feasible. One reason for this pessimistic conclusion is that speech recognition was used to generate the cues. Our approach bypasses full-blown speech recognition because accurate automatic speech recognition (ASR) is optimized for recognizing words, not acoustic features, and requires huge computational resources and is limited to less than real-time performance. (Best performance occurs with at least a 3-GHz processor, recognizing after each complete sentence is available. Successful systems carry out something like a cepstral analysis or similar technique with about 60 to 90 spectral features—with little relationship to linguistically-relevant features.) All three of these limitations preclude our use of ASR because the requirements for our approach are the tracking of acoustic features, close to real-time performance, and a lightweight portable device with limited computing power. Our proposed alternative is to simply detect a few robust acoustic features that can be mapped into visual cues simultaneously with their detection.

To compensate for the delay required for full-blown speech recognition, Duchnowski et al. (2000), recorded a video of the talking face and replayed this video to the listener simultaneously with the Cued Speech with a 2-second delay. This solution would be functional in televised broadcast or played on a video monitor. The system would not be practical in a face-to-face encounter whereas our envisioned system, on the other hand, would be highly functional in all foreseeable applications.

In summary, the widespread use of Cued Speech and the research with visual cueing systems show that automatically supplementing speech with visual features is a worthwhile research objective. Our future research will test improvements in such a manner that will lead to

a successful system. The requirements of a successful system include a light footprint for a wearable device, operation in near real time, accurate tracking of acoustic features, learnable visual features, and integration of these features with auditory and visual speech.

Research from the Perceptual Science Laboratory

We have carried out pilot research to investigate how to supplement talking faces with information that is ordinarily conveyed by auditory means. We now describe our initial work on this problem of supplementing visual speech. We have separated this research into two areas, which will be discussed in the next two sections: (1) developing a neural network to perform real-time analysis of certain acoustic features for visual display, and (2) determining how quickly subjects can learn to use these selected cues and how much they benefit from them when combined with speechreading.

Acoustic Feature Analysis

The goal of feature analysis is to track certain acoustic features in real time and to transform them into continuous visual displays. In pilot research, we developed and trained a neural network to recognize three auditory speech characteristics: nasality, voicing, and frication. The training database was a sample of 23 words, containing 2,607 analysis frames from in the Bernstein & Eberhardt (1986) corpus. Each frame was 7.8 ms (Hanning windowed) and a new frame was sampled every 1.6 ms. These words were Viterbi aligned in order to determine the phoneme segments. In previous research, we developed a computer-animated talker trained on real speech to produce accurate speech with appropriate coarticulation (Massaro et al., 2005). To improve speech perception for hard-of-hearing individuals, Massaro et al. (2007) patented a set of supplementary visible speech features to provide additional information not seen on the face, and these features were shown to be effective in training speech perception and production in hard-of-hearing children (Massaro & Light, 2004). Baldi could now be aligned with the natural speech in the database to give subphonemic features describing the moment-to-moment changes in voicing, frication, and nasality.

The neural net included 22 input units, 8 hidden-layer units, and 3 output units. A fast Fourier transform (FFT) computed the amount of energy in each of 20 Bark frequency bands (the Bark scale is nonlinear to match the properties of the peripheral auditory system). These measures, together with overall amplitude and number of zero-crossings, gave a 22-valued input vector. The feedback to the three output nodes were the subphonemic values computed in the alignment process. The weights on the connections among the units in the neural net were adjusted to minimize the differences between the actual and predicted features. Training gave a 0.057 root mean square deviation (RMSD) between the actual and predicted feature values on a 0 to 1 scale. To summarize, the neural net model was successfully trained to provide moment-by-moment outputs for the three features on the basis of acoustic input.

Thus in principle, we have learned that we can use a network to transform the Bark scale energies from each speech frame into continuous visual features for presentation. Extensions of this work to obtain a functional, effective, and real-time system are described later in this chapter.

Visual Feature Perception

Our studies of the perception of supplementary visual feature information were done using simulated rather than real-time analysis of acoustic features. We wished to see how difficult it would be for subjects to learn to effectively use the visual features we had selected to supplement speechreading. A table giving the mapping between the phonemes and the visual features, as well as phonetic and coarticulatory information, was provided in written form to the subjects. For example, vowels are voiced, fricatives have frication, frication can occur during the onset of stop consonants, and the nasal following a vowel can produce nasality during the vowel as well as during the nasal segment. In a five-day experiment, subjects speechread 318 one-syllable words from the Bernstein and Eberhardt (1986) corpus presented visually. The visual speech was presented by a human speaker whose facial image was 13.7 degrees (deg) horizontal and 20.4 deg vertical on a 30.5 cm diagonal screen 50 cm from the viewer. One group of 4 subjects was presented with feature information along with this silent talking head, whereas a control group of three subjects received only the silent talking face and no feature information.

For the feature group, the features nasal, voiced, and fricative were presented at the left side of the screen (centered 10.2 deg from face midline) in the form of intensity (saturation) of colored bars (5.1 deg horizontal by 2.0 deg vertical in size, spaced 2.9 deg apart vertically). Figure 22–1 gives an example of the dis-

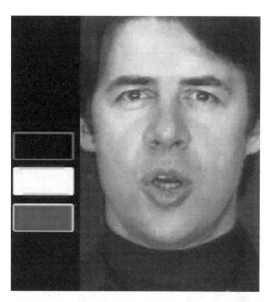

Figure 22–1. An example of the video display with the visual features. The top nasal bar indicates the nasals by lighting up orange during the period they occur. The middle voicing bar indicates voiced sounds by lighting up white and the bottom frication bar lights up when there is frication noise. The intensity of each cue corresponded to the degree to which the corresponding acoustic feature was present in the speech signal.

play with the features. A series of trials is given on Band 14.8 in Massaro (1998), and is available online at http://mambo.ucsc.edu/psl/mmc/14_8.mov. It shows the continuous nature of the colored features during the speech input.

The top bar indicated the nasal sounds by lighting up orange during the period they occurred. The middle bar indicated voiced sounds by lighting up white when they occurred and remaining off when they did not. Two bars could light up at the same time as during a voiced fricative, for example. Silence would be indicated when all three features are dark. The bottom bar corresponded to frication, which lit up during the frication in fricatives and the burst/aspiration period in stop consonants. In all cases, the intensity of each of the three cues corresponded to the degree to which the corresponding acoustic feature was present in the speech signal. The cues were generated based on the phonetic labels of the acoustic speech as determined by Viterbi alignment (when knowledge of the words was provided). This is described in more detail below. Subjects made their responses by typing a word on a keyboard, which was followed by feedback during which presenting the word (with features for the feature group) was presented again, with the sound on, and the word shown in print on the left side of the screen.

Several analyses were carried out including accuracy of word identification; accuracy in identifying initial consonants, vowels, and final consonants; consonant and vowel confusions; and accuracy of feature identification for initial and final consonants. The left panel of Figure 22–2 shows the proportion of words correctly identified as a function of the five successive experimental blocks. Both groups improved with experience, but the feature group was significantly better overall and improved faster. The center and right panels of Figure 22–2 show a d-prime measure of accuracy for identification of initial voicing and nasality respectively for the two groups. (The d-prime measure is bias free and measured in z-scores. Note that these two panels have different scales, given the different ranges of performance.) Relative to the control group, the feature group was able to improve quickly by utilizing the supplementary visual feature information. It should be noted that word accuracy was still below perfect performance. This could mean either that

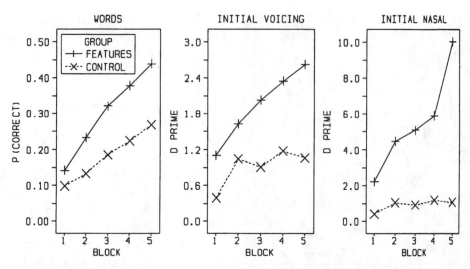

Figure 22–2. Proportion correct word identification (*left panel*), identification (d-prime) of initial voicing (*center panel*), and identification (d-prime) of initial nasality (*right panel*) as a function of experimental block, for feature and control groups.

the speechreading and features together were still insufficient to disambiguate the words, or the subjects had not yet learned to use the information to achieve perfect word recognition.

Analyzing the consonant confusions for the control and feature groups indicated that the feature group was able to make discriminations that were not possible for the controls. For example, within the labial stops /b, m, p/, the feature group could discriminate between the three members of the class, whereas the control group split their responses equally among the three alternatives. This experiment demonstrates that speechreading with these visual features is learnable and greatly improves speechreading accuracy. However, it is necessary to extend the research to more challenging situations, including scenarios with conversational speech and multiple speakers. In the next

two sections, we outline plans for our ongoing and future work towards the goals of determining suitable acoustic features to extract from the speech, transforming them to present on the wearable supplement, and evaluating the prototype system.

Acoustic Feature Analysis

Evaluating Different Approaches to the Extraction of Features

The success of our approach is critically dependent on successfully extracting informative acoustic features from the speech signal. Several recent investigations have found that the use of abstract phonetic features is advantageous as a preliminary stage of automatic speech recognition (ASR) (King & Taylor, 2000). Typically, investigators have used TIMIT sentences with a preliminary Mel frequency cepstral coefficient (MFCC) analysis with a 25.6-ms window moving in 10-ms steps. This representation, sometimes with additional sets of first and second time derivatives (delta and double delta features) are then analyzed using neural nets (NNs), hidden Markov models (HMMs), support vector machines (SVMs), or decision trees. Chang, Greenberg, and Wester (2001), for example, use an NN solution with separate networks for each phonetic feature with a mechanism for using only high-confidence results. Eide (2001) instead used a Gaussian-mixture (GM) approach. Frankel, Wester, and King (2004) compared dynamic GM models with NNs but found no advantage for either. Abu-Amer and Carson-Berndsen (2003) used independent HMMs. Our research will focus on designing and training neural networks to extract three or four acoustic (rather than phonetic) features: voicing, frication, nasality, and sonorant.

Extracting Voicing

Relevant research for this aspect of our work comes from a study by Aioanei, Carson-Berndsen, and Kanokphara (2006). They developed two phonetic feature-extraction engines for voicing and frication, similar to two of the four acoustic features we evaluate. The output of their engine was the presence or absence of a feature. "The TIMIT training set was parameterized into 13 dimensional MFCCs, energy and their delta and acceleration (39 length front-end parameters)." The feature models were trained from these parameters. Performance for voicing was very good, averaging about 90% accuracy.

Extracting Frication

In contrast to the good performance for voicing, the overall accuracy for fricative was only about 37% correct because, although fricatives were usually recognized, the burst and aspiration phases of stops were also erroneously recognized as fricatives. Although this type of false alarm is problematic for phonetic features, it is not in our proposed system because the acoustic feature frication occurs in both fricatives and stops. Our supplementary visual feature frication conveys the acoustic feature frication, not the phoneme fricative. Participants are told and learn that frication is a characteristic of stop bursts and voiceless transitions. We found in our visual feature perception study that perceivers benefited from this source of information in identifying both stops and fricatives. That is, when perceivers learn the appropriate mapping, activation of the acoustic feature frication during the stop onset is informative, as it is during fricatives. Supporting this analysis, when accuracy was recomputed for frication occurrence for both stops and fricatives in the Aioanei et al. (2006) study, feature extraction performance improved to over 80%.

Extracting Nasality

Frankel et al. (2007) trained multilayer perceptrons (MLPs) for feature classification on close to 2,000 hours of telephone speech. A context window of 9 to 10-ms frames (central frame plus 4 frames each of left and right context) was used on the input layer for all MLPs. Given the 39 dimensional input feature, this amounts to 351 input units. The number of units on the output layer of each MLP corresponded to the number of levels of the feature group. For the nasality feature, the system achieved an accuracy of 90% correct. This study provides initial support for the feasibility of accurately tracking the acoustic feature nasality in our application.

Extracting Sonorant

This feature categorizes "+ sonorant" for vowels, semivowels, and nasals, and "– sonorant" for fricatives, stops, and non-speech. Shutte and Glass (2005) implemented a support vector machine to detect sonorant features in TIMIT sentences. For each utterance, 14 Mel-frequency cepstral coefficients (MFCCs) were computed every 10 ms over a 25.6-ms Hamming window, with cepstral-mean subtraction performed over each 500-ms window. After training, a fairly accurate performance was obtained even when a moderate amount of noise was added to the speech.

Discrete Features with Continuous Outputs

King and Taylor (2000) pointed out that although the feedback data used to train the feature-detection mechanism (e.g., an NN) might be discrete, the output features of the NN may be continuous in value. In our prior use of visual features for supplementing speechreading this type of continuous output is explicitly the case. Figure 22–3, a screen shot from our development system, shows an illustration of the mapping of the acoustic signal to the fricative indicator for the phrase "he then sat."

We generated the display intensity in the same way as other synthesis control parameters for a computer animated talking face (Massaro, 1998; Massaro & Cohen, 1993) using coarticulation blending functions with specific target values and coarticulation dominance functions for each phoneme. Although the occurrence of

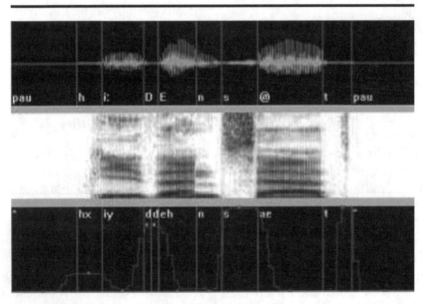

Figure 22–3. Frication display intensity (*bottom panel*) for the phrase "he then sat" for the speech signal in the top panel, and the spectrogram in the middle panel.

frication at each moment is coded as either present or absent, the coarticulation blending function produces continuous outputs. For example, in Figure 22–3, the output of frication for /h/ is computed as having weaker frication than the output for /s/. In addition, the amount of frication changes dynamically at the transitions between successive phonemes. Figure 22–3 also shows that a short frication is displayed during the consonant release burst of /t/.

In evaluating competing approaches to the signal analysis, a critical factor will be the requirement of real-time performance because there should not be too much of a time lag between the visual facial information and the feature displays. Research in auditory/visual speech perception suggests that some delay (e.g., up to 50-100 ms) would be acceptable (Grant, 2002; Grant & Greenberg, 2001; Grant, Greenberg, Poeppel, & van Wassenhove, 2004; Massaro, 1998).

Other Continuous Features

The previous features of voicing, frication, nasality, and sonorant are derived from prior knowledge of phonetics, and as such are likely to be highly effective for determining phoneme identity when combined with the facial display. However, (1) these may not necessarily be the most discriminable of all possible features and (2) these 4 features may not be completely independent, and may be jointly redundant with the facial display. Furthermore, the number of visual features should be kept to a minimum because of limits in the number of visual cues that the glasses can accommodate (probably limited to 3), and due to limits in the number of visual cues that a subject may reasonably be able to learn. This suggests using machine learning techniques to determine the opti-

mal visual features, where we roughly define "optimal features" as the 3 functions of the acoustic vector that, when augmented with the face, best classify the acoustics into phonemes. Although these features will likely lack a straightforward interpretation as, say, frication, this may not necessarily result in an increased difficulty for a subject to learn them.

We now explore different specific methods to determine the optimal visual features. One possibility is to extract informative features from each acoustic frame (13-D MFCCs) using dimensionality reduction methods. These methods look, in an unsupervised way, for a small number of continuous features that preserve information about the acoustic vector. Many methods exist in the machine learning and statistics literature, including linear methods (such as PCA, factor analysis and independent component analysis) and nonlinear methods (such as autoencoders, nonlinear latent variable models, Isomap, LLE, Laplacian eigenmaps, and others) (Carreira-Perpiñán, 2001; Saul, Weinberger, Ham, Sha, & Lee, 2007). For our task, which requires us to extract three latent features and to extract features from test data unseen during training, we plan to use a recently introduced nonlinear method, the Laplacian Eigenmaps Latent Variable Model (LELVM; Carreira-Perpiñán & Lu, 2007). This method has the advantages of scaling well to latent spaces of three dimensions or greater, having no local optima, and providing both continuous mappings (for dimensionality reduction and reconstruction) and probability densities (for the data and latent features); no other nonlinear method that we know of possesses all these simultaneously.

A more direct approach that actively looks for features that maximize discrimination ability jointly with the face display is as follows. Consider for simplicity visual features $\mathbf{W^*x}$ that are a linear projection of the 13-D MFCCs $\mathbf{x}$ (where $\mathbf{W}$ is a matrix of weights); and assume we can extract a face-feature vector $\mathbf{y}$ from the face image, say the lip and tongue contours (note these face features are only used in an offline analysis to determine the best visual features, not in real-time use with the glasses). Now, we can use the joint vector $(\mathbf{W^*x,y})$ of linear visual features and face features as inputs to a neural-net classifier that maps its input to its corresponding phoneme. By minimizing the classification error over the neural-net weights and the linear projection weights $\mathbf{W}$, we can find the best linear projection. "Best" here means optimal for classification, and the projection may differ from the PCA projection that we would obtain in an unsupervised training. Thus, this would be a form of supervised dimensionality reduction. Clearly, we can also use a nonlinear projection (e.g., another neural net) of the acoustic vector $\mathbf{x}$ instead of a linear one $\mathbf{W^*x}$. The classification error would also allow a comparison with the phonetic features of voicing, frication, nasality, and sonorant.

Labeling New Data Sets

Our pilot training was fairly limited, and in future work we will extend training and testing to include several new more ecologically valid and comprehensive databases. We also chose these corpora because they have the advantages of being publicly available for the research community, having time-aligned word transcription and phonetic transcription, as well as a variety of speakers.

We use the well-known TIMIT sentences, which are available in two different multimodal databases. Hazen, Sanko, La, and Glass (2004) provide the 450 SX TIMIT sentences read by 223 talkers. The VidTIMIT database (Sanderson, 2002), recently made available by the Linguistic Data Consortium (LDC), consists of 43 subjects reciting 10 different TIMIT sentences each. Fortunately, there is now an ideal database available for training on face-to-face spontaneous speech (Pitt et al., 2007). Forty speakers, all natives of central Ohio, contributed about 300,000 words of spontaneous speech in interviews in which they expressed their opinions in conversation. The speech of central Ohioans is fairly representative of American speech without the accents of the Northeast or Southeast.

Although these databases have been orthographically transcribed and phonetically aligned, this markup is not adequate for the training of our acoustic features. We therefore will first select a subset of each of these databases and mark up the presence or absence of our four targeted acoustic features. The existing database contains the waveform and spectrum, the phoneme labels and boundaries, and the written transcription. We mark up each acoustic frame of the waveform as plus (1) or minus (0) on each of the four acoustic features voicing, frication, nasality, and sonorant. The markup is guided by both the phoneme markup and the acoustic properties, which are evaluated by both listening and visual inspection. These analyses will be carried out using readily available applications such as Wavesurfer (http://www.speech.kth.se/wavesurfer/).

Training and Testing Neural Networks

We train and test neural networks on the corpora in order to determine whether the acoustic features can be accurately tracked by a neural network and to determine which acoustic features give the most accurate performance. We use feed-forward neural networks with a single layer of hidden units, which can approximate most of the useful functions to a high degree of precision when a sufficient number of hidden units are used. Several different configurations of the acoustic input and the number of hidden units are used to converge on a successful representation. As an example, there would be 9 input frames, consisting of a center frame and four frames preceding and following the center frame, each corresponding to 10 ms of speech. For each input frame, the neural net would have 22 input units, 8 hidden-layer units, and 4 output units. The amount of energy in each of 20 Bark frequency bands together with overall amplitude and number of zero-crossings would give a 22-valued input vector. The target value for the four output nodes would be the subphonemic values computed in the proposed alignment process. The networks are trained using backpropagation to minimize the prediction error on the training set, with weight decay to improve generalization. The best network architecture (i.e., the number of hidden units and the number of frames in the input window) are determined by cross-validation. Training and test data come, for example, from the TIMIT database (e.g., 12 sentences sampled from 12 speakers for a total of 144 sentences). Analogous training regimes is employed for the conversation database.

Remote Recordings of the Speech

To succeed, the envisioned system requires the recording of the acoustic speech in face-to-face conversations by a microphone worn by the listener. The biggest sources of potential error using a remote

microphone on the listener include background noise and room reverberation during the conversation. Most ASR systems have the luxury of the talker speaking into a lapel microphone or a telephone for the recording. Given that the microphone will be worn by the listener, the best performance should occur when the system is trained on remote recordings of the acoustic speech. In this case, the signal processing will be on live presentations of the acoustic speech rather than on the original digital representation of the speech database. Thus, we repeat the previous training of the neural networks on sentences and conversational speech when the speech is processed by a microphone at distances resembling those in face-to-face conversation.

Goal of Neural Network Training

Our goal is to test the feasibility of our proposed feature analysis. Given previous successes in phonetic feature analysis reviewed above and our pilot research, we expect this aspect of our work to be successful. Apart from the trained neural networks themselves (needed for the real-time computation of the features), another outcome will be a direct measure of how accurately each of the four acoustic features can be tracked by a neural network. This information will partially indicate which visual features would most likely be effective in representing the input in face-to-face communication.

Visual Feature Perception

Participant Population

Participants will include normal-hearing as well as deaf and hard-of-hearing persons, who have a vested interest in enhancing their communication interactions. We also attempt to recruit persons who are skilled in Cued Speech to assess to what extent this experience and skill facilitates or inhibits performance with the supplementary visual features.

Use Neural Network Outcome to Choose Visual Features

The outcome of the neural network experiments will provide direct measures of how accurately each of the four acoustic features can be tracked by a neural network. We use this information to choose the three visual features to be used in these experiments. Ideally, all four visual features might be tested and compared with all combinations of three features. Given that each experiment requires some significant amount of learning, however, these 4 independent experiments (i.e., the 4 combinations ABC, ABD, ACD, BCD of 4 acoustic features A, B, C, D) would be too time consuming. Furthermore, if one of the acoustic features proves to be too difficult to track accurately, then it would not be functional and, in fact, could be disruptive for performance. For these reasons, the design of the experiments on visual feature processing contingent on the outcome of the neural network experiments.

Extend Presentation of the Visual Features to LED Eyeglasses

Our pilot research indicated that perceivers were able to use the supplementary visual features presented in the periphery while still attending to the speaker's lips. Performance improved significantly with about 40 minutes of practice per day across 5 days of training. This improvement might have been due to the presentation of facial as well as visual feature information on the same computer display monitor. Therefore, it is important to replicate this study in a situation that more accurately approximates our envisioned real-world application. In this study, we will replicate our initial experiment so that the participants look through the instrumented eyeglasses to see the talking face on a computer monitor, with visual features displayed on LEDs in their peripheral vision. The supplementary feature displays are computer-generated and their output is displayed on the eyeglasses-mounted LEDs. All other procedural details and data analyses will be similar to our pilot study. It is necessary to build and configure eyeglass frames to hold the LED display. Figure 22–4 shows a picture of our first mockup of the specialized eyeglasses. The display is mounted at the periphery of each lens. We will evaluate whether the LED display can be processed adequately or whether it must be moved closer to the center. It also may be necessary to adjust the forward-back location of the display for some users, to maximize comfort and view-ability.

We will assess whether it is valuable to have the LED display on both sides or whether one is sufficient. Eyeglasses with LEDs on just a single side would significantly streamline the design. If just a single side is sufficient, the side of the eyeglasses that holds the display may be an important variable, since this determines whether the visual features well be seen to the right or left of the talking face. There is a large literature on hemifield effects in visual perception and language processing, and although the research is not conclusive (Smeele et al., 1998), it would be advantageous to choose the side that leads to best performance. Thus, we will systematically vary whether the LED display is shown on the left side of the left lens or on the

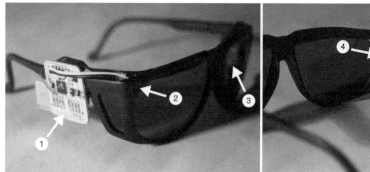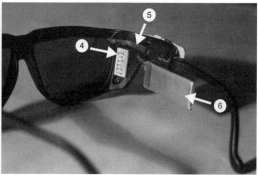

Figure 22–4. Picture of the first version of a mockup of the eyeglasses that would hold the processor (1), microphone (2), LED display (3, 4), vibrator (5), and battery (6).

right side of the right lens. We expect that performance with the LED display will improve speech perception, as it did in our pilot study. If it does not, we will explore the differences between these two situations in order to better design an effective wearable display.

Figure 22–4 shows that the microphone, the processor, the battery, and the LED display can be placed together on just one side of the eyeglasses. We have mounted a small vibrator because we will also investigate the efficacy of transforming one of the acoustic features such as sonorant into a slight vibration of the frame of the eyeglasses.

Evaluate Speechreading and Feature Perception with Sentences and Conversational Speech

Our pilot research indicated that the supplementary visual features positively influenced the perception and recognition of words presented in isolation. Natural dialogue provides continuous speech, and we will test the functionality of our system with complete sentences. It is important to extend the testing to continuous sentences as opposed to isolated words used in the pilot research. This comparison is important because with isolated words, subjects may be able to employ perceptual strategies that are difficult with longer materials. Martony (1974) reports a supplementary feature advantage for recognition of whole sentences, which were previously trained with a closed response set method. For sentences not previously trained, however, only a small nonsignificant advantage over unaided speechreading was observed. Therefore, it is important to test whether we observe a positive contribution of supplementary visual features with sentences from multiple speakers in our application.

The test materials consist of 144 sentences from the TIMIT database. The sentences are presented both with and without the supplementary features. Subjects are asked to type in as much of the sentence as they can. The results are analyzed in terms of the number of words correctly reported under the two conditions. With the exception of continuous sentences as opposed to isolated words, all other procedural details and data analyses are similar to our initial pilot study described above. The same evaluation task is extended to include the perception of speech from the corpus of conversational speech.

An important aspect of these studies involves learning. Our pilot study indicated that participants do indeed learn to take advantage of the supplementary visual features. Even though learning occurred, there are potentially alternative learning regimens that can increase the rate and asymptote of learning. One possible training situation is to practice just a single supplementary visual feature at a given time. After achieving good learning on one feature, the presentation could be made more challenging by adding a second feature and then a third in like manner. Another technique to facilitate learning would be to present a practice period on each feature directly rather than in the context of words and sentences. In this case, the test materials would consist of simply consonant-vowel syllables so participants will be able to focus on the visual features for just a single consonant. Another possibility is to practice the participants on the features without the face present so they can directly learn the supplementary features. If we observe that the benefit from the supplementary features is acquired slowly in our standard testing paradigm, we experiment with optimizing the learning process by instantiating some or all of these potential learning aids.

Combine Visual Feature Perception and Acoustic Feature Analysis in Real Time

Having completed the research on visual feature perception and acoustic feature analysis in real time, an experiment will be carried out to test their combination. In this case, the acoustic feature analysis and visual feature presentation are combined during the evaluation testing. To implement this experimentation, it will be necessary to add a microphone and a wearable processor to the eyeglasses with the LED display. The microphone will capture the speaker's conversational surroundings and an analog audio circuit transmit the acoustic signal to the processor where it will be digitized. Given that the neural networks have already been trained offline, it is only necessary to program the processor with any necessary signal processing for the sampled digital signal, the feed forward network with the learned weights from the learning phase, and the output generation algorithm to drive the LED display. Running on the processor, the trained neural networks will process the digitized speech sounds in real time and directly drive the LED display on the eyeglasses. All other procedural details follow that given in the previous tests with sentences and conversational speech.

Evaluation Summary

Normally, there are three mostly sequential activities that can evaluate the quality of the pedagogy and technology: (1) exploratory research, (2) formative evaluation, and (3) summative evaluation. Our exploratory research has already been carried out along with specified procedures for formative evaluation: accuracy of acoustic feature analysis and the speech perception benefit of supplementary visual features. The summative evaluation will assess the effectiveness these two components in the context of a complete system of supplementing talking faces with visual features. The quality of the proposed system will be directly measured by the extent to which perceivers benefit from the supplementary visual displays.

Extensions to Real World Performance

Given a successful outcome, participants will be chosen to wear the eyeglasses throughout their typical day. Participants will include deaf and hard-of-hearing persons, who have a vested interest in enhancing their communication interactions. These participants will be monitored to determine how functional the system is in typical interlocutor situations. Based on these observations and participant reports, we can determine the positive and negative aspects of the system. Modifications can then be made, if possible, to improve the system and the resulting quality of the face-to-face conversations.

Significance and Concomitant Advantages of our Current and Future Work

The technology we are developing would be ideally designed for wearable computing so a person could have a face-to-face conversation while wearing a pair of simple glasses, which could also be fitted with the person's normal eye prescription. The wearable product would process primitive characteristics of the speech signal such as voicing (the presence of energy at the fundamental frequency such as heard in vowel sounds); frication (high frequency noise like energy characteristic of various consonants such as [s], [z], and [sh]; and nasality (which is a unique resonance characteristic as in [m], [n], and [ŋ]). These characteristics would be tracked in near real time, and the output displayed on the glasses (Costanza et al., 2006).

Our envisioned system holds much promise because the proposed system does not replace auditory information with the supplementary cues but rather supplements the auditory speech that is normally available to the listener. People naturally integrate auditory and visual information so they should necessarily benefit from having both visible and audible speech. In addition, this strategy is particularly effective because of the complementarity of auditory and visual speech. The acoustic speech that is robust in the signal and fairly easy to automatically recognize is exactly that which is not visible on the face. This serendipitous occurrence makes it more likely to succeed at automatically recognizing the robust acoustic characteristics and simultaneously presenting them visually as supplementary cues.

The proposed technology qualifies as a transparent information appliance that adds perceptual and cognitive resources to the listener (Clark, 2003; Norman, 1999; Weiser, 1991). We have developed a requirements analysis, a conceptual design, and possible physical designs for this appliance. It consists of a very affordable noninvasive device that is seamlessly integrated with normal dress, adding a pair of glasses (which might be used regardless). This qualifies as an augmented-reality device, supplementing the wearer's experience of the world around them, available for use around the clock, and requiring very little maintenance.

Usability for All Individuals

The system we propose is naturally available to all individuals who can wear a pair of eyeglasses. The device does not require literate speakers because no written information is presented as would be the case in a captioning system. It is also age independent in that it can be used by toddlers, adolescents, and throughout the life span. There is evidence that very young children can learn sign language and even fingerspelling of the spoken language. The same should be true for the proposed supplementary cues. The phonetic basis for the speech driven cues should also reinforce an understanding of the phonology of the language (Morais & Kolinsky, 1994). Studies have shown that deaf and hard-of-hearing children who have mastered Cued Speech have internalized much of the phonology of their language and learn to read naturally. Thus, with our system, we expect that children will learn vocabulary and grammar and will gain meta-awareness of the structure of the community's spoken language.

Available to All Language Groups

One of the major advantages of our envisioned system is that it is language independent because all languages share the same fundamental acoustic characteristics. Other non-automated systems such as Cued Speech and Sign Language are language dependent. Thus, all language groups can use the proposed system without compromising their normal language processing in other domains such as in signing or Cued Speech conversations. The device would be primarily functional in the frequent case when the listener is faced with oral language of a person who does not use Cued Speech.

Significant Help for People with Hearing Aids and Cochlear Implants

There have been substantial improvements in the technology of hearing aids and cochlear implants, which now provide significant help for many individuals. However, these persons are still challenged in many natural environments such as those with background noise and reverberation, and in challenging conversations. The technology we propose will provide exactly the additional supplement to speechreading that will allow communication in these situations.

Extended Reach of the Research

The benefits of this research extend beyond the deaf and hard-of-hearing community. There are many individuals, including autistic children and persons recovering from brain trauma, who have difficulty processing acoustic speech. Many of them successfully communicate by alternative communication methods. Our research will improve the state of the art in transforming acoustic speech into other forms on information, which will offer a larger number of potential communication methods for these individuals.

Benefits to Pedagogy of Reading

It is well-known that there are substantial out-of-the-ordinary problems that a number of children encounter in learning to read and spell. Children who have much more difficulty in reading and spelling than would be expected from their other perceptual and cognitive abilities are labeled as dyslexic (Fleming, 1984; Willows, Kruk, & Crocos, 1993). Psychological science has established a tight relationship between the mastery of written language and the child's ability to process spoken language (de Gelder & Morais, 1995; Morais & Kolinsky, 1994; Taylor & Olson, 1994). That is, it appears that many dyslexic children also have deficits in spoken language perception. The difficulty with spoken language can be alleviated through improving children's perception of phonological distinctions in their spoken language, which in turn improves their ability to read and spell (National Reading Panel, 2000). Experience with the wearable system should help these children gain insights into the spoken language and therefore improve their reading skill.

Potential Limitations of the Research Agenda

A potential limitation of our system is that some nonvisible acoustic features of consonants but not vowels are mapped into visible features to help disambiguate the spoken message. Cueing vowels would obviously provide more potential information for the listener. As in all applications, however, there are tradeoffs that have to be considered. Cueing vowels would have a number of possible negative effects. First, recognizing vowels or vowel features from the waveform would be highly fallible relative to recognizing the other features being analyzed in our system. Second, there is a limit on the number of features that the listener can process in parallel with the audible and visible speech input. Adding several vowel features would probably exceed that limit. Third, vowels carry less a priori information than consonants in English. Thus, vowels are more predictable in word contexts than consonants. Fourth, with partial hearing due to hearing loss, noise, or cochlear implants, vowels appear to be less perceptually degraded and therefore more intelligible than consonants. In this case, the listener will probably benefit more from the acoustic signal for vowels than for consonants, making any visible feature for vowels less informative. Fifth, the visible speech from the speaker is relatively informative for vowels, much more than it is for the voicing, frication, nasality, and sonorant features currently in the proposed system. Vowel information is perceived fairly accurately from just the face alone, however. Montgomery and Jackson (1983) and Massaro (1998) found about 75% correct lipreading among eight vowel categories. Our research will determine whether consonant cues are sufficient for accurate performance when a reasonable amount of training is given. If so, the case can be made that a robust system of augmented communication can be implemented even though no additional supplementary cues are provided for vowels.

It might be proposed that automatic speech recognition (ASR) by machine will improve sufficiently in the near future so that a full captioning of the speech being spoken can be accurately rendered. Although this significant breakthrough is always possible, it seems unlikely to occur in the near future. ASR recognition can be expected to be reasonably functional when there is a limited vocabulary and grammatical structure as input, if the system is speaker dependent—that is, trained on a single speaker, and/or used in a completely noise-free environment. We also have described how accurate ASR requires less than real-time performance and huge computational resources. These constraints exist because most ASR systems do a poor job of recognizing phonemes (Greenberg, 2006; Greenberg & Chang, 2000), and must use sophisticated word models (usually bi- or tri-gram models) to deduce words from a flawed recognition of the phonemes. Our device, on the other hand, is functional in natural settings of open dialogs and conversations from multiple speakers. Most importantly, however, our approach has five important advantages: (1) it supplements rather than replaces the acoustic signal, (2) it can be carried out in real time, (3) it requires relatively few computational resources, (4) it conveys a continuous analysis rather than a discrete categorization of the speech input, and (5) it is language independent because the acoustic features that will be analyzed should vary relatively little across different languages.

Another potential limitation of our approach is the recording of the acoustic speech in face-to-face conversations. Most ASR systems have the luxury of having the talker speak into a lapel microphone or a telephone for the recording. In our system, the microphone will be worn by the listener. This challenge is anticipated in the present project by training the system on somewhat remote recordings. In addition, because it is simply necessary to transmit acoustic features, the challenge of remote recording is diminished significantly. The most likely sources of potential error using a remote microphone on the listener include background noise and room reverberation in the location of verbal exchange and the speech of others who are not in the conversation. In addition to the challenge of having the microphone distant from the speaker, it would also be somewhat variable because the distances and directions will vary in typical face-to-face conversations. Techniques are available to adjust for these sources of degradation of the acoustic spectrum. By training our neural-net acoustic-feature recognition system on remote recordings, the potential sources of degradation will be reduced.

Regardless of the advances or lack of advances in speech-recognition technology, it will always be more accurate and effective to automatically pick off features than phonemes. First, there are typically only two to five alternatives for features, as opposed to roughly 40 to 60 phonemes. Second, the features (voicing, frication, nasality, and sonorant) are relatively straightforward to recognize automatically. We do not attempt to analyze the most difficult acoustic feature place of articulation, which is exactly the information that is so easily seen on the face.

It might be argued that the tactile modality might be more appropriate for the presentation of the supplementary features. For example, instead of providing three colored bars, the same information could be mapped into three vibratory transducers. There are well-known commonalities between the visual and tactile sensory systems (Freides, 1974; Hirsh & Sherrick, 1961; Lederman & Klatzky, 2004; Loomis & Lederman, 1986; Loveless, Brebner, & Hamilton, 1970; Sherrick & Cholewiak, 1986), and it may be that observers will be at a disadvantage dividing their attention between two visual sources of information relative to coordinating two sources from separate modalities. However, it is also known that the tactile modality has much poorer spatial and temporal resolution than vision. In an experiment with CV syllables, better performance was found for visual than for tactile presentation of features (Martony, 1974). For voiced stops, there was no improvement with tactile, but a significant improvement with visual feature presentation. Martony suggested that this was due to an inability of subjects to perceive the exact temporal relation between the visual and tactile information. Thus, there may be an advantage to using two sources from the visual modality because of an enhanced ability to perceive the temporal relationship between speechreading and visual cues. With two visual sources listeners should more easily detect temporal relation cues, such as voice onset time (a cue to voicing which in this case would be realized as a relation between some visible facial articulation and the activation of the supplementary voicing bar).

Summary and Conclusion

The need for language aids is pervasive in today's world. Millions of individuals with language and speech challenges require additional support for language understanding and learning. Currently, however, these needs are not being met because there are not enough skilled teachers, interpreters, and professionals to give them the one on one attention that they need. Speechreading allows deaf and hard of hearing individuals to perceive and understand oral language and even to speak. Speechreading seldom disambiguates all of the spoken input, however, and other techniques have been used to allow a richer input. Cued Speech, for example, is one solution to having a limited auditory input and consists of hand gestures while speaking that provide the perceiver with extra information to supplement what is seen on the face. Our research, influenced, in part, by Cued Speech, will advance engineering research and speech science by developing a real-time system to automatically detect robust characteristics of auditory speech and to transform these acoustic features into supplementary visible features. This information combined with watching the speaker's face provides enough information for a person with lim-ited hearing to perceive and understand what is being said. This new technology will allow a wearable computing device to recognize primitive characteristics of the speech signal in real time and to display the supplementary features on a pair of eyeglasses. This system improves upon Cued Speech because it is directly based on acoustic and phonetic properties of speech and gives continuous rather than only categorical information.

Pilot research has demonstrated that it is possible to recognize robust characteristics of isolated auditory words and to transform them into visible features in real time. Our ongoing work extends this research to sentences from multiple speakers, along with tests of different feature detectors and automatic recognition models. It is being carried out by a team with expertise in psychology, speech science, machine learning, and embedded system engineering. This research will advance the state of the art in human machine interaction, speech, machine learning, and assistive technologies, and will benefit society by providing a research and theoretical foundation for a system that would be naturally available to almost all individuals at a very low cost. It does not require literate users because no written information is presented (as would be the case in a captioning system); it is age-independent in that it might be used by toddlers, adolescents, and throughout the life span; it is functional for all languages because it is language independent given that all languages share the same phonetic features with highly similar corresponding acoustic characteristics; it would provide significant help for people with hearing aids and cochlear implants; and it would be beneficial for many individuals with language challenges and even for children learning to read. Finally, regardless of the advances or lack of advances in speech recognition technology, it will always be more accurate and effective to pick off features than phones.

Acknowledgments. This research was supported (in part) by the National Science Foundation under a SBIR grant (NSF IIS 0839802 to Animated Speech Corporation). Any opinions, findings, and conclusions or recommendations expressed in this material are those of the authors and do not necessarily reflect the views of the National Science Foundation.

References

Abu-Amer, T., & Carson- Berndsen, J. (2003). *HARTFX: A multi-dimensional system of HMM based recognisers for articulatory features extraction.* Proceedings from NOLISP '03, ITRW on Non-Linear Speech Processing, Le Croisic, France.

Aioanei, D., Carson-Berndsen, J., & Kanokphara, S. (2006). *Diagnostic evaluation of phonetic feature extraction engines: A case study with the Time Map model.* Proceedings from IEA/AIE '06: The 19th International Conference on Industrial, Engineering, & Other Applications of Applied Intelligent Systems. LNAI 4031, Annecy, France, pp. 691–700.

Bernstein, L. (2005). Some principles of the speech perceiving brain. In D. Pisoni & R. Remez (Eds.), *Handbook of speech perception* (pp. 79–98). Oxford, UK: Blackwell.

Bernstein, L., Demorest, M., & Tucker, P. (2000). Speech perception without hearing. *Perception & Psychophysics, 62,* 233–252.

Bernstein, L., & Eberhardt, S. (1986). *Johns Hopkins Lipreading Corpus Videodisk Set.* Baltimore, MD: Johns Hopkins University.

Better Hearing Institute. (2009). Retrieved February 8, 2009, from http://www.betterhearing.org/research/factoids.cfm

Blei, D., Ng, A., & Jordan, M. (2003). Latent dirichlet allocation. *Journal of Machine Learning Research, 3,* 993–1022.

Breslaw, P., Griffiths, A., Wood, D., & Howarth, C. (1981). The referential communication skills of deaf children from different educational environments. *Journal of Child Psychology, 22,* 269–282.

Carreira-Perpiñán, M. (2001). *Continuous latent variable models for dimensionality reduction and sequential data reconstruction* (Ph.D. thesis). University of Sheffield, UK.

Carreira-Perpiñán, M., & Lu, Z. (2007). *The Laplacian Eigenmaps Latent Variable Model.* 11th International Workshop on Artificial Intelligence and Statistics (AISTATS'2007), pp. 59–66.

Chang, S., Greenberg, S., & Wester, M. (2001). *An elitist approach to articulatory-acoustic feature classification. Proceedings from Eurospeech '01.* The 7th European Conference on Speech Communication and Technology, Aalborg, Denmark.

Clark, A. (2003). *Natural-born cyborgs: Minds, technologies, and the future of human intelligence.* New York, NY: Oxford University Press.

Cooke, M., Barker, J., Cunningham, S., & Shao, X. (2006). An audio-visual corpus for speech perception and automatic speech recognition. *Journal of the Acoustical Society of American, 120*(5). Retrieved October 17, 2008, from http://www.dcs.shef.ac.uk/spandh/gridcorpus/

Cornett, R. O. (1967). Cued Speech. *American Annals of the Deaf, 112,* 3–13.

Cornett, R., Beadles, R., & Wilson, B. (1977). Automatic Cued Speech. In J. Pickett (Ed.), *papers from the research conference on speech processing aids for the deaf* (pp. 224–239). Washington DC: Gallaudet College.

Costanza, E., Inverso, S., Pavlov, E., Allen, R., & Maes, P. (2006). *Eye-Q: Eyeglass peripheral display for subtle intimate notifications.* Proceedings from Mobile HCI '06: The 8th International Conference on Human-Computer Interaction with Mobile Devices and Services, Espoo, Finland.

de Gelder, B., & J. Morais (Ed.). (1995). *Speech and reading: A comparative approach.* Hove, England: Erlbaum (UK) Taylor & Francis, Publishers.

Denes, P., & Pinson, E. (1963). *The speech chain: The physics and biology of spoken language.* New York, NY: Bell Telephone Laboratories.

Duchnowski, P., Lum, D. S, Krause, J., Sexton, M., Bratakos, M., & Braida, L. (2000). Development of speechreading supplements based on automatic speech recognition. *IEEE Transactions on Biomedical Engineering, 47,* 487–495.

DuMouchel, W. (1994). *Hierarchical bayes linear models for meta-analysis.* Technical Report #27. National Institute of Statistical Sciences.

Eide, E. (2001). *Distinctive features for use in an automatic speech recognition system.* Proceedings from Eurospeech '01: The 7th European Conference on Speech Communication and Technology, Aalborg, Denmark.

Erber, N. (1972). Auditory, visual, and auditory-visual recognition of consonants by children with normal and impaired hearing. *Journal of Speech and Hearing Research, 15,* 423–422.

Flaush, D., Stephens, M., & Pritchard, J. (2003). Inference of population structure using multilocus genotype data: Linked loci and correlate allel frequencies. *Genetics, 164,* 1567–1587.

Fleming, E. (1984). *Believe the heart.* San Francisco, CA: Strawberry Hill Press.

Frankel, J., Magimai-Doss, M., King, S., Livescu, K., & Cetin, Ö. (2007). *Articulatory feature classifiers trained on 2000 hours of telephone speech.* Proceedings from Interspeech '07: The 8th Annual Conference in the Annual Series of INTERSPEECH events. Antwerp, Belgium.

Frankel, J., Wester, M., & King, S. (2004). *Articulatory feature recognition using dynamic bayesian networks.* Proceedings from ICLSP '04: The 8th International Conference on Spoken Language Processing, Jeju Island, Korea.

Freides, D. (1974). Human information processing and sensory modality: Cross-modal functions, information complexity, memory, and deficit. *Psychological Bulletin, 81,* 284–310.

Friedman, D., Massaro, D., Kitzis, S., & Cohen, M. (1995). A comparison of learning models. *Journal of Mathematical Psychology, 39,* 164–178.

Gengel, R. (1976). Upton's wearable eyeglass speechreading aid: History and current status. In S. K. Hirsh, D. Eldredge, I. Hirsh, & S. Silverman (Eds.), *Hearing and Davis: Essays honoring Hallowell Davis* (pp. 291–299). St. Louis, MO: Washington University Press.

Grant, K. (2002). Measures of auditory-visual integration for speech understanding: A theoretical perspective. *Journal of the Acoustical Society of America, 112,* 30–33.

Grant, K., & Greenberg, S. (2001): Speech intelligibility derived from asynchronous processing of auditory-visual information. *Proceedings from AVSP '01: Audio-Visual Speech Processing* (pp. 132–137). Scheelsminde, Denmark.

Grant, K., Greenberg, S., Poeppel, D., & van Wassenhove, V. (2004). Effects of spectro-temporal asynchrony in auditory and auditory-visual speech processing. *Seminars in Hearing, 25,* 241–255.

Greenberg, S. (2006). A multi-tier theoretical framework for understanding spoken language. In S. Greenberg & W. Ainsworth (Eds.), *Listening to speech: An auditory perspective* (pp. 411–433). Mahwah, NJ: Lawrence Erlbaum Associates.

Greenberg, S., & Chang, S. (2000). *Linguistic dissection of switchboard-corpus automatic speech recognition system.* Proceedings from ISCA '00: The International Speech Communication Association Workshop on Automatic Speech Recognition: Challenges for the New Millennium (pp. 195–202). Paris, France.

Hage, C., & Leybaert, J. (2006). The effect of Cued Speech on the development of spoken language. In P. Spencer & M. Marschark (Eds.), *Advances in the spoken language development of deaf and hard-of-hearing children* (pp. 193–211). New York, NY: Oxford University Press.

Hazen, T., Saenko, K., La, C., & Glass, J. (2004). *A segment based audio-visual speech recognizer: Data collection, development, and initial experiments*. Proceedings from ICMI '04: IEEE International Conference on Multimedia and Expo, Taipei, Taiwan.

Hirsh, I., & Sherrick, C. (1961). Perceived order in different sense modalities. *Journal of Experimental Psychology, 62*, 423–432.

Holt, J., Traxler, C., & Allen, T (1997). *Interpreting the scores: A user's guide to the 9th Edition Stanford Achievement Test for educators of deaf and hard-of-hearing students*. Washington, DC: Gallaudet Research Institute.

Jesse, A., Vrignaud, N., & Massaro, D. (2000/01). The processing of information from multiple sources in simultaneous interpreting. *Interpreting, 5*, 95–115.

King, S., & Taylor, P. (2000). Detection of phonological features in continuous speech using neural networks. *Computer Speech and Language, 14*, 333–353.

Kisor, H. (1990). *What's that pig outdoors?: A memoir of deafness*. New York, NY: Hill and Wang.

Kitzis, S., Kelley, H., Berg, E., Massaro, D., & Friedman, D. (1998). Broadening the tests of learning models. *Journal of Mathematical Psychology, 42*, 327–355.

Lederman, S., & Klatzy, R. (2004). *Multisensory texture perception. Handbook of multisensory processes* (pp. 107–122). Cambridge, MA: MIT Press.

Loomis, J., & Lederman, S. (1986). Tactual perception. In K. Boff, L. Kaufman, & J. Thomas (Eds.), *Handbook of perception and human performance, Vol. 2: Cognitive processes and performance* (pp. 31–41). New York, NY: John Wiley & Sons.

Loveless, N., Brebner, J., & Hamilton, P. (1970). Bisensory presentation of information. *Psychological Bulletin, 73*, 161–199.

Martony, J. (1974). Some experiments with electronic speechreading aids. *KTH Speech Transmission Laboratory: Quarterly Progress and Status Report, 2–3*, 34–56. Stockholm: Royal Institute of Technology.

Massaro, D. (1984). Children's perception of visual and auditory speech. *Child Development, 55*, 1777–1788.

Massaro, D. (1987). *Speech perception by ear and eye: A paradigm for psychological inquiry*. Hillsdale, NJ: Erlbaum.

Massaro, D. (1998). *Perceiving talking faces: From speech perception to a behavioral principle*. Cambridge, MA: MIT Press.

Massaro, D. (1999). From theory to practice: Rewards and challenges. Proceedings from ICPhS '07: *The International Conference of Phonetic Sciences*, San Francisco, CA.

Massaro, D. (2004). Symbiotic value of an embodied agent in language learning. Proceedings from HICSS '04: *The 37th Annual Hawaii International Conference on System Sciences*. Computer Society Press, 2004. Retrieved October 19, 2008, from http://mambo.ucsc.edu/pdf/ETSIB10.pdf

Massaro, D. (2006). Embodied agents in language learning for children with language challenges. Proceedings from ICCHP '06: *The 10th International Conference on Computers Helping People with Special Needs* (pp. 809–816). University of Linz, Austria. Berlin, Germany: Springer.

Massaro, D., & Bosseler, A. (2003). Perceiving speech by ear and eye: Multimodal integration by children with autism. *Journal of Developmental and Learning Disorders, 7*, 111–144.

Massaro, D., & Cohen, M. (1993). Perceiving asynchronous bimodal speech in consonant-vowel and vowel syllables. *Speech Communication, 13*, 127–134.

Massaro, D., & Cohen, M. (1999). Speech perception in hearing-impaired perceivers: Synergy of multiple modalities. *Journal of Speech, Language, and Hearing Science, 42*, 21–41.

Massaro, D., Cohen, M., & Beskow, J. (2007). *Visual display methods for in computer-animated speech production models*. United States Patent 7,225,129, May 29, 2007.

Massaro, D., & Light, J. (2004). Using visible speech for training perception and production of speech for hard-of-hearing individuals. *Journal of Speech, Language, and Hearing Research, 47*(2), 304–320.

Massaro, D., & Stork, D. (1998). Sensory integration and speechreading by humans and machines. *American Scientist, 86,* 236–244.

Miller, J., Engebretson, A., & DeFillipo, C. (1974). Preliminary research with a three channel vibrotactile speech-reception aid for the deaf. In G. Fant (Ed.), *Speech communication (Vol. 4) Speech and hearing deficits and aids.* Proceedings from the Speech Communication Seminar '74. Stockholm, Sweden. New York, NY: John Wiley & Sons.

Mirrielees, D. (1947). *Education of the young deaf child: Special subjects and methods.* Chicago, IL: University of Chicago Home Study Department.

Montgomery, A., & Jackson, P. (1983). Physical characteristics of the lips underlying vowel lipreading performance. *Journal of the Acoustical Society of America, 73,* 2134–2144.

Morais, J., & Kolinsky, R. (1994). Perception and awareness in phonological processing: The case of the phoneme. *Cognition, 50,* 287–297.

Munhall, K., Kroos, C., Jozan, G., & Vatikiotis-Bateson, E. (2004). Spatial frequency requirements for audiovisual speech perception. *Perception and Psychophysics, 66,* 574–583.

Munhall, K., & Vatikiotis-Bateson, E. (2004). Spatial and temporal constraints on audiovisual speech perception. In G. Calvert, J. Spence, & B. Stein (Eds.), *Handbook of multisensory processes* (pp. 177–188). Cambridge, MA: MIT Press.

National Reading Panel (2000). *Teaching children to read.* U.S. Department of Health and Human Services, Public Health Service, National Institutes of Health, National Institute of Child Health and Human Development, NIH Pub. No. 00-4769.

Neto, J., Almeida, L., Hochberg, M., Martins, C., Nunes, L., Renals, S. Robinson, T. (1995). *Speaker adaptation for hybrid HMM-ANN continuous speech recognition system.* Proceedings from Eurospeech '95: The 4th European Conference on Speech Communication and Technology, pp. 2171–2174.

Norman, D. (1988). *The psychology of everyday things.* New York, NY: Basic Books.

Norman, D. (1999). *The invisible computer.* Cambridge, MA: MIT Press.

Pickett, J., Gengel, R., Quinn, R., & Upton, H. (1974). Research with the Upton eyeglass speechreader. In G. Fant *Speech communication (Vol. 4) Speech and hearing defects and aids.* Proceedings of the Speech Communication Seminar '74. Stockholm, Sweden. New York, NY: John Wiley & Sons.

Pitt, M., Dilley, L., Johnson, K., Kiesling, S., Raymond, W., Hume, E., & Fosler-Lussier, E. (2007). *Buckeye Corpus of Conversational Speech* (2nd release). Columbus, OH: Department of Psychology, Ohio State University (Distributor). Retrieved, October 7, 2008, from www.buckeyecorpus.osu.edu

Sanderson, C. (2002). *The VidTIMIT Database.* IDIAP Communication 02-06. Martigny, Switzerland.

Saul, L., Weinberger, K., Ham, J., Sha, F., & Lee, D. (2006). Spectral methods for dimensionality reduction. In O. Chapelle, B. Schoelkopf, & A. Zien (Eds.), *Semisupervised learning.* Cambridge, MA: MIT Press..

Schutte, K., & Glass, J. (2005). *Robust detection of sonorant landmarks.* Proceedings from Interspeech '05: The 9th European Conference on Speech Communication and Technology (pp. 1005–1008), Lisbon, Portugal.

Sherrick, C., & Cholewiak, R. (1976). Cutaneous sensitivity. *Handbook of perception and human performance, 2 Cognitive processes and performance* (pp. 12–58). New York, NY: John Wiley & Sons.

Smeele, P., Massaro, D., Cohen, M., & Sittig, A. (1998). Laterality in visual speech perception. *Journal of Experimental Psychology: Human Perception and Performance, 24,* 1232–1242.

Summerfield, Q. (1987). Some preliminaries to a comprehensive account of A/V speech perception. In B. Dodd & R. Campbell (Eds.), *Hearing by eye: The psychology of lipreading.* Hillsdale, NJ: Lawrence Erlbaum Associates.

Tager-Flusberg, H. (2000). Language development in children with autism. In L. Menn & N. Bernstein Ratner (Eds.), *Methods for studying language production* (pp. 313–332). Mahwah, New Jersey: Lawrence Erlbaum Associates.

Taylor, I., & D. Olson (Eds.). (1995). *Scripts and literacy: Reading and learning to read alphabets, Syllabaries and characters.* Dordrecht, Netherlands: Kluwer Academic Publishers.

Upton, H. (1968). Wearable eyeglass speech-reading aid. *American Annals of the Deaf, 113,* 222–229.

Wandel, J. (1998). *Use of internal speech in reading by hearing and hearing-impaired students in oral, total communication, and Cued Speech programs.* Unpublished Ph.D. Dissertation, Columbia University Teacher's College.

Weiser, M. (1991). The computer for the 21st century. *Scientific American, 265,* 94–104.

Williams, J., Massaro, D., Peel, N., Bosseler, A., & Suddendorf, T. (2004). Visual-auditory integration during speech imitation in autism. *Research in Developmental Disabilities, 25,* 559–575.

Willows, D., Kruk, R., & Corcos, E. (Eds.). (1993). *Visual processes in reading and reading disabilities.* Hillsdale, NJ: Lawrence Erlbaum.

Zigoris, P., & Zhang, Y. (2006) *Bayesian adaptive user profiling with explicit & implicit feedback.* Proceedings from CIKM '06: The Conference on Information Knowledge Management, Arlington, VA.

Chapter 23

A VERSION OF THE EDUCATIONAL INTERPRETER PERFORMANCE ASSESSMENT FOR CUED SPEECH TRANSLITERATORS: PROSPECTS AND SIGNIFICANCE

Jean C. Krause, Brenda Schick, and Judy Kegl

Introduction

Soon after Cued Speech was developed (Cornett, 1967), the need for Cued Speech transliterators in educational settings began. This need intensified in 1975 when Public Law 94-142 was passed, mandating education in the "least restrictive environment" for all children with disabilities. Large numbers of deaf and hard-of-hearing children, who previously would have been educated in residential programs, began moving to local public schools (Moores, 1992). Many of these children required interpreters or transliterators for

access to classroom communication, and those children who used Cued Speech were no exception. Today, the exact number of children using Cued Speech in the public schools is unknown, but a national survey conducted annually by the American Annals of the Deaf (Anon., 1999) showed that 14% of educational programs for deaf students offered a Cued Speech component in 1999. Moreover, the National Cued Speech Association reports that the vast majority of children currently using Cued Speech are mainstreamed. For these children, Cued Speech transliterators serve an important role in providing access to classroom communication.

In recognition of the important role of all individuals involved in the education of children, the No Child Left Behind Act (2001) specifies that only "highly qualified" staff can work with children in the public schools. For classroom interpreters, the motivation behind such a law is clear. If interpreters who work in public school settings do not have sufficient skills to afford deaf and hard-of-hearing students adequate access to classroom communication, the value of inclusive education for these students is greatly diminished. As the Commission on Education of the Deaf (COED, 1988) pointed out in a 1988 report to Congress, federal law requires that "deaf students be integrated into regular classroom settings to the maximum extent possible, but if quality interpreting services are not provided, that goal becomes a mockery" (p. 103). As a result, tools are needed to assess the skills of all interpreters who work with children, including transliterators who use Cued Speech, in order to ensure that no child is left behind.

To date, the most widely used tool for evaluating educational interpreters and transliterators is the Educational Interpreter Performance Assessment (EIPA; Schick & Williams, 1992). The EIPA is used by more than 25 state departments of education to evaluate interpreters in the public schools and was recently adopted as a certification option by the national Registry of Interpreters for the Deaf. The EIPA also serves as an important research tool for examining the quality of educational interpreters, and research studies using the EIPA have reported data for more than 2,000 educational interpreters nationwide. These studies (Schick, Williams, & Bolster, 1999; Schick, Williams, & Kupermintz, 2006) have been instrumental in identifying areas of need in the field of educational interpreting. If a Cued Speech version of the EIPA were available, research investigations equivalent to those that have been conducted with signing interpreters could be extended to Cued Speech transliterators. Such research is not only important from a scientific standpoint but also essential to the process of gaining wider acceptance for Cued Speech and cued language transliteration as a profession. It is also likely that the extension of the EIPA to Cued Speech in and of itself would raise visibility of both Cued Speech transliteration as a profession and Cued Speech as a communication option.

In this context, this chapter discusses a pilot Cued Speech version of the EIPA, recently developed, which shows great promise as a valid and reliable tool for evaluating Cued Speech transliterators. After a review of general issues in evaluating educational interpreters and transliterators, this new EIPA instrument for Cued Speech transliterators is described in detail, and feasibility of its implementation as an official version of the EIPA is analyzed. The case is then made that these steps toward an official Cued Speech version of the EIPA represent a significant advance in the field of Cued Speech transliteration that ultimately should lead to better services for children who use Cued Speech.

Methods of Assessment for Interpreters and Transliterators

In order to discuss methods of assessment for interpreters and transliterators, it is first worth noting that even though American Sign Language (ASL) is the preferred language of many deaf adults, it is rarely used in public schools. Instead, surveys suggest that most K–12 sign interpreters/transliterators use Pidgin Sign English (PSE), a form of nativized English signing used by the deaf community (e.g., Jones, Clark, & Soltz, 1997). EIPA assessments are consistent with such surveys in that 79% of the EIPA evaluations are in PSE, and only 11% are in ASL and 9% in manually coded English (MCE).

Depending on the communication option used, interpreting professionals are required to function quite differently in order to facilitate communication effectively. Given the functional differences that interpreting professionals face as a result of differences in communication options, the terms *interpreter* and *transliterator* have developed rather specific meanings in the field: the function of an interpreter is to transfer information between two languages (e.g., spoken English and ASL), whereas the function of a transliterator is to transfer information between two modes of the same language (e.g., spoken English and signed English). Given this distinction, the term "transliterator" is most appropriate for referring to an interpreting professional who uses Cued Speech (specifically, *Cued Speech transliterator* or *cued language transliterator*, for reasons discussed throughout this volume), because this individual transfers information between spoken English and cued English.

In addition, "interpreter" is also sometimes used as a general term to refer to an individual who works in the interpreting profession, either as an interpreter or a as a transliterator. This usage stems in part from the fact that the role of a transliterator goes beyond direct rendering of English grammatical structures and vocabulary. In fact, elements of a transliterator's job require some of the same (or similar) skills as those used by interpreters; both groups must interpret situations and make judg-

ments regarding how best to paraphrase fast speech, which information to convey when multiple talkers speak simultaneously, when and how to represent sounds in the environment, and so forth. In light of this more general term, this chapter distinguishes between interpreters who use sign communication (a nearly general usage of the term "interpreter") and transliterators who use Cued Speech. Conveniently, the use of "interpreter" in this largely general sense is consistent with EIPA terminology and with terminology currently used in the national certification of interpreters by the National Council on Interpreting (NCI). Finally, when a completely generic term is needed to refer to both of these groups collectively in this chapter, the term *interpreting professionals* is used.

Interpreters and Interpreter Assessments

Interpreters have always served an important role in facilitating communication between members of the Deaf community and members of the hearing community. In educational settings, their role dates back at least to the early 1800s when Thomas Hopkins Gallaudet served as an educational interpreter for Laurent Clerc (Frishberg, 1990). Yet until recent decades, most interpreting work was performed without compensation by relatives, friends, or other individuals who could claim some degree of signing competence. Beginning in the early 1970s, however, interpreting began to emerge more formally as a profession. In part, this change was stimulated by federal legislation, as Section 504 of the Rehabilitation Act of 1973 guaranteed all "handicapped individual[s]" the right to access "any program or activity receiving Federal financial assistance." The result was a sharp increase in the demand for interpreters, an acknowledgment that the work of interpreters should be financially compensated, and an increased need for assessment of interpreter skills.

In response to these issues, the Registry of Interpreters for the Deaf (RID), established in 1964, began to test and certify the qualifications of interpreters in 1972. The RID certification test was pass/fail and examined an individual's skills in both interpreting and transliterating. Designed for adult community interpreters, the test included a written component and a performance component that was videotaped for review by an evaluation team. Some problems with reliability ultimately became apparent, however, and RID opted to release a new test in 1988, emphasizing the new test's psychometric validity and reliability. Meanwhile, the National Association of the Deaf (NAD) membership had voted in 1986 to explore the feasibility of establishing an alternative certification system for community interpreters, and NAD established its own interpreter certification program in 1991. The NAD test did not distinguish between transliteration and interpreting. Instead, candidates were presented with a range of signers and were expected to make a determination on their own concerning the nature of the interpretation to be provided. The test was conducted in a live format and included an oral examination and interview. Interpreters completing the NAD test were provided with a profile indicating specific strengths and weaknesses and assigned a score from Level I (novice) to Level V (master), with Levels III, IV, and V receiving NAD certification. Other quality assurance (QA) tests aimed at assessing the skills of community interpreters also were developed during this time period, such as the Kansas Quality Assurance Skills (KQAS) test. Although such QA tests were, and continue to be, widely used for state and regional purposes, the national certification mechanisms have remained the gold standards for assessing the qualifications of community interpreters.

In 2005, the NAD and RID tests were replaced by a single national certification mechanism, the National Interpreter Certification (NIC) test. This test was developed jointly by the NAD and RID via the National Council on Interpreting (NCI) and consists of a written test followed by an interview and performance assessment. In contrast with the prior test, which separately assessed skills in transliteration and interpretation, the new NIC test parallels the former NAD test in requiring a range of interpretation styles within a single test. Individuals who pass attain certification at one of three levels: NIC, NIC Advanced, or NIC Master. For those who wish to specialize, RID continues to develop and maintain specialty certificates for areas such as oral transliterating and legal interpreting. However, no specialty certificate had ever been available for educational interpreting, even though it is generally accepted that interpreting for children in educational settings differs substantially from interpreting for adults, particularly when children are young and still acquiring language.

To address the need for assessment tools specific to interpreting in educational settings, the Educational Interpreter Performance Assessment was established in 1992. Recognizing that many aspects of classroom communication are unique to K–12 education (see Schick, 2004), the EIPA evaluates an interpreter's ability to convey pragmatic and prosodic information (why and how a message is delivered, respectively) as well as lexical information (what the message is), in both voice-to-sign and sign-to-voice situations. A Likert scale is used to assess specific skills, with scores ranging from 0 (no skills demonstrated) to 5 (advanced native-like skills). In addition, the EIPA Written Test (pass/fail) was released in 2005 as a mechanism for testing a set of knowledge standards pertaining to educational interpreting. Besides the EIPA, other tests specific to educational interpreting have been developed at the state level, such as Florida's Educational Interpreter Evaluation (EIE), and such state tests continue to be used to some degree. However, the EIPA has become the gold standard for assessing the qualifications of educational interpreters, and in 2006, the RID Board of Directors opted to grant certified member status (ED: K-12 certification) to those individuals who have (1) passed the EIPA Written Test, and (2) obtained a level of 4.0 or higher on the EIPA performance test. This move not only recognized that the EIPA written and performance examinations for their high validity and reliability but also signified a major paradigm shift in how educational interpreters were viewed in the RID organization. As RID President Angela Jones explained at the time, "Interpreters in the educational setting have been organizationally disenfranchised since their introduction into the profession, and it is time to recognize their importance to the profession and to the Deaf community" (RID, 2006).

Cued Speech Transliterators and Transliterator Assessments

In the 1970s and early 1980s, transliterators followed a path that was not all that different from interpreters. Early transliterators were friends, family members or other individuals with cueing skills. They transliterated informally, as needed, without compensation, in a variety of settings, including the educational setting. In these early years of Cued Speech, it was also not uncommon for teachers and interested classmates to learn how to cue in order to facilitate direct communication with deaf children who used Cued Speech in their classrooms (Cornett & Daisey, 2001). Between 1971 and 1976, it was in this type of classroom environment that one of the earliest forms of educational Cued Speech transliteration occurred: when teachers in Leah Henegar's elementary school classrooms did not cue or did not cue clearly, Leah's classmates would cue information that she missed for her (M. Daisey, personal communication, 2007).

From these beginnings, a confluence of factors helped transliterating begin to emerge more formally as a profession in the latter half of the 1970s. Most notably, federal legislation again played a key role in changing the face of the field, as it had for interpreting. Section 504 of the Rehabilitation Act of 1973 was followed by Public Law 94-142 in 1975, which mandated education in the "least restrictive environment" for all children with disabilities. As a result, parents of children with disabilities could demand that school systems provide "appropriate" support services, and many parents argued that a transliterator was an appropriate service for deaf children who used Cued Speech. Based on this law, Leah Henegar's mother approached Prince George's County Public Schools (Maryland) in 1976 and requested the first Cued Speech "interpreter" for Leah's seventh grade classroom. Although this request was denied (M. E. Daisey, personal communication, 2007), the effect of Public Law 94-142 on schools had begun. Linda Balderson became the first professional Cued Speech transliterator in the fall of 1978, when she was hired by Montgomery County Public Schools (for a different child). Soon after, Wake County Public Schools (North Carolina) provided a Cued Speech transliterator for Leah's final three years of high school from 1979 to 1982 (Cornett & Daisey, 2001). By 1980, Cued Speech transliterators were employed by school districts in Milwaukee, WI, Montgomery County, MD, and Raleigh, NC (National Cued Speech Association, 1980).

Another factor that helped shape the development of the transliterating profession throughout the late 1970s was that more children continued to be introduced to Cued Speech. The small but steady influx of children who used Cued Speech further increased demand for transliterators and thus gave additional legitimacy to Cued Speech transliteration as a stable and viable occupation, particularly in certain parts of the country where Cued Speech was most popular (e.g., Montgomery County, Maryland).

Finally, a concomitant explosion in the number of interpreters—RID membership shot from roughly 500 members in 1974 to well over 2,000 members in 1980 (Cokely, 2005)—brought increased recognition to interpreting professionals on the whole and more formal descriptions of the profession in general; both developments allowed the work performed by Cued Speech transliterators to be more readily understood.

In the wake of these developments in the interpreting community, it is perhaps not surprising that transliterators would soon initiate a systematic and introspective examination of transliteration services provided to the cueing community. Barbara Williams-Scott and Earl Fleet-

wood led the effort in 1981, documenting the techniques of Cued Speech transliterators and analyzing how such techniques facilitated mainstreaming (Fleetwood & Metzger, 1990). Their initial investigation was continued by the staff of the Cued Speech Interpreter Training Programs (CSITP) at Gallaudet University, which set forth guidelines for the transliterating profession and offered the first formal transliterator training courses in the summer of 1985 (National Cued Speech Association, 1985). Shortly thereafter, the National Cued Speech Association (NCSA) formed a group to assess transliterators, and the first Cued Speech Transliterator Certification Examination was administered to eight individuals on November 12 to 13, 1988, in Williamsburg, Virginia (National Cued Speech Association, 1988). The group, soon known as the Training, Evaluation, and Certification Unit (TECUnit), originally operated as a division of the NCSA before becoming its own organization in the early 1990s. Subsequently renamed the *Testing, Evaluation, and Certification Unit*, the TECUnit continues to administer the transliterator certification exam nationally.

Revised in 1991, the TECUnit's certification exam currently serves as the only nationally recognized certification process for transliterators. Now known as the Cued Language Transliterator National Certification Exam, or CLTNCE, the exam consists of six components: two prerequisite tests that measure basic expressive and receptive proficiency, a written exam, a commentary that assesses ethical decision-making and familiarity with the Cued Language Transliterator Code of Conduct, a syllables-per-minute fluency test, and a performance component. Prior to 1997, transliterators who completed the exam were assigned a level; the top three levels were fully or partially certified, with level 4 indicating "expert" skills, level 3 indicating "competent" skills, and level 2 indicating "functional" skills. Since 1997, however, the exam has been offered to transliterators on a pass/fail basis only, and transliterators who pass are awarded a Transliterator Skills Certificate (TSC).

In some states, another evaluation mechanism available to transliterators is the Cued Language Transliterator State Level Assessment, or CLTSLA. Developed in 1991, the CLTSLA Package can be purchased by state agencies from TECUnit and used as a mechanism for assessing transliterators within a state. The purchasing agency administers the exam, which may be offered under a different name (in Virginia, for example, the test is called the Virginia Quality Assurance Screening, or VQAS), and sends performance assessment videos to the TECUnit for rating. The exam consists of (1) a written test covering basic knowledge of the field, ethical decision-making, and familiarity with the Transliterator Code of Conduct, and (2) a performance assessment including five expressive tasks from a variety of settings (both community and educational settings: a dialogue, a first-grade story with environmental sounds, a freelance lecture, a freelance situation requiring use of paraphrase, and foreign language in an educational setting) and two receptive tasks. Transliterators receive either pass/fail scores or levels (0, I, II, III, IV), depending on the state. The CLTSLA is currently offered in Louisiana, North Carolina, Virginia, and Utah.

Beyond these four states and the state of Minnesota, which requires transliterators to pass the CLTNCE, most states have not established minimum performance standards for transliterators pertaining to actual transliteration skills. Although many states have no performance standards for transliterators at all, some states do use one or more tests of cueing proficiency to monitor the general cueing skills of transliterators. Two such evaluation mechanisms with the longest history in the cueing community are the BCSPR and the CSRT, developed by Walter J. Beaupre at the University of Rhode Island in 1983 and 1986, respectively. The BCSPR, or Basic Cued Speech Proficiency Rating (Beaupre, 1985), measures expressive proficiency, requiring test-takers to cue syllables, words, short phrases, and a written story. Based on this sample, numerical ratings between 0.0 (proficient) and 7.0 (nonproficient) are assigned, and diagnostic feedback is provided. The CSRT, or Cued Speechreading Test (Beaupre, 1987), measures receptive proficiency at the sentence level, requiring cuers to speechread one set of short sentences and to cueread another set of similar sentences. A pass/fail score is assigned based on the cuereading score and the amount of improvement between cuereading and speechreading conditions. Both tests were used as prerequisites to the national certification exam until 2002 and remain in limited use for purposes within the National Cued Speech Association, such as providing feedback to individuals wishing to become certified instructors of Cued Speech. Since 2002, two other evaluation mechanisms that have been used widely for assessing general cueing proficiency are the TECUnit's Cued American English Competency Screenings, or CAECS-E (Expressive) and CAECS-R (Receptive). Developed in 2001, the CAECS-E evaluates expressive skills and assigns cuers a rating of 0.0 to 4.0; a rating of 3.4 or higher is considered acceptable. Developed in 2002, the CAECS-R evaluates receptive skills at the word level: cuers speechread two lists of words and cueread two lists of words; a passing score is awarded to individuals who achieve at least 85% accuracy in the cuereading condition. The CAECS-E and CAECS-R tests are offered by the TECUnit and currently serve as prerequisites for the CLTNCE.

Yet even when states that opt to use these proficiency tests (rather than tests designed explicitly to assess transliteration skill such as the CLTNCE or CLTSLA) are included, the number of states that have established minimum performance standards for transliterators is fewer than ten. In contrast, more than 25 states require minimum performance standards for educational interpreters who sign, and this number has dramatically increased since the No Child Left Behind (NCLB) Act was passed in 2001. Among states with standards currently in place, 21 require a specified level of performance on the EIPA; in most of these states, a minimum score of 3.5 on the 5.0 scale is required. As the EIPA is fast becoming the most widely adopted mechanism for evaluating educational interpreters, several states (e.g., Maine, Louisiana, New York) have expressed interest in a Cued Speech version of the EIPA.

Educational Interpreter Performance Assessment

The Educational Interpreter Performance Assessment (EIPA) was developed in 1992 at Boys Town National Research Hospital (BTNRH). For the first several years after its development, the EIPA was used to evaluate interpreters filmed in their own classrooms. Since 1999, however, the EIPA has relied upon standardized test materials in order to conduct evaluations of interpreters. The test materials consist of video recordings of classroom situations that are appropriate for evaluation of interpreters who use (1) American Sign Language (ASL), typically viewed as the sign language of the adult deaf community; (2) Pidgin Sign English (PSE), the type of English signing found among the adult deaf community; or (3) Manually Coded English (MCE; see Bornstein, 1990). In addition, two versions of the EIPA test materials are available for each communication option: one version is applicable to interpreters who work in elementary settings, and the other version is applicable interpreters who work in secondary settings.

In an EIPA evaluation, the test materials are used to collect two samples of an interpreter's work: a voice-to-sign sample of the interpreter translating or transliterating spoken English in the classroom environment into sign communication, and a sign-to-voice sample of the interpreter translating or transliterating what a deaf child signs into spoken English. The samples are then submitted to the EIPA Diagnostic Center[1] for evaluation. A 3-member evaluation team, one of whom is deaf, rates the interpreter using a Likert scale of 0 (*no observable skills*) to 5 (*advanced skills*) in each of 37 skill areas (Appendix 23–A). These skill areas are organized into four broad evaluation domains: (1) voice-to-sign production (syntax, spatial grammar, and nonmanual aspects of prosody), (2) sign-to-voice production, (3) vocabulary (range and depth of vocabulary, fingerspelling, and numbers), and (4) overall factors

---

[1]Contact information for the EIPA Diagnostic Center: Boys Town National Research Hospital, 555 North 30th Street, Omaha, NE 68131, 402-452-5033 or E-mail: eipa@boystown.org

(aspects of interpreting that are discourse based, such as discourse mapping and cohesion). The interpreter receives ratings in each skill area and evaluation domain, as well as an overall average score that is generated from these ratings. In addition, the interpreter receives diagnostic feedback which explains areas of strength and areas that should be targeted in professional development for each of the four evaluation domains. For a complete description of the EIPA tool and procedures, see www.classroominterpreting.org or Schick and Williams, 2004.

Since its inception, the EIPA has become an established research tool with good validity and reliability (Schick et al., 2006). It covers many of the situations encountered by educational interpreters, and the availability of a Cued Speech version of the EIPA would increase its applicability to an even greater number of educational interpreters. Such a development would be particularly useful for states seeking to evaluate Cued Speech transliterators in educational settings and would help ensure that an additional population of educational interpreters is held to appropriate competency standards.

Adaptations of EIPA for Cued Speech

In order to adapt the EIPA to include Cued Speech (CS), it was first necessary to modify the existing EIPA test materials and scoring sheet to accommodate issues specific to Cued Speech transliteration. The resulting Cued Speech EIPA pilot test (EIPA-CS) was then administered to 25 transliterators. Using these pilot tests as a basis for discussion, experts were con-

sulted to establish appropriate evaluation procedures and to pilot rating procedures. These consultants served as one EIPA evaluation team and also assisted in the development of materials that were used to train additional raters.

Test Materials

The EIPA comprises two types of videotaped test materials: (1) classroom materials designed to elicit the interpreting professional's expressive product (usually voice-to-sign, or for CS transliterators, voice-to-cue), and (2) student materials designed to elicit the interpreting professional's receptive product (usually sign-to-voice, or for CS transliterators, cue-to-voice). Because the types of classroom communications that must be conveyed are the same for all interpreting professionals, regardless of the communication option used to transmit information to the deaf student, no modification to the existing classroom materials was needed. The classroom video recordings that were in use by the EIPA Diagnostic Testing Center in 2005 (Elementary Classroom—Options A and B, Secondary Classroom—Options A and B) were used as the classroom materials for the Cued Speech pilot test.

The student materials, however, are specific to the communication option used by the interpreting professional. Therefore, it was necessary to develop new student materials that were appropriate for Cued Speech transliterators. To create these materials, three deaf elementary students (0 girls, 3 boys; ages: 10 years) and three deaf secondary students (3 girls, 0 boys; ages: 13-16 years) whose primary mode of communication was Cued Speech were recruited from Cued Speech communities in the Midwest and in New England. Following the format that was used in creating the previous EIPA student materials for signing, an adult cuer interviewed each child for 60 to 90 minutes. In order to ensure that the look and feel of the EIPA student materials would be achieved, BTNRH provided the EIPA backdrop and a videographer experienced in eliciting student materials for EIPA.

The interview was conducted in two parts. In the first part of the interview, the child spoke and cued simultaneously, and in the second part, the child communicated in CS only (using cues synchronized with mouth movements, but without accompanying speech). The reason for eliciting both of these modes was so that the EIPA-CS pilot test could reflect the varied nature of receptive cueing tasks facing educational CS transliterators today. On the one hand, most CS users have typically also had oral goals, and any receptive training that CS transliterators receive usually is based on the expectation that they will have access to audiovisual (AV) information, that is, that students will speak and cue simultaneously. On the other hand, there is now growing support for using Cued Speech to convey English in bilingual-bicultural programs (LaSasso & Metzger, 1998), where speech is not necessarily the primary goal (see Chapter 10 by Kyllo in this volume for a description of a bilingual-bicultural program that uses Cued Speech). Consequently, some settings will require educational CS transliterators who are capable of voicing CS presented in a visual-only (VO) modality, that is, students who cue with only silent mouth movements rather than with audible speech accompanying the cues. Nonetheless, CS transliterators who do not possess this skill but have strong audiovisual cue-to-voice

skills are still adequate for many settings, and some settings (in which deaf student who use CS have oral goals) may not require cue-to-voice skills at all. By evaluating both AV and VO cue-to-voice performance, the EIPA-CS pilot test provides a mechanism for ensuring that a given CS transliterator has competencies in the receptive tasks necessary for his or her job.

After reviewing the quality and quantity of language samples elicited from each child as well as his or her presence on-camera, it was determined that the materials elicited from one elementary boy (age: 10 years) and one secondary girl (age: 16 years) were best-suited for use in the student test materials. The materials from the other children were excluded for a variety of reasons: one child was shy on-camera, and his materials lacked language samples of adequate length and complexity; two children had very intelligible speech, such that no materials of adequate difficulty were available for the audio visual cue-to-voice portion of the test; and one child's age (13 years) was borderline, and her language samples were thus neither appropriate for the elementary nor secondary level. For each of the two children who were selected, warmup and test materials were developed. Both sets of materials contained an AV and a VO segment that was created following the format and procedures previously established for signing versions of the EIPA. In addition, minor modifications to the EIPA instructions (written and spoken) were required: references to "signing" were replaced with "cueing," and instructions were added to facilitate the transition between AV and VO segments. Because the tapes contained two cue-to-voice segments (i.e., AV and VO materials), the CS student test materials were somewhat longer in duration than their signing counterparts: the warmup video materials were approximately 8 minutes (signing versions: ~5 minutes) in length, and the test video materials were approximately 40 minutes (signing versions: 25 to 30 minutes) in length.

So that the final tapes could match the look and feel of other EIPA test materials, BTNRH provided all necessary audio files as well as the EIPA music and EIPA video graphics to the Media Innovation Team at the University of South Florida, who performed the final video editing. Two complete sets of video materials were produced: (1) Elementary—Option A: warm-up and Elementary—Option A: test, and (2) Secondary—Option A: warm-up and Secondary—Option A: test. Although only one option was developed at each level, the materials were labeled "Option A" for two reasons. First, this naming scheme parallels the naming scheme for the classroom materials as well as for the student materials on signing versions of the EIPA. Secondly, it allows "Option B" tapes to be introduced seamlessly (with no additional editing of pre-existing tapes required) whenever resources become available to develop additional student materials.

Score Sheets

The primary purpose of the EIPA score sheet is to itemize all skills that are assessed (on a scale of 0 to 5) in an EIPA evaluation. It also provides a mechanism for providing feedback to the interpreting professional. Because the skill set required of Cued Speech transliterators is not identical to the skill set required of interpreters, modifications to the existing EIPA score sheet were required for the EIPA-CS pilot test.

On the score sheet for the signing version of the EIPA, 37 skills are organized under four general domains, Roman I to Roman IV (see Appendix 23–A). In constructing the EIPA-CS score sheet, these skills were reviewed and any that were not applicable to Cued Speech transliteration (e.g., "Use of verb directionality/pronominal system" in the Roman I domain), including the entire Roman III (Vocabulary) domain of skills, were eliminated. Other skills, however, were deemed applicable to Cued Speech transliteration and were not changed (particularly skills related to conveying prosody in the expressive, Roman I, and receptive, Roman II, cueing domains, e.g., "Stress/emphasis for important words or phrases" as well as some skills in the overall factors, Roman IV domain (e.g., "Demonstrates process decalage appropriately"). Finally, a number of Cued Speech-related transliteration skills (e.g., "Appropriate use of alternate cueing hands") were introduced to the score sheet, and the name for the Roman III domain was changed to "Intelligibility." In addition, Roman II was subdivided into two domains, so that AV cue-to-voice and VO cue-to-voice performances could be evaluated separately.

After constructing the initial draft of the EIPA-CS score sheet in this manner, three consultants (2 transliterators, 1 consumer; all were certified Instructors of Cued Speech, and all were either pursuing or had completed masters degrees) provided additional input to ensure that the final list of skills on the EIPA-CS score sheet was comprehensive. A replica of the final version of the EIPA-CS score sheet is shown in Table 23–1. For reference, the standard EIPA score sheet for evaluations of sign interpreters is summarized in Appendix 23–A.

Table 23–1. Summary of the Score Sheet for the EIPA-CS Pilot Test

I. Interpreter Product: Voice-to-Cue	II(AV). Interpreter Product: AudioVisual Cue-to-Voice	II(VO). Interpreter Product: Visual-Only Cue-to-Voice
Prosodic information: A. Stress/emphasis for important words or phrases B. Affect/emotions C. Register D. Sentence/clausal boundaries E. Sentence types indicated Other supporting information: F. Use of space, natural gestures, eye gaze, and body shifts G. Identification of speaker and other sound sources H. Communication of meaningful environmental sounds I. Appropriate use of alternate cueing hands Interpreter performance: J. Awareness and self-correction of cueing errors	Can read and convey student's: A. Cued words B. Proper names, unusual vocabulary C. Register (if applicable) Vocal/Intonational features: D. Speech production E. Sentence/clausal boundaries indicated F. Sentence types G. Emphasize important words, phrases, affect/emotions Interpreter performance: H. Adds no extraneous words/sounds to message	Can read and convey student's: A. Cued words B. Proper names, unusual vocabulary C. Register (if applicable) Vocal/Intonational features: D. Speech production E. Sentence/clausal boundaries indicated F. Sentence types G. Emphasize important words, phrases, affect/emotions Interpreter performance: H. Adds no extraneous words/sounds to message

III. Intelligibility	IV. Overall Factors
Cue accuracy: A. Appropriate selection of cues B. Representation of dialects (if applicable) C. No extraneous cues Clarity of cues: D. Appropriate formation of handshapes E. Appropriate locations for placements F. Appropriate execution of specified movements G. No extraneous movements or distracting physical features Clarity of oral information: H. Visibility of articulators I. No inappropriate oral mannerisms or distracting facial features Timing: J. Fluency (rhythm and rate) K. Synchronization of cues and mouth movements	Message processing voice-cue (V-C): A. Preserves a sense of the whole message V-C B. Keeps pace with speaker V-C C. Uses verbatim transliteration and paraphrasing appropriately V-C Message processing cue-voice (C-V): D. Preserves a sense of the whole message C-V E. Demonstrates process decalage appropriately C-V F. Uses verbatim transliteration and paraphrasing appropriately C-V

Development of Evaluation Procedures

After modifications to the test materials and score sheet were complete, 25 EIPA-CS pilot tests (14 elementary, 11 secondary) were administered to educational CS transliterators from four states. In order to rate the pilot tests, evaluation procedures were developed with input from the same three consultants who provided feedback on the score sheet. In particular, it was necessary to (1) develop evaluation procedures for each Cued Speech-based transliteration skill that was added to the EIPA-CS score sheet and (2) adapt existing evaluation procedures for any skills that were identical or analogous to skills on the standard EIPA score sheet (for signing versions of the EIPA). In order to promote discussion of each evaluation procedure, the consultants and facilitator viewed roughly 15 pilot tests, looking for common features associated with transliterators at specific skill levels in each of the areas to be evaluated. The observations and discussions generated from viewing these tests led to precise written descriptions of transliterator behavior (i.e., rubrics, measurable and quantifiable whenever possible) that were associated with each of six scores available to evaluators (0, 1, 2, 3, 4, 5) for each skill to be evaluated. Table 23–2 describes what each of these scores corresponds to in terms of overall skill level, with standard EIPA skill descriptions (for signing versions of the EIPA) provided for reference in Appendix 23–B.

After specifying the details of the evaluation procedures in this manner, the consultants then served as the first evaluation team and began rating tests. During this period, the team rated a number of tests at both the elementary and the secondary level. From the experience gained through using the rubrics that had been developed, modifications were made to the evaluation procedure. When a modification was made to an evaluation procedure for a particular skill, all tests that had been scored previously were re-rated in that skill area.

Rater Training

With evaluation procedures in place, a 1½-day workshop was designed to train a second team of evaluators. The workshop consisted of a lecture intermixed with opportunities for participants to practice evaluating sample materials. The consultants assisted with the development of the lecture materials that were used in the workshop, incorporating their experiences as the first EIPA-CS evaluation team. Participants received a copy of the lecture materials as well as a rater's manual specifying the details of the evaluation procedures, which was developed to serve as a reference manual both during and after the workshop. Two consultants also attended the workshop and were available to answer any questions that arose, as well as to provide personal insights on the evaluation process. The format of the workshop was designed so that it can be repeated in the future, in the event that the CS pilot test is permanently adopted by the EIPA Diagnostic Center and additional teams of evaluators are needed.

Prospects for Adoption

Results from EIPA-CS pilot testing (see Krause, Kegl, & Schick, 2007) have shown that the instrument has good face validity and test-retest reliability. In addition, intrarater reliability was quite high, demonstrating that the EIPA-CS pilot test can be

Table 23–2. EIPA-CS Profile of Skills at Each Rating Level

Level 1: Beginner. Demonstrates very limited intelligibility with frequent errors in production. At times, cue production may be incomprehensible and lacks prosody and other supporting information. Individual is only able to interpret very simple voice-to-cue communication. Individual has difficulty conveying, comprehending and interpreting cued messages; single words may be comprehended/interpreted, but effective communication is lost. An individual at this level is not appropriate for classroom interpreting.

Level 2: Advanced Beginner. Demonstrates only basic intelligibility. Limitations in cueing speed and intelligibility interfere with successful communication. More fluent than a Beginner, but lack of fluency still greatly interferes with communication. In cue production, frequent errors and/or unclear cues and mouth movements are apparent. Some use of prosody and supporting information, but use is inconsistent and often inappropriate. Individual is able to read cues at the word level, but complete sentences often require repetitions and repairs. Both voice-to-cue and cue-to-voice interpreting demonstrates serious deficiencies in the message conveyed. Without considerable mentoring, an individual at this level is not recommended for classroom interpreting.

Level 3: Intermediate. Demonstrates moderate intelligibility, yet cueing speed and clarity would most likely be insufficient for complex interpreting situations. Some aspects of cue production may be incorrect even though it may not interfere with communication. Production of prosodic and other supporting information is emerging, but may still be incorrect. Technical topics will most likely pose a great problem. May comprehend a cued message but may need repetition and assistance at times. Both voice-to-cue and cue-to-voice interpretations generally contain all of the key points, but parts of the message may be missing. An individual at this level would be able to interpret basic classroom content but would demonstrate great difficulty conveying all information in the message and may have difficulty with interpreting rapid or technical information. An individual at this level needs supervision and additional training.

Level 4: Advanced Intermediate. Demonstrates high intelligibility at most speaking rates with cue production generally correct. Individual demonstrates paraphrasing strategies for conveying information when a speaker's rate exceeds his or her maximum cueing rate. Cued messages are generally clear and consistent but complex interpreting situations may still pose problems. Prosody is acceptable. Consistently includes other supporting information. Fluency may deteriorate when rate or complexity of input increases. Comprehension of most cued messages at a normal rate is good and cue-to-voice message convey all keys points. An individual at this level would be able to interpret most classroom content but may still have difficulty clearly or accurately conveying information in some complex situations involving rapid speech, technical vocabulary, and multiple speakers.

Level 5: Advanced. Demonstrates high intelligibility at a wide variety of speaking rates, with paraphrasing strategies for communicating extremely high rates of speech. Prosody is skillfully conveyed. Individual correctly uses space and other techniques to incorporate fully all supporting information. Complex interpreting situations do not pose a problem. Comprehension of cued messages is very good. An individual at this level is capable of clearly and accurately conveying the vast majority of classroom interactions.

rated as reliably as signing versions of the EIPA. Although continued work (described in Krause et al., 2007) could improve the EIPA-CS, the results of pilot testing suggest that the EIPA-CS is already in a position to provide reasonable information regarding skill levels of educational transliterators. Therefore, Boys Town National Research Hospital is making plans (at the time this chapter is written) to offer the Cued Speech version of the EIPA nationwide, through the EIPA Diagnostic Center. It is expected that EIPA-CS will be adopted officially in early 2010 and formally offered as an option of the EIPA for a one-year trial period shortly thereafter.

Significance

The inclusion of Cued Speech in the EIPA has a number of potentially important ramifications. One significant consequence, for example, is likely to be an increased visibility of CS transliteration as a profession and of CS as a communication option. Currently, the EIPA is used to some extent in at least 38 states (see www.classroom interpreting.org), and BTNRH conducts more than 2,500 EIPA evaluations per year. Those states and individuals, as well as their corresponding educational administrators, presumably will take notice of the fact that Cued Speech is formally included as a communication option on the EIPA and listed on all EIPA materials. Because the EIPA is widely regarded in the educational interpreting community as the gold standard in assessment, such increased visibility is likely to have a legitimizing effect for transliterators and may elevate their status among members of the interpreting community. As the stature of

CS transliteration is raised, it is possible that administrators of other interpreter assessments (e.g., NCI) might become interested in developing CS versions of their tests at some point in the future, particularly if the size of the market for a CS version of the EIPA suggests that such ventures would prove financially prudent.

For transliterators, a more direct consequence of including CS in the EIPA is the increased opportunity to obtain assessment and diagnostic feedback. Prior to the development of the EIPA-CS, the only assessment tool available to transliterators in most states was the CLTNCE, and in many cases, taking that exam involved traveling a considerable distance. In contrast, transliterators will be able to arrange to take the EIPA-CS with the EIPA Local Test Administrator in their area (since the existing infrastructure for interpreters can be leveraged). As a result of this added convenience, more transliterators should be able to obtain information regarding the skills they need to target for improvement. Moreover, the diagnostic feedback that they receive will be specifically geared to transliterating in educational settings. Armed with this information, educational transliterators may be empowered to demand additional training and/or professional development opportunities from their school districts.

In some cases, the availability of EIPA-CS results *at the state level* could be the source of benefit for transliterators. Depending on how a given state opts to use the EIPA, educational administrators may have access to EIPA scores and diagnostic feedback for transliterators across the state. Such aggregate data collected specifically on the skill levels of Cued Speech transliterators would be important for determining the typical quality of their services. This information is essential for states because so little data concerning the actual skills of these individuals is currently available. This type of data would also be helpful in assessing what special types of training are needed for transliterators or whether the current training methods are adequate. Such data could likely be used, for example, to justify the creation of transliterator training programs at universities and to provide an evidence-base for the curriculum design. Part of this evidence-base has already begun to form, as analysis of pilot testing data indicates that most transliterators are in need of voice-to-cue training (Krause et al., 2007). Thus, receptive training materials, such as those described elsewhere in this volume, are urgently needed.

Finally, the availability of a CS version of the EIPA provides states with another mechanism for establishing minimum performance standards for transliterators. Although a few states already have such standards in place via the CLTNCE or CLTSLA, most do not. In some states with only a handful of transliterators, the prospect of managing a separate evaluation instrument for these individuals could have been a factor in prohibiting the establishment of standards. For these states, the EIPA-CS instrument should be especially attractive, because the same mechanism already in use for sign interpreters can be applied seamlessly to CS transliterators. Given the prevalence of the EIPA, it may also be a convenient option for other states seeking to establish performance standards for transliterators. For these reasons, it seems likely that the availability of a Cued Speech version of the EIPA will allow more states to evaluate transliterators on a regular basis in order to ensure that minimum performance

standards are met. Such developments would help more states make certain that no child is left behind.

Differences Between EIPA-CS and Other Transliterator Assessments

Before concluding, it is worth noting that the EIPA-CS differs from other transliterator assessments in a few respects. First, the EIPA-CS evaluation focuses entirely on the basic transliterating competencies necessary to convey classroom discourse. It does not evaluate Cued Speech transliteration skills in specialty areas such as music, foreign languages, and regional dialects. In addition, the EIPA-CS does not require transliterators to cue expressively for the AV cue-to-voice and VO cue-to-voice portions of the test. Although transliterators are not explicitly downgraded for cueing expressively while voicing, their skills are judged on the quality of the spoken English output alone, reflecting our belief that the natural prosody of spoken English must be the priority for situations in which the primary consumers of the transliterator's output are hearing individuals (i.e., cue-to-voice situations).

The exclusion of the expressive cueing requirement in the receptive portion of the EIPA-CS assessment was purposeful and is a major distinguishing factor between the EIPA-CS and other transliterator assessments. The goal of transliteration is naturalness and message equivalence for the consumer of the transliterator's product. When a transliterator is voicing, the hearing consumer should, ideally, be able to close his or her eyes and receive the message without realizing it was being mediated by a transliterator. When expressive cueing accompanies speech, the speech frequently has a different rhythm, and in some cases, a different intonation, than typical spoken English. If such disruptions in the natural prosody of a transliterator's spoken English were to occur during the EIPA-CS evaluation, that transliterator's cue-to-voice score would be negatively affected. A related issue is the likelihood that the quality of a cue-to-voice transliteration is also frequently degraded by the increased cognitive load of expressively cueing while performing an already difficult task. This possibility should be explored in future research, in order to assess the advantages and disadvantages of this practice.

Summary and Conclusions

The Educational Interpreter Performance Assessment (EIPA) is an important tool for examining the quality of interpreters who use American Sign Language or a sign system in classroom settings. This chapter describes an effort to broaden the applicability of the EIPA to include Cued Speech. As a research tool, the EIPA-CS pilot test has already begun to advance our knowledge regarding typical skill levels of CS transliterators. Given its good validity and reliability, it is also likely that the Cued Speech version of the EIPA will be adopted by Boys Town National Research Hospital in the latter half of 2010. For Cued Speech to be included in an instrument as widely used as the EIPA represents a significant advance for the transliteration profession. The inclusion not only advances the status of Cued Speech as a communication option but also increases the likeli-

hood that transliterators will be held to appropriate performance standards. Such outcomes will help ensure that, indeed, no child is left behind.

References

Anonymous. (1999). Schools and Programs in the United States. *American Annals of the Deaf, 144*, 122–147.

Beaupre, W. (1985). A test for Cued Speech proficiency. *Cued Speech Annual, 1*, 38–45.

Beaupre, W. (1987). The cued speechreading test: An analysis of results. *Cued Speech Annual, 3*, 32–40.

Bornstein, H. (Ed.). (1990). *Manual communication: Implications for education.* Washington DC: Gallaudet University Press.

Cokely, D. (2005). Shifting positionality: A critical examination of the turning point in the relationship of interpreters and the Deaf community. In M. Marschark, R. Peterson, & E. Winston (Eds.), *Sign language interpreting and interpreter education: Directions for research and practice* (pp. 3–28). Oxford, UK: Oxford University Press.

Cornett, R. O. (1967). Cued Speech. *American Annals of the Deaf, 112*(1), 3–13.

Cornett, R. O., & Daisey, M. (2001). Cued Speech. *The Cued Speech resource book for parents of deaf children.* Cleveland, OH: National Cued Speech Association.

Commission of Education of the Deaf. (1988). *Toward equality: Education of the deaf.* Washington, DC: U.S. Government Printing Office.

Fleetwood, E., & Metzger, M. (1990). *Cued Speech transliteration: Theory and application.* Silver Spring, MD: Calliope Press.

Frishberg, N. (1990). *Interpreting: An introduction.* Silver Spring, MD: RID Publications.

Jones, B., Clark, G., & Soltz, D. (1997). Characteristics and practices of sign language Interpreters in inclusive education programs. *Exceptional Children, 63*, 257–268.

Krause, J., Kegl, J., & Schick, B. (2008). Towards extending the Educational Interpreter Performance Assessment to Cued Speech. *Journal of Deaf Studies and Deaf Education, 13,* 432–450.

LaSasso, C., & Metzger, M. (1998). An alternate route for preparing deaf children for BiBi programs: The home language as L1 and Cued Speech for conveying traditionally spoken languages. *Journal of Deaf Studies and Deaf Education, 3,* 265–289.

Moores, D. (1992). A historical perspective on school placement. In T. Kluwin, D. Moores, & M. Gaustad (Eds.), *Toward effective public school programs for deaf students: Context, process, and outcomes* (pp. 7–29). New York, NY: Teachers College, Columbia University.

National Cued Speech Association. (1980). Interested in becoming a Cued Speech interpreter? *Cued Speech News, XIII*(1), 3.

National Cued Speech Association. (1985). Get in on a new field—Be innovative—Be a Cued Speech interpreter. *Cued Speech News, XVIII*(1), 12–13.

National Cued Speech Association. (1988). CST Column. *Cued Speech News, XXI*(4), 7.

No Child Left Behind Act. (2001). Pub. L. 107-110, Statute 1425.

Registry of Interpreters for the Deaf. (September 6, 2006). *News Release: RID To Grant Certified Member Status To EIPA-Evaluated Interpreters—Appoints Members To Educational Interpreting Committee.* Retrieved April 7, 2007, from http://www.rid.org/EIPAnews-release0906.pdf

Rehabilitation Act. (1973). Pub. L. 93-112, 87 Statute 394.

Schick, B. (2004). How might learning through an educational interpreter influence cognitive development? In E. Winston (Ed.), *Educational interpreting: How it can succeed* (pp. 73–87). Washington, DC: Gallaudet University Press.

Schick, B., & Williams, K. (1992). *The educational interpreter performance assessment: A tool to evaluate classroom performance.* Paper presented at the issues in Language and Deafness: The use of sign language in educational settings: Current concepts and controversies, Omaha, NE.

Schick, B., & Williams, K. (2004). The Educational Interpreter Performance Assessment: Current structure and practices. In E. Winston (Ed.), *Educational interpreting: How it can succeed.* Washington, DC: Gallaudet University Press.

Schick, B., Williams, K., & Bolster, L. (1999). Skill level of educational interpreters working in public schools. *Journal of Deaf Studies and Deaf Education, 4,* 144–155.

Schick, B., Williams, K., & Kupermintz, H. (2006). Look who's being left behind: Educational interpreters and access to education for deaf and hard-of-hearing students. *Journal of Deaf Studies and Deaf Education, 11,* 3–20.

Appendix 23–A

SUMMARY OF STANDARD EIPA SCORE SHEET (SIGNING VERSION)

I. Interpreter Product: Voice-to-Sign
   A. Stress/emphasis for important words or phrases
   B. Affect/emotions
   C. Register
   D. Sentence boundaries
   E. Sentence types/clausal boundaries indicated
   F. Production and use of nonmanual markers
   G. Use of verb directionality/pronominal system
   H. Comparison/contrast, sequence, and cause/effect
   I. Location/relationship using ASL classifier system
   J. Follows grammar of ASL or PSE (if appropriate)
   K. Use of English morphological markers (if appropriate)
   L. Clearly mouths speaker's English (if appropriate)

II. Interpreter Product: Sign-to-Voice
   A. Can read and convey the student's signs
   B. Can read and convey fingerspelling and numbers
   C. Register
   D. Nonmanual behaviors and ASL morphology
   E. Speech production (rate, rhythm, fluency, volume)
   F. Sentence/clausal boundaries indicated
   G. Sentence types

   H. Emphasize important words, phrases, affect/emotions
   I. Correct English word selection
   J. Adds no extraneous words/sounds to message

III. Vocabulary
   A. Amount of sign vocabulary
   B. Signs made correctly
   C. Fluency
   D. Vocabulary consistent with the sign language or system chosen for testing
   E. Key vocabulary represented
   F. Production of fingerspelling
   G. Words spelled correctly
   H. Appropriate use of fingerspelling
   I. Production of numbers
   J. Variety of strategies for compensating for unknown signs
   K. Sign invention appropriate

IV. Overall Factors
   A. Appropriate eye contact/movement
   B. Developed a sense of the whole message (voice to sign)
   C. Developed a sense of the whole message (sign to voice)
   D. Demonstrated process decalage appropriately (voice to sign)
   E. Demonstrated process decalage appropriately (sign to voice)
   F. Follows principles of discourse mapping
   G. Indicates who is speaking

Appendix 23–B

STANDARD EIPA PROFILE OF SKILLS (SIGNING VERSIONS)

Level 1: Beginner. Demonstrates very limited sign vocabulary with frequent errors in production. At times, production may be incomprehensible. Grammatical structure tends to be nonexistent. Individual is only able to communicate very simple ideas and demonstrates great difficulty comprehending signed communication. Sign production lacks prosody and use of space for the vast majority of the interpreted message. An individual at this level is not recommended for classroom interpreting.

Level 2: Advanced Beginner. Demonstrates only basic sign vocabulary, and these limitations interfere with communication. Lack of fluency and sign production errors are typical and often interfere with communication. The interpreter often hesitates in signing, as if searching for vocabulary. Frequent errors in grammar are apparent, although basic signed sentences appear intact. More complex grammatical structures are typically difficult. Individual is able to read signs at the word level and simple sentence level, but complete or complex sentences often require repetitions and repairs. Some use of prosody and space, but use is inconsistent and often incorrect. An individual at this level is not recommended for classroom interpreting.

Level 3: Intermediate. Demonstrates knowledge of basic vocabulary, but may lack vocabulary for more technical, complex, or academic topics. Individual is able to sign in a fairly fluent manner using some consistent prosody, but pacing is still slow with infrequent pauses for vocabulary or complex structures. Sign production may show some errors but generally will not interfere with communication. Grammatical production may still be incorrect, especially for complex structures, but in general is intact for routine and simple language. Comprehends signed messages but may need repetition and assistance. Voiced translation often lacks depth and subtleties of the original message. An individual at this level would be able to communicate very basic classroom content but may incorrectly interpret complex information resulting in a message that is not always clear. An interpreter at this level needs continued supervision and should be required to participate in continuing education in interpreting.

Level 4: Advanced Intermediate. Demonstrates broad use of vocabulary with sign production generally correct. Demonstrates good strategies for conveying information when a specific sign is not in their vocabulary. Grammatical constructions are generally clear and consistent, but complex information may still pose occasional problems. Prosody is good, with appropriate facial expression most of the time. May still have difficulty with the use of facial expression in complex sentences and adverbial nonmanual markers. Fluency may deteriorate when rate or complexity of communication increases. Uses space consistently most of the time, but complex constructions or extended use of discourse cohesion may still pose problems. Comprehension of most signed messages at a normal rate is good, but translation may lack some complexity of the original message. An individual at this level would be able to convey much of the classroom content but may have difficulty with complex topics or rapid turn taking.

Level 5: Advanced. Demonstrates broad and fluent use of vocabulary, with a broad range of strategies for communicating new words and concepts. Sign production errors are minimal and never interfere with comprehension. Prosody is correct for grammatical, nonmanual markers, and affective purposes. Complex grammatical constructions are typically not a problem. Comprehension of signed messages is very good, communicating all details of the original message. An individual at this level is capable of clearly and accurately conveying the majority of interactions within the classroom.

Chapter 24

HOW CUED SPEECH IS PROCESSED IN THE BRAIN: DIRECTIONS FOR FUTURE RESEARCH

Mario Aparicio, Philippe Peigneux, Brigitte Charlier, and Jacqueline Leybaert

In Chapter 12, LaSasso and Crain discuss the view of Chomsky and others that humans are biologically predisposed to acquire language as long as they have early, clear, complete exposure to the (presumably auditory) "continuous phoneme stream" of the language and opportunities to interact with fluent users of the language. In Chapter 3, Metzger and Fleetwood report findings from their research showing that Cued Speech clearly and completely conveys the continuous phoneme stream of language entirely via the visual modality. In this chapter, we support our view that that our brains are biologically predisposed to process speech information *multimodally*. That is, humans can process speech information entirely either auditorily or visually (see Alegria, Chapter 5). We first provide a brief overview of the multimodal processing of oral language

by hearing individuals. Then we discuss how Cued Speech is processed by deaf individuals. As background for this discussion, we first present behavioral data, including findings from memory, speech perception, and cerebral lateralization experiments, and next, we present data from brain activation, linked to visual speech perception, together with some preliminary results of brain activity linked to the perception of Cued Speech.

Audiovisual Speech Integration in the Brain

Empirical data collected during the last 25 years show that speech perception is *multimodal* in individuals with normal hearing. That is, during face-to-face conversations, speech perception is substantially improved when the receiver has the opportunity to watch the lips of the speech producer, especially when the words are pronounced in noise (Sumby & Pollack, 1954). The receiver is generally not conscious of the influence of visual cues upon auditory perception of speech; however, this influence becomes obvious when the visual cues are not synchronous with the heard speech. This is the case when we watch a dubbed film. This phenomenon also is exemplified experimentally by the McGurk effect (McGurk & MacDonald, 1976). In a McGurk laboratory experiment, subjects watch a video clip with a face repeatedly pronouncing the syllable /ga/ (or /ka/), while the sound track delivers the syllable /ba/ (or /pa/). The percept of the subjects consists predominantly into a /da/ (see: http://www.cee.hw.ac.uk/~cmj/projects/McGurk/download.html for a demonstration of the McGurk effect). Inversely, when the face in the video pronounces the syllable /ba/ (or /pa/), which begins with a highly visible bilabial consonant, most of the time, subjects experience an audiovisual combination: /bga/ (or /pka/). Although the time point at which visual cues exert an influence on speech perception has not yet been precisely identified, evidence provided by behavioral studies suggests that it occurs very early in audiovisual processing, before the word identification stage, and very likely before the phonetic categorization stage (Green, 1998; Summerfield, 1987). It is theorized that the two stimuli sources (i.e., acoustic and visual) specify the same physical events, and the observers integrate auditory and visual information " . . . before phonetic or lexical categorization takes place; the two streams are analogue at their conflux . . . " (Summerfield, 1987, p. 16).

Studies in cerebral imagery might reveal the possible neuroanatomic basis of the interactions between visual and auditory information in speech processing in hearing individuals. A number of studies of hearing subjects have examined the cortical area activated by speechreading. Using functional magnetic resonance imaging (fMRI) methods, Calvert et al. (1997) showed that identification of numerals (1 to 9) presented in a speechreading condition activates areas belonging to the visual primary cortex, and more interestingly, to the primary and secondary auditory cortices (see also MacSweeney et al., 2000). The primary auditory cortex consists of Heschl's transversal gyri (or Brodmann area 41). The regions near this area, the areas BA 42, and BA 22, 21, 20, and 37 constitute the secondary auditory cortices. The neural projections are prewired from the inner ear to the primary auditory cortex; the secondary auditory cortex is the locus of crossmodal interactions. Visual speech, thus, has the power to activate parts of the neural circuitry which were considered up to the mid-1990s as being devoted exclusively to the processing of the auditory input. More recent studies have clarified that when visual speech activates auditory areas, and more particularly, the superior temporal sulcus (STS), it does not activate the primary auditory cortex (Bernstein et al., 2002; see also Chapter 18, this volume).

Several teams have investigated the areas of the brain activated by audiovisual speech by exploiting the incongruent stimuli designed by McGurk and MacDonald. Using magnetoencephalography, Sams et al. (1991) showed that the presentation of incongruent audiovisual stimuli, among a series of congruent stimuli (like auditory /ba/ coupled with a visual /ba/) entails a differential activation at the level of supratemporal auditory cortex. The involvement of this region in audiovisual speech integration, and more particularly of the STS, has been confirmed by several teams (Calvert et al., 1999; Calvert, Campbell, & Bramer, 2000; Jones & Callan, 2003; Macaluso, George, Dolan, Spence, & Driver, 2004). This activation is less pronounced, however, when the auditory and visual signals are incongruent (Calvert et al., 2000; Wright, Pelphrey, Allison, McKeown, & McCarthy, 2003), which confirms the role of this region in the processing of stimuli that have social pertinence. In contrast, the activation is more pronounced for auditory signals presented in noise (Callan, Callan, Kroos, & Vatiokis-Bateson, 2001; Sekiyama, Kanno, Miura, & Sugita, 2003), supporting the behavioral observation that speechreading contributes even more to speech perception when the auditory signal is masked by noise (Sekiyama & Tohkura, 1991; Sumby & Pollack, 1954). Therefore, it is not surprising that activation in the left superior posterior temporal gyrus appears to be modulated by speechreading skills in normally hearing participants, as a positive correlation exists between activation of this region and speechreading ability (Hall, Fussell, & Summerfield, 2005).

How Phonological Information Is Processed in Memory by Hearing Individuals Perceiving Audiovisual Speech

The first investigations of how the brain processes visual speech stimuli employed short-term memory experiments. Memory for speech stimuli can be measured by use of primacy, recency, and suffix effects.

In such studies, subjects are presented with lists of stimuli (e.g., lexical items, digit spans) to be recalled in the same order they were presented. A subject who more readily recalls items occurring at the beginning of a list is exhibiting a *primacy effect*. A subject who more readily remembers items occurring at the end of a list is exhibiting a *recency effect*. Finally, a subject who experiences difficulty remembering items at the end of a list when that item is followed by an extraneous stimulus (e.g., a sound, an unrelated lexical item) is exhibiting a *suffix effect*. Results of such studies constitute strong evidence of the processing of phonological information by the memory circuits of the brain.

In a classical memory experiment, participants are presented orally a list of items (digits or words) to be recalled in the same order as they were presented. The length of the list is classically 9 items (but can be 6 to 8 for younger subjects), meaning that the participants could not reasonably recall all the items of the lists. The recall performance is structured so that the subject will have good performance for the items presented at the beginning of the lists (i.e., the primacy effect), worse performance for the items of the middle of the list, and good performance again for the items at the end of the lists (i.e., the recency effect). The recency effect has *not* been found to occur for graphically-presented word lists, which suggests that it may be particular to auditory stimuli (Crowder, 1971; Crowder & Morton, 1969). In addition, the auditory presentation of the last stimulus that has *not* been recalled by the subjects (e.g., "zero") reduces the advantage for the last to be recalled items: the *suffix* effect, which is interpreted to mean that the suffix erases the trace left by the last to be recalled items (Spoehr & Corin, 1978).

A number of studies have revealed that the recency and suffix effects are *cross-modal* in hearing subjects (Campbell & Dodd, 1980; Gathercole, 1986; Spoehr & Corin, 1978). Specifically, it has been shown that: (1) lists of stimuli which are lipread (but not heard) give rise to a recency effect (Campbell & Dodd, 1980), (2) a spoken suffix, which is heard but not seen, reduces the recency effect obtained on lists which are lipread (Campbell & Dodd, 1980); (3) a suffix which is lipread (but not heard) reduces the auditory recency (Spoehr & Corin, 1978); and (4) a suffix which is lipread impairs recall of lipread lists (Gathercole, 1986), whereas a nonspeech lip movement suffix does not interfere with lipread recency (Campbell & Dodd, 1982). These data collectively support that speech that is received *visually* (i.e., seen speech), and speech that is received *auditorily* (i.e., heard speech) share a common representation in the brain processes involved in immediate memory in hearing subjects. This should not surprise us as the visual signal that we read from the lips is shaped by the same physical events as the acoustic signal that we hear; that is, the shared representation is structurally isomorphic with the talker's articulations.

How Phonological Information Is Processed in Memory by Deaf Individuals Perceiving Visual Speech or Cued Speech

Similar to verbal memory studies conducted with hearing subjects, Dodd, Hobson, Brasher, and Campbell (1983) investigated recency and suffix effects of deaf individuals. They found that for deaf students:

(1) lists of stimuli that are lipread create a recency effect that was not observed in the recall of graphically presented lists; and (2) a lipread suffix abolishes the lipread recency effect whereas, in contrast, a tongue protrusion presented as suffix does not abolish the recency effect, meaning that a facial gesture has an effect only when it corresponds to articulation. This was observed for youngsters who were good articulators as well as for those who were poor articulators (Dodd, Hobson, Brasher, & Campbell, 1983). It was concluded that deaf subjects do not differ from hearing subjects in the way they remember the lipread stimuli, and that lipread stimuli is coded phonologically by deaf subjects.

Leybaert, Alegria, Hage, and Charlier (1998; see also Leybaert & Lechat, 2001) demonstrated that the presentation of word lists via Cued Speech provokes a recency effect in both deaf subjects exposed to Cued Speech, as well as for hearing subjects who are familiar with Cued Speech (e.g., parents of a deaf child, interpreters, speech therapists). The presentation of a list of cued items also left a trace that is processed in a particular way by the brain. Interestingly, hearing cuers displayed a *larger* recency effect when lists were presented in Cued Speech + sound condition than when they were presented via Cued Speech without sound. The trace left by auditory stimuli seems to be stronger than that left by visually cued stimuli. Leybaert and Lechat (2001) concluded that the recency advantage of Cued Speech with sound over Cued Speech without sound in hearing subjects cannot be attributed to a phonetically "richer" trace, because the phonetic content was identical in both conditions. Rather, what provokes a stronger recency effect for lists with an auditory component seems to be acoustic spectral energy of the vowels. This makes auditory vowels perceptually very salient and creates a longer "echo" (Leybaert & Lechat, 2001, p. 961). To conclude, these data suggest that there are common processes to audiovisual speech processing (for hearing subjects) and for the processing of Cued Speech for both hearing and deaf subjects.

Integration of Lipread and Manual Information in Cued Speech

Our hypothesis related to what is occurring in the brain when cuers perceive cued language is that lip movements and hand cues of Cued Speech may be interpreted as unitary *phonological gestures* (and induce an activity in the language-related neural circuits of the brain)—at least in those individuals who experienced Cued Speech early and intensively as a primary mode of communication. The theoretical question related to how manual cues and lipreading combine to produce a unitary percept in Cued Speech receivers has been addressed mainly by Alegria and colleagues (Alegria, Charlier, & Mattys, 1999; Alegria & Lechat, 2005; Alegria, Leybaert, Charlier, & Hage, 1992) who distinguished two kinds of possible models: (1) lipreading information provides the core phonological information, and the manual information resolves the remaining lipreading ambiguities or (2) a true integration of the manual information and lip information occurs: "The lipreading/cues compound would produce a unique amodal phonemic percept con-

ceptually similar to Summerfield's (1987) 'common metric' which integrates auditory and lip-reading information to generate a vocal tract filter function" (Alegria et al., 1999, p. 468; see Chapter 5).[1]

Alegria et al. (1992) discuss the question of integration in light of two kinds of observations: misperceptions of cued gestures and the effect of incongruent manual cues/labial movements on speech perception by deaf Cued Speech users. Phonological misperceptions induced by the structural characteristics of cues might be substitutions based on the similarity between cues (i.e., perceiving /da/ for /ʒa/) which might result from the fact that /d/ and /ʒ/ share the same handshape. They could also be intrusions of extra syllables in lexical items requiring a number of cued units greater than the number of syllables. An example of this is the English word *red*, which requires two cued units (i.e., /re/ at the chin and /d/ at the side), but contains only one syllable. Psycholinguists are interested in observing and computing such cue misperceptions because the child has to pay attention to the lips posture in order to discriminate between /dra/ and /dara/, for example. Thus, the very fact of perceiving /dara/ for /dra/ indicates that the processing of the manual cues has taken priority compared to the processing of the lip gestures.

Alegria et al. (1999) used a pseudo-word identification task presented via Cued Speech (CS) or in lipreading alone. They measured the number of "CS errors," (i.e., errors based on the interpretation of the manual cues without taking into account the lipreading). An example of

---

[1]Note that the second model proposed by Alegria et al. (1999) is compatible both with the Metzger/Fleetwood view that Cued Speech can function entirely in the visual modality and a model in which Cued Speech refers to spoken language articulation.

these CS errors is when the presentation of a CCV syllable (e.g., *tra*) or a CVC syllable (e.g., *cam*) via Cued Speech provokes the judgment that there were two syllables presented instead of one. The late CS-users made more errors, generally speaking; however, the proportion of CS-errors based on over-reading of the hand cues was larger in the early Cued Speech-users than in the late Cued Speech-users, indicating that the former tend to pay more attention to the hand cues than the latter.

To explore the question of integration in more detail, Alegria and Lechat (2005) subjected deaf youngsters to a situation where lipread information could be either *congruent* or *incongruent* with Cued Speech information. An example of incongruent stimulus is the lipread syllable /va/ accompanied by the /p, d, ʒ/ handshape. The rationale was based on the McGurk effect, which shows that the perceptual system exposed to incongruous information will be forced to adopt a phonological solution. The premise of this study was that the nature of the response given by the subject would inform us about the perceptual weights the subject attributes to each source. If the subject were to respond /va/, this could be interpreted to mean that the subject is more attuned to process the lipread information. If the subject were to respond /pa/ or /da/ or /ʒa/, it could be interpreted that the subject is more tempted to read the manual cues and ignore the lips. Early and late Cued Speech-users were included in the experiment. Findings from this study indicate that with incongruent cues, performance decreased relative to lipreading only, indicating that the cues were not ignored. Regarding the comparison between the two subgroups, the results showed that the total number of errors was greater in the "late" group. An important observa-

tion was that the proportion of Cued Speech misperceptions relative to the total number of errors was larger in the "early Cued Speech" group. These data show that early Cued Speech-users do exploit visual information conveyed via Cued Speech, especially when the lipread information is ambiguous and/or is more difficult to extract.

Hemispheric Specialization for Reading and Exposure to Cued Speech

Another source of evidence about how the brain deals with Cued Speech consists of looking to hemispheric specialization for the processing of cued information. Lateralized cerebral function for speech perception develop during the first three years of life of hearing children, and seems more dependent on linguistic experience than on chronological age per se (Mills, Coffey-Corina, & Neville, 1993, 1997).

In his "Theory of Neurolinguistic Development," Locke (1997) distinguishes a phase of initial storage of utterances in a holistic way, which mainly depends on resources located in the right hemisphere. The next phase involves the development of analytical language processes, around the age of two years. These analytical processes would be housed in the left hemisphere. According to Locke, "Children who are delayed in the second phase have too little stored utterance material to activate their analytic mechanism at the optimum biological moment, and when sufficient words have been learned, this modular capability has already begun to decline" (p. 266). It might thus be the case that the explanation for better phonological processing is that early Cued Speech users, compared to late Cued Speech users, have stored many perceptually distinct cued utterances during the first years of life, which would allow the analytical mechanism, housed in the left hemisphere, to function during the appropriate period. In contrast, late Cued Speech users may have experienced the first critical years in linguistically-deprived situations resulting in the initial bias for left hemisphere specialization for language disappearing or at least being lessened. The implication of this, of course, is that to the extent possible, Cued Speech should be introduced early to deaf children.

The lateralization of those aspects of the processing that are directly dependent on perception of Cued Speech as a first language have been investigated by D'Hondt (2001) (see also Leybaert & D'Hondt, 2003). Two questions were addressed. First, is the linguistic processing of Cued Speech stimuli better performed by the left hemisphere? Second, if there is a left hemisphere advantage for linguistic processing, is it modulated by the time in their development in which deaf children received formal linguistic input? In an experiment conducted by D'Hondt (2001), subjects had to compare two sets of video stimuli, the first presented in the central visual field (the standard), and the second presented, very briefly, in either the left or right visual hemifield (the target). In the linguistic condition, subjects had to decide whether the same word in Cued Speech was produced in the two videos, irrespective of the hand which produced the stimuli. In the nonlinguistic condition, they had to decide whether the cue was produced with the same hand, irrespective of the word cued. In this way, subjects were known to be attending to the linguistic aspects of cueing in one condition, and not in the other. A sample of subjects with early exposure to Cued Speech was com-

pared to a sample of subjects with late exposure to Cued Speech. The results were clear cut. Specifically, in the linguistic condition, the early-Cued Speech group obtained an accuracy advantage for stimuli presented in the right visual field, while the subjects of the late-Cued Speech group did not show any hemifield advantage. In the nonlinguistic condition, no visual advantage was observed in either group (Leybaert & D'Hondt, 2003). These results confirmed the already existing evidence that the left cerebral hemisphere is specialized for language, regardless of the nature of the language medium. They also suggest that the neural systems, which mediate the processing of linguistic information, are modifiable in response to language experience. The left hemisphere superiority for language processing appears more systematically in children exposed early to a structured linguistic input than in children exposed only late to this input.

The next question we recently addressed relates to the neural activation of Cued Speech in deaf subjects with early exposure to Cued Speech. Specifically, we were interested in whether the neural activation would be similar to that in hearing subjects in audiovisual languages. Furthermore, how would hand cues and lips be integrated in Cued Speech? In the next section, we present some neuroanatomofunctional data from visual speech and Cued Speech perception in order to address these questions.

Neural Circuits of Visual Speech and Cued Speech Perception in Deaf Subjects

In order to better understand the processing of linguistic information by deaf individuals, we deemed it important to examine their functional activity in the brain during speech perception. Before doing that, however, it was important to determine whether there are neuroanatomical differences in the auditory cortex when it is not stimulated by auditory information. The auditory cortex includes the gyri transverse Heschl (site of the primary auditory cortex), the superior temporal sulcus, and the planum temporal. The volume of the planum temporal and of the gyri transverse Heschl is, in deaf as in hearing subjects, more developed in the left hemisphere. In the case of congenital deafness, the temporal areas keep their macroanatomy and their level of glucose metabolism (Kujala, Alho, & Näätänen, 2000). The volume of grey matter in the regions normally devoted to auditory processing is similar in congenital deaf and hearing subjects (Emmorey, Allen, Bruss, Schenker, & Damasio, 2003; Penhune, Cismaru, Dorsain-Pierre, Pettito, & Zatorre, 2003). However, auditory deprivation seems to entail a functional reorganization of auditory cortical areas, as Neville, Schmidt, and Kutas (1983) have observed visual evoked potentials (ERP) in temporal cortical areas that are thought to be devoted to auditory processing.

Deaf people have been found to outperform hearing people in comprehending seen speech from the lips (i.e., lipreading) (Bernstein, Demorest, & Tucker, 2000; Mohammed, Campbell, MacSweeney, Barry, & Coleman, 2006). However, MacSweeney et al. (2001) found that whereas lipreading provokes a bilateral activation of temporal cortex in hearing subjects, no significant activation of this region is observed in the deaf subjects taken as a group. The largest difference between hearing and deaf subjects is located in the left temporal cortex. In this area, hearing subjects show a larger activation than deaf subjects, which extends from medium temporal gyrus (BA 21) up to contiguous areas of superior temporal gyrus (including areas BA 22 and BA 42) and the inferior parietal lobe (BA 40). However, an individual analysis reveals that a left temporal activation is observed in most of the deaf individuals, but with a more dispersed pattern than in hearing individuals. MacSweeney et al. (2001) conclude that hearing speech helps to develop a coherent speech perception system inside the lateral areas of left temporal lobe; however, when this input has been absent since birth, this region does not show the expected pattern of focal specialization. In contrast to this data, Capek et al. (2008) found recently greater activation *in deaf subjects than in hearing subjects,* in the left middle and posterior portions of superior temporal cortex during lipreading. The pattern of activation survived after control for speechreading skills, which were still more developed in deaf than in hearing participants. The authors explain the discrepancy by suggesting that the previous study of MacSweeney et al. (2001) either lacked power (they had only six subjects per group) or there were differences in stimulus factors that systematically affected the extent to which temporal regions are recruited during silent speechreading in deaf subjects (MacSweeney et al. [2001] used *single numbers* as stimuli whereas Capek et al. [2008] used *words*). In any case, the significance of this finding by Capek et al. (2008) is that classical auditory regions, in the absence of stimuli acoustic experience, might be activated by silent speech in the form of speechreading, which gives access to spoken language structure by eye. It is an illustrative example of functional brain plasticity.

Results from the studies considered above, taken collectively, allow the following hypotheses related to the perception of Cued Speech in the brain of a deaf individual with early, intense exposure to Cued Speech:

1. Cued Speech has the power to activate parts of the neural circuitry considered up to now as devoted solely to the processing of auditory input. The left middle and posterior portions of superior temporal cortex could be activated by the processing of lip movements in deaf as well as in hearing participants. These regions could also be activated by the manual components (handshape and hand placement) of Cued Speech, at least in those deaf individuals who have experienced early and intense exposure to Cued Speech.

2. The posterior superior temporal sulcus has been proposed as a key binding site, responsible for integration of audiovisual speech processing (Calvert et al., 2000). Capek et al. (2008) showed a greater activation in deaf subjects than in hearing subjects in the posterior superior temporal sulcus while lipreading suggesting that in deaf subjects this region surely has become sensitive to the dominant visual speech modality. Is this region also a key binding site for integration of cues and lipreading in CS? In that case, CS should increase the activation of the posterior supratemporal sulcus compared to lipreading only.

3. There could be a convergence between labial and manual information at a prelexical level, before the word identification stage, and possibly, before the phonetic categorization stage. Indeed, the two sources, *labial* and *manual*, specify the same phonological gesture.

The first two hypotheses are currently being tested in our laboratory using fMRI methods. In a neuroanatomofunctional study, we are comparing lexical perception of Cued French, in deaf early users of Cued Speech, with lexical perception of audiovisual French in hearing French speakers. In the speech perception task, deaf participants watch a videotape of a woman producing words in Cued French. The speaker's full face and torso are shown. Hearing participants watch and hear a videotape of the same female producing words in French. Participants press a button only when they perceive a target (e.g., the word "daddy") from a word list. Similarly, in the control condition, subjects watch a videotape of the same female at rest. The participants are instructed to press a button only when they detect a small cue (red circle) digitally superimposed on the woman's chin. Therefore, both conditions are rather passive and the target is included in order to ensure that participants perceive and process the stimuli, paying attention to them. At the moment, 15 hearing but only five deaf subjects have been evaluated, and it is not possible to make a consistent group comparison analysis between deaf and hearing. However, preliminary results of individuals in deaf group show maximal foci of activation in same regions as the hearing group: superior and middle temporal lobe bilaterally and the left inferior frontal gyrus. These regions are also activated during speech perception with signs (MacSweeney et al., 2002), suggesting that these regions might constitute the "core language system" of spoken language regardless of modality and hearing status.

Regarding the second hypothesis about lips and hands integration, we found activation of posterior superior temporal sulcus in all deaf participants.

There also was activation in the MT/V5 region in 4 of the 5 deaf participants; this region was not activated in the hearing group. Activation of MT/V5 may simply reflect processing of movement when using Cued Speech (Zeki et al., 1991). However, this may also be linked to linguistic integration of visual information in Cued Speech (i.e., cues and lipreading), as it was already shown in spoken audiovisual language when the speech signal was made difficult to perceive by experimentally increasing noise to the signal (Sekiyama, Kanno, Miura, & Sugita, 2003; see Chapter 4 by Koo & Supalla in this volume).

The third hypothesis might be tested by comparing Cued Speech activity with both lipreading-only and manual cues-only. If the common activity is found in posterior parts of the brain, around fusiform gyrus or MT/V5, we could suggest that integration is taking place at early stages of speech perception.

Conclusion

The bulk of data related to early cuers indicates very clearly that deaf children are equipped with a biological predisposition to perceive human communicative signals and to linguistically and symbolically process the combination of manual cues and lipreading. Our expectation, to be confirmed by additional research, is that the brain areas responsible for the processing of cued information in early cuers would be similar to those involved in sign language processing for early signers and audiovisual speech for hearing subjects. Indeed, our preliminary results from fMRI data support our initial hypotheses.

More practically, parents, speech therapists, and transliterators who use Cued Speech with deaf children should be aware of the enormous potential of using cues for the development of cognitive architecture of deaf children. Providing clear, complete, and visual access to traditionally oral language via Cued Speech for young deaf children of nonsigning hearing parents enables the development of the child's home language according to biological predispositions, meaning that Cued Speech favors the tendency of the left hemisphere to process language, to create pieces of phonology. The long-term theoretical consequences of this cerebral organization are very important, notably on reading acquisition (see Chapters 11 to 14 in this volume).

References

Alegria, J., Charlier, B., & Mattys, S. (1999). The role of lipreading and Cued Speech in the processing of phonological information in French-educated deaf children. *European Journal of Cognitive Psychology, 11,* 451–472.

Alegria, J., & Lechat, J. (2005). Phonological processing in deaf children: When lipreading and cues are incongruent. *Journal of Deaf Studies and Deaf Education, 10,* 122–133.

Alegria, J., Leybaert, J., Charlier, B., & Hage, C. (1992). On the origin of phonological representations in the deaf: Hearing lips and hands. In J. Alegria, D. Holender, J. Morais, & M. Radeau (Eds.), *Analytic approaches to human cognition.* Brussels: Elsevier Science Publishers.

Bernstein, L., Auer, E., Moore, J., Ponton, C., Don, M., & Singh, M. (2002). Visual speech perception without primary auditory cortex activation. *NeuroReport, 13,* 311–315.

Bernstein, L., Demorest, M., & Tucker, P. (2000). Speech perception without hearing. *Perception & Psychophysics, 62,* 233–252.

Callan, D., Callan, A., Kroos, C., & Vatikiotis-Bateson, E. (2001). Multimodal contribution to speech perception revealed by independent component analysis: A single-sweep EEG case study. *Cognitive Brain Research, 10,* 349–353.

Calvert, G., Brammer, M., Bullmore, E., Campbell, R., Iversen, S., & David, S. (1999). Response amplification in sensory-specific cortices during crossmodal binding. *NeuroReport, 10,* 2619–2623.

Calvert, G., Bullmore, E., Brammer, M., Campbell, R., Williams, S., McGuire, P., . . . David, A. S. (1997). Activation of auditory cortex during silent lipreading. *Science, 276,* 593–595.

Calvert, G., Campbell, R., & Brammer, M. (2000). Evidence from functional magnetic resonance imaging of crossmodal binding in the human heteromodal cortex. *Current Biology, 10,* 649–657.

Campbell, R., & Dodd, B. (1980). Hearing by eye: The psychology of lipreading. *Quarterly Journal of Experimental Psychology, 32,* 85–99.

Campbell, R., & Dodd, B. (1982). Some suffix effects on lipread lists. *Canadian Journal of Psychology, 36,* 509–515.

Capek, C., MacSweeney, M., Woll, B., Waters, D., McGuire, P., David, A., Brammer, M., & Campbell, R. (2008). Cortical circuits for silent speechreading in deaf and hearing people. *Neuropsychologia, 46,* 1233–1241.

Crowder, R. (1971). The sound of vowels and consonants in immediate memory. *Journal of Verbal Learning and Verbal Behavior, 10,* 587–596.

Crowder, R., & Morton, J. (1969). Precategorical acoustic storage (PAS). *Perception and Psychophysics, 5,* 365–371.

D'Hondt, M. (2001). *Spécialisation hémisphérique pour le langage chez la personne à déficience auditive effet de l'expérience linguistique précoce.* Unpublished doctoral dissertation, Université libre de Bruxelles.

Dodd, B., Hobson, P., Brasher, J., & Campbell, R. (1983). Deaf children's short-term memory for lip-read, graphic and signed stimuli. *British Journal of Developmental Psychology, 1,* 353–364.

Emmorey, K., Allen, J., Bruss, J., Schenker, N., & Damasio, H. (2003). A morphometric analysis of auditory brain regions in congenitally deaf adults. *Proceedings of the National Academy of Sciences, 100,* 10049–10054.

Gathercole, S. (1986). The Modality effect and articulation. *Quarterly Journal of Experimental Psychology, 38A,* 461–474.

Green, K. (1998). The use of auditory and visual information during phonetic processing: Implications for theories of speech perception. In R. Campbell, B. Dodd, & D. Burnham (Eds.), *Hearing by eye: The psychology of lipreading* (Vol. II, pp. 3–25). Hove, UK: Psychology Press.

Hall, D., Fussell, C., & Summerfield, A. (2005). Reading fluent speech from talking faces: Typical brain network and individual differences. *Journal of Cognitive Neuroscience, 17,* 939–953.

Jones, J., & Callan, D. (2003). Brain activity during audiovisual speech perception: An fMRI study of the McGurk effect. *NeuroReport, 14,* 1129–1133.

Kujala, T., Alho, K., & Näätänen, R. (2000) Cross-modal reorganization of human cortical functions. *Trends in Neurosciences, 3,* 115–120.

Leybaert, J., Alegria, J., Hage, C., & Charlier, B. (1998). The effect of exposure to phonetically augmented lipspeech in the prelingual deaf. In R. Campbell, B. Dodd, & D. Burnham (Eds.), *Hearing by eye (Vol. II): The psychology of speechreading and auditory-visual speech* (pp. 281–299) Hove, UK: Psychology Press.

Leybaert, J., & D'Hondt, M. (2003). Neurolinguistic development in deaf children. *International Journal of Audiology, 42,* (Supp. 1), S34–S40.

Leybaert, J., & Lechat, J. (2001). Phonological similarity effects in memory for serial order for Cued Speech. *Journal of Speech, Language, and Hearing Research, 44,* 949–963.

Locke, J. (1997). A theory of neurolinguistic development. *Brain and Language, 58,* 265–326.

Macaluso, E., George, N., Dolan, R., Spence, C., & Driver, J. (2004). Spatial and temporal factors during processing of audiovisual speech: A PET study. *NeuroImage, 21,* 725–732.

MacSweeney, M., Amaro, E., Calvert, G., Campbell, R., David, A., McGuire, P., et al. (2000). Silent speechreading in the absence of scanner noise: An event-related fMRI study. *NeuroReport, 11*, 1729–1733.

MacSweeney, M., Campbell, R., Calvert, G., McGuire, P., David, A., Suckling, J., . . . Brammer, M. J. (2001). Dispersed activation in the left temporal cortex for speech-reading in congenitally deaf people. *Proceedings of the Royal Society of London, 268*, 451–457.

MacSweeney, M., Woll, B., Campbell, R., McGuire, P., David, A., Williams, S., . . . Brammer, M. (2002). Neural systems underlying British Sign Language and audiovisual English processing in native users. *Brain, 125*, 1583–1593.

McGurk, H., & MacDonald, J. (1976). Hearing lips and seeing voices. *Nature, 264*, 746–748.

Mills, D., Coffey-Corina, S., & Neville, H. (1993). Language acquisition and cerebral specialization in 20 months-old infants. *Journal of Cognitive Neuroscience, 5*, 317–334.

Mills, D., Coffey-Corina, S., & Neville, H. (1997). Language comprehension and cerebral specialization from 13 to 20 months. *Developmental Neuropsychology, 13*, 397–445.

Mohammed, T., Campbell, R., MacSweeney, M., Barry, F., & Coleman, M. (2006). Speechreading and its association with reading among deaf, hearing and dyslexic individuals. *Clinical Linguistics & Phonetics, 20*, 621–630.

Neville, H., Schmidt, A., & Kutas, M. (1983). Altered visual-evoked potentials in congenitally deaf adults. *Brain Research, 266*, 127–132.

Penhune, V., Cismaru, R., Dorsaint-Pierre, R., Petito, L., & Zatorre, R. J. (2003). The morphometry of auditory cortex in the congenitally deaf measured using MRI. *Neuroimage, 20*, 1215–1225.

Sams, M., Aulanko, R., Hämäläinen, M., Hari, R., Lounasmaa, O., Lu, S., Simola, J. (1991). Seeing speech: Visual information from lip movements modifies activity in the human auditory cortex. *Neuroscience Letters, 127*, 141–145.

Sekiyama, K., Kanno, I., Miura, S., & Sugita, Y. (2003). Auditory-visual speech perception examined by fMRI and PET. *Neuroscience Research, 47*, 277–287

Sekiyama, K., & Tohkura, Y. (1991). McGurk effect in non-English listeners: Few visual effects for Japanese subjects hearing Japanese syllables of high auditory intelligibility. *Journal of Acoustical Society of America, 90*, 1797–1805.

Spoehr, K., & Corin, W. (1978). The stimulus suffix effect as a memory coding phenomenon. *Memory and Cognition, 6*, 583–589.

Sumby, W., & Pollack, I. (1954). Visual contribution to speech intelligibility in noise. *Journal of the Acoustical Society of America, 26*, 212–215.

Summerfield, A. (1987). Some preliminaries to a comprehensive account of audiovisual speech perception. In B. Dodd & R. Campbell (Eds.), *Hearing by eye: The psychology of lipreading* (pp. 3–51). Hove, UK: Lawrence Erlbaum Associates.

Wright, T., Pelphrey, K., Allison, T., McKeown, M., & McCarthy, G. (2003). Polysensory interactions along lateral temporal regions evoked by audiovisual speech. *Cerebral Cortex, 13*, 1034–1043.

Zeki, S., Watson, J., Lueck, C., Friston, K., Kennard, C., & Frackowiak, R. (1991). A direct demonstration of functional specialization in human visual cortex. *Journal of Neuroscience, 11*, 641–649.

INDEX